Textbook of
BIOCHEMISTRY
for Paramedical Students

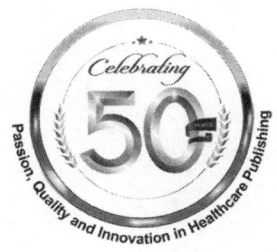

Textbook of
BIOCHEMISTRY
for Paramedical Students

(Based on the Latest Syllabi of Biochemistry for Allied Health Sciences Courses)

Second Edition

P Ramamoorthy
PhD (Biochemistry, Faculty of Medicine)
Ex-Professor
Department of Biochemistry
ACS Medical College and Hospital
Dr MGR University
Chennai, Tamil Nadu, India

Ex-Professor and Head
Department of Biochemistry
Mahatma Gandhi Medical College and Research Institute
Pondicherry University
Puducherry, India

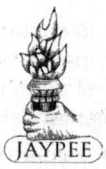

JAYPEE BROTHERS MEDICAL PUBLISHERS
The Health Sciences Publisher
New Delhi | London

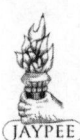

Jaypee Brothers Medical Publishers (P) Ltd

Headquarters
EMCA House
23/23-B, Ansari Road, Daryaganj
New Delhi 110 002, India
Landline: +91-11-23272143, +91-11-23272703
+91-11-23282021, +91-11-23245672
E-mail: jaypee@jaypeebrothers.com

Corporate Office
Jaypee Brothers Medical Publishers (P) Ltd.
4838/24, Ansari Road, Daryaganj
New Delhi 110 002, India
Phone: +91-11-43574357
Fax: +91-11-43574314
E-mail: jaypee@jaypeebrothers.com

Overseas Office
JP Medical Ltd.
83, Victoria Street, London
SW1H 0HW (UK)
Phone: +44-20 3170 8910
Fax: +44(0)20 3008 6180
E-mail: info@jpmedpub.com

Website: www.jaypeebrothers.com
Website: www.jaypeedigital.com

© 2021, Jaypee Brothers Medical Publishers

The views and opinions expressed in this book are solely those of the original contributor(s)/author(s) and do not necessarily represent those of editor(s) of the book.

All rights reserved. No part of this publication may be reproduced, stored or transmitted in any form or by any means, electronic, mechanical, photocopying, recording or otherwise, without the prior permission in writing of the publishers.

All brand names and product names used in this book are trade names, service marks, trademarks or registered trademarks of their respective owners. The publisher is not associated with any product or vendor mentioned in this book.

Medical knowledge and practice change constantly. This book is designed to provide accurate, authoritative information about the subject matter in question. However, readers are advised to check the most current information available on procedures included and check information from the manufacturer of each product to be administered, to verify the recommended dose, formula, method and duration of administration, adverse effects and contraindications. It is the responsibility of the practitioner to take all appropriate safety precautions. Neither the publisher nor the author(s)/editor(s) assume any liability for any injury and/or damage to persons or property arising from or related to use of material in this book.

This book is sold on the understanding that the publisher is not engaged in providing professional medical services. If such advice or services are required, the services of a competent medical professional should be sought.

Every effort has been made where necessary to contact holders of copyright to obtain permission to reproduce copyright material. If any have been inadvertently overlooked, the publisher will be pleased to make the necessary arrangements at the first opportunity. The **CD/DVD-ROM** (if any) provided in the sealed envelope with this book is complimentary and free of cost. **Not meant for sale.**

Inquiries for bulk sales may be solicited at: jaypee@jaypeebrothers.com

Textbook of Biochemistry for Paramedical Students
First Edition: 2015
Second Edition: **2021**
ISBN 978-93-90595-54-9

Printed at Nutech Print Services - India

Dedicated to

My parents and teachers

Preface to the Second Edition

The importance of biochemistry is unquestionable for all paramedical (Allied Health Science) students. It gives me great pleasure to bring out the second edition of the book *Textbook of Biochemistry for Paramedical Students*. This edition has been revised basis constructive suggestions from the students and teachers.

This book is divided into six sections with special topics and appendices containing useful information for clear understanding of the subject to paramedical students belonging to Nursing, Pharmacy, Physiotherapy, Medical Laboratory Technology, Nutrition and other Allied Health Science Courses.

I have added several new features in this edition which are as follows:
- All chapters are completely revised
- Written in simple language and easy-to-understand style
- Chapters arranged as followed for regular lecture classes
- Clinical importance (in boxes)
- Description of some important diseases, instruments and techniques
- More than 200 figures, 75 tables and 40 color figures
- Simplified metabolic pathways/cycles/charts
- Chapterwise exam-orientated questions, with answers for MCQs
- Simple clinical cases with diagnosis
- Biochemistry practical guide

This book is designed to improve the teaching and learning of biochemistry for paramedical (Allied Health Sciences) students. The book will create an impression among the students that biochemistry is not a difficult subject but an easy subject to read and understand.

Suggestions for further improvement of the book can be sent to my email: prmoorthipvm@gmail.com

P Ramamoorthy

Preface to the First Edition

Textbook of Biochemistry for Paramedical Students has been written for Nursing, Pharmacy, Physiotherapy, Medical Laboratory Technology, Nutrition and several other Allied Health Sciences courses.

It is based on the latest syllabi of Biochemistry for Paramedical Students (Allied Health Sciences courses). Most of the textbooks available in biochemistry satisfy mostly the requirements of medical students in biochemistry. Nowadays, very few books on biochemistry written for paramedical students are available. However, the number of paramedical courses is large and each course is a specialty of its own. As such, subject coverage also differs in some aspects among different specialties. I have attempted to give subject coverage to the maximum extent.

This book has been written in simple language and easily understandable style suited for all paramedical students. The book has been divided into five sections, and in each section, individual chapters have been arranged as followed for regular classroom lectures by the teachers. I have given much importance, especially, to the examination-oriented topics and questions in biochemistry.

I shall be pleased to receive the comments, suggestions and constructive criticism from the students and teachers regarding the book.

P Ramamoorthy

Acknowledgments

I am thankful for the faculty, students, and friends for the feedback of first edition which prompted me to bring out second edition of this book. This book would not have been completed without the help and support of my former colleagues in various medical and paramedical colleges.

I am grateful to M/s Jaypee Brothers Medical Publishers (P) Ltd., New Delhi, India, especially Shri Jitendar P Vij (Group Chairman) for his personal advice, and Mr Ankit Vij (Managing Director), Mr MS Mani (Group President) for their encouragement during preparation of the second edition of this book.

I wish to thank Dr Madhu Choudhary (Publishing Head-Education), Ms Pooja Bhandari (Production Head), Ms Sunita Katla (Executive Assistant to Group Chairman and Publishing Manager), Ms Samina Khan (Executive Assistant to Publishing Head-Education), Mr Rajesh Sharma (Production Coordinator), Ms Seema Dogra (Cover Visualizer), Ms Geeta Barik (Proofreader), Mr Ajeet Rathore (Typesetter), and Mr Pappu Kumar (Graphic Designer) of M/s Jaypee Brothers Medical Publishers (P) Ltd., New Delhi, India for their excellent work to bring out the second edition of the book in a well-designed form within short time.

I also thank Mr Maran (Regional Business Manager-South), M/s Jaypee Brothers Medical Publication (P) Ltd, Chennai Branch, Tamil Nadu, for his motivational help to bring out this book.

Contents

SECTION 1: Introduction to Biochemistry

1. **The Cell (Biochemical and Biophysical Aspects)**   1
   Biochemical Aspects   1
   The Eukaryotic Cell   1
      Cytoplasm   1; Nucleus   4; Cell Membrane (Plasma Membrane)   5
   Biophysical Aspects   5
      Water   5; pH   6; Acid, Base, and Buffer   6; Diffusion   7; Osmosis   7; Dialysis   7; Gibbs–Donnan Membrane Equilibrium   8; Surface Tension   8; Viscosity   8; Colloids   8; Adsorption   9; Absorption   9
   Radioactivity/Radioactive Isotopes   9
      Definition   9; Types of Radiation   9; Isotopes   9; Unit of Measurement   9; Applications   10
   Membrane Transport   10
      Transport Mechanisms for Small Molecules   10; Transport System   11; Transport of Macromolecules   11; Additional Information   12

SECTION 2: Chemistry of Biomolecules

2. **Chemistry of Carbohydrates**   13
      Definition   13; Alternative Name   13; Occurrence   13; Composition   13; Biomedical Importance/Functions   13; Classification   13; Additional Information   30

3. **Chemistry of Lipids**   31
      Definition   31; Alternative Name   31; Occurrence   31; Composition   31; Biomedical Importance/Functions   31; Classification   31; Related Terms in Lipid Chemistry   46

4. **Chemistry of Proteins**   47
   Amino Acids   47
      Definition   47; Occurrence   47; Composition   47; Biomedical Importance/Functions   47; Classification of Amino Acids   48; Properties   50
   Proteins   51
      Definition   51; Meaning   51; Composition   51; Occurrence   51; Biomedical Importance/Functions   52; Classification   52; Structural Organization of Proteins   54; Properties   56; Estimation of Proteins (in Blood)   57; Criteria for Purity of Proteins   57; Methods of Separation of Proteins   57
   Plasma Proteins   58
      Biomedical Importance/Functions   58; Method of Separation   58; Individual Plasma Proteins   58; Abnormalities in Plasma Proteins (Clinical Importance)   59
   Immunoglobulins   59
      Definition   59; General Function   59; Classification   59; Structure of Immunoglobulins   60

Peptides 60
Definition 60; Composition 60; Formation 61; Structure 61; Properties 61; Biomedical Importance/Functions 61; Miscellaneous Proteins/Peptide 61

5. **Chemistry of Nucleic Acids**   63
Definition 63; Discovery 63; Types 63; Occurrence 63; Biomedical Importance/Functions 63; Composition 63; Nucleosides 64; Nucleotides 65; Nucleic Acids 66; Biologically Important Nucleotides 69; Nucleoproteins 72; Additional Information 72

6. **Chemistry of Hemoglobin**   73
Definition 73; Biomedical Importance/Functions 73; Composition 73; Porphyrin 73; Normal Human Hemoglobins 75; Spectroscopic Analysis of Hemoglobin and its Derivatives 78; Hemoglobinopathies 78; Technique for Identification (Separation) of Hemoglobins 80; Estimation of Hemoglobin in Blood 80; Test for Hemoglobin in Abnormal Urine 80

Other Hemoproteins 80
Myoglobin 80

7. **Enzymes**   81
Definition 81; Discovery 81; Meaning 81; Biomedical Importance/Functions 81; Commercial Uses 81; Composition 81; Properties 82; Substrate 82; Naming Enzymes 82; Classification of Enzymes 83; Numbering Enzyme 84; Enzyme Specificity 84; Cofactors 84; Mechanism of Enzyme Action 85; Factors Affecting Activity of Enzymes or Velocity of Enzymatic Reaction (Enzyme Kinetics) 86; Regulation of Enzyme Activity 89; Expression of Enzyme Activity 90; Application of Enzymes in Medicine 90; Isoenzymes 91; Additional Information 92

8. **Vitamins**   93
Definition 93; Alternative Name 93; Discovery 93; Biomedical Importance/Functions 93; Classification 93

Fat-soluble Vitamins (Lipid-soluble Vitamins) 93
Vitamin A 93; Vitamin D 97; Vitamin E 100; Vitamin K 101

Water-soluble Vitamins 102
B-complex Vitamins 103; Non B-complex Vitamin 113; Vitamin-like Compounds 115; Antivitamins 116

SECTION 3: Metabolism

9. **Introduction to Metabolism**   119
Definition 119; Phases of Metabolism 119; Importance 119; Methods of Studying (Investigating) Metabolism 119; Type of Reactions in Metabolic Pathways 120; Additional Information 120

10. **Biological Oxidation, Electron Transport Chain, and Bioenergetics**   121
Biological Oxidation 121; Electron Transport Chain 122; Oxidative Phosphorylation 123; Bioenergetics 124; Additional Information 125

11. **Digestion, Absorption, and Metabolism of Carbohydrates**   126
Digestion 126; Absorption 127; Metabolism of Glucose 128; Alternative Pathways of Glucose Catabolism 134; Glucose Tolerance Test (GTT) 146; Additional Information 147

12. Digestion, Absorption, and Metabolism of Lipids — 148
Digestion   148; Absorption   148; Transport and Storage   149; Metabolism   149

13. Digestion, Absorption, and Metabolism of Proteins — 164
Digestion   164; Absorption   165; Metabolism of Amino Acids (General Pathways)   165; Urea Cycle (Urea Biosynthesis)   168; Metabolism of Nonessential Amino Acids   169; Metabolism of Essential Amino Acids   176; Additional Information   184

14. Integration of Metabolism — 186
Definition   186; Metabolic Pathways   186; Integration of Metabolism   186

15. Digestion, Absorption, and Metabolism of Nucleic Acids — 189
Digestion   189; Absorption   189; Metabolism   189

16. Metabolism of Hemoglobin — 195
Biosynthesis of Hemoglobin   195; Catabolism of Hemoglobin   196; Jaundice   198

17. Mineral Metabolism — 200
Definition   200; Alternative Name   200; Biomedical Importance/Functions   200; Classification   200; Abnormal States   200; Macrominerals   200; Sodium (Na^+)   202; Potassium (K^+)   202; Chloride (Cl^-)   203; Calcium (Ca)   203; Phosphorus (P)   205; Magnesium (Mg)   206; Sulfur (S)   207; Microminerals (Trace Elements)   207; Iron (Fe)   208; Iodine (I)   211; Copper (Cu)   212; Zinc (Zn)   213; Manganese (Mn)   214; Molybdenum (Mo)   214; Fluoride (F)   215; Cobalt (Co)   215; Chromium (Cr)   216; Selenium (Se)   216; Nonessential Trace Elements   217

18. Metabolism of Xenobiotics (Detoxication) — 218
Sources   218; Importance   218; Alternative Names   218; Definition   218; Site   218; Mechanism   218; Types of Detoxication Mechanism   218

19. Excretion — 221
Urine   221; Feces   221; Proteinuria   222; Microalbuminuria   222; Glycosuria   222; Sweat   222

SECTION 4: Miscellaneous Topics of Biochemical Importance

20. Energy Metabolism — 223
Energy   223; Calorific Value of Foods   223; Respiratory Quotient   224; Energy Expenditure   224; Energy Requirement   226

21. Food and Nutrition — 227
Food   227; Energy-yielding Foods (Primary Foods)   227; Body-building Foods   228; Protective Foods   229; Balanced Diet   230; Milk   231; Diet and Public Health   231; Nutrition   232; Related Terms in Food and Nutrition   233

22. Water (Fluid) and Electrolyte Balance — 235
Water   235; Electrolytes   236; Regulation of Water and Electrolyte Balance   236

23. Acid–Base Balance — 238
Sources of Acids in the Blood   238; Sources of Bases in the Blood   238; Mechanisms for Maintaining Acid–Base Balance   238; Disturbances in Acid–Base Balance (Acid–Base Imbalance)   241

24. Organ Function Tests — 243

Liver Function Tests 243; Renal Function Tests 245; Pancreatic Function Tests 247; Thyroid Function Tests 247; Gastric Function Tests 247; Cardiac Function Tests 249

25. Hormones — 250

Definition 250; Biomedical Importance/Functions 250; Classification 251; Individual Hormones 253

SECTION 5: Applied Biochemistry

26. Molecular Biology — 267

Definition 267; Historical Background 267; Nucleus 267; Gene 267; Cell Cycle 268; Central Dogma of Molecular Biology 268; Replication (DNA Synthesis) 268; DNA Replication in Prokaryotes 269; DNA Replication In Eukaryotes 270; DNA Damage 270; DNA Repair 270; Mutations 271; Transcription (RNA Synthesis) 272; Transcription in Prokaryotes 272; Post-transcriptional Modifications (mRNA in Eukaryotes) 272; Transcription in Eukaryotes 273; Genetic Code 273

Translation (Protein Biosynthesis) 274
Translation in Prokaryotes 274; Translation in Eukaryotes 276; Regulation of Gene Expression 277; Molecular Biological Techniques 277; Human Genome Project 281

27. Immunology — 282

Definitions 282; Organization of the Immune System 282; Monoclonal Antibodies 284

28. Clinical Biochemistry — 285

Definition 285; Historical Background 285; Instrumentation and Techniques in Clinical Biochemistry 286; Types of Biochemical Tests 289; Normal Values (Reference Range) 290

29. Instrumentation and Techniques in Biochemistry — 291

Colorimetry 291; Spectrophotometer 292; Electrolyte Analyzer 292; Autoanalyzers 294; Glucometer 295; Blood Gas Analyzers 295; Hormone Analyzers 296; pH Meter 296; Clinical Centrifuge 297; Chromatography 297; Electrophoresis 298; Radioimmunoassay 300; Enzyme-linked Immunosorbent Assay 300 Biochemical Laboratory Instruments 301

30. Biochemistry in Medical and Paramedical Specialties — 303

Definition 303; Historical Background 303; Objectives 303; Branches 303; Biochemistry in Medicine 303; Biochemistry in Paramedical Specialties (Allied Health Sciences Courses) 304

SECTION 6: Special Topics

31. Eicosanoids (Prostaglandins) — 307

Definition 307; Classification 307

32. Lipid Peroxidation—Free Radicals and Antioxidants — 309

Definition 309; Formation 309; Mechanism of Lipid Peroxidation 309; Assessment 309; Harmful Effects 309; Antioxidants 309; Types 309

33. Environmental Biochemistry — 311

Definition 311; Classification 311; General Effects 311; Types 311

34. Cancer — 314
Definition 314; Types 314; Causative Factors of Cancer 314; Chemical Carcinogens 314

35. Acquired Immune Deficiency Syndrome — 316
Causes 316; Epidemiology 316; Structure of HIV 316; Abnormal Activities 316; Clinical Symptoms 316; Diagnosis 316; Treatment 316

36. Biotechnology — 317
Definition 317; Historical Development 317; Branches (Divisions) 317; Scope/Importance 317; Process 317; Applications 317; Risks, Hazards, and Ethics 318; Related Terms in Molecular Biology 318; Stem Cells 318; Mitochondrial DNA (mtDNA/mDNA) 318

Appendices

Appendix A: Questions (Chapter-wise) — 319
Appendix B: Clinical Cases — 335
Appendix C: Inborn Errors of Metabolism — 337
Appendix D: Isomerism — 339
Appendix E: Abbreviations used in this Book — 340
Appendix F: List of Paramedical Courses (Allied Health Science Courses) [BSc (UG) Level] — 342
Appendix G: Normal Value Chart — 343
Appendix H: Biochemistry Practical Guide — 344

Index — 347

Plate 1

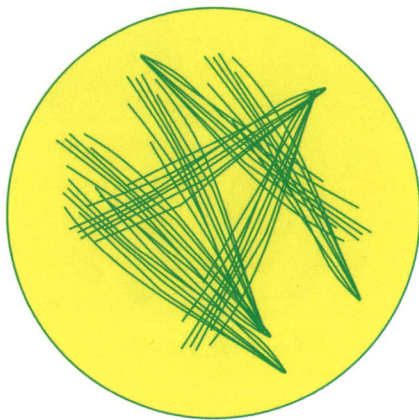

Fig. 2.2: Glucosazone/fructosazone.

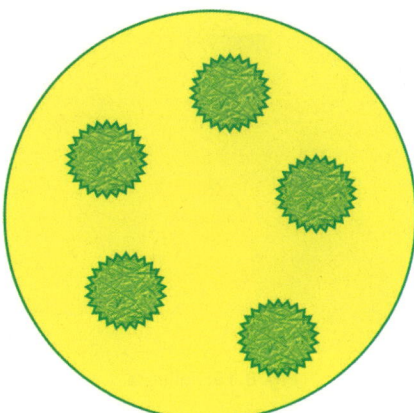

Fig. 2.3: Lactosazone.

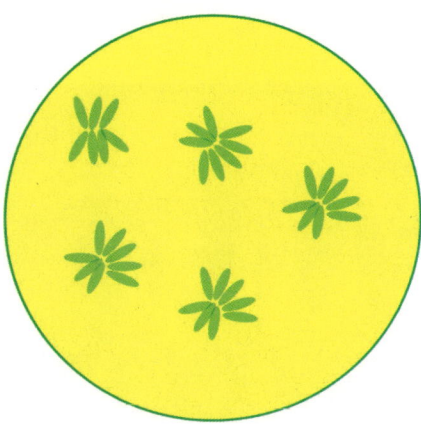

Fig. 2.4: Maltosazone.

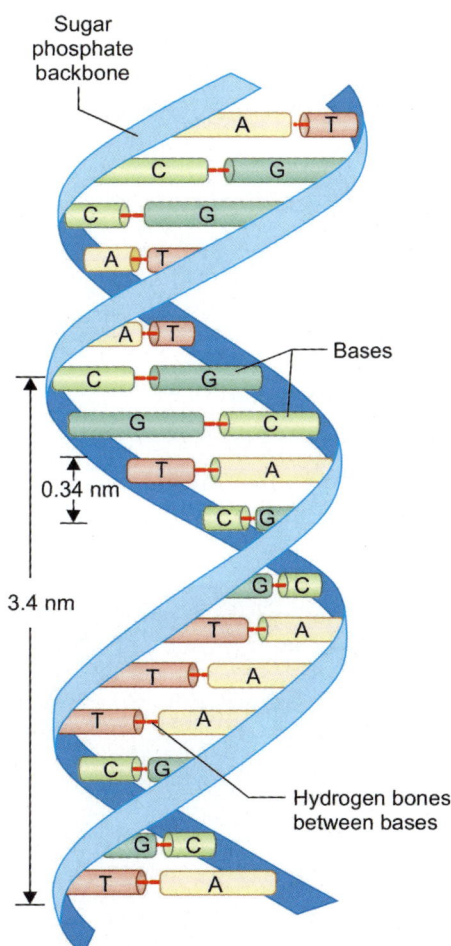

Fig. 5.9: DNA double helix.

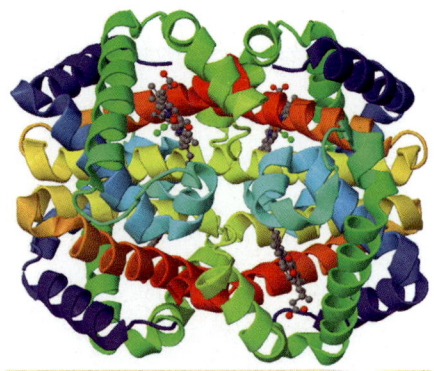

Fig. 6.3: Hemoglobin structure.

Plate 2

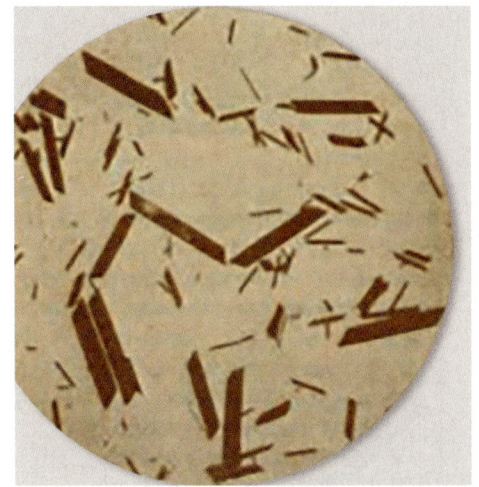

Fig. 6.5: Hemin crystals.

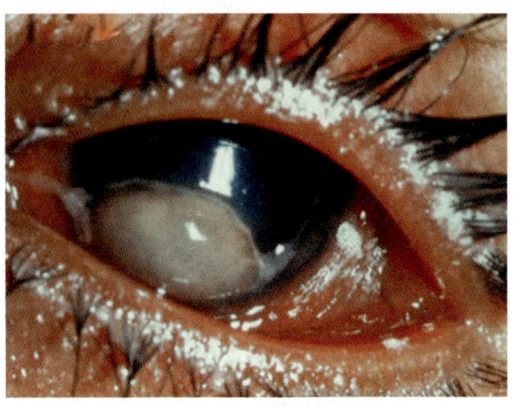

Fig. 8.4: Xerophthalmia

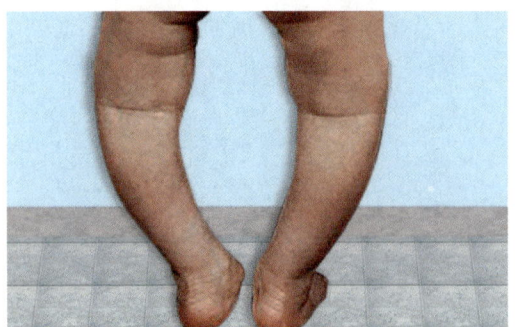

Fig. 8.8: Rickets.

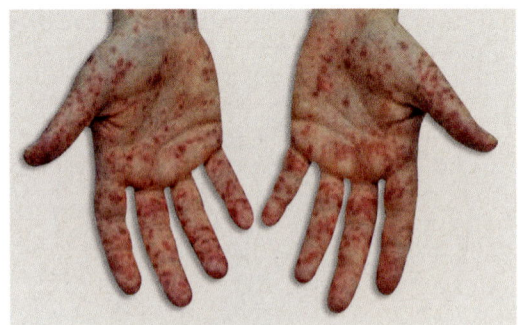

Fig. 8.13: Beriberi.

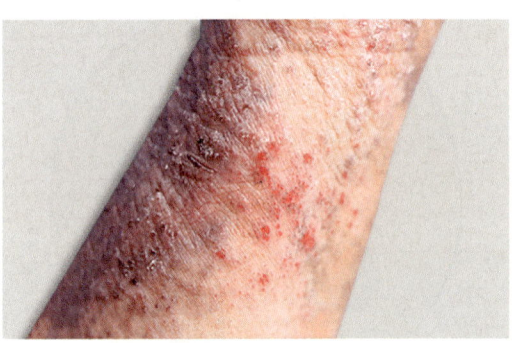

Fig. 8.16: Pellagra.

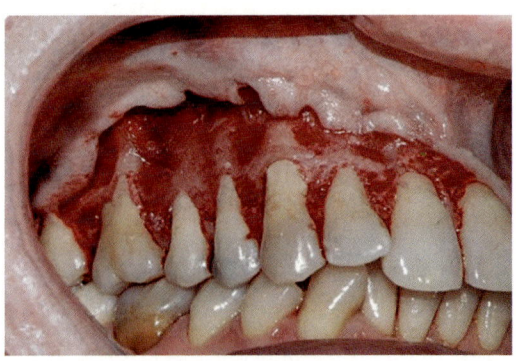

Fig. 8.24: Scurvy.

Plate 3

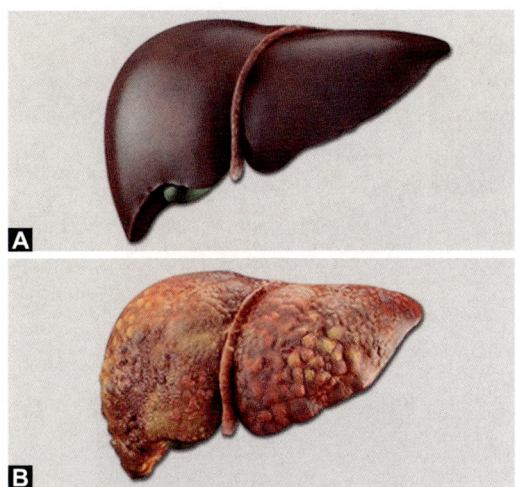

Figs. 12.10A and B: (A) Healthy liver and (B) Fatty liver.

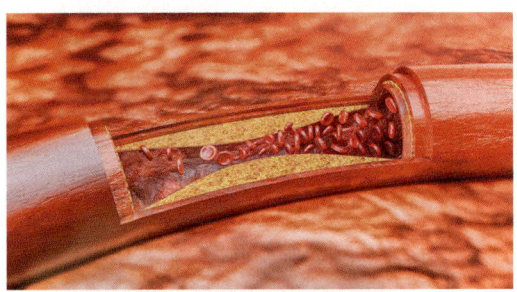

Fig. 12.15: Atherosclerosis.

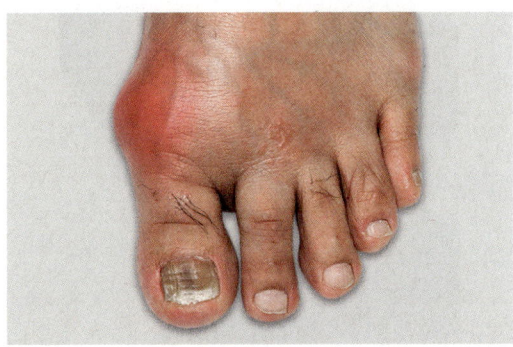

Fig. 15.4: Gout.

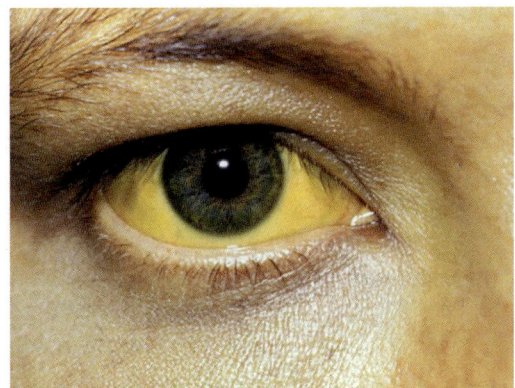

Fig. 16.3: Jaundice.

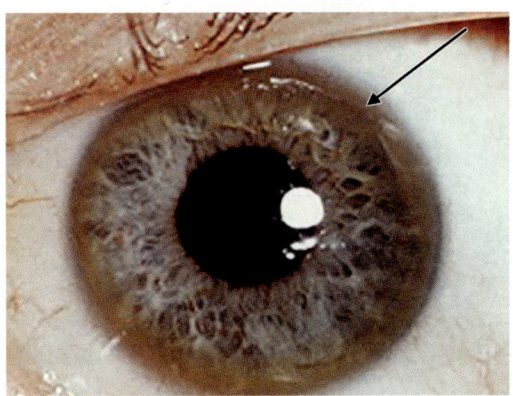

Fig. 17.6: Wilson's disease.

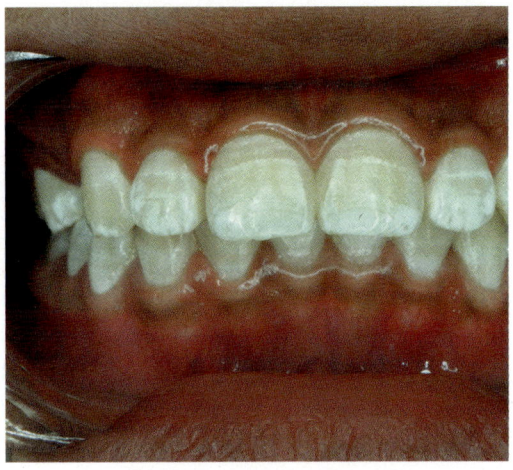

Fig. 17.7: Dental fluorosis.

Plate 4

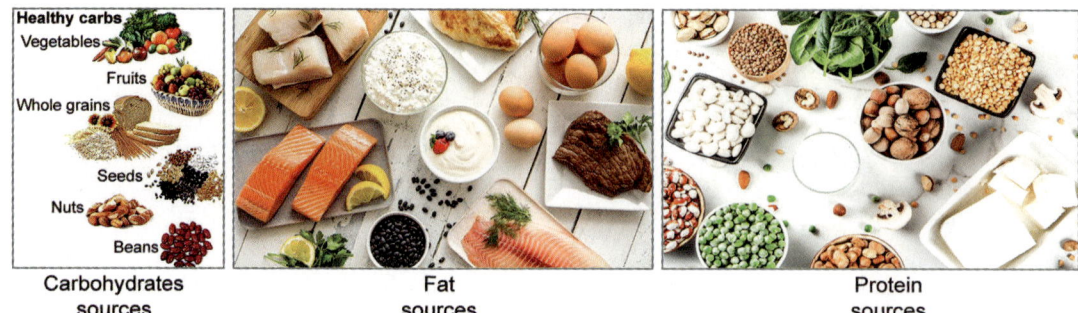

Fig. 21.2: Energy-yielding foods.

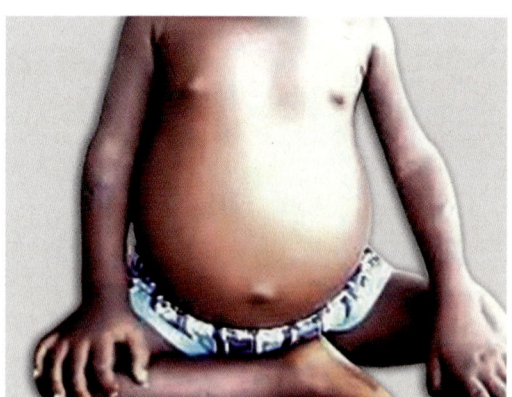

Fig. 21.3: Kwashiorkor.

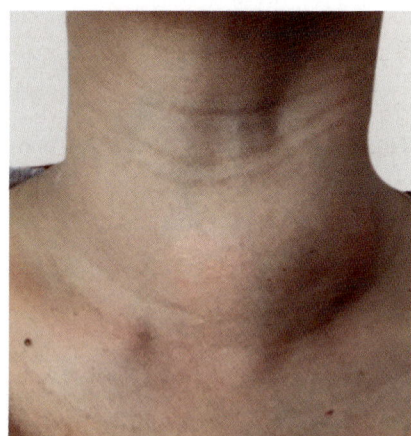

Fig. 25.5: Goiter.

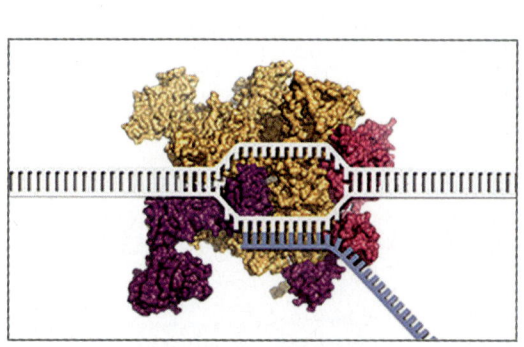

Fig. 26.1: Molecular biology.

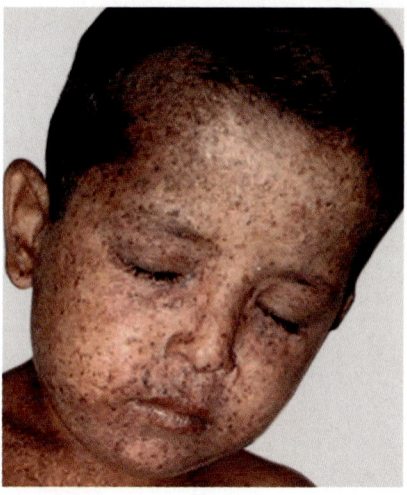

Fig. 26.7: Xeroderma pigmentosum.

Plate 5

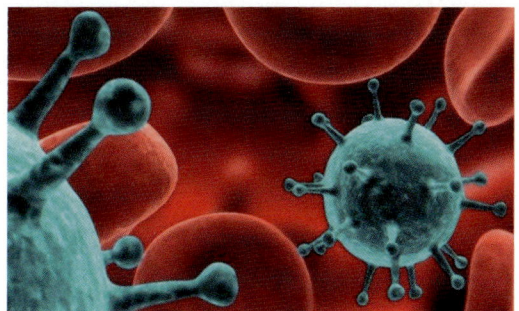

Fig. 27.1: Immunology.

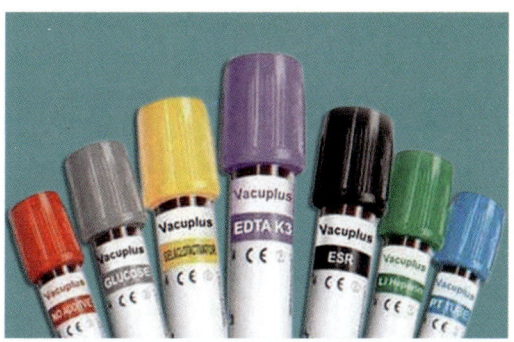

Fig. 28.4: Vacutainer tubes.

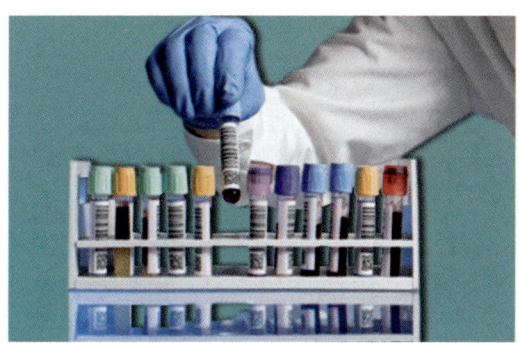

Fig. 28.1: Clinical biochemistry.

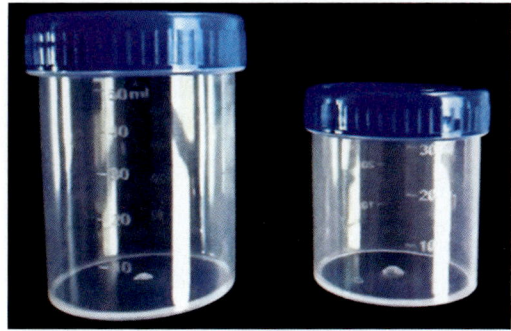

Fig. 28.5: Urine containers.

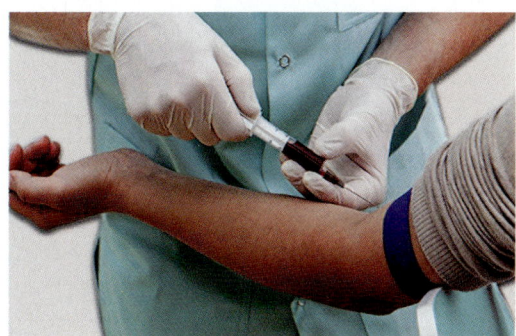

Fig. 28.3: Blood collection.

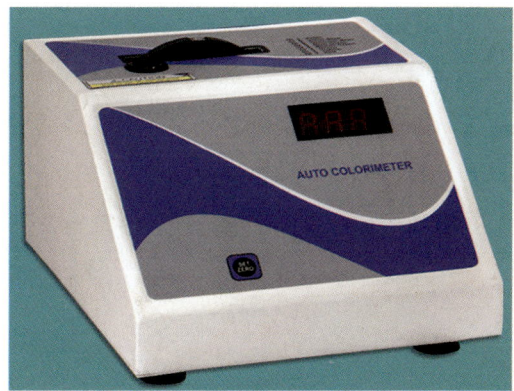

Fig. 29.15: Colorimeter.

Plate 6

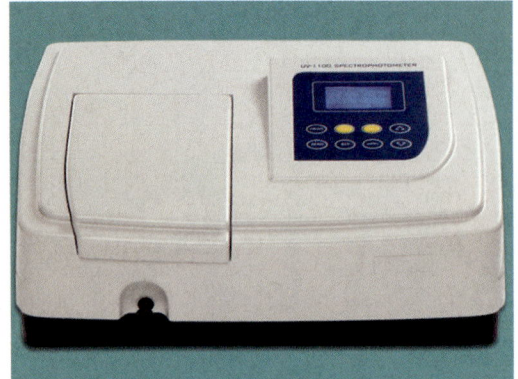

Fig. 29.16: Spectrophotometer.

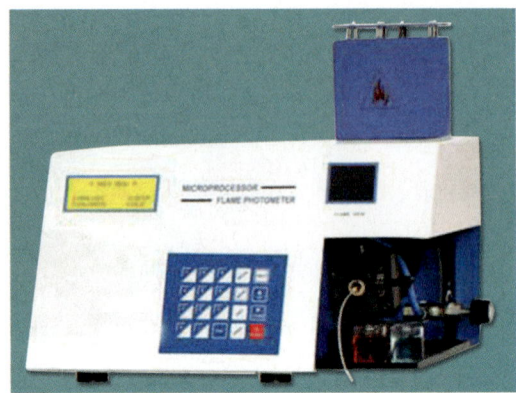

Fig. 29.19: Flame photometer.

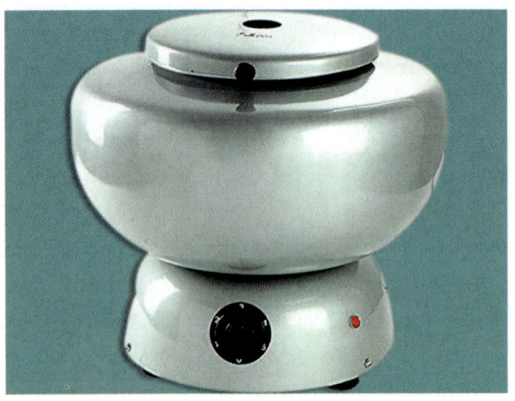

Fig. 29.17: Clinical centrifuge.

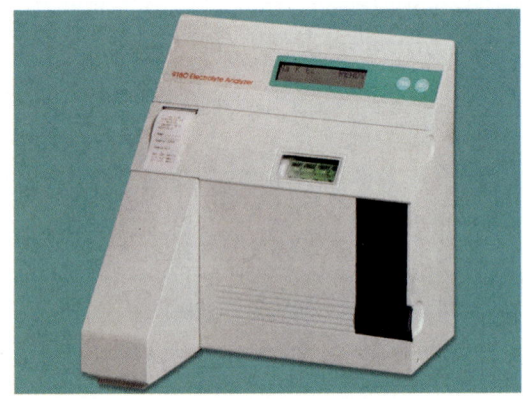

Fig. 29.20: Electrolyte analyzer.

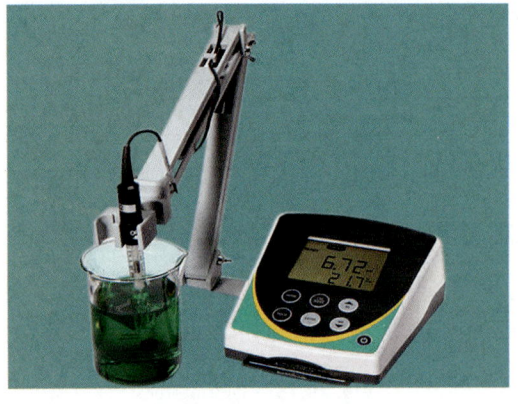

Fig. 29.18: pH meter.

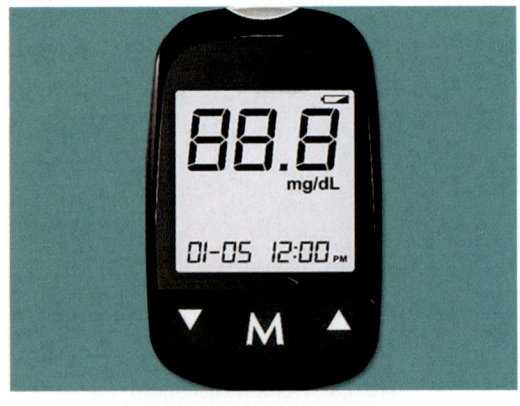

Fig. 29.21: Glucometer.

Plate 7

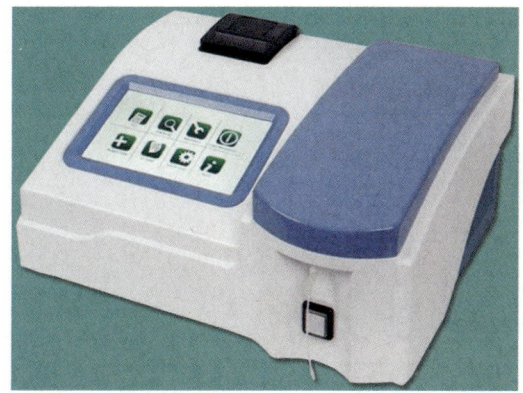

Fig. 29.22: Semiautoanalyzer.

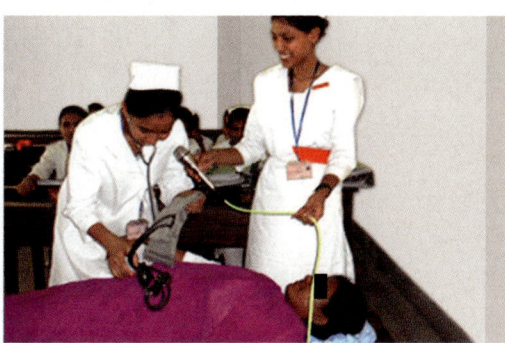

Fig. 30.4: Nursing.

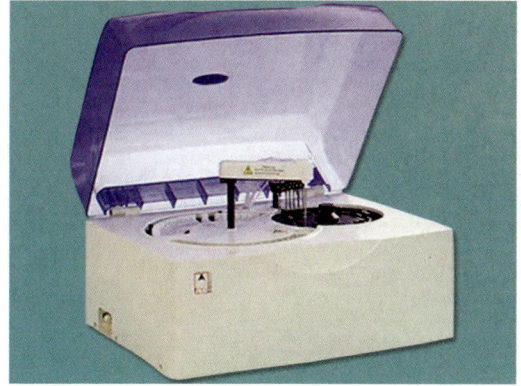

Fig. 29.23: Fully automatic analyzer.

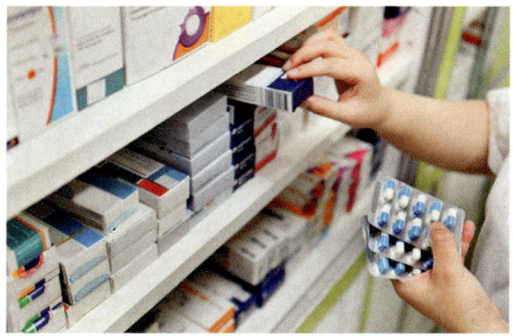

Fig. 30.5: Pharmacy.

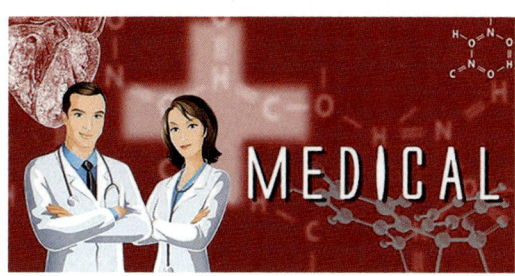

Fig. 30.2: Medical.

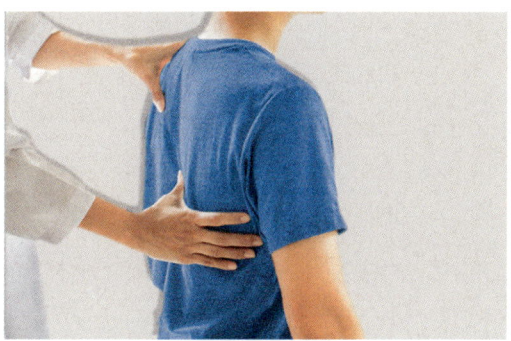

Fig. 30.6: Physiotherapy.

Plate 8

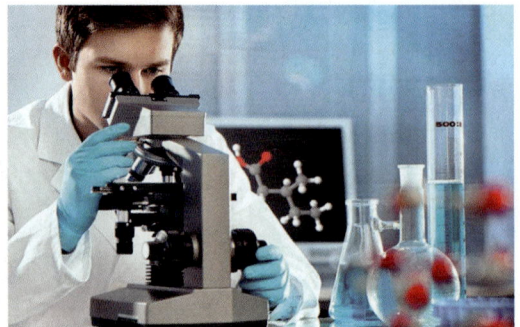

Fig. 30.7: Medical laboratory technology.

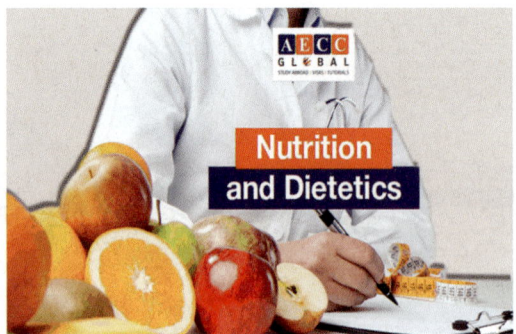

Fig. 30.8: Nutrition and dietetics.

Section 1: Introduction to Biochemistry

1. The Cell (Biochemical and Biophysical Aspects)

Chapter Outline

Biochemical Aspects
The Eukaryotic Cell
- Cytoplasm
- Nucleus
- Cell Membrane (Plasma Membrane)

Biophysical Aspects
- Water
- pH
- Acid, Base and Buffer
- Diffusion
- Osmosis
- Dialysis
- Gibbs–Donnan Membrane Equilibrium
- Surface Tension
- Viscosity
- Colloids
- Adsorption
- Absorption

Radioactivity/Radioactive Isotopes
- Definition
- Types of Radiation
- Isotopes
- Unit of Measurement
- Applications

Membrane Transport
- Transport Mechanisms for Small Molecules
- Transport System
- Transport of Macromolecules
- Additional Information

BIOCHEMICAL ASPECTS

The cell is the basic structural and functional unit of the living organisms. Cells are composed of characteristic parts which coordinate together to perform a specific role. They are divided into two categories based on their organizational features.

1. *Prokaryotes:* They have relatively simple structure and lack a well-defined nucleus, e.g., bacteria (**Fig. 1.1**).
2. *Eukaryotes:* They are very complex in structure and function. They possess a well-defined nucleus surrounded by cell membrane, e.g., humans, animals, plants (**Table. 1.1**).

THE EUKARYOTIC CELL

The eukaryotic cell has three important parts (**Fig. 1.2**):
1. Cytoplasm
2. Nucleus
3. Cell membrane

■ CYTOPLASM

The cytoplasm is composed of:

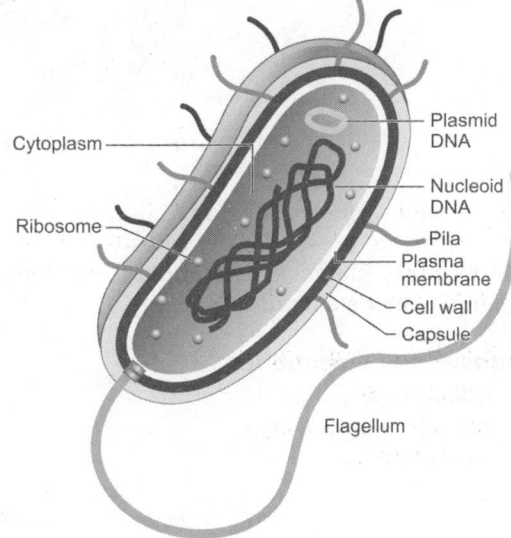

Fig. 1.1: Prokaryote.

1. Cytosol
2. Subcellular organelles
3. Subcellular fractions

Cytosol

It is the soluble portion of the cell (cell sap). Several enzymes, coenzymes, inorganic ions,

Section 1: Introduction to Biochemistry

Table 1.1: Differences between prokaryotic cell and eukaryotic cell.

Sl. No.	Features	Prokaryotic cell	Eukaryotic cell
1.	Size	Small	Large
2.	Nucleus	Not well defined, present as nuclear, no nuclear membrane	Well-defined nucleus surrounded by nuclear membrane
3.	Cellular organelles	Very few	Distinct cell organelles present
4.	Organization	• Single cell • Cell is enveloped by cell membrane and surrounded by cell wall	Multicellular, enveloped by flexible cell membrane
5.	Cell division	Usually fission	Mitosis
6.	Ribosomes	70s	80s

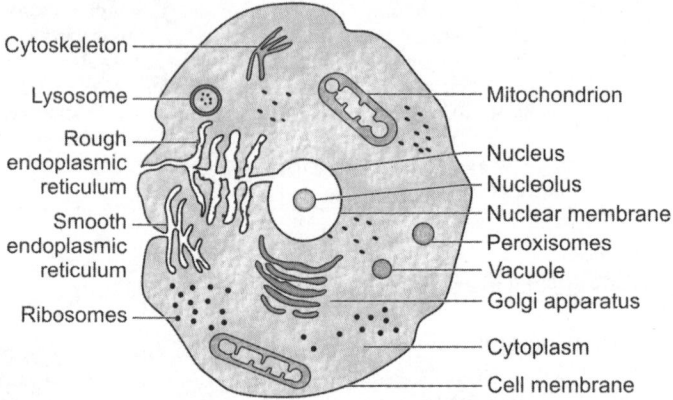

Fig. 1.2: Structure of an eukaryotic cell.

amino acids, nucleotides, metabolites, RNA molecules are present in the cytosol. It is the site of many chemical (metabolic) reactions required for existence of cells.

Subcellular Organelles

1. Mitochondria
2. Endoplasmic reticulum
3. Golgi complex
4. Lysosomes
5. Peroxisomes

Mitochondria (Fig. 1.3)

Mitochondria are membrane bound cell organelles. Each cell contains few to several thousand number of mitochondria. They vary from cell to cell, more in metabolic active cells, such as liver, kidney, etc. They

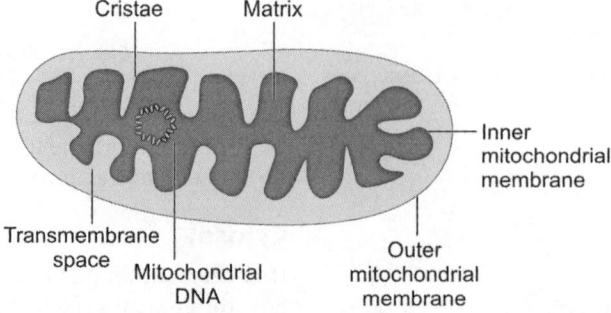

Fig. 1.3: Mitochondria.

Chapter 1: The Cell (Biochemical and Biophysical Aspects)

are spherical, oval, rod-shaped and vary in size.

Structure
It consists of two membranes—
1. *Inner membrane:* It is arranged in a series of folds known as cristae enclosing the matrix which is fluid in nature containing enzymes for chemical reactions occurring in metabolism.
2. *Outer membrane:* It is unwrinkled and surrounds the organelle. It consists mostly of phospholipids and considerable amount of cholesterol.

Functions
- They are called as power houses of the cell, because they are involved in producing adenosine triphosphate (ATP) in electron transport chain. ATP is a high energy compound.
- They contain enzymes for TCA cycle, β oxidation of fatty acids, ketone body formation, urea cycle, etc.
- They also contain specific DNA (mtDNA) which encodes information for synthesis of certain mitochondrial proteins.

Note
☞ Erythrocytes (RBCs) do not contain mitochondria.

Endoplasmic Reticulum (ER)
It is a network of membranes that form flattened sacs or tubules called cisterne. It is of two types:

Structure
1. *Rough endoplasmic reticulum (RER):* It is continuous with nuclear membrane. The outer surface of RER is studded with ribosomes, the sites of protein synthesis.
   Functions: It synthesizes secretory proteins and membrane lipids.
2. *Smooth endoplasmic reticulum (SER).*
   It extends from RER to form a network of membrane tubules. It does not contain ribosomes on the outer surface of its membrane.

Functions
- It is the site of synthesis of phospholipids, fats, steroids.
- It is involved in the metabolism of certain drugs and toxic compounds and also in modification and transport of proteins synthesized in RER.

Golgi Complex
(Golgi bodies/Golgi apparatus)

Structure
It consists of 3–20 flattened membrane sacs with bulging edges called Golgi sacs. It was named after its discoverer Camillo Golgi. Each cell may have one or more Golgi complexes.

The Golgi sacs differ in size and shape. Its convex side faces RER and the exit side faces plasma membrane. Between these are medial cisternae.

Functions
- Protein sorting
- Glycosylation reaction
- Sulfuration

Lysosomes

Structure
Lysosomes are spherical vesicles surrounded by membranes. They are present in all cells except erythrocytes. They are derived from Golgi complex. They may vary in number and are 0.4—0.9μ in diameter. They contain a variety of hydrolytic and degradative enzymes. Acid phosphatase is a marker enzyme of lysosomes **(Table 1.2)**. They are called as suicidal bags of the cell, e.g., lipases, ribonuclease, etc.

Functions
- Digestion of substances that enter a cell (endocytosis)
- Digestion of worn out organelles (autophagocytosis)
- Digestion of entire cell (autolysis)

Table 1.2: Marker enzymes of subcellular organelles.

Sl. No.	Subcellular organelles	Marker enzymes
1.	Mitochondria	Succinate dehydrogenase
2.	Golgi bodies	Galactosyltransferase
3.	Endoplasmic reticulum	Glucose 6-phosphatase
4.	Lysosomes	Acid phosphatase
5.	Peroxisomes	Catalase
6.	Nucleus	DNA polymerase, RNA polymerase
7.	Cell membrane	5, Nucleosidase
8.	Cytosol	Lactate dehydrogenase (LDH)

❏ Extracellular digestion. Acrosome (present in head of spermatozoa) is a specialized lysosome. It penetrates ovum.

Clinical Importance

* Enzymes released from ruptured lysosomes may damage tissue as in allergy, gout, etc. Some inborn errors of metabolism occur due to absence of specific acid hydrolases in lysosomes.
* I-cell disease occurs due to absence of all normal lysosome enzymes.

Peroxisomes
Structure
Peroxisomes are also membrane bound vesicles. They are smaller and spherical 0.5–1.5μ in diameter.

Functions
❏ They contain enzymes, such as peroxidase, catalase which can oxidize various organic substances, and
❏ Modified β oxidation of fatty acids.
❏ Clinical importance: Absence of peroxisomes leads to Zellweger's syndrome.

Subcellular Fractions
Cytoskeleton
It is a network of three different kinds of protein filaments which extend throughout the cell in the cytosol:
1. Microfilaments
2. Intermediate filaments
3. Microtubules

Functions
❏ It provides a structural framework of the cell.
❏ It is responsible for cell movements including:
  • The internal cell organelles attachment
  • The movement of chromosomes during cell division
  • The movement of whole cell such as phagocytosis.

Ribosomes
Ribosomes are tiny cell fractions which are packages of ribosomal RNA (rRNA) and proteins. They are not membrane bound. Each ribosome has two subunits bigger and smaller. They are produced in nucleolus present in the nucleus separately, exit the nucleus and join together in the cytosol.

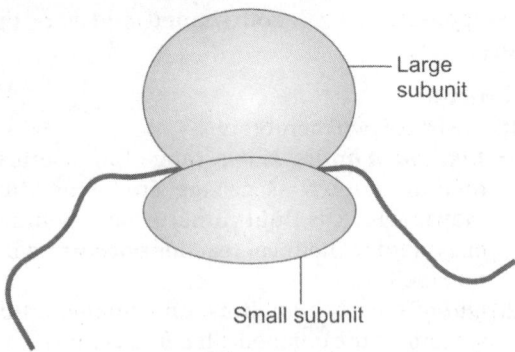

Fig. 1.4: Ribosome.

Type
There are two types of ribosomes:
1. *Free ribosomes:* These are not attached to any structure in the cytoplasm. They synthesize protein used within the cell.
2. *Membrane ribosomes:* These are attached to the nuclear membrane and also rough endoplasmic reticulum. They synthesize proteins for insertion in the plasma membrane or for export from the cell.

Ribosomes may join together in a string-like arrangement called polysomes (polyribosome).

Note

☞ Ribosomes are also located within mitochondria where they are involved in synthesizing mitochondrial proteins.

Composition (Fig. 1.4)
Prokaryotes: Its ribosomes (70s) have two subunits:
1. 50s (large subunits)
2. 30s (small subunits)

Eukaryotes: Its ribosomes (80s) also have two subunits:
1. 60s subunits (large subunits)
2. 40s subunits (small subunits)

Functions
They are sites of protein synthesis.

■ NUCLEUS
It is the largest cellular organelle. It contains DNA which possesses the genetic information.

Structure
Nuclear envelope: It is a double membrane structure. It separates the nucleus from the

cytoplasm. It contains nuclear pores which permit the movement of RNAs and protein across the nuclear envelope.

Nucleolus: It is a dense body and is the site of synthesis of rRNAs.

Nucleoplasm: It is the ground material of the nucleus. It contains various enzymes, such as DNA polymerases and RNA polymerases.

Functions
- Center of genetic control
- Replication (DNA → DNA) and transcription (DNA → RNA) occur in the nucleus.
- Humans have 46 chromosomes packed in the nucleus.

CELL MEMBRANE (PLASMA MEMBRANE)

It is an envelope covering the cell. It separates cellular contents from the external environment.

Structure/Composition (Fig. 1.5)

It is composed of lipid, protein and carbohydrates. Its structure was described as *fluid mosaic model* by Singer and Nicolson in 1972. It is essentially composed of a lipid bilayer. The lipids present are phospholipids, glycolipids and cholesterol. The hydrophobic (nonpolar) regions of the lipids face each other at the core of the bilayer, and hydrophilic (polar) regions face outside. Proteins are irregularly embedded in the lipid bilayer. Proteins are globular proteins and are of two types:
1. *Extrinsic (peripheral) membrane proteins:* These are loosely attached to the surface of the bilayer, e.g., cytochrome C.
2. *Intrinsic (integral) membrane proteins:* These are tightly bound to the lipid bilayer, e.g., hormone receptors.

The membrane appears as a mosaic and freely changes and hence known as *fluid mosaic model.*

Functions
- Transport of molecules in and out of cells
- Intercellular communication
- Protection of cell contents from external environment
- Gives shape and size to the cell
- Separates intracellular fluid (ICF) from extracellular fluid (ECF).

BIOPHYSICAL ASPECTS

Fundamental laws of chemistry and physics apply equally well to biological systems. Hence related biophysical principles are described here.

WATER

Water is the most abundant component of the body. It contains about 60% of total body weight. The cell contains approximately 80% of water. Molecular formula of water is H_2O and its molecular weight is 18. Its structure resembles an irregular tetrahedron with oxygen in the center. It is a polar molecule. It is an ideal biological solvent and modifies the properties of biomolecules. It is very essential to life and water balance should be maintained to have normal and healthy life (*refer* Chapter 22).

Water molecules have slight tendency to dissociate to form hydroxide ions and hydrogen ions. This is known as dissociation of water. It can be represented by the following equation:

$$H_2O \rightleftarrows H^+ + OH^-$$

Water behaves as a weak electrolyte establishing a chemical equilibrium by the reaction as shown above.

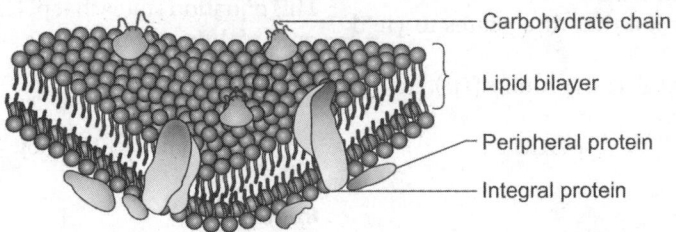

Fig. 1.5: Structure of cell membrane (fluid mosaic model).

pH

Acidic or basic nature of a solution is measured by H⁺ ion concentration. It is expressed as pH.

Definition

It refers to the negative log of the hydrogen ion concentration.

$$pH = -\log [H^+]$$

The term pH was introduced by Sorensen in 1909, who defined pH as mentioned above. It refers to relative acidity. pH scale is 1–14. pH of water is 7. pH lower than 7 denotes high concentration of H^+ (acidic). pH higher than 7 denotes lower concentration of H^+ (alkaline).

Determination

pH of any solution can be determined by several methods:
- pH meter (*refer* Chapter 28)
- pH paper
- Indicators

Biomedical Importance

- Various body fluids maintain a specific pH for the reaction to occur. pH of blood is 7.4; pH of normal urine is 6.0. Acid-base balance should be maintained to have normal and healthy life (*refer* Chapter 23).
- Amino acids and protein exist as Zwitterions at isoelectric pH (*refer* Chapter 4)
- Change in pH may result in impairment of acid-base balance.

ACID, BASE, AND BUFFER

Concept of acid-base chemistry is based on Lowry Bronsted theory.

Acid

Definition

An acid may be defined as:
- A substance or ion that dissociates to yield hydrogen.
- A substance that gives of protons (H^+). Acid is a proton donor.

$$H_2CO_3 \rightarrow H^+ + HCO_3^-$$

Base

Definition

A base can be defined as:
- A substance that yields OH^- ions.

$$NaOH \rightarrow Na^+ + OH^-$$

- A substance that combines with protons (H^+). Base is a proton acceptor.

Salt

It is a combination of acid and base.

Definition

A salt is a compound of a metal radical (or a metal acting radical) and an acid radical.

$$\underset{\text{Base}}{2NaOH} + \underset{\text{Acid}}{H_2SO_4} \rightarrow \underset{\text{Salt}}{Na_2SO_4} + \underset{\text{Water}}{2H_2O}$$

Buffer

Definition

A buffer is one that tends to maintain constant hydrogen ion concentration when acid or alkali is added to it, i.e., it resists a change in pH on addition of acid or alkali.

Composition

It is a mixture of:
- A weak acid and its conjugate base (salt)
- A weak base and its conjugate acid (salt).

Examples (refer Chapter 23)

Principal physiological buffers:
- Bicarbonate buffer
- Hemoglobin buffer
- Phosphate buffer
- Protein buffer

Uses

- To maintain pH of blood and other body fluids (acid-base balance)
- To resist change in pH of any solution

Henderson–Hasselbalch Equation

Definition

This equation states that pH is dependent on the ratio of the concentration of the base to acid.

Henderson–Hasselbalch equation for any buffer can be written as:

$$pH = PKa + \log \frac{[base]}{[acid]}$$

Importance

- To determine pH of any buffer solution
- To determine pH of blood or any body fluid

☐ To express the relationship between pH, pK and ratio of base to acid.

■ DIFFUSION

Definition

It is the movement of solute molecules across a permeable membrane from high concentration to lower concentration until they get uniformly distributed.

Process

When NaCl (solute) is added to water (solvent), it rapidly spreads and forms a homogeneous solution. Diffusion is more rapid in gases than in liquids.

Biomedical Importance

☐ Exchange of gases (O_2 and CO_2) in lungs and tissues occurs through diffusion.
☐ Nutrients, such as pentoses, some mineral ions and water soluble vitamins are absorbed by diffusion in GI tract.
☐ Passage of the waste products, such as ammonia, urea in the renal tubules occurs through diffusion.

■ OSMOSIS

Definition

Osmosis is the passage of solvent (water) to the solution through semipermeable membrane.

Process

Flow of solvent occurs from a solution of low concentration to a solution of high concentration through a semipermeable membrane. It occurs in the direction opposite to that of diffusion.

Osmotic Pressure

Definition

It is the excess pressure that must be applied to a solution to prevent the passage of solvent into the solution when both are separated by a semipermeable membrane. It is the force required to oppose osmosis.

Characteristics

It depends on the number of solute particles and not on their nature (colligative property).

☐ *Iso-osmotic:* Solution that exerts the same osmotic pressure. When a cell is in direct contact with an iso-osmotic solution (0.9% NaCl), it is said to be isotonic
☐ *Hypertonic:* Solution with greater osmotic pressure
☐ *Hypotonic:* Solution with lower osmotic pressure
☐ *Oncotic pressure:* It represents the osmotic pressure of colloidal substances, e.g., albumin.
  • *Instrument to measure osmotic pressure:* Osmometer
  • *Unit of measurement:* Milliosmoles/L
  • Osmotic pressure of plasma = 280–300 milliosmoles/L.

Biomedical Importance

☐ *Fluid balance:* Fluid balance of the various compartments of the body and blood volume are maintained due to osmosis.
☐ *Fragility of RBC:* RBC undergoes hemolysis when kept in hypotonic solution. It is increased in hemolytic jaundice and decreased in certain anemias.
☐ *Transfusion:* Isotonic solutions (0.9% NaCl or 5% glucose) or a suitable mixture of both are used in transfusion to treat burns, dehydration, etc.
☐ *Edema:* It occurs due to reduced oncotic pressure of plasma leading to accumulation of excess fluid in tissue spaces as in hypoalbuminemia.
☐ *Osmotic diuresis:* It occurs in diabetes mellitus due to loss of water, electrolytes and glucose in the urine.

■ DIALYSIS

Definition

It is a technique for separating colloidal particles from small ions using a cellophane, collodion or parchment dialyzing membrane.

Biomedical Importance

☐ Dialysis of blood of patients with renal failure helps to remove small solutes, such as urea, creatinine from blood, while retaining plasma proteins and blood cells. It is applied in medicine in the 'artificial kidney'.
☐ It is used to separate proteins from a mixture with salts.

GIBBS–DONNAN MEMBRANE EQUILIBRIUM

Definition

Nondiffusible ions occurring on one side of semipermeable membrane increase the concentration of oppositely charged diffusible ions, by decreasing their diffusion to the other side. They decrease similarly charged diffusible ions on the same side by increasing their diffusion to the opposite side. But the total cations and anions are equal on either side at equilibrium. This is known as Gibbs–Donnan membrane equilibrium.

Biomedical Importance

Gibbs–Donnan effect is observed in the following:
- Difference in ionic concentrations in various fluid compartments of the body.
- Low pH in RBC
- Osmotic imbalance
- Chloride shift
- Concentration of Na^+/K^+ in renal glomerular filtrate

SURFACE TENSION

Definition

The force with which the surface molecules are held together and form a membrane over the surface of the liquid is known as 'surface tension' of the liquid.

Measurement

Drop weight method using stalagmometer.

Factors affecting surface tension:
- Bile salts, soaps, detergents, lipids and proteins decrease surface tension.
- Most inorganic salts (NaCl, KCl) slightly raise surface tension.

Biomedical Importance

- *Hay's test for bile salts:* It is used to detect bile salts in urine of patients suffering from jaundice. Bile salts in urine lower surface tension which is responsible for sulfur to sink.
- *Digestion and absorption of fats:* Bile salts lower surface tension of fat droplets and form emulsification. This is important for digestion and absorption of lipids.
- *Surfactants in lung function:* Surfactants (e.g., dipalmitoyl lecithin) is responsible for maintaining low surface tension in the alveoli. Its deficiency causes respiratory distress syndrome in the infants.

VISCOSITY

Definition

It is the internal resistance offered by a liquid or a gas to flow.

Determination

By using Ostwald's viscometer.

Unit

Poise.

Biomedical Importance

- *Viscosity of blood:* Blood is more viscous than water. It is due to suspended blood cells and colloidal plasma proteins. It is high in polycythemia and low in chronic anemia. Blood viscosity helps in the streamlining the blood flow.
- *Viscosity of synovial fluid:* Hyaluronic acid present in synovial fluid imparts viscosity which helps in the lubricating function of joints.

COLLOIDS

Solutes (substances) can be divided into two groups based on their passage through membrane.
1. *Crystalloids:* Substances which diffuse readily through membrane (e.g., sugar, salts, etc.). They usually exist in crystalline form.
2. *Colloids:* Substances which cannot diffuse (or diffuse at a very slow rate) are called as colloids, e.g., albumin, gelatin, starch, etc. These are noncrystallizable.

Classification

Colloids are of two types depending on their ability to take up the dispersion medium.
1. *Emulsoids (lyophilic colloids):* This type of colloids have great affinity for water. They carry electric charges—positive and negative of proteins. They are stable and not easily precipitated.

2. *Suspensoids (lyophobic colloids):* These colloids are not hydrated. They carry definite electric charge. They are easily precipitated.

Properties

- *Brownian movement:* It is the continuous and haphazard movement of colloidal particles.
- *Tyndall effect:* It refers to scattering of light when passed through a colloidal solution.
- *Electrical property:* Colloidal particles carry electric charge which may be positive or negative. They can be separated by electrophoresis.
- *Osmotic pressure:* Colloids exert low osmotic pressure.

Biomedical Importance

- *Donnan membrane equilibrium:* Nondiffusible colloids (protein) in biological system influence the concentration of diffusible ions across the membrane.
- *Adsorption:* Emulsoids can imbibe good amount of water. Adsorption is a colloidal phenomenon.
- Biological compounds, complex molecules, such as protein, lipids and polysaccharides exist in colloidal state.
- *Biological fluids:* Blood, cerebrospinal fluid and milk exist as colloids.
- *Protective colloids:* Colloids which prevent precipitation are known as protective colloids. Bile salts act as protective colloids and prevent precipitation of cholesterol and bile salts (gallstone). Protective colloids present in urine prevent formation of urinary stones.

■ ADSORPTION

Definition

It is the process of accumulation of a substance on the surface of another substance.

Biomedical Importance

- It is used for the separation and purification of compounds, such as enzymes.
- Drugs and poisons exert their action on adsorption at the cell surface.
- *Catalysis:* It occurs due to adsorption of substrate on the enzyme forming enzyme substrate complex.

■ ABSORPTION

Definition

It is a process by which a substance is not only retained on the surface, but also penetrates to the interior of the material.

Biomedical Importance

Some compounds bring about water insoluble substances soluble in water by absorption. For example, soaps of higher fatty acids, benzoic acid. These compounds are known as hydrotropic substances.

RADIOACTIVITY/RADIOACTIVE ISOTOPES

■ DEFINITION

The phenomenon by which unstable atomic nucleus of some elements emits ionizing radiation during decay, is known as radioactivity.

■ TYPES OF RADIATION

There are three types of radiations: α rays, β rays and γ rays.

■ ISOTOPES

Definition

The elements with the same atomic number, but different atomic weight.

Types

There are two types of isotopes:
1. *Nonradioactive (stable) isotopes:* They are naturally occurring isotopes and do not emit radiations, e.g., ^2H (deuterium/heavy hydrogen).
2. *Radioactive isotopes (unstable isotopes):* These compounds continuously disintegrate with spontaneous emission of radiation (α, β or γ rays).

Instruments to measure radioactivity:
- Geiger–Muller counter
- Liquid scintillation counter

■ UNIT OF MEASUREMENT

Curie (Ci)

APPLICATIONS

Biochemical/Metabolic

Used as tracers:
- ^{14}C, ^{15}N, ^{32}P, etc., are used as tracers to study intermediary metabolism.
- ^{59}Fe, ^{45}Ca, ^{131}I, etc., are used to study mineral metabolism.
- To elucidate drug metabolism
- To study metabolic pools and tumors

Medical/Therapeutic

Used for treatment of some diseases:
- ^{131}I for thyroid cancer
- ^{32}P for polycythemia vera
- ^{48}Au for pleural/peritoneal effusion

Diagnostic

Used to estimate hormones by radioimmunoassay, e.g., T_3, T_4, TSH, etc.

Hazards

Exposure to radioactivity is harmful for living organisms.
- It affects bone marrow, GI tract and CNS.
- It produces carcinogenesis and genetic effects.
- It shortens the life span.

MEMBRANE TRANSPORT

The role of the cell membrane is to allow compounds to enter or leave the cells in an orderly manner for the normal functions of the cell. It operates by various mechanisms and systems.

TRANSPORT MECHANISMS FOR SMALL MOLECULES

There are two main types of mechanisms for the transport of solutes (small molecules) through the membrane.

1. **Passive transport:** The solute passes from high concentration to lower concentration along concentration gradient. It is of two types:
   a. *Simple (passive) diffusion:* It occurs from higher concentration to lower concentration. It does not require carrier protein or energy. It is a slow process and operates unidirectionally, e.g., passage of gases, pentoses, water into the cells.

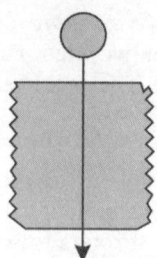

   b. *Facilitated diffusion:* It also allows solutes along concentration gradient (higher concentration to lower concentration). It requires carrier protein, but does not require energy. It operates bidirectionally. Its mechanism can be explained by ping-pong model, e.g., transfer of fructose into intestinal mucosal cells.

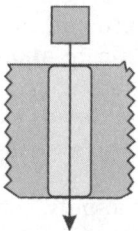

2. **Active transport:** It occurs against concentration gradient (lower concentration to higher concentration) and electrical gradient. Thus, it requires energy and also carrier protein, e.g., Transport of glucose into intestinal mucosal cells is mediated by sodium pump (Na^+-K^+ ATPase). It is of two types:
   a. *Primary active transport:* It requires metabolic energy provided by the direct hydrolysis of ATP, e.g., Na^+/k^+. ATPase (sodium pump) **(Fig. 1.6)**.
   b. *Secondary active transport:* It uses free energy of the electrochemical gradient generated, e.g., amino acid transport system, electron transport system.

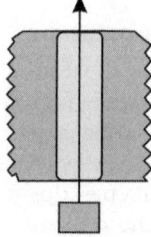

Chapter 1: The Cell (Biochemical and Biophysical Aspects)

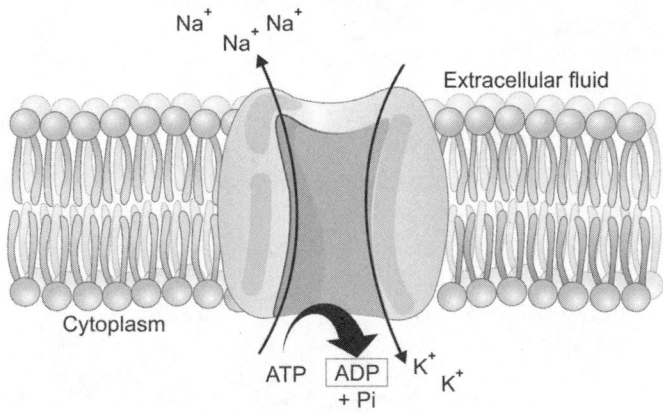

Fig. 1.6: Sodium-pump.

> **Note**
> Membranes of host cells contain specific channels or ionophores. Channels are specific for inorganic ions like sodium, potassium, chloride, etc. Ionophores are specific for sufficiently small organic molecules, such as antibiotics.

■ TRANSPORT SYSTEM

The transport system is mainly divided into two types:
1. **Uniport system:** It refers to the movement of a single molecule through the membrane, e.g., transport of glucose into RBCs.

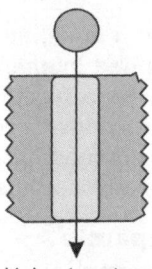

Uniport system

2. **Cotransport system:** It is divided into two subtypes:
   a. *Symport system:* It refers to the simultaneous transport of two different molecules

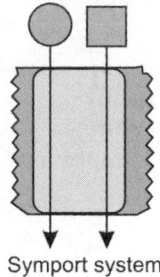

Symport system

in the same direction, e.g., transport of sodium and glucose into the intestinal cells.

b. *Antiport system:* It refers to the simultaneous transport of two different molecules in the opposite directions, e.g., exchange of chloride and bicarbonate in RBCs.

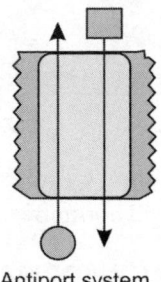

Antiport system

> **Clinical Importance**
> - *Hartnup disease:* Transport of amino acids in the intestine is defective
> - *Cystinuria:* Renal absorption of cysteine is defective.

■ TRANSPORT OF MACROMOLECULES

The transport of macromolecules, e.g., polysaccharides, proteins and polynucleotides through the membrane is brought about by the two different mechanisms **(Figs. 1.7A and B)**.
1. **Endocytosis:** It indicates entry of macromolecules into the cells through the membrane, e.g., uptake of low-density lipoproteins (LDL) by the cells.
2. **Exocytosis:** It refers to the exit of macromolecules from the cells through the membrane,

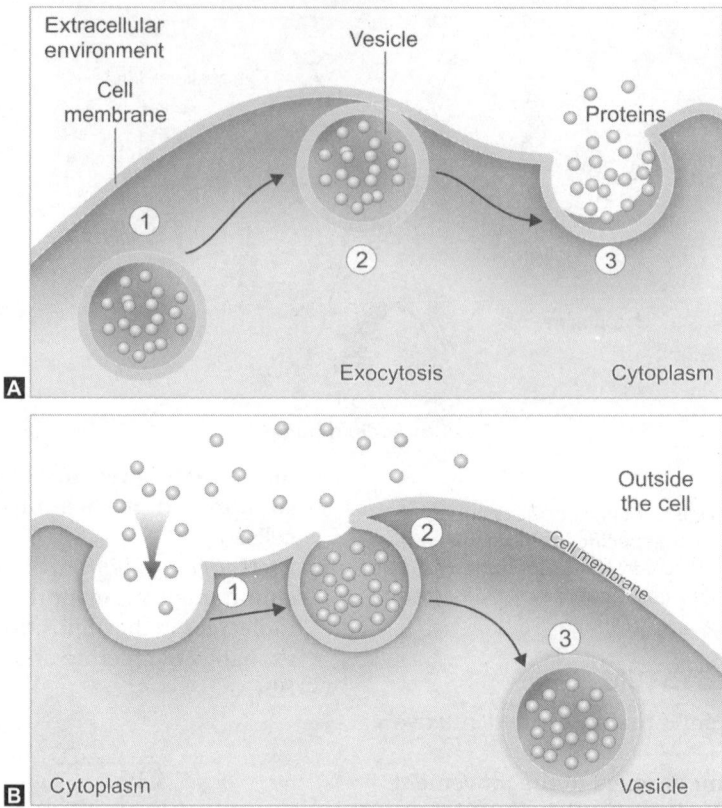

Figs. 1.7A and B: (A) Exocytosis; (B) Endocytosis.

e.g., secretion of hormones, such as insulin and parathyroid hormone.

■ ADDITIONAL INFORMATION

Composition of human body:
- *Major elements:* Carbon, hydrogen, oxygen and nitrogen.
- *Other elements:* Calcium, phosphorus, sodium, potassium, chloride, magnesium, iron, zinc, copper, etc.
- *Water:* The major constituent of the human body (60%).
- *Biomolecules:* Five major complex biomolecules are polysaccharides, complex lipids, proteins, nucleic acids. (DNA and RNA).
- *Microsomes (microsomal fraction):* It is mostly a mixture of RER, SER and free ribosomes formed during cell fractionation.
- *Cell organelle:* It is defined as subcellular entity surrounded by membrane and can be isolated by centrifugation. According to this definition, cytosol, cytoskeleton and ribosomes are not subcellular organelles, but are considered as subcellular fractions.

Methods to Separate Subcellular Organelles

Subcellular fractionation: It consists of three procedures:
1. Extraction
2. Homogenization
3. Differential centrifugation (using ultracentrifuge)

Methods to determine biomolecular structure:
- NMR spectroscopy
- Mass spectrometry
- X-ray crystallography, etc.

Section 2: Chemistry of Biomolecules

2. Chemistry of Carbohydrates

Chapter Outline
- Definition
- Alternative Name
- Occurrence
- Composition
- Biomedical Importance/Functions
- Classification
  - Monosaccharides
  - Oligosaccharides
- Polysaccharides
- Additional Information

DEFINITION

Carbohydrates are polyhydroxy alcohols having aldehyde/keto group or their derivatives which yield such compounds on hydrolysis. They are organic compounds.

ALTERNATIVE NAME

Saccharides (Saccharide = Derived from Greek word 'Sakcharon' meaning sugar).

OCCURRENCE

Carbohydrates are widely distributed in nature. They are synthesized in plants from carbon dioxide and water by photosynthesis. Though humans and animals can synthesize carbohydrates from fat and protein to a little extent, mostly they are derived from plants.

COMPOSITION

Carbohydrates may be considered as hydrates of carbon. Hence, general molecular formula for carbohydrate was given as $C_n(H_2O)_n$. According to this formula, ratio of carbon, hydrogen and oxygen in carbohydrates is 1:2:1.

BIOMEDICAL IMPORTANCE/FUNCTIONS

1. *Energy:* Carbohydrates are the major source of energy. They provide 55–65% of total energy needed for the body.
2. *Storage:* Starch in plants and glycogen in humans and animals serve as stores of glucose.
3. *Structural components:* They serve as structural and supportive elements in cells. They mediate much of the intercellular communication.
4. *Biochemical compounds:* They are constituents of glycolipids, glycoproteins, proteoglycans, nucleic acids, etc.
5. *Drugs:* Some of the carbohydrate derivatives are used as drugs.
   - Antibiotics (streptomycin, erythromycin)
   - Cardiac glycosides (digitonin)
6. They spare protein and fat for other purpose.
7. *Miscellaneous:* They act as:
   - Dietary fiber, e.g., cellulose
   - Lubricant and intercellular cement, e.g., mucopolysaccharides
   - Anticoagulant, e.g., heparin
   - Pharmacopeial product, e.g., dextrose
   - Food sweetener, e.g., glucose.

Clinical Importance
- Defective metabolism of glucose will result in diabetes mellitus.
- Deficiency of specific enzymes in metabolic pathways of carbohydrates can cause inborn errors of metabolism, e.g., glycogen storage diseases, galactosemia, etc.

CLASSIFICATION (FIG. 2.1)

Carbohydrates can be divided into three major classes depending on the number of saccharide units (sugar units).

Section 2: Chemistry of Biomolecules

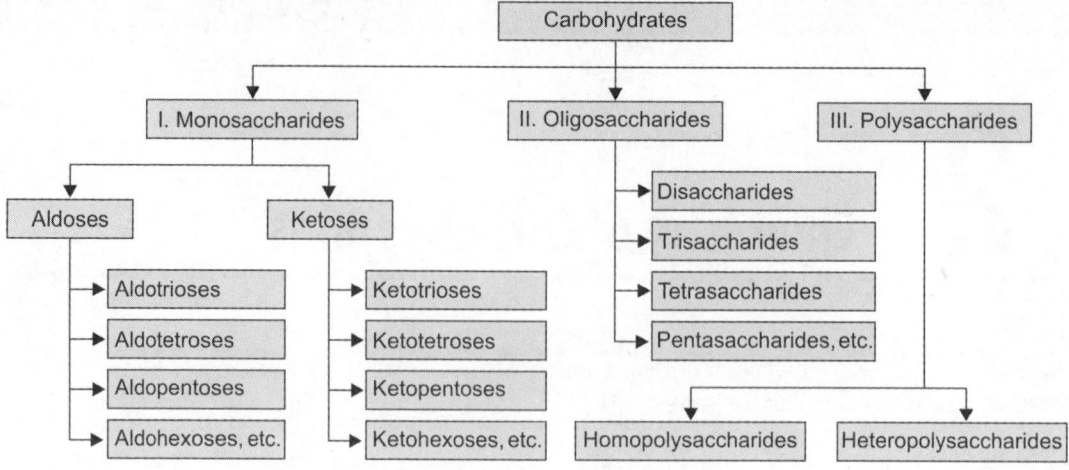

Fig. 2.1: Classification of carbohydrates.

I. Monosaccharides *(contain one saccharide unit)*
II. Oligosaccharides *(contain two to ten monosaccharide units)*
III. Polysaccharides *(contain more than ten monosaccharide units).*

Each major class is further divided into many subclasses as given below:

I. Monosaccharides (Table 2.1)

Monosaccharides have only one saccharide unit. They are also called as simple sugars. They have low molecular weight. They are polyhydroxy alcohols containing aldehyde or keto group. They cannot be hydrolyzed further to simpler sugars.

Subclasses

They are subdivided depending on:
- The number of carbon atoms
- The presence of aldehyde group (–CHO) or keto group (–CO)

The smallest monosaccharides are three carbon sugars, e.g.,

- *Glyceraldehyde (aldotriose):* All other aldosugars are derived from it. They may be D or L forms (*refer* p. 17).

$$\begin{array}{c} ^1CHO \\ | \\ ^2H-C-OH \\ | \\ ^3CH_2OH \end{array} \qquad \begin{array}{c} ^1CHO \\ | \\ ^2HO-C-H \\ | \\ ^3CH_2OH \end{array}$$

D-glyceraldehyde   L-glyceraldehyde

- *Dihydroxyacetone (ketotriose):* All other ketosugars are derived from it. Except dihydroxyacetone, all other ketosugars exist as D and L isomers.

$$\begin{array}{c} ^1CH_2OH \\ | \\ ^2CO \\ | \\ ^3CH_2OH \end{array}$$

Structural Aspects
Structure of Glucose
Glucose is a monosaccharide and an aldohexose. Its molecular formula is $C_6H_{12}O_6$.

Subclasses	No. of carbon atoms	Aldoses (aldosugars)	Ketoses (ketosugars)
Trioses	3	Aldotrioses	Ketotrioses
Tetroses	4	Aldotetroses	Ketotetroses
Pentoses	5	Aldopentoses	Ketopentoses
Hexoses	6	Aldohexoses	Ketohexoses

Chapter 2: Chemistry of Carbohydrates

Table 2.1: Examples (monosaccharides of biomedical importance).

Aldoses (aldosugars)		
Examples	Sources	Biomedical Importance
Aldotrioses D-Glyceraldehyde	Glyceraldehyde 3-phosphates are intermediate compounds in glycolysis and hexose monophosphate shunt (carbohydrate metabolism).	
Aldotetroses D-Erythrose	Erythrose phosphates are intermediate compounds in hexose monophosphate shunt	
Aldopentoses D-Ribose	A constituent of ribonucleic acid (RNA), coenzymes, etc.	Structural element of RNA and coenzymes (NAD, NADP, ATP, etc.) Ribose in hexose monophosphate shunt
2-Deoxy D-ribose	A constituent of deoxy ribonucleic acid (DNA)	Structural element of DNA
D-Arabinose	Present in gum arabic	A constituent of glycoprotein. It is used in bacterial testing
D-Xylose	Present in wood gums	A constituent of proteoglycans and glycosaminoglycans. Also used in bacterial testing
D-Lyxose	Present in heart muscle	A constituent of lyxoflavin
L-Fucose	Present in glycoproteins	A constituent of blood group substances
Aldohexoses D-Glucose	Present in fruits. A constituent of disaccharides (lactose, maltose and sucrose) and polysaccharides (starch, glycogen, dextrin, etc.)	The major sugar used for energy in the body; Stored as glycogen in liver and muscles. Known as blood sugar. Defective metabolism leads to diabetes mellitus. Present in the urine of diabetic patients
D-Galactose	Synthesized in the mammary gland to form lactose of milk. Also a constituent of glycolipids and glycoproteins	Converted to glucose in the liver. Defective metabolism of galactose leads to galactosemia
D-Mannose	Present in plant gums	A constituent of glycoproteins
Ketoses (ketosugars)		
Examples	Sources	Importance
Ketotrioses Dihydroxyacetone	Dihydroxyacetone phosphates are intermediate compounds in glycolysis	
Ketotetroses D-Erythrulose	A natural product	
Ketopentoses L-xylulose	Xylulose phosphates are intermediate compounds in uronic acid pathway	Found in urine of patients with essential pentosuria
D-Ribulose	Ribulose phosphates are intermediate compounds in hexose monophosphate shunt.	
Ketohexose D-Fructose	It occurs in honey and fruits. It is present in seminal fluid. A constituent of sucrose and inulin, known as fruit sugar	Also used for energy. Its abnormal metabolism leads to hereditary fructose intolerance and essential fructosuria

It has three types of structures:
1. Straight (open/linear) chain forms.
2. Ring (cyclic) forms.
3. Boat and chair forms.

Straight (open/linear) chain forms
Glucose is a straight chain polyhydroxy alcohol containing a free aldehyde group. It has six carbon atoms. Aldehyde group is represented

at the top. Rest of the hydrogen atoms and hydroxyl groups are attached to each carbon atom as shown in the figure.

```
   ¹CHO              ¹CHO
H—²CO—OH        H—²C—OH
HO—³C—H         HO—³C—H
H—⁴C—OH         H—⁴C—OH
H—⁵C—OH         HO—⁵C—H
   ⁶CH₂OH            ⁶CH₂OH
  D-glucose         L-glucose
```

It has 4 asymmetric carbon atoms ($C_{2,3,4,5}$) because to each of these carbon atoms are attached different atoms or groups. So glucose will have 16 stereoisomers according to the formula 2^n.

Ring (cyclic) forms
Straight chain structures of glucose are unable to explain some of its reactions, e.g., mutarotation. Hence, ring (cyclic) structures have been proposed.

Types
Two types of ring structures of glucose are possible.
1. Pyranose ring
2. Furanose ring

They can be represented by:
- Fischer projection
- Haworth projection

Pyranose ring
Glucose is predominantly present in the pyranose ring form (99%). It is a six-membered ring form. (It resembles 'pyran' - a six-membered compound).

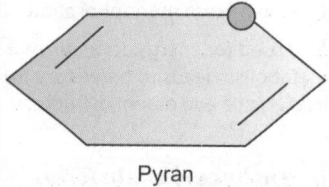
Pyran

Pyranose ring is formed by intramolecular hemiacetal linkage between carbonyl group at C_1 and hydroxyl group at C_5. Pyranose ring of glucose in various forms is given below:

D-glucose: It can exist as:
- α-D-glucopyranose
  - *Fischer projection:* OH at C_1 is on the right and H on the left.

```
   ¹
H—C—H
H—²C—OH
HO—³C—H
H—⁴C—OH
H—⁵C
   ⁶CH₂OH
```

- *Haworth projection:* OH at C_1 below and H above the plane of the ring.

- β-D-glucopyranose
  - *Fischer projection:* OH at C_1 is on the left and H is on the right.

```
HO—C—H
H—C—OH
HO—C—H
H—C—OH
H—C
   CH₂OH
```

- *Haworth projection:* OH at C_1 above and H below

Furanose ring

Glucose also exists as furanose ring (1%). It is a five-membered ring (It resembles a five-membered ring compound namely 'Furan').

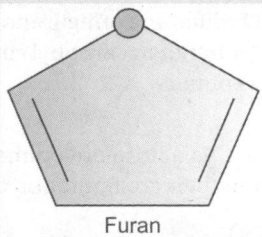
Furan

This ring is formed by intramolecular hemiacetal linkage between aldehyde group at carbon atom 1 with hydroxyl group at carbon atom 4. It can also be represented by:
- Fischer projection
- Haworth projection

Various forms of furanose ring of glucose are given below.
- α-D-glucofuranose
  - *Fischer projection:* OH on C_1 is on the right, and H on the left.

```
    1
H—C—OH
    2
H—C—OH
    3
HO—C—H
    4
H—C———
    5
H—C—OH
    6
   CH₂OH
```

- *Haworth projection:* OH on C_1 down and H up

- β-D-Glucofuranose
  - *Fischer projection:* OH on C_1 is on the left and H on the right.

- *Haworth projection:* OH on C_1 is above and H below.

Boat and chair forms have also been proposed to explain the stability of sugars.

Isomerism in Sugars (Refer Appendix D)

Optical isomers
Glucose may exist as optical isomers because it contains asymmetric carbon atoms. They exhibit:

Dextrorotatory (+) or (d)
Rotating plane polarized light to right, (or)

Levorotatory (−) or (l)
Rotating plane polarized light to left.

D or L isomers
Orientation of H and OH groups around the carbon atom (C_5) adjacent to primary alcoholic carbon atom determines whether the sugar is D or L form.
- In D isomer - OH on C_5 is on the right.
- In L isomer - OH on C_5 is on the left.
- D and L isomers are mirror images to each other (Enantiomers).
- D isomer may be dextrorotatory (+) or levorotatory (−).
- L isomer may be dextrorotatory (+) or levorotatory (−).
- Most of the monosaccharides occurring in nature are of *D* configuration.

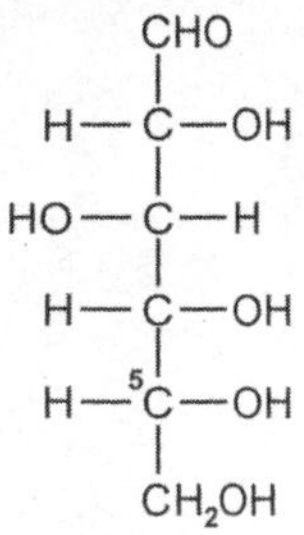

D-glucose

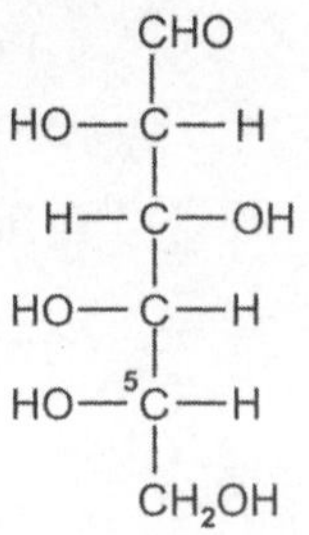

L-glucose

Anomers

Definition

Two isomers which differ only in the configuration at C_1 (as in aldoses) or C_2 (as in ketoses) are known as *anomers*. Such carbon atoms are anomeric carbon atoms or carbonyl carbon atoms.

Examples:

- α-D-Glucose and β-D-Glucose are anomers of glucose.

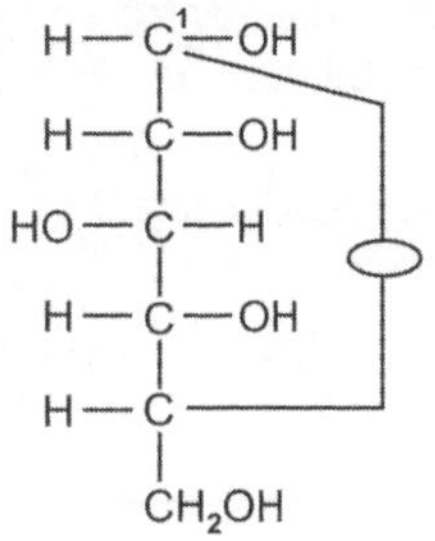

α-D-glucose

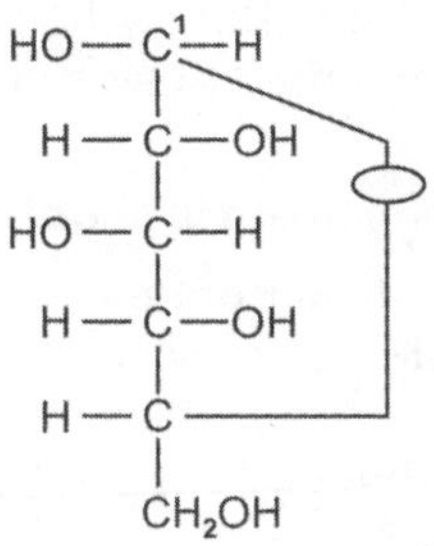

β-D-glucose

- α-D-Fructose and β-D-Fructose are anomers of fructose.

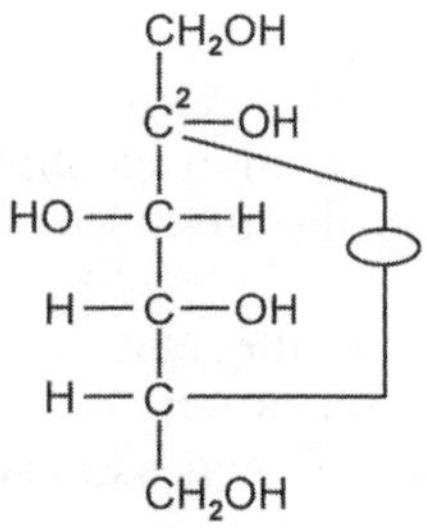

α-D-fructose

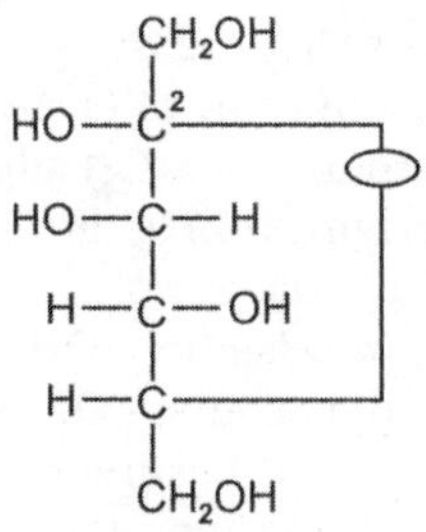

β-D-fructose

Importance

- Anomers differ in certain physical and chemical properties.
- They have different optical rotation.
- Mutarotation represents interconversion of α and β anomers.

Epimers

Definition

Isomers which differ in configuration at carbon atoms ($C_{2,3,4}$) other than carbonyl carbon atoms are known as epimers.

Examples:

- Glucose and galactose are epimers because they differ in their configuration at C_4.

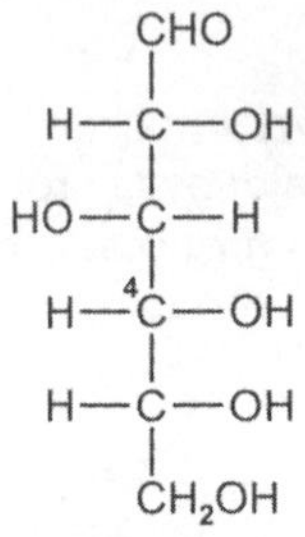

D-glucose

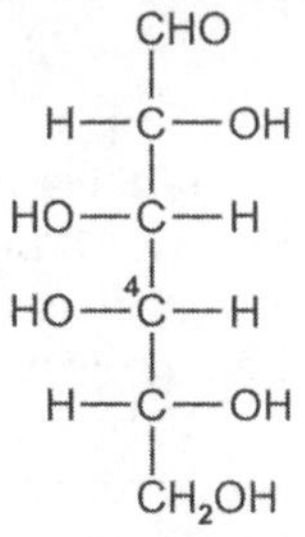

D-galactose

- Glucose and mannose are epimers due to difference in their configuration at C_2.

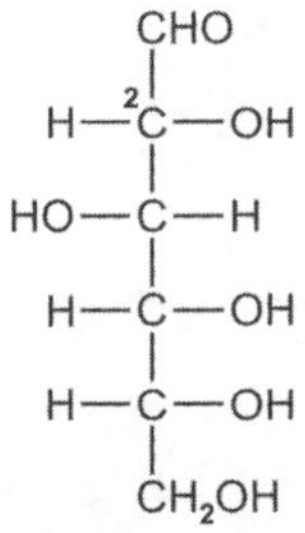

D-glucose

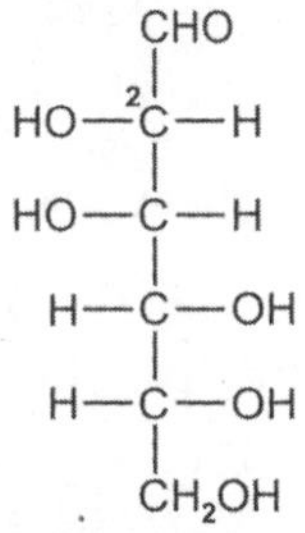

D-mannose

Importance

- Interconversion of epimers is known as epimerization and is catalyzed by epimerase.
- Galactose is converted to glucose in the body by epimerization.

Structures of fructose

Fructose is a monosaccharide and a ketohexose. Its molecular formula is $C_6H_{12}O_6$.

It can also exist as the following structures:

Straight chain

It has 6 carbon atoms and a keto group as specific functional group. Naturally occurring form of fructose is D(-) and so called as levulose. It has 3 asymmetric carbon atoms ($C_{3,4,5}$) and can exist as 8 isomers.

Chapter 2: Chemistry of Carbohydrates

```
  ¹CH₂OH              ¹CH₂OH
   |                    |
  ²CO                  ²CO
   |                    |
HO—³C—H              HO—³C—H
   |                    |
 H—⁴C—OH             H—⁴C—OH
   |                    |
 H—⁵C—OH            HO—⁵C—H
   |                    |
  ⁶CH₂OH              ⁶CH₂OH
 D-fructose          L-fructose
```

Ring forms
- Pyranose ring
- Furanose ring

Properties

Physical properties
- *State:* Colorless, crystalline compounds
- *Solubility:* Readily soluble in water
- *Taste:* Sweet
- *Optical activity:* All monosaccharides except dihydroxyacetone are optically active. They exhibit mutarotation.

Mutarotation
Definition: It refers to change in specific rotation of an optically active solution due to interconversion of α and β anomers of sugars.

Examples: Glucose and other reducing sugars except few ketoses exhibit this property.

Mechanism
It was proposed by Tanret using polarimeter.
   When α D-glucopyranose is dissolved in water, its specific rotation is +112° at first. Then it decreases slowly with time and finally becomes steady at +52.5°. β-D-glucopyranose first shows specific rotation +19° but slowly increases and becomes steady at +52.5°. This solution giving specific rotation +52.5° is an equilibrium mixture of two cyclic forms α and β. In this process, ring form opens to the linear form and then closes to give α and β cyclic forms and open chain form.

α-D-glucopyranose → Equilibrium mixture
     +112°   + 52.5°
← β-D-glucopyranose
     + 19°

$$\begin{pmatrix} \alpha \text{ - D - Glucopyranose 36\%} \\ \beta \text{ - D - Glucopyranose 63\%} \\ + \\ \text{Open chain 1\%} \end{pmatrix}$$

This change is catalyzed by the enzyme mutarotase. Alkali also catalyzes this reaction.

Importance
- Glucose exists in straight and ring forms.
- Three forms of glucose are interconvertible in aqueous solution.
- All reducing sugars except few ketoses undergo mutarotation

Chemical properties
Carbohydrates contain functional groups which are responsible for their chemical properties.
- Aldehyde (CHO) or Keto (CO) group
- Hydroxyl (OH) groups
- Both CHO/CO and OH groups

Reactions due to aldehyde (CHO) or keto (CO) group

Action of alkalis
- With dilute alkali (NaOH) and on standing, glucose is isomerized to D-fructose and D-mannose. These three sugars are in equilibrium through an intermediate enediol form. The same transformation also takes place with fructose or mannose.

```
              Mannose
                ↕
Glucose ⇌ H–C–OH ⇌ Fructose
           ‖
          C–OH
           |
        HO–C–H
           |
         H–C–OH
           |
         H–C–OH
           |
          CH₂OH     Enediol
```

- On boiling with *strong* alkalis, sugar undergoes caramealization, i.e., solution turns yellow and then brown as a result of formation of a series of resinous products.

Reducing action
Monosaccharides act as effective reducing agents.
Definition: Sugar containing a free aldehyde or keto group, (i.e., carbonyl group of a sugar not attached to any other structure) is called reducing sugar.
Mechanism: Monosaccharides readily reduce oxidizing agents, such as cupric ion. Thus,

glucose is oxidized to aldonic acid and cupric ion becomes reduced to cuprous ion.

Importance/applications: This principle is the basis of the following tests which are used for identification of reducing sugars in solutions or urine.

Tests to identify reducing sugars
Benedict's test: It is used to identify all reducing sugars.
Procedure: When a reducing sugar is treated with alkaline copper reagent (Benedict's qualitative reagent), sugar is converted to enediol form which is a powerful reducer. This reduces cupric ion of copper sulfate to cuprous ion of cuprous oxide (red in color). Simultaneously sugar is also oxidized to sugar acid (aldonic acid).

Glucose + Alkali → Enediol
$\downarrow Cu^{2+}$
CuOH (Cuprous hydroxide) + Sugar acid
$\downarrow$
Cu_2O (Cuprous oxide)

Clinical Importance

It is mainly used in the clinical laboratory to detect glucose in the urine to diagnose diabetes mellitus. It is a semiquantitative tests.

Fehling's test: It is also used to identify all reducing sugars.

Barfoed's test: It is used to identify (reducing) monosaccharides.

Reduction
The monosaccharides are reduced to their corresponding alcohols by reducing agents, such as sodium amalgam.

Glucose $\xrightarrow{(CHO \to CH_2OH)}$ Sorbitol

Mannose $\xrightarrow{(CHO \to CH_2OH)}$ Mannitol

Galactose $\xrightarrow{(CHO \to CH_2OH)}$ Dulcitol

Fructose $\xrightarrow{(CO \to CHOH)}$ Sorbitol and Mannitol

Importance: Sorbitol and dulcitol accumulation in tissue and may cause cataract, nephropathy and neuropathy. Mannitol is used to reduce intracranial tension.

Formation of osazones
Definition
Glucose when heated with phenylhydrazine and a buffer (glacial acetic acid and sodium acetate) yellow crystalline compounds are formed. These are called as osazones.

Shape
They have needle-shaped appearance when observed under microscope.

Mechanism
It was proposed by Weygand through Amadori rearrangement.
❐ One molecule of glucose condenses with one molecule of phenylhydrazine to form gluco-phenylhydrazone.
❐ Second molecule of phenylhydrazine enters the reaction and an intermediate compound is formed.
❐ Third molecule of phenylhydrazine reacts with intermediate compound to produce glucosazone **(Fig. 2.2)**.

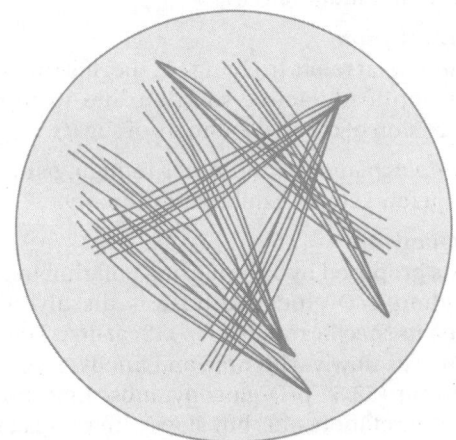

Fig. 2.2: Glucosazone/fructosazone.
(For color version, see Plate 1)

Glucose + Phenylhydrazine → Gluco-phenylhydrazone
(NH$_2$—NH—C$_6$H$_5$)

H—C=N—NHC$_6$H$_5$
|
C=N—NHC$_6$H$_5$ ← Phenylhydrazine — Intermediate compound
|
R
Glucosazone

Applications
❐ To identify various reducing sugars
❐ To determine the structural configurations of sugars.

> **Note**
> - Fructose also forms needle-shaped osazones (Fructosazones)
> - During osazone formation, structural dissimilarity at C_1 and C_2 of glucose and fructose disappears and both form same type of osazones.

Fermentation
Glucose, fructose and mannose can be fermented by zymase present in yeast to produce alcohol and carbon dioxide.

$$C_6H_{12}O_6 \xrightarrow{\text{Zymase}} 2C_2H_5OH + 2CO_2$$
Glucose $\quad\quad\quad\quad\quad\quad$ Ethyl alcohol

Reactions due to hydroxyl groups
Formation of esters
- Hexoses are converted to their phosphoric acid esters in carbohydrate metabolism.
  Glucose → Glucose 6-phosphate
- Fructose forms fructose 6-phosphate
  Fructose → Fructose 6-phosphate
- Ribose forms ribose 6-phosphate which is involved in the formation of nucleic acids.
  Ribose → Ribose 5-phosphate.

Formation of Glycosides (refer below)
Reactions due to both CHO/CO and OH groups
Action of acids
- Weak acids have no significant action on sugars.
- On treatment with strong acids, such as HCl or H_2SO_4 and heating, sugars undergo dehydration to form furfural or its derivatives. These compounds develop characteristic colors with alcoholic solution of α Naphthol.
  Glucose → 5-hydroxymethylfurfural
  Ribose → Furfural
  This reaction is the basis for Molisch's test, Seliwanoff's test, and Bial's test which are used for identification of sugars.

Oxidation
Products of oxidation of glucose depend on the nature of oxidizing agents.
- Glucose is oxidized to gluconic acid (aldonic acid) when treated with bromine water (CHO is converted to COOH).

$$\text{Glucose} \xrightarrow{Br_2 + H_2O} \text{Gluconic acid}$$

- Glucose is oxidized to glucuronic and (uronic acid) when treated with platinum carbon catalyst (CH_2OH is converted to COOH group).

$$\text{Glucose} \xrightarrow{\text{Catalyst}} \begin{array}{c} CHO \\ | \\ H-C-OH \\ | \\ HO-C-H \\ | \\ H-C-OH \\ | \\ H-C-OH \\ | \\ COOH \end{array}$$
Glucuronic acid

Glucuronic acid is used as a conjugating agent in detoxication of toxic substances in the liver. It is a constituent of mucopolysaccharides.
- Glucose is oxidized to saccharic acid (aldaric acid) when treated with conc. nitric acid (both CHO and CH_2OH are oxidized to COOH groups).

$$\text{Glucose} \xrightarrow{\text{Conc. } HNO_3} \text{Saccharic acid}$$

Derivatives
Glucose forms several useful derivatives.

Glycosides
Definition: Glycosides are compounds formed by condensation between hydroxyl group of anomeric carbon of a monosaccharide and hydroxyl group of another monosaccharide or noncarbohydrate (aglycone), such as methyl alcohol, sterol, etc.

Composition:

Carbohydrate/
Carbohydrate + Noncarbohydrate = Glycoside
(aglycone)

The bond which connects these two compounds is called as glycosidic linkage. If carbohydrate portion (hemiacetal) is glucose, the resulting compound is called as glucoside.

Occurrence: They are naturally occurring derivatives of carbohydrates.

Formation: Glycoside is formed when a solution of glucose is boiled with methyl alcohol using HCl as a catalyst.

Glucose + Methyl alcohol $\xrightarrow{\text{HCl}}$

Methyl α-D-glucoside   Methyl β-D-glucoside

Properties: They are crystalline colorless bitter compounds. They are soluble in water and alcohol. They do not show reducing properties and do not exhibit mutarotation.

Important uses (Table 2.2)

Aminosugars
Definition: Sugars containing an amino group (–NH$_2$) are called as amino sugars. They are formed by the replacement of hydroxyl group attached to carbon atom 2 of the sugar by an amino group.

D-glucosamine   D-galactosamine

Importance: They are present as N-acetyl derivatives in many biologically important substances.

	Examples	Importance
a.	N-acetyl D-glucosamine	Occurs in certain mucopolysaccharides, such as hyaluronic acid and also in blood group substances
b.	N-acetyl D-galactosamine	Occurs in mucopolysaccharides, such as chondroitin sulfates which are present in cartilages, tendons and heart valve
c.	Aminosugar	Erythromycin (antibiotic)

Aminosugar acid: For example—
- *Neuraminic acid:* It is formed by aldol condensation between an aminosugar and an organic acid.
  - Mannosamine + Pyruvic acid → Neuraminic acid
- *Sialic acid:* (N-acetyl neuraminic acid - NANA)

It is present in glycoproteins and gangliosides (glycolipids).

Deoxysugars
They represent sugars in which the oxygen of an OH group has been removed, leaving the hydrogen.

Deoxysugars of biological importance are:
- *2-deoxy-D-ribose:* It is present in deoxyribonucleic acid (DNA) which contains the genetic message (*refer* Chapter 5).

Table 2.2 : Importance: Glycosides function as drugs.

Examples	Sources	Importance
• Cardiac glycosides, e.g., Digitonin = Xylose + Galactose + Digitogenin	Leaves and seeds of digitalis	They act on heart and are used in heart insufficiency
• Ouabain (Glucose + Steroid)	Strophanthus	It inhibits active transport of Na$^+$ in cardiac muscle in vivo (Sodium pump inhibitor)
• Phlorizin (Glucose + Phloretin)	Roots and bark of apple tree	It blocks the transport of sugar across the mucosal cells of small intestine and also renal tubular epithelium and produces glycosuria
• Antibiotic (Streptomycin)	Genus *Streptomyces*	It is used to treat tuberculosis

Chapter 2: Chemistry of Carbohydrates

```
        CHO
         |
      H—C—H
         |
      H—C—OH
         |
      H—C—OH
         |
       CH₂OH
```
2-deoxy-D-ribose

- *6-deoxy-L-galactose:* It is a constituent of glycoproteins and blood group substances.
- *Vitamin C (ascorbic acid):* Its structure resembles to that of a monosaccharide. It is a water soluble vitamin (*refer* Chapter 8).

II. Oligosaccharides

Definition
Oligosaccharides consist of short chain of 2–10 monosaccharide units joined together by glycosidic linkages. Their general molecular formula is $C_n(H_2O)_{n-1}$ (Oligo = few).

Subclasses
Depending on the number of monosaccharide units, they are subdivided as:

Disaccharides: (2 monosaccharide units), e.g., lactose, maltose, sucrose.

Trisaccharides: (3 monosaccharide units), e.g., raffinose.

Tetrasaccharides: (4 monosaccharide units), e.g., stachyose.

Pentasaccharides: (5 monosaccharide units), e.g., verbascose and so on.

Importance
- Cell membrane proteins contain oligosaccharides.
- Secretory proteins, such as antibodies (immunoglobulins) coagulation factors, peptide hormones contain oligosaccharides.
- Many oligosaccharides are present in glycoproteins.

Disaccharides
Disaccharides are the most important common oligosaccharides. They are composed of 2 monosaccharide units joined by a glycosidic linkage. If one of the carbonyl carbon atoms is free, the disaccharide is a reducing sugar. If both carbonyl carbon atoms are involved in the linkage, the disaccharide is a nonreducing sugar. They are crystalline substances, sweet and soluble in water. Their general molecular formula is $C_n(H_2O)_{n-1}$.

Examples: The physiologically important disaccharides are:
- Lactose
- Maltose
- Sucrose

Lactose
Alternative name
Milk sugar.

Sources
It is synthesized in mammary gland and is present in milk.

Composition: Galactose + Glucose = Lactose.

Structure
Its molecular formula is $C_{12}H_{22}O_{11}$. Each lactose molecule contains 1 molecule of glucose and

β-D-galactopyranosyl (1 → 4) β-D-glucopyranose
(*Simplified:* Galactose ←―――――― β1 → 4 glycosidic linkage ――――――→ Glucose)

1 molecule of galactose. Carbon atom 1 of galactose is linked to carbon atom 4 of glucose by β-1, 4 glycosidic linkage.

Properties
It is a white crystalline substance. It is less soluble in water. It is less sweet than sucrose. It is dextrorotatory (+). It is a reducing sugar, because it has a free aldehyde group in glucose molecule. It shows reducing properties. It answers Molisch's test. It exhibits mutarotation. It can exist in α and β forms. It forms osazone (Lactosazone) having hedgehog/badminton ball/powder puff shape crystals (**Fig. 2.3**).

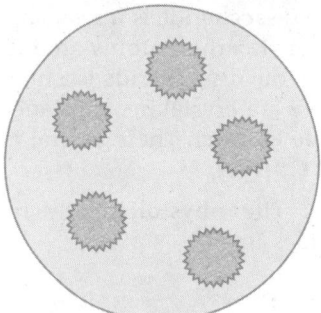

Fig. 2.3: Lactosazone.
(*For color version, see Plate 1*)

Biomedical importance
- It serves as a nutrient especially in infants.
- Indigestion of lactose due to deficiency of enzyme lactase may result in *lactose intolerance* in children. Its symptoms are diarrhea and flatulence (*refer* Chapter 11).

Maltose
Alternative name
Malt sugar.

Sources
It is present in germinating seeds and malt. It is also obtained when starch is hydrolyzed by acid or digested by maltase.

Composition: Glucose + Glucose = Maltose.

Structure
Its molecular formula is $C_{12}H_{22}O_{11}$. It is made up of 2 molecules of glucose. Carbon atom 1 of first glucose molecule is linked to carbon atom 4 of second glucose molecule through α-1, 4 glycosidic linkage.

Properties
It is a white crystalline substance. It is sweeter in taste. It is a reducing sugar because the aldehyde group in second glucose molecule is free and shows reducing properties. It can exist in α and β forms. It exhibits mutarotation. It is fermentable. It forms osazone (maltosazone) which looks like petals of sunflower (**Fig. 2.4**).

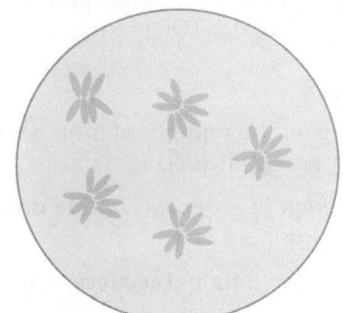

Fig. 2.4: Maltosazone.
(*For color version, see Plate 1*)

Biomedical importance
It serves as a nutrient.

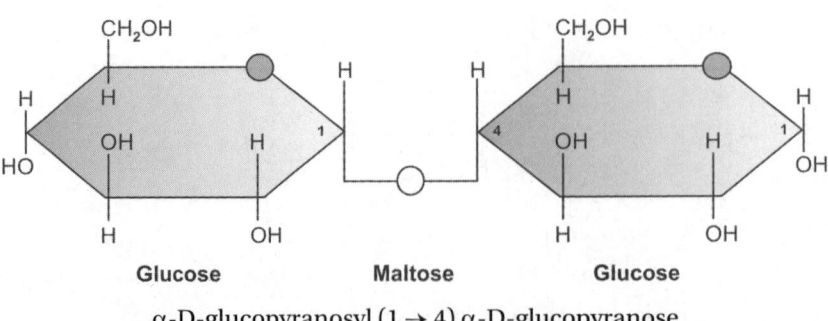

α-D-glucopyranosyl (1 → 4) α-D-glucopyranose
(*Simplified:* Glucose ←——— α1 → 4 glycosidic linkage ———→ Glucose)

α-D-glucopyranosyl (1 → 2) β-D-fructofuranoside
(*Simplified:* Glucose $\xleftarrow{\alpha 1 \to \beta 2 \text{ glycosidic linkage}}$ Fructose)

Sucrose
Alternative names: Table sugar, cane sugar.

Sources
It is present in sugar cane, pine apple, carrot roots, potato and honey.

Composition
Glucose + Fructose = Sucrose

Structure
Its molecular formula is $C_{12}H_{22}O_{11}$. It is composed of one molecule of glucose and one molecule of fructose. Carbon atom 1 (CHO) of glucose is joined to carbon atom 2 (CO) of fructose by ($\alpha 1 \to \beta 2$) glycosidic linkage. So it has no free aldehyde or keto group and thus it is a non-reducing sugar.

Properties
It is a white crystalline solid. It is soluble in water. It is more sweet than other two disaccharides. It does not show reducing properties. It cannot exist as α and β forms. It does not exhibit mutarotation. It cannot form osazone.

Importance
- It serves as a nutrient.
- It is a sweetening agent.
- It can be converted to *invert sugar*.
- It produces dental caries.

Inversion and invert sugar
Sucrose undergoes inversion to produce invert sugar.

Definition
The process by which sucrose (dextrorotatory) (+) is converted to a mixture of glucose and fructose which is (levorotatory) (−) is called as inversion.

Process
Sucrose is dextrorotatory (+66.5°). But when sucrose is treated with dilute acid or *sucrase (invertase)*, it gives equal amount of glucose and fructose. This mixture is levorotatory (−), as levorotation of fructose (−92°) is higher than dextrorotation of glucose (+52.5°). Since dextrorotation of sucrose is converted to levorotatory mixture with inversion of optical rotation, the process is called as *inversion*. The mixture of glucose and fructose is called as *invert sugar*.

Sucrose $\xrightarrow{\text{Sucrase (Invertase)}}$ Glucose + Fructose
+66.5°   +52.5°   −92°

Biomedical importance:
- Invert sugar is more sweet than sucrose itself. Honey is mostly invert sugar and the presence of fructose accounts for the greater sweetness of honey.
- Inversion of sucrose is an important reaction in jam making.

III. Polysaccharides

Definition
They consist of long chain of more than 10 monosaccharide units. They are high molecular weight compounds. They are not crystalline substances. They are not soluble in water. They are not sweet. Their general molecular formula is $(C_6H_{10}O_5)_n$.

Alternative name: Glycans.

Functions
- Storage
- Nutrition
- Structural component
- Lubrication
- Corneal transparency
- Anticoagulant

Subclasses

They are subdivided into two types, depending on whether they contain same or different type of sugars or their derivatives.
- Homopolysaccharides
- Heteropolysaccharides

Homopolysaccharides

Definition
If a polysaccharide is made up of only same type of monosaccharide, it is called as a homopolysaccharide.

Alternative name: Homoglycans.

Examples:
- Starch
- Dextrins
- Glycogen
- Dextran
- Cellulose
- Inulin

Starch

Occurrence
It is present in cereals (wheat, rice), potatoes, legumes and other vegetables.

Structure
It is composed of glucose molecules only (glucosan). It is highly branched with α-1, 4 linkage at straight chain and α-1, 6 linkage at branch points **(Fig. 2.5)**.

Starch is made up of two structurally different units:
1. Amylose (linear)
2. Amylopectin (branched).

Differences between amylose and amylopectin is shown in **Table 2.3**.

Table 2.3: Differences between amylose and amylopectin.

Amylose	Amylopectin
15–20%	80–85%
Low molecular weight	High molecular weight
About 300 glucose units	About 1,000 units
Not branched	Branched
Soluble in water	Sparingly soluble in water
Gives blue color with iodine	Gives violet color with iodine

Properties
It is a nonreducing polysaccharide. It gives blue color with iodine. It has a characteristic shape which is used in identification of starch. It forms various dextrins on hydrolysis **(Fig. 2.6)**.

Biomedical importance
- It is the major carbohydrate present in our food
- It is the storage form of carbohydrate in plants.

Dextrins

Occurrence
Dextrins occur in the leaves of all starch containing plants. They are present in honey also.

Formation
Various dextrins are formed by partial hydrolysis of starch by enzyme salivary amylase or dilute mineral acid.

Starch → Amylodextrin → Erythrodextrin → Achrodextrin → Maltose → Glucose

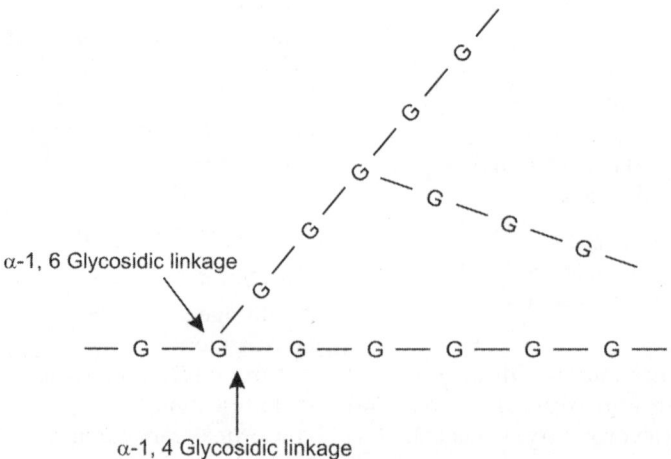

Fig. 2.5: Structure of starch.

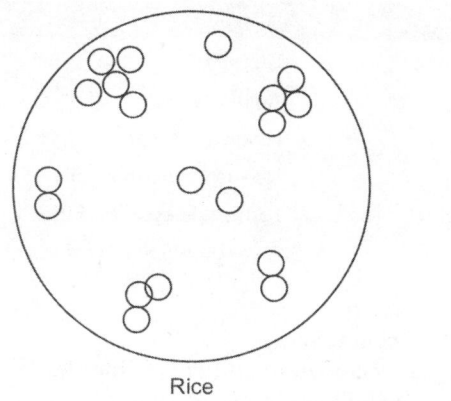
Rice

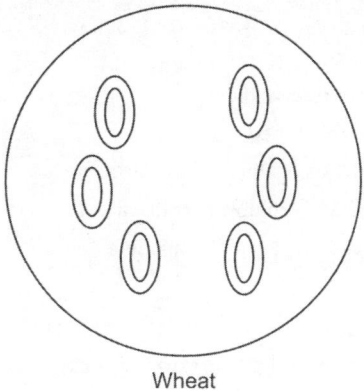
Wheat

Fig. 2.6: Starch granules.

Structure
Dextrins have glucose molecules only (glucosan). May be linear or branched.

Properties
They are less sweet. They have slight reducing properties due to presence of free aldehyde groups. They give red color with iodine. They form paste when mixed with water.

Biomedical importance
They are constituents of various food products, such as corn syrups.

Glycogen
Alternative name: Animal starch.

Occurrence
It is the reserve carbohydrate in liver and muscles of animals and human beings.

Structure
It is highly branched, such as a tree with D-glucose units only (Glucosan). Straight chain is linked through α-1, 4 glycosidic linkage and at branching points, the bond is by α-1, 6 glycosidic linkage (**Fig. 2.7**).

Properties
It is water soluble. It is nonreducing. It gives red color with iodine.

Biomedical importance
- It is the storage form of carbohydrate in humans and animals.
- Its abnormal metabolism leads to glycogen storage diseases, e.g., von Gierke's disease.
- Differences between starch and glycogen are shown in **Table 2.4**.

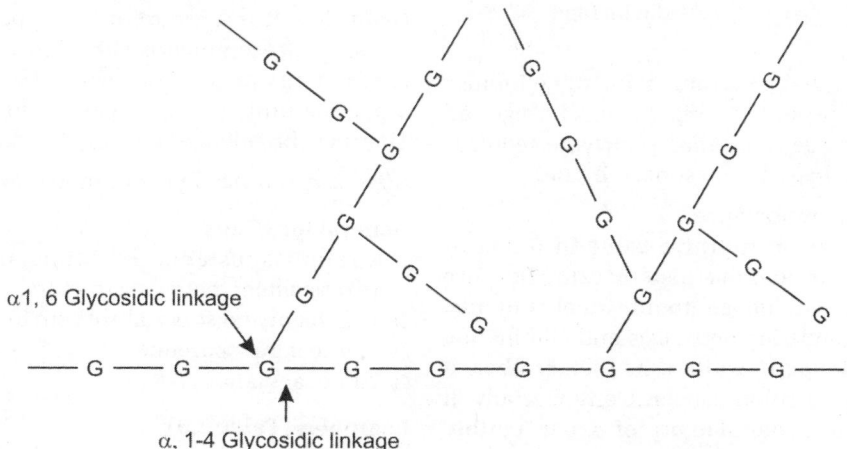

Fig. 2.7: Structure of glycogen.

Section 2: Chemistry of Biomolecules

Table 2.4: Differences between starch and glycogen.

Sl. No.	Starch	Glycogen
1.	Plant reserve food	Animal reserve food
2.	Less branched	Highly branched
3.	Consists of amylose and amylopectin	No such structural units
4.	Sparingly soluble in cold water forms paste with hot water	Forms opalescent solution with water
5.	Gives violet color with iodine	Gives brown to red color with iodine

Dextrans

Occurrence
They are produced by certain bacteria.

Structure
They have D-glucose units (Glucosan) and are branched.

Properties
They have various molecular weights. They can absorb water and form viscous colloidal solutions.

Biomedical importance
They are used:
❑ As plasma expander in treatment of shock
❑ In chromatography

Cellulose

Occurrence
Cellulose is the chief constituent of the fibrous parts of plants.

Structure
It is a straight chain with D glucose units (Glucosan).

–G–G–G–G–G–G–G–G–
↑
β-1, 4, glycosidic linkage

Properties
It is hydrolyzed by strong acids to cellobiose (disaccharide) and glucose. It cannot be digested by humans due to absence of enzyme cellulase (hydrolase) in gastrointestinal (GI) tract.

Biomedical importance
Cellulose has no nutritive value in humans. But it has considerable dietetic value because it adds bulk (roughage) to intestinal contents, thereby stimulating peristalsis and eliminating indigestible food residues. As dietary fiber, it protects from colon cancer. Commercially, it is used in the manufacture of paper, cotton, explosives, photographic film, etc.
(Dietary fiber: *refer* Chapter 21)

Inulin

Occurrence
It occurs in the tubers of chicory, dahlia and in the bulbs of onion and garlic.

Structure
It consists of D-fructose units only and so called as fructosan. It is a straight chain structure.

–F –F –F –F –F –F–

Properties
It is a white crystalline powder. It gives no color with iodine.

Biomedical importance
It is used in 'Inulin clearance test' (renal function test) for determining glomerular filtration rate (GFR). It has no dietary value.

Heteropolysaccharides

Definition: Polysaccharides containing different sugars or their derivatives are called as heteropolysaccharides.

Alternative name: Heteroglycans

Examples: Mucopolysaccharides.

Mucopolysaccharides

Definition: It is a group of heteropolysaccharides. They are mucous substances. They are components of proteoglycans. They contain repeating units (–Sugar acid – Amino sugar). They may be sulfated or nonsulfated.

Alternative name: Glycosaminoglycans (GAG).

General functions
❑ Ground substance in connective tissue (extracellular matrix)—structural component
❑ Lubricant and shock absorbent in joints
❑ Corneal transparency
❑ Anticoagulant.

Examples (Table 2.5)
Several types of mucopolysaccharides have been isolated.

Table 2.5: Mucopolysaccharides.

Sl. No.	Examples	Locations	Structure (repeating unit)	Importance/Functions
1.	Hyaluronic acid	Synovial fluid of joints, vitreous humor of eyes, connective tissue, umbilical cord	D–Glucuronic acid—N–Acetyl D-glucosamine (Nonsulfated)	Lubricant, shock absorbent, ground substance (biological cement) in connective tissue. Hydrolyzed by hyaluronidase which (a) helps spermatozoa to penetrate ova; (b) renders toxic substances to enter into cells
2.	Chondroitin sulfate: A (Chondroitin 4 - sulfate)	Cartilage, bones, tendons	D–Glucuronic acid—N–Acetyl galactosamine 4 sulfate	Role in corneal transparency, lipid clearing factor, slight, anticoagulation action (β-heparin)
	Chondroitin sulfate: B (Chondroitin 6 - sulfate)	Valves, tendons, lung	N–Acetyl galactosamine 6 sulfate D–Glucuronic acid	
3.	Dermatan sulfate	Skin, cornea, bone	D–Glucuronic acid/D–Iduronic acid—N–Acetyl galactosamine 4 sulfate	Role in corneal transparency
4.	Heparin (α-Heparin)	Blood, liver, kidney, lung, spleen thymus	D–Glucuronic acid/D–Iduronic acid—D–Glucosamine (sulfated and acetylated)	Anticoagulant, lipid clearing factor
5.	Heparan sulfate	Aortic vessel wall, brain	D–Glucuronic acid—D–Glucuronic acid sulfate	Component of the cell surface
6.	Keratan sulfate I	Cornea	D–Galactose—N–Acetyl glucosamine sulfate	Role in corneal transparency
7.	Keratan sulfate II	Connective tissue	D–Galactose—N–Acetyl glucosamine sulfate	Ground substance

Clinical significance: Defective metabolism of mucopolysaccharides leads to inborn error of metabolism (mucopolysaccharidosis), e.g., Hurler's syndrome, Hunter's syndrome. They produce joint stiffness, corneal clouding, etc.

ADDITIONAL INFORMATION

- *Dextrose:* It is D-Glucose. It is used as a nutrient and in fluid therapy.
- *Diastereoisomers:* Sugars which are not mirror images are known as diastereoisomers.
- *Isomaltose:* It contains 2 glucose units linked through α-1, 6 linkage.
- *Chitin:* It is also a homopolysaccharide. It is present in seaweeds. It is used in culture of bacteria. It is also used as laxative.
- *Maltotriose:* It consists of three molecules of glucose linked by α1–4 linkage.
- *Artificial sweetener:* Aspartame, saccharin sucralose
- *Carbohydrates in cell membrane:* The mammalian cell contains carbohydrates as glycoproteins and glycolipids.
- *Isomerism:* It refers to the compounds having same molecular formula but different structures (*refer* Appendix D: Isomerism).
  - *Glycoconjugates* (complex carbohydrates): Glycoproteins and proteoglycans.
- *Blood group substances:* They consist of galactose, galactosamine, N-acetyl glucosamine, sialic acid and fucose. They are used to determine blood grouping.

3 Chemistry of Lipids

Chapter Outline
- Definition
- Alternative Name
- Occurrence
- Biomedical Importance/Functions
- Classification/Examples
- Related Terms in Lipid Chemistry

DEFINITION
Lipids are a heterogeneous group of organic compounds. They are oily or greasy substances. They are relatively insoluble in water but considerably soluble in organic solvents, such as chloroform, benzene and ether, etc.

ALTERNATIVE NAME
Fat.

OCCURRENCE
They are widely distributed throughout the plant and animal kingdoms.

COMPOSITION
They contain fatty acid(s), alcohol and/or related substances.

BIOMEDICAL IMPORTANCE/FUNCTIONS
1. *Energy:* The lipids are important constituents of the diet because of their high calorific value (9C/g) and due to fat soluble vitamins and essential fatty acids present in them. They provide about 25% of energy to the body.
2. *Storage:* They are stored mainly in adipose tissue (stored fat is called as fat depots).
3. *Structural components:* Lipoproteins and phospholipids present in cell membrane are essential for maintaining cell integrity.
4. *Insulation:* They serve as thermal insulator in the subcutaneous tissues and as electrical insulators in neurons. They act as padding material around certain internal organs.
5. *Biochemical compounds:* Vitamin D, steroid hormones and bile acids are all synthesized from cholesterol. Prostaglandins are fatty acid derivatives.
6. *Transport:*
   - They help in the absorption and transport of fat soluble vitamins.
   - Lipoproteins are used as transport forms of certain metabolic fuel in the blood.
7. *Miscellaneous:* They act as:
   - Lung surfactant (dipalmitoyl lecithin)
   - Lipotropic factor to prevent formation of fatty liver (inositol)
   - Emulsifying agent in digestion and absorption (bile salts).
   - Metabolic regulation (prostaglandins)

Clinical Importance
- Lipids are the causative agents in obesity, atherosclerosis, etc.
- Defective metabolism of lipids due to enzyme deficiency may lead to inborn errors of metabolism, e.g., Gaucher's disease, Tay-Sachs disease.

CLASSIFICATION (FIG. 3.1)
According to Bloor's modified classification, lipids are divided into four major groups based on their composition:
1. Simple lipids
2. Compound lipids
3. Derived lipids
4. Miscellaneous lipids

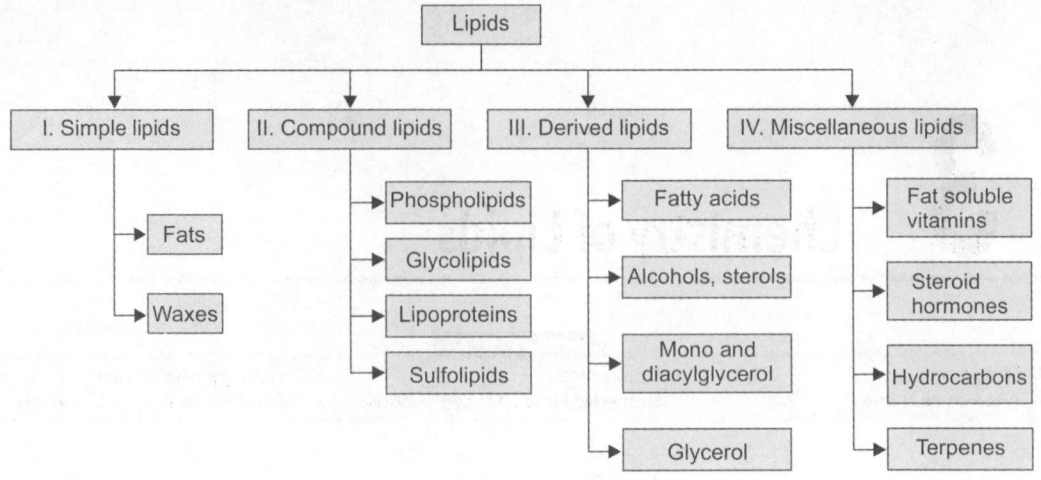

Fig. 3.1: Classification of lipids.

I. Simple Lipids

Definition
Simple lipids are esters of fatty acids with various alcohols.

Composition
Simple lipid = Fatty acids + Alcohol

Subclasses
They are divided into two subclasses:
1. Fats
2. Waxes

I. Fats
Alternative names:
- Triacylglycerols
- Triglycerides
- Neutral fats

Definition
Fats are the esters of fatty acids with glycerol.

Composition
Fat = Fatty acids + Glycerol

Structure

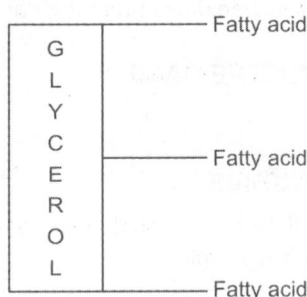

Examples
Simple triacylglycerol: If three molecules of same fatty acid combine with one molecule of glycerol, the resulting fat is a simple *triacylglycerol*, e.g., tripalmitin.
- *Mixed triacylglycerol:* If fatty acids are different, the resulting fat is a mixed *triacylglycerol*.

$$\begin{array}{c} CH_2OH \\ | \\ CHOH \\ | \\ CH_2OH \end{array} + 3C_{15}H_{31}COOH \longrightarrow \begin{array}{c} CH_2-OOC-C_{15}H_{31} \\ | \\ CH-OOC-C_{15}H_{31} \\ | \\ CH_2-OOC-C_{15}H_{31} \end{array} + 3H_2O$$

Alcohol   Fatty acid   Simple triacylglycerol
(glycerol)   (palmitic acid)   (tripalmitin)

$$\begin{array}{l} CH_2-O-OC-R_1 \\ | \\ CH\ -O-OC-R_2 \\ | \\ CH_2-O-OC-R_3 \end{array}$$

Mixed triacylglycerol

Functions

The fats serve several physiological functions in the body.
- They are storage lipids in adipose tissue.
- They provide insulation against the loss of body heat.
- They act as padding material of support and protect internal organs.

Sources

Fats represent the most common and widespread class of lipids in nature.

Plant fats

Coconut oil, olive oil, gingelly oil, cotton seed oil, groundnut oil, and soya bean oil.

They contain mostly unsaturated fatty acids such as oleic acid, linoleic acid and linolenic acid.

Animal fats

Butter, fish oil, lard, milk, eggs and tallo (ox/sheep fat)

They mostly contain saturated fatty acids such as palmitic acid and stearic acid.

Properties

Physical properties
- *State:* They are greasy in nature. Animal fats are solid at room temperature. Plant fats are liquids at room temperature and are known as plant oils.
- *Solubility:* They are insoluble in water, but are readily soluble in organic solvents, such as chloroform, ether, etc.
- *Color, odor, and taste:* Pure fats are colorless, odorless and tasteless. But they develop flavor and color due to presence of certain foreign substances or bacterial flora.
- *Reaction:* Neutral. But after exposure to air, they become acidic.
- *Specific gravity:* They have less specific gravity than water and therefore they float on water.
- *Melting point:* Fats containing saturated fatty acids have higher melting point. Those containing unsaturated fatty acids have lower melting point.
- *Spreading:* Liquid fats spread uniformly over the surface of water when it is placed on it. This property called spreading is to reduce surface tension of water and help transport of fat.
- *Emulsification*
  - *Definition:* It is the process by which lipid mass is converted into a number of small lipid droplets.
  - *Process:* Fats may be emulsified by shaking either with water or with emulsifying agents, such as soaps, gums, proteins, etc.
  - *Importance:* The process of emulsification has great metabolic significance. Emulsification greatly increases the surface area of fats. Fats are emulsified by bile salts before they are absorbed by the intestinal wall.

Chemical properties
- **Hydrolysis**
  - Alkali hydrolysis (*Saponification*)
    - *Definition:* The hydrolysis of a fat by an alkali is called as saponification. The resulting products are glycerol and alkali salts of fatty acids.
    - *Importance:* Soaps consist largely of sodium or potassium salts of palmitic or stearic acids.

$$\begin{array}{l} CH_2-OOC-C_{17}H_{35} \\ | \\ CH\ -OOC-C_{17}H_{35} + 3KOH \longrightarrow \\ | \\ CH_2-OOC-C_{17}H_{35} \end{array}$$

$$\begin{array}{l} \phantom{3\ C_{17}H_{35}COOK\ \ } CH_2\ OH \\ 3\ C_{17}H_{35}COOK | \\ \phantom{3\ C_{17}H_{35}COO} CH\ OH \\ \text{Potassium stearate} + \\ \phantom{3\ C_{17}H_{35}COOK\ \ } CH_2\ OH \end{array}$$

Triacylglycerol   Alkali   Soap   Glycerol

- *Enzymatic hydrolysis:* The fats are hydrolyzed by the enzyme lipase of pancreatic juice to yield first diacylglycerol, then monoacylglycerol and finally fatty acids and glycerol.
- ❏ *Auto-oxidation:* Some of the natural oils containing unsaturated fatty acids when exposed to atmosphere and light absorb oxygen and undergo auto-oxidation. This process is used in the manufacture of paints and varnishes.
- ❏ *Rancidity:*
  - *Definition:* Auto-oxidation occurring in natural edible fats is called rancidity. The rancidity develops disagreeable odor and taste and becomes unfit for consumption.
  - *Causes/types:* Rancidity may be caused by the following:
    - *Hydrolytic rancidity:* It involves partial hydrolysis of triacylglycerol to mono or diacylglycerol, glycerol and fatty acids, by the influence of moisture, warmth and enzymes-like lipases. Butter becomes rancid in summer due to liberation of volatile fatty acids, (e.g., Butyric acid).
    - *Oxidative rancidity:* (Lipid peroxidation) (*refer* Chapter 32).

      The unsaturated fatty acids may be oxidized to form peroxides which then decompose to form aldehydes and ketones giving objectionable odor and taste. This type of rancidity is known as lipid peroxidation. It occurs more frequently in animal fats.

      Causes: It may be initiated by *free radicals* (ROO.) formed in the body. It will affect integrity of biomembranes leading to cell death, aging, cancer, atherosclerosis, inflammatory diseases, etc.
  - *Prevention (antioxidants)*
    - Addition of antioxidants, such as vitamin C, A and E, phenols, gallic acid, etc.
    - Storing fats in air-tight nonmetallic vessels and keeping away from light, moisture and warmth.
    - Refrigeration
- ❏ *Addition reactions:* The unsaturated fatty acids present in fat undergo all the addition reactions, e.g., hydrogenation, halogenation, etc.

Hydrogenated oils and refined oils: The unsaturated fatty acids of fats may be hydrogenated in the presence of nickel catalyst.

$$\text{Olein} \xrightarrow{H} \text{Stearin}$$
(unsaturated fat) (saturated fat)

This process is used to prepare cooking fat and margarine in food industry. Oils which are liquids at ordinary temperature become solids on hydrogenation. This is the basis of manufacture of vanaspathi.

Tests for purity of fats (Characterization of fats)

Fats and oils form essential constituents of diet. So, it is necessary to detect the impurities and adulterations in food fat and also to determine the proportions of different types of fat in a mixture. Following tests are employed:

$$\begin{array}{l} CH_2-OOC-R_1 \\ | \\ CH-OOC-R_2 \\ | \\ CH_2OOC-R_3 \\ \text{Triacylglycerol} \end{array} \xrightarrow{H_2O} \begin{array}{l} CH_2-OOC-R_1 \\ | \\ CH-OOC-R_2 \quad + R_3COOH \\ | \qquad\qquad\qquad \text{Fatty acid} \\ CH_2OH \\ \text{Diacylglycerol} \end{array}$$

$$\downarrow H_2O$$

$$\begin{array}{l} R_1COOH \\ \text{Fatty acid} \end{array} + \begin{array}{l} CH_2OH \\ | \\ CHOH \\ | \\ CH_2OH \\ \text{Glycerol} \end{array} \xleftarrow{H_2O} \begin{array}{l} CH_2OOCR_1 \\ | \\ CHOH \qquad + R_2COOH \\ | \qquad\qquad \text{Fatty acid} \\ CH_2OH \\ \text{Monoacylglycerol} \end{array}$$

Physical methods
- Specific gravity
- Refractive index
- Melting point
- Solidification point

Chemical methods
- *Saponification number (SN):* It is the number of mg of KOH required to saponify (hydrolyze) 1 g of fat or oil. It gives a measure of their molecular weight and size of the fatty acid chain in the fat.
  SN of butter   =   233–240
  SN of coconut oil =   250–264
- *Iodine number (IN):* It is the number of grams of iodine absorbed by 100 g fat or oil. Thus, it is a measure of degree of unsaturation of fat.
  - Oils have higher iodine number because they contain more unsaturated fatty acids. Fats have lower iodine number because they contain more saturated fatty acids.
    IN of butter   = 26–28
    IN of sunflower oil   = 125–135
  - Certain iodized oils (e.g., iodized poppy seed oil) are used in medicine for injection into body cavities to be X-rayed.
- *Acid number (AN):* It is the number of mg of KOH required to neutralize the free fatty acids present in 1 g fat or oil.
  - It is of value in determining rancidity due to free fatty acids. The edibility of fat is inversely proportional to the acid number.
    AN of butter = 0.35–0.45

> **Note**
> Other chemical methods are also used, e.g., acetyl number.

II. Waxes
Definition
Waxes are the esters of higher fatty acids with long chain alcohol.

Composition
Waxes = Higher fatty acids + Long-chain alcohol
        C_{24} to C_{31} (myricyl alcohol)

Examples
- *Common wax:* This is cholesterol ester (cholesterol palmitate) found in human blood plasma and sebaceous glands.
- *Lanolin (or) woolwax:* It is used for making ointments and cosmetics.
- *Carnauba wax:* It is plant wax used for manufacture of polishes.
- *Bees wax:* This is secreted by honey bee to form honey comb. Its chief ingredient is myricyl palmitate.

Properties
They are not easily hydrolyzed and hence no nutritional value.

Biomedical importance/functions
- Used as protective coatings of the skins and furs of animals.
- Presence of wax on feathers and hairs of birds helps to keep them soft and flyable.
- Highly resistant to atmosphere oxidation. Hence used in polishing furniture and automobiles and in manufacture of wax coat paper to preserve perishable food products.

II. Compound Lipids (Complex Lipids)
Definition
Compound lipids are esters of fatty acids with alcohol containing additional groups.

Composition
Compound lipid = Fatty acid + Alcohol + Other group(s).

Subclasses
They are subdivided into:
- Phospholipids
- Glycolipids
- Lipoproteins
- Sulfolipids

Phospholipids
Definition
They are esters of fatty acids with glycerol or other alcohols containing phosphoric acid, nitrogenous base and other constituents.

Composition
Phospholipid = Fatty acid + Glycerol/Other alcohol + Phosphoric acid + Nitrogenous base + Other constituent

Section 2: Chemistry of Biomolecules

Biomedical importance/functions

- *Structure:* They are components of lipoprotein complexes, which constitute the matrix of cell walls and membranes, microsomes, mitochondria and myelin sheath.
- *Absorption:* Lecithin aids in emulsification of lipid-water mixture for digestion and absorption of lipids from GI tract.
- *Transport:*
  - They take an active part in the transport of triglycerides as chylomicrons.
  - They are required for the formation of very low-density lipoprotein (VLDL) which carries endogenous triacylglycerol from liver to various tissues.
- *Blood coagulation:* They play an essential role in blood coagulation.
  - In conversion of prothrombin to thrombin
  - In the activation of factor VIII
- *Insulation:* Phospholipids present in myelin sheaths provide insulation around nerve fibers.
- *Lipotropic action:* Lecithin provides choline which acts as a lipotropic factor to prevent the formation of fatty liver.
- *Hormone action:* Phosphatidylinositol acts as second messenger in hormone action.

Clinical Importance

- Deficiency of dipalmitoyl lecithin in premature babies may produce respiratory distress syndrome.
- Lecithin/sphingomyelin ratio can be used as an indicator for evaluation of fetal lung maturity.

Sources

They are present in large amounts in nerve tissue, brain (white matter), liver, kidney, pancreas, heart, egg yolk and soya bean oils.

Subclasses

They are divided into three subgroups based on the type of alcohol present:
1. Phosphoglycerides
2. Phosphoinositides
3. Phosphosphingosides

Phosphoglycerides

Definition
These are triesters of glycerol 3-phosphate and a nitrogenous base. They are derivatives of phosphatidic acid.

Composition

$$\underbrace{\text{Fatty acids} + \text{Glycerol} + \text{Phosphoric acid}}_{\text{Phosphatidic acid}} + \text{Nitrogenous base}$$

Examples
1. Lecithin
2. Cephalin
3. Plasmalogens
4. Cardiolipin

Lecithin:
Alternative name: Phosphatidyl choline.

Composition:
Lecithin = Fatty acids + Glycerol + Phosphoric acid + Choline

Sources:
- *Animal:* Nerve tissue, glandular tissue, egg yolk
- *Plant:* Soyabean oil, yeasts.

Structure

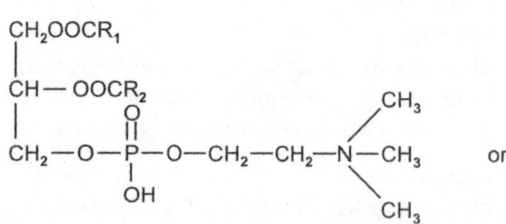 or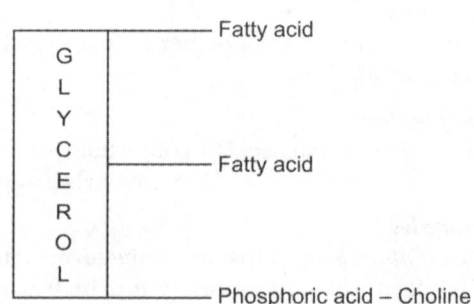

Chapter 3: Chemistry of Lipids

Properties
- It is a waxy white substance when pure but turns brown on exposure to air and light due to auto-oxidation and decomposition.
- Soluble in all fat solvents except acetone.
- Exists as zwitterions
- *Hydrolysis:* Lecithins can be hydrolyzed by dilute acids, alkalis or enzymes called *lecithinases (phospholipases)*. Complete hydrolysis of lecithin yields glycerol, phosphoric acid, choline and fatty acids. But partial hydrolysis of lecithins by lecithinases yields various products, such as lysolecithins which are potent *hemolytic poisons*.

There are mainly four types of lecithinases (phospholipases):

Types	Present in
• Phospholipase A2	Cobra, spider venom and poisonous stings
• Phospholipase A1	Penicillium notatum, pancreas
• Phospholipase C	Snake venom, human brain, plants
• Phospholipase D	Carrots, cabbages, cotton seed

Action of Lecithinases on Lecithins (*refer Chapter 12*): They hydrolyze lecithin in a characteristic way.

Lecithin $\xrightarrow{A_2}$ Fatty acid + Lysolecithin

Lecithin $\xrightarrow{A_1}$ Fatty acid + Glyceryl phosphoryl choline

Lecithin $\xrightarrow{C}$ Diglyceride + Phosphoryl choline

Lecithin $\xrightarrow{D}$ Choline + Phosphatidic acid

Biomedical importance:
- Lecithins are necessary for normal transport and utilization of other lipids especially in liver. In their absence, accumulation of lipids occurs in liver leading to a disorder called fatty liver. Choline is a lipotropic factor which prevents fatty liver formation.
- Maintain cell integrity
- They act:
  • As a store of labile methyl groups, e.g., choline
  • As emulsifying agent in digestion and absorption of fats.
- Involved in transmission of nerve impulses, e.g., acetylcholine

Clinical Importance

Respiratory distress syndrome: Dipalmitoyl lecithin acts as lung surfactant and lowers surface tension in lung alveoli. Its absence in premature babies may result in collapse of lung alveoli producing respiratory distress syndrome (RDS). Its symptoms are rapid and shallow breathing, and blue skin. Patient should be given breathing support and oxygen therapy.

Cephalin

Alternative name: Phosphatidylethanolamine/phosphatidylserine.

Composition: Cephalin resembles lecithin except that choline is replaced by ethanolamine or serine.

Cephalin = Glycerol + Fatty acids + Phosphoric acid + Ethanolamine/serine.

Structure

```
            ┌──── Fatty acid
G           │
L           │
Y           │
C           │
E           ├──── Fatty acid
R           │
O           │
L           │
            └──── Phosphoric acid – Ethanolamine/Serine
```

Occurrence: Cephalins are present in brain, spinal cord, soya bean oil.

Properties: They have characteristic properties similar to lecithins. They are more acidic and less soluble in alcohol than lecithins.

Biomedical importance/functions: It is a part of enzyme thromboplastin and so it has thromboplastic activity.

Plasmalogens

They resemble lecithin or cephalin, but one fatty acid molecule is replaced by an unsaturated ether. The nitrogenous base is usually ethanolamine or choline.

Composition:
Plasmalogen = Fatty acid + Unsaturated ether + Glycerol + Phosphoric acid + Ethanolamine/Choline

Structure

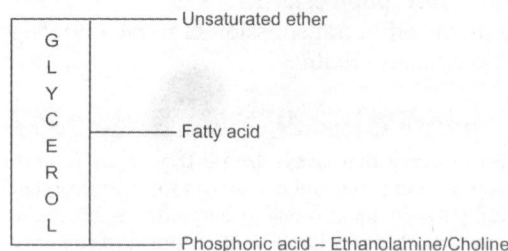

e.g., 1. Phosphatidylcholine
2. Phosphatidylethanolamine

Occurrence: Present in brain and muscle.

Importance: Platelet activating factor is a plasmalogen.

Cardiolipin

Composition:
Cardiolipin = Glycerol + Fatty acid + Phosphoric acid,
e.g., Diphosphatidylglycerol

Structure:
Phosphatidic acid — Glycerol — Phosphatidic acid

Occurrence: Present in mitochondria and mainly in myocardium.

Biomedical importance:
- Used as an antigen in serological test (VDRL) for syphilis.
- Essential for mitochondrial function. Its deficiency produces cardiomyopathy.

Phosphoinositides

These are phospholipids where a cyclic hexa-hydroxy alcohol called inositol (as myoinositol) replaces base, e.g., phosphatidylinositol.

Composition:
Fatty acids + Glycerol + Phosphoric acid + Inositol

Structure

```
       ┌── Fatty acid
G      │
L      │
Y      │
C      ├── Fatty acid
E      │
R      │
O      │
L      └── Phosphoric acid – Inositol
```

Occurrence: Brain and nerve tissues, tubercle bacilli, soya beans.

Importance: Involved in transport process in cell; Acts as a precursor of second messenger in hormone action.

Phosphosphingosides

These are phospholipids which do not contain glycerol but an amino alcohol called sphingosine along with fatty acid, phosphoric acid and choline, e.g., *sphingomyelins*.

Composition

$$\underbrace{\text{Fatty acids} + \text{Sphingosine}}_{\text{Ceramide}} + \text{Phophoric acid} + \text{Choline}$$

Structure
Sphingosine - Fatty acid
|
Phosphoric acid - Choline

Sources
Brain and nerve tissue especially in the myelin sheath.

> **Clinical Importance**
>
> **Niemann–Pick disease:** It is an inherited disorder of sphingomyelin metabolism (inborn error of lipid metabolism). It is a lipid storage disease. In this disease, sphingomyelin is not degraded due to absence of enzyme sphingomyelinase. Hence large quantity of sphingomyelin accumulates in brain and also in liver and spleen especially in children. The clinical symptoms are enlargement of abdomen, liver, spleen and mental retardation.

Glycolipids

Definition
Lipids containing carbohydrate moiety are called glycolipids.

Composition
Similar to sphingolipids but base is replaced by a sugar. Also they do not contain phosphoric acid.
Fatty acid + Sphingosine + Sugar.

Classification
They are classified into two types:
1. Cerebrosides
2. Gangliosides.

Cerebrosides

Occurrence:
- *High:* Brain (white matter and myelin sheath)
- *Low:* Gray matter and other tissues

Composition: They contain galactose (instead of choline) and sphingosine and a higher molecular weight fatty acid. They do not contain phosphoric acid.

Structure:
Sphingosine–Fatty acid
|
Galactose

Properties: They mostly resemble sphingomyelins in properties.

Types: Four types of cerebrosides have been identified.

Examples	Fatty acid component
1. Nervon	Nervonic acid
2. Oxynervon	Oxynervonic acid
3. Kerosin	Lignoceric acid
4. Cerebron	Cerebronic acid

Clinical Importance

Gaucher's disease: It is a lipid storage disease. It is an inborn error of lipid metabolism due to deficiency of enzyme β *Glucosidase*. Galactose in cerebrosides is replaced by glucose. Glucose cerebrosides accumulate in liver and spleen. Cerebronic acid is the major fatty acid increased in this condition. The clinical symptoms are enlarged liver and spleen, osteoporosis and mental retardation.

Gangliosides

Occurrence: Present in ganglions and hence the name gangliolipids. High in gray matter of brain.

Composition: They are similar to cerebrosides in structure but also contain N-acetyl galactosamine and neuraminic acid. e.g., GM_1, GM_2, GM_3.

Structure
Fatty acid – Sphingosine – Glucose – Galactose
 – N-acetylgalactosamine
N-acetylneuraminic acid (NANA)

Clinical Importance

Tay–Sachs disease: It is an inborn error of lipid metabolism due to deficiency of the enzyme hexosaminidase A. It is also a lipid storage disease. Concentration of gangliosides increases in brain and nervous tissue in this disorder. The clinical symptoms are muscular weakness, blindness and mental retardation.

Lipoproteins

Definition
They are macromolecular complexes of lipids and proteins (also called as conjugated proteins).
Lipid + Protein = Lipoprotein

Classification (types)
They are classified into many subclasses depending on ultracentrifugation and electrophoresis.

Sl. No.	Ultracentrifugation	Electrophoresis
1.	Chylomicrons	Chylomicrons
2.	Very low-density lipoproteins (VLDL)	Pre β-lipoproteins
3.	Intermediate density lipoproteins (IDL)	–
4.	Low-density lipoproteins (LDL)	β-lipoproteins
5.	High-density lipoproteins (HDL)	α-lipoproteins

Composition (Table 3.1)
❏ They have characteristic density, mol.wt and size.
❏ They differ in their composition.

Table 3.1: Composition of lipoproteins.

Sl. No.	Fraction	Protein %	Total lipid %	Triglycerides %	Phospholipids %	Cholesterol %	Cholesterol esters %	Free fatty acids %
1.	Chylomicrons	1–2	98–99	88	8	3	1	-
2.	VLDL	7–10	90–93	56	20	15	8	1
3.	IDL	11	89	29	26	34	9	1
4.	LDL	21	79	13	28	48	10	1
5.	HDL	33	67	16	43	31	10	–

Note: LDL contains more cholesterol.

Lipids present in lipoproteins
Triacylglycerol, phospholipids, cholesterol, cholesterol esters.

Proteins present in lipoproteins
Apoproteins (A, B, C, E with subclasses) (*refer* Chapter 4)

Biomedical importance/functions
- Maintain structural integrity of cellular membranes, mitochondria, microsomes.
- Involved in transport and metabolism of lipids (*refer* Chapter 12).

Clinical Importance

Lipoproteins present in plasma are of *clinical importance*. They may alter in:
- Atherosclerosis
- Hyperlipoproteinemia
- Hypolipoproteinemia

(*refer* Chapter 12)

Sulfolipids
Composition
They resemble cerebrosides but galactose is sulfated.

Structure
Sphingosine-Fatty acid
|
Galactose-Sulfate

Occurrence
Present in high concentration in white matter of brain and also in liver, kidney, testes and tumors. Widely distributed in plants (chloroplast).

Biomedical importance
Accumulates in metachromatic leukodystrophy due to deficiency of enzyme aryl sulfatase A.

III. Derived Lipids
Definition
They are derivatives obtained by the hydrolysis of simple or compound lipids.

Examples
1. Fatty acids
2. Alcohols (glycerol, sterols)
3. Monoacylglycerol and diacylglycerols

Fatty acids
Definition
Fatty acids are characteristic building block components of the most of the lipids. Most of the fatty acids are monocarboxylic acids. They have a single ionizable carboxyl group and a long nonpolar hydrocarbon chain.

$$CH_3 - CH_2 - CH_2 - CH_2 - CH_2 - COOH$$

Biomedical importance/functions
- They act as fuel molecules. They are stored as triacylglycerols and catabolized to generate energy.
- They are components of cell membranes
- Derivatives of fatty acids serve as:
  - Local hormones (prostaglandins)
  - Second messenger (diacylglycerol).

Numbering of carbon atoms (Table 3.2)
It is by two ways:
1. *Delta system:* The position of carbon atoms in the fatty acids chain is indicated by numbering. In this case, carboxyl carbon is numbered as C_1. The carbon adjacent to C_1 is C_2 and so on.
2. *ω system:* Position of carbon atoms in the fatty acid chain may be indicated by Greek letters. The carbon atom adjacent to carboxyl group is α carbon. Next to α carbon is β carbon. ω carbon is farthest from the carboxyl group.

Indicating position of double bonds
Various conventions are in use for indicating the number and position of double bonds.
- A widely used convention is to indicate the number of carbon atoms, the number of double bond(s) and the position of the double bond(s). Position of a double bond is indicated by the lower number of two carbon

Table 3.2: Numbering of carbon atoms in fatty acids.

Methyl terminus/ω terminus							Carboxyl terminus				
	CH_3-	CH_2-	CH_2-	CH_2-	CH_2-	CH_2-	CH_2-	CH_2-	CH_2-	CH_2-	COOH
Numbering	10	9	8	7	6	5	4	3	2	1	
Letter											
Designation ω	ω						γ	β	α		

atoms included in double bond, e.g., oleic acid : 18 : 1 : 9 (or) 18 : 1 : Δ9

$CH_3(CH_2)_7 CH = CH(CH_2)_7 COOH$

(It has 18 carbon atoms and one double bond between 9 and 10 carbon atoms).

❐ Alternative method to name the unsaturated fatty acid is to write first the position of double bonds in numerals and then the total number of carbon atoms in Roman followed by the suffice 'enoic acid'.

For example: Oleic Acid: 9 Octadecenoic acid.

Classification/types
They are classified as:

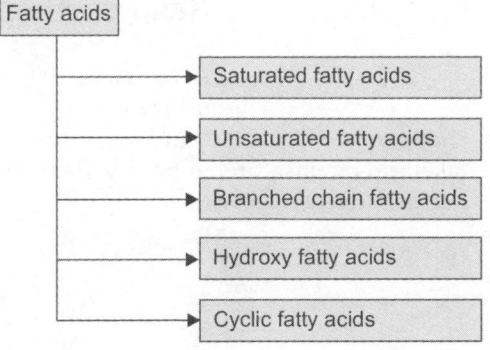

Saturated fatty acids
They do not contain double bond(s). Their general molecular formula is $C_nH_{2n+1}COOH$. They are built from acetic acid which is the first member of the series, e.g.,
❐ Palmitic acid $C_{15}H_{31}COOH$
❐ Stearic acid $C_{17}H_{35}COOH$

They contain generally even number of carbon atoms, but few odd carbon fatty acids are also present. Animal fats contain saturated fatty acids. Presence of saturated fatty acid makes the fat solid, but there are some exceptions, e.g., coconut oil is a liquid fat containing saturated fatty acids.

Unsaturated fatty acids
They are characterized by having one or more double bonds. Their general molecular formula is $C_nH_{2n-1}COOH$. They are usually liquids (plant oils).

They are subdivided based on the degree of unsaturation, (i.e., according to number of double bonds).

❐ *Monounsaturated fatty acids* (only one double bond), e.g., oleic acid

(9 octadecenoic acid) $C_{17}H_{33}COOH$

$CH_3(CH_2)_7CH = CH(CH_2)_7COOH$

❐ *Polyunsaturated fatty acids* (more than one double bond)—PUFA
  • Fatty acid with two double bonds, e.g., linoleic acid (9, 12, octadecadienoic acid) $C_{17}H_{31}COOH$

  $CH_3-(CH_2)_4-CH = CH-CH_2-CH= CH-(CH_2)_7 COOH$

  • Fatty acid with three double bonds, e.g., linolenic acid
  (9, 12, 15 Octadecatrienoic acid) $C_{17}H_{29}COOH$

  $CH_3-CH_2-CH = CH-CH_2 - CH = CH - CH_2$
  $CH = CH(CH_2)_7 - COOH$

  • Fatty acid with four double bonds, e.g., arachidonic acid
  (5, 8, 11, 14 eicosatetraenoic acid) $C_{19}H_{31}COOH$

  $CH_3(CH_2)_4 CH = CH CH_2 CH = CH$
  $- CH_2CH = CH CH_2 CH = CH (CH_2)_3 COOH$

All three polyunsaturated fatty acids are essential fatty acids.

Isomerism in unsaturated fatty acids:
Unsaturated fatty acids exhibit cis-trans isomerism (geometrical isomerism) depending on the orientation of atoms or groups around double bond.

In cis-isomer, acyl chains are on the same side of the bond, e.g., oleic acid.

All the naturally occurring unsaturated fatty acids are cis isomers.

In trans-isomer, acyl chains are on the opposite sides of the bond, e.g., elaidic acid.

```
CH_3 (CH_2)_7    –    C – H              CH_3 (CH_2)_7  –  C – H
                      ||                                    ||
HOOC (CH_2)_7    –    C – H                           H – C – (CH_2)_7 COOH
    Oleic acid (cis)                          Elaidic acid (trans)
```

Transfatty acids
They are a type of unsaturated fatty which occur in small amount in meat, milkfat, and fastfoods. Artificial trans fats are also formed during hydrogenation of oils. They raise LDL (bad cholesterol) which may lead to heart disease.

Branched chain fatty acids
- They are present in certain foods, e.g., phytanic acid in butter.
- Sebum contains branched chain fatty acids.
- Tuberculostearic acid (C_{19}). It is found in Bacillus tuberculosis.

Hydroxy fatty acids
For example,
- *Ricinoleic acid:* It occurs in castor oil.
- *Cerebronic acid:* It is present in glycolipids.

Cyclic fatty acids
For example,
- Chaulmoogric acid
- Hydnocarpic acid

Both are present in chaulmoogra oil which is used to treat leprosy.

Properties
Physical properties
- *State:* Lower fatty acids from butyric acid (C_4) to capric acid (C_{10}) are liquids at ordinary temp. Higher fatty acids above C_{10} are solids.
- *Solubility:* Lower fatty acids are soluble in water. Higher fatty acids are insoluble in water.
- *Specific gravity:* Except acetic acid, all other fatty acids are lighter than water.
- *Melting point:* Increases with increase in chain length. Decreases with increase in unsaturation.
- *Boiling point:* Increases with increase in chain length.
- *Volatility:* The short chain fatty acids are steam volatile. Volatility decreases with increase in chain length.
- *Spreading: Refer* properties of "Fats".

Chemical properties
Due to carboxyl group
- *Alcohol or aldehyde formation:* A fatty acid can be reduced to alcohol or aldehyde at high temperature in the presence of hydrogen. The sodium salts of these derivatives are used as detergents.

$$RCOOH \rightarrow RCHO \text{ or } RCH_2OH$$

- *Salt formation:* Fatty acids form salts with alkalis. The alkali salts of fatty acids are called as soaps.

$$RCOOH + NaOH \rightarrow RCOONa + H_2O$$

- *Ester formation:* Fatty acid condenses with alcohol to form esters.

$$RCOOH + CH_3OH \rightarrow RCOOCH_3 + H_2O$$

For example, triacylglycerols, cholesterol esters.

Due to hydrocarbon chain
- *Addition reaction:* Hydrogenation of unsaturated fatty acids using nickel as catalyst yields saturated fatty acids.

$$CH_3(CH_2)_7 CH = CH-(CH_2)_7 COOH$$
Oleic acid
$$\xrightarrow{+2H} CH_3(CH_2)_{16} COOH$$
Stearic acid

- *Halogenation:* Iodine and bromine are taken up by unsaturated fatty acids to give halogenated derivatives.

$$CH_3(CH_2)_4 CH = CH\ CH_2\ CH = CH\ (CH_2)_7 COOH$$
Linoleic acid
$$\downarrow 2I_2$$
$$CH_3(CH_2)_4-CH-CH-CH_2-CH-CH(CH_2)_7 COOH$$
| | | | |
I I I I
Tetraiodostearic acid

This reaction is the basis of calculating iodine number.

- *Oxidation:*
  - *With atmospheric oxygen:* Unsaturated fatty acids are oxidized to form unstable peroxides which are later decomposed into a mixture of short-chain fatty acids and aldehydes. These give rancid taste and odor to the fats. This process is called as auto-oxidation or rancidity.

$$—CH=CH—$$
$$\downarrow$$
$$—CH—CH—$$
$$|\quad\ \ |$$
$$O—O$$

- *Biological oxidation:* In living systems, the fatty acids are enzymatically oxidized mainly by β oxidation.

Essential fatty acids (EFA)

Definition

They are long chain polyunsaturated fatty acids which cannot be synthesized by the body. They have to be obtained from diet. They are essential constituents of diet (ω-group).

Examples
- Linoleic acid
- Linolenic acid
- Arachidonic acid

Sources

Animal fats contain more saturated fatty acids, Vegetable fats contain more unsaturated fatty acids which are rich in EFA.

Vegetable oils: Sunflower oil—75%, Corn oil—50%, Cotton seed oil—45%, Peanut oil—25%.

Animal fats: Egg—9%, Lard—9%.

Biomedical importance/functions
- Required for growth and reproduction
- Prolong clotting time
- Diet containing animal fat (saturated fatty acid) tends to increase serum cholesterol.
- Diet containing vegetable oil (unsaturated fatty acids + EFA) tends to lower serum cholesterol. This property of EFA is important in the management of hypercholesterolemia, which is accompanied by atherosclerosis.
- Arachidonic acid and some related C20 fatty acids with double bonds give rise to a group of physiologically and pharmacologically active compounds:
  For example, prostaglandins, thromboxanes and leukotrienes.

Deficiency symptoms

Animals

Poor growth, dermatitis, decreased capacity to reproduce, impaired transport of lipids.

Human

Phrynoderma (toad skin): Characterized by scaly dermatitis on limbs, loss of hair, poor wound healing, and growth impairment, defective transport of lipids, fatty liver, degeneration changes in arterial wall.

Treatment

By EFA intake of 1–2% of total caloric requirement.

ω-Fatty Acids (Omega Fatty Acids)

Definition

Fatty acids may also be numbered starting from ω end (methyl end). According to this classification, unsaturated fatty acids are divided into 3 groups.

1. ω-3 Fatty Acids

It is unsaturated fatty acid with double bond between C_3 and C_4 from omega end of hydrocarbon chain. It is found in fish oils especially salamon and other cold water fish, flax seeds. It lowers LDL cholesterol and BP, e.g., linolenic acid.

2. ω-6 Fatty Acids

It is unsaturated fatty acid, e.g., linoleic acid: It has double bond between C_6 and C_7 from ω end of hydrocarbon chain. It is present in, sunflower oil, corn, soyabean. They have anti-inflammatory effects. Mainly used for energy.

3. ω-9 Fatty Acids

For example, oleic acid: Present in olive oil. It has double bond between 9–10 position from methyl end of hydrocarbon chain. It increases HDL cholesterol (good cholesterol) and decreases. LDL cholesterol (bad cholesterol). They help eliminate plaque buildup in the arteries which causes heart attack and stroke.

Derivatives of fatty acids

Eicosanoids (*refer* **Chapter 31**)

Definition

Eicosanoids are the derivatives of eicosanoic fatty acids (C_{20}), namely—arachidonic acid.
- *Discovered by:* Von Euler
- *Sources:* All tissues especially seminal fluid.

Classification/types (Fig. 3.2)

Eicosanoids are divided into two major classes which are further subdivided.

Biomedical importance/functions

Prostaglandins:
- Induce labor, abortion
- Act as contraceptives
- Prevent aggregation of platelets
- Lower blood pressure
- Affect membrane permeability
- Used to treat gastric ulcer, asthma
- Induce inflammation

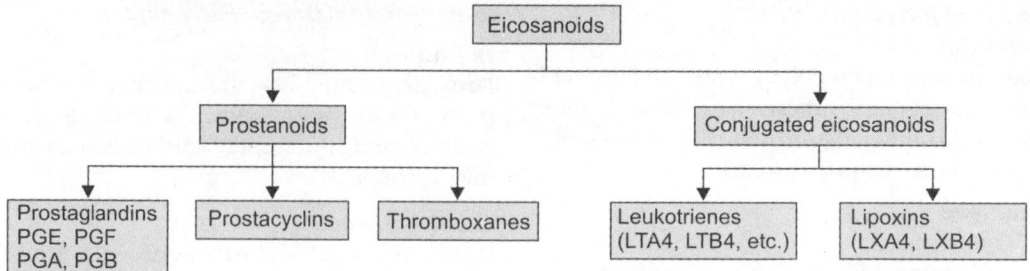

Fig. 3.2: Types of eicosanoids.

Thromboxanes:
Increase—
- Vasoconstriction
- Platelet aggregation
- Lymphocyte proliferation
- Bronchoconstriction.

Leukotrienes: Involved in chemotaxis, inflammation and allergic reactions.

Alcohols
Glycerol
Structure: It is a trihydroxy saturated alcohol.

CH$_2$OH
|
CHOH
|
CH$_2$OH

Properties: It is a colorless heavy fluid. It is a byproduct of soap manufacture. It is a component of triacylglycerol, lecithin, etc. It is obtained from lipolysis of fat in adipose tissue. It can be converted to glucose by gluconeogenesis in the body and thus possesses nutritional value.

Importance: Glycerol therapy is used in cerebrovascular disease. Nitroglycerin is a vasodilator. Glycerol is used in the preparation of culture medium and in manufacture of cosmetics.

Test: It can be detected by *Acrolein test*.

Sterols
They are a class of steroids characterized by: Cyclopentanoperhydrophenanthrene ring (Fig. 3.3).

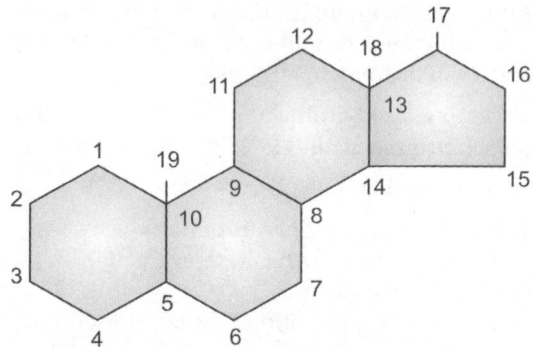

Fig. 3.3: Steroid nucleus (cyclopentanoperhydrophenanthrene ring).

Types:
- Animal sterols
- Plant sterols

Animal sterols
- **Cholesterol:** It is the most important sterol present in mammalian body. It is absent in plants, but widely distributed in all animal tissues.
  Alternative name: Solid bile alcohol (first isolated from bile).

Sources

High	Moderate
Brain and nervous tissues	Liver
Adrenal cortex	Kidney
Corpus luteum	Spleen
Testes	Skin
Egg yolk	Plasma

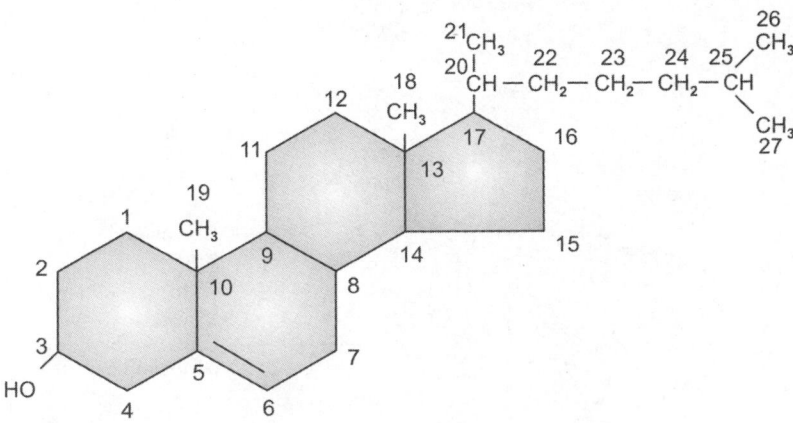

Fig. 3.4: Structure of cholesterol.

Structure (Fig. 3.4)
- Its molecular formula is $C_{27}H_{45}OH$.
- It has cyclopentanoperhydrophenanthrene ring.
- An aliphatic side chain attached to C-17.
- A secondary alcoholic hydroxyl group attached to C_3.
- A double bond between C_5 and C_6.
- Two methyl groups (one at C_{10} and another at C_{13}).

Properties
Physical properties:
- *Shape:* It is a white shinning crystal. It looks like rhombic plates with characteristics notches at its corner **(Fig. 3.5)**.
- *Taste and odor:* Tasteless, odorless
- *Solubility:* It is insoluble in water but soluble in fat solvents, soap solution and bile salt solution.

Chemical properties:
- *Addition and hydrogenation:* It is an unsaturated alcohol and hence its chemical properties are mostly based on these characteristics.
- *Oxidation:* On oxidation, it gives various ketones, hydroxy compounds and acids, depending on oxidizing agents used and experimental conditions involved.
- *Esterification:* It forms esters with acids, e.g., cholesterol acetate, cholesteryl palmitate.
- *Hydroxylation:* OH group in cholesterol reacts with digitonin to form an insoluble digitonide. This property is used to separate cholesterol from its esters.
- *Color reactions/tests:*
  - Liebermann Burchard reaction
  - Salkowski reaction

Biomedical importance/functions
- *Membrane fluidity:* It helps in maintaining the structure of membrane by providing fluidity.
- *Insulation:* It functions as an electrical insulator in brain neurons and spinal cord, because it is a poor conductor of electricity.
- *Precursors of bile acids, steroid hormones and vitamin D:* It is the precursor of other biologically important sterols, such as bile acids and steroid hormones and vitamin D.
- It is an important constituent of lipoproteins.

Clinical Importance
❖ Normal level in blood 150–200 mg/100 mL.
❖ If it exceeds its normal level in blood, it will lead to hypercholesterolemia resulting in atherosclerosis (*refer* Chapter 12).

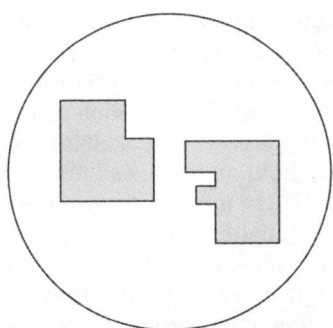

Fig. 3.5: Cholesterol crystals.

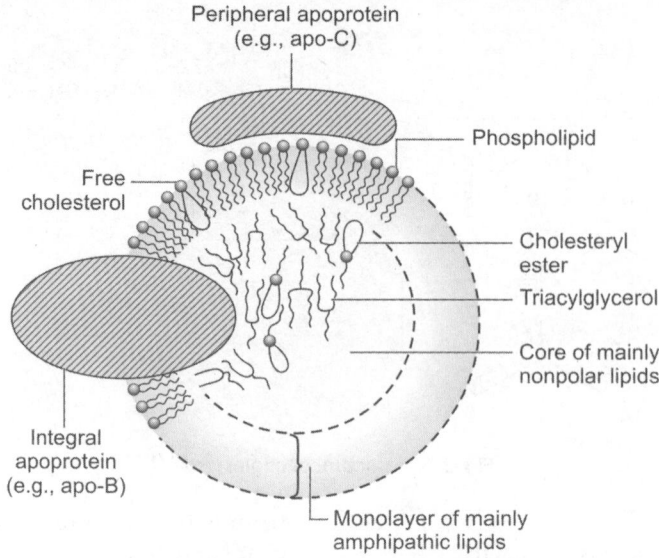

Fig. 3.6: Lipoprotein structure.

Coprosterol

It occurs in feces due to reduction of cholesterol by bacterial action.

7-dehydrocholesterol (provitamin D3)

It is present in skin.

Plant sterols

Examples	Sources
a. Stigmasterol	Soya bean oils
b. Sitosterol	Wheat germ oil
c. Ergosterol (provitamin D_2)	Ergot

IV. Miscellaneous Lipids

Definition

These compounds have characteristics of lipids.

Examples

- Fat soluble vitamins A, D, E and K (*refer* Chapter 8)
- Steroid hormones (*refer* Chapter 25)
- Hydrocarbons
- Terpenes

RELATED TERMS IN LIPID CHEMISTRY

- *Amphipathic lipids:* Lipids which contain both hydrophobic and hydrophilic groups are called as amphipathic lipids, e.g., fatty acids, phospholipids, sphingolipids, bile salts, cholesterol.
- *Micelles:* When amphipathic lipids are mixed in water in particular concentration, micelles are formed. They are small particles (lipids droplets). They aid in lipid digestion and absorption facilitated by bile salts.
- *Emulsions:* They are much larger particles formed by nonpolar lipids in aqueous medium. They are stabilized by emulsifying agents.
- *Neutral lipids:* The uncharged lipids are neutral lipids, e.g., cholesterol, cholesteryl esters, glycerides (acylglycerols).
- *Lipid bilayer:* It is basic structural feature of biological membranes. In this form, polar head orient towards outer aqueous phase on either side and the nonpolar tail into the interior.
- *Liposomes:* When amphipathic lipids in aqueous medium are subjected to sonification, liposomes are formed. They are used as carriers of drugs to target tissues.
- *Lipoprotein molecule (structure) (Fig. 3.6):* Lipoprotein is a complex molecule consisting of both lipids and proteins. It is a compound/complex lipid. It is also called as conjugated protein. There are mainly four types of lipoproteins (chylomicrons, VLDL, LDL, HDL). The outer shell of all lipoprotein consists of apolipoproteins and amphiphilic lipids—unesterified cholesterol and phospholipids. The interior part contains triacylglycerols and cholesterol esters (neutral lipids).

4 Chapter — Chemistry of Proteins

> **Chapter Outline**
>
> **Amino Acids**
> - Definition
> - Occurrence
> - Composition
> - Biomedical Importance/Functions
> - Classification of Amino Acids
> - Properties
>
> **Proteins**
> - Definition
> - Meaning
> - Composition
> - Occurrence
> - Biomedical Importance/Functions
> - Classification
> - Structural Organization of Proteins
> - Properties
> - Estimation of Proteins (In Blood)
> - Criteria for Purity of Proteins
> - Methods of Separation of Proteins
>
> **Plasma Proteins**
> - Biomedical Importance/Functions
> - Method of Separation
> - Individual Plasma Proteins
> - Abnormalities in Plasma Proteins
>
> **Immunoglobulins**
> - Definition
> - General Function
> - Classification
> - Structure of Immunoglobulins
>
> **Peptides**
> - Definition
> - Composition
> - Formation
> - Structure
> - Properties
> - Biomedical Importance/Functions
> - Miscellaneous Proteins/Peptide

AMINO ACIDS

DEFINITION

Amino acids are the building blocks of proteins. They are linked through peptide bonds to form proteins/peptides.

OCCURRENCE

Though there are more than 300 amino acids in nature, only 20 different amino acids are constituents of mammalian proteins. They are called as *standard amino acids*. They are present in proteins from all forms of life-plant, animal and microorganisms.

COMPOSITION

Each amino acid has an amino group and a carboxyl group attached to the same carbon atom (α carbon). The side chain varies from one amino acid to other.

```
R — CH - COOH    COOH   - Carboxyl Group
     |           NH2    - Amino Group
     NH2         R      - Side Chain
```

BIOMEDICAL IMPORTANCE/FUNCTIONS

- *Constituents of proteins and peptides:* Amino acids are the constituents of proteins and peptides which serve a variety of functions in the living systems.
- *Biosynthesis of carbohydrates, fat or both:* Some amino acids can be converted to glucose or ketones or both.
- *Specialized compounds:* Some amino acids give rise to specialized compounds, e.g.,
  - Tryptophan forms vitamin niacin
  - Tyrosine forms hormones, e.g., thyroid hormones (T_3, T_4) and adrenal medullary hormones (Epinephrine and Norepinephrine)
  - Glycine produces several compounds, such as heme, creatinine, purines, bile acids, etc.
  - The catabolism of amino acids gives rise to many compounds of biomedical importance, e.g., decarboxylation of some amino acids produces the corresponding amines, e.g., histamine, GABA, etc.

❏ *Detoxication:* Glycine and cysteine are used in detoxification of specific compounds.

> **Clinical Importance**
> ❖ Abnormal metabolism of amino acids leads to inborn errors of metabolism, e.g., phenylketonuria, albinism, etc.
> ❖ A number of diseases arise due to abnormalities in the transport of amino acids, e.g., Hartnup disease.
> ❖ Changes in protein structure produces prion disease.

■ CLASSIFICATION OF AMINO ACIDS

Amino acids are classified in several ways.

A. Classification (Fig. 4.1)

Amino acids are classified into three groups depending on their reaction in solution.

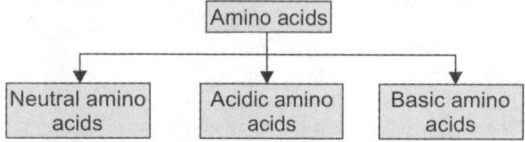

Fig. 4.1: Classification of amino acids (A).

Neutral Amino Acids

They have one COOH group and one NH_2 group. They are neutral in reaction. They are further subdivided depending on the presence of side chains (structure).

❏ Amino acids with aliphatic side chains
 • Glycine $\quad CH_2-COOH$
  $\qquad\qquad\;\;\; |$
  $\qquad\qquad\; NH_2$
 • Alanine $\quad CH_3-CH-COOH$
  $\qquad\qquad\qquad\;\; |$
  $\qquad\qquad\qquad NH_2$
 • Valine $\quad H_3C$
  $\qquad\qquad\;\;\;\; \backslash$
  $\qquad\qquad\;\;\;\;\; CH-CH-COOH$
  $\qquad\qquad\;\;/\qquad\quad |$
  $\qquad\;\; H_3C\qquad\quad NH_2$
 • Leucine H_3C
  $\qquad\qquad\;\; \backslash$
  $\qquad\qquad\;\;\; CH-CH_2-CH-COOH$
  $\qquad\;\;/\qquad\qquad\quad |$
  $\;\; H_3C\qquad\qquad\quad NH_2$
 • Isoleucine CH_3
  $\qquad\qquad\quad\; |$
  $\qquad\qquad\; CH_2$
  $\qquad\qquad\;\;\;\; \backslash$
  $\qquad\qquad\qquad CH-CH-COOH$
  $\qquad\qquad\;\;/\qquad\quad |$
  $\qquad\;\; H_3C\qquad\quad NH_2$

• Serine $CH_2-CH-COOH$
 $\qquad\quad |\qquad\;\; |$
 $\qquad\; OH\quad NH_2$

• Threonine $H_3C-CH-CH-COOH$
 $\qquad\qquad\qquad\quad |\qquad\; |$
 $\qquad\qquad\qquad\; OH\quad NH_2$

❏ Amino acids with side chains containing sulfur
 • Cysteine $CH_2-CH-COOH$
  $\qquad\qquad\;\; |\qquad\;\; |$
  $\qquad\qquad\; SH\quad NH_2$
 • Methionine $CH_2-CH_2-CH-COOH$
  $\qquad\qquad\qquad\; |\qquad\qquad |$
  $\qquad\qquad\qquad S-CH_3\quad NH_2$

❏ Amino acids containing aromatic side chains
 • Phenylalanine

  ⟨benzene ring⟩$-CH_2-CH-COOH$
  $\qquad\qquad\qquad\qquad\quad |$
  $\qquad\qquad\qquad\qquad NH_2$

 • Tyrosine

  $HO-$⟨benzene ring⟩$-CH_2-CH-COOH$
  $\qquad\qquad\qquad\qquad\qquad\quad |$
  $\qquad\qquad\qquad\qquad\qquad NH_2$

 • Tryptophan

  ⟨indole ring⟩$-CH_2-CH-COOH$
  $\qquad\qquad\qquad\qquad\quad |$
  $\qquad\qquad\qquad\qquad NH_2$

❏ Imino acid
 • Proline $H_2C\;\cdots\cdots\; CH_2$
  $\qquad\qquad |\qquad\qquad\quad |$
  $\qquad\; H_2C\qquad\qquad CH$
  $\qquad\qquad\; \backslash\qquad\qquad /\; \backslash$
  $\qquad\qquad\;\;\; NH\qquad\qquad COOH$

Acidic Amino Acids

❏ These amino acids have two COOH groups and one $-NH_2$ group. They are acidic in reaction:
 • Aspartic acid
  $HOOC-CH_2-CH-COOH$
  $\qquad\qquad\qquad\quad |$
  $\qquad\qquad\qquad\; NH_2$

- Glutamic acid

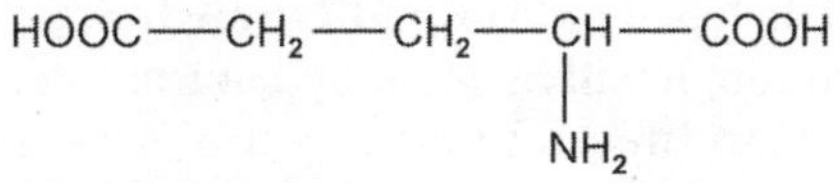

$$HOOC-CH_2-CH_2-CH(NH_2)-COOH$$

❑ Amino acids containing amide group
  - Asparagine

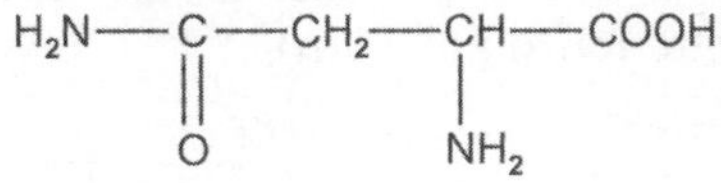

$$H_2N-C(=O)-CH_2-CH(NH_2)-COOH$$

  - Glutamine

$$H_2N-C(=O)-CH_2-CH_2-CH(NH_2)-COOH$$

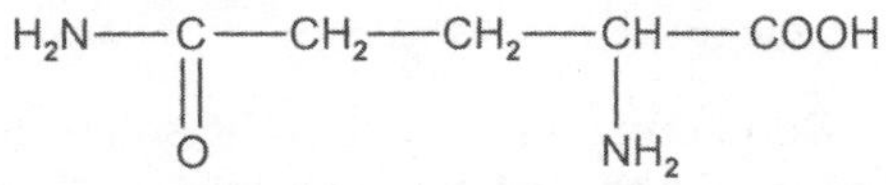

Basic Amino Acids

They contain one —COOH group and two —NH$_2$ groups. They are basic in reaction.

❑ Arginine

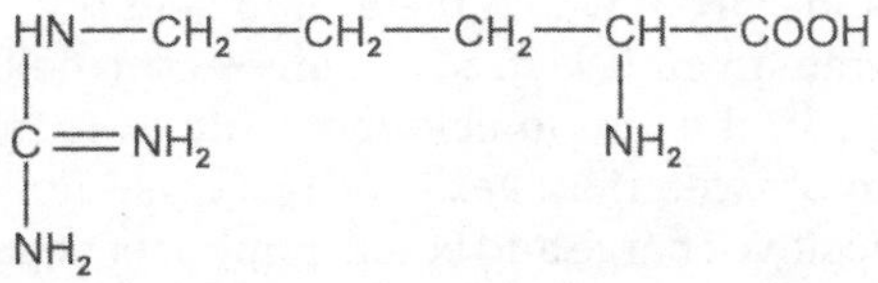

$$HN(C(=NH_2)NH_2)-CH_2-CH_2-CH_2-CH(NH_2)-COOH$$

❑ Lysine

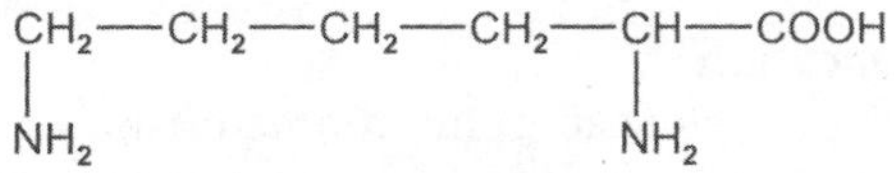

$$CH_2(NH_2)-CH_2-CH_2-CH_2-CH(NH_2)-COOH$$

❑ Histidine

(imidazole ring)—CH_2—$CH(NH_2)$—COOH

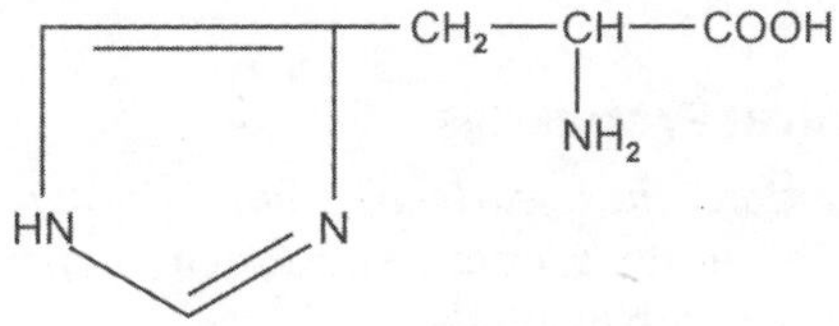

B. Classification

Based on metabolic products formed, amino acids are of three groups:

1. Glucogenic amino acids (produce precursors for glucose)
   - Alanine
   - Arginine
   - Aspartic acid
   - Asparagine
   - Cysteine
   - Glutamic acid
   - Glutamine
   - Glycine
   - Histidine
   - Methionine
   - Proline
   - Serine
   - Threonine
   - Valine
2. Ketogenic amino acids (produce ketone bodies)
   - Leucine
   - Lysine
3. Glucogenic and ketogenic amino acids (produce both)
   - Isoleucine
   - Phenylalanine
   - Tyrosine
   - Tryptophan

C. Classification

Nutritionally standard amino acids are of two types:

Essential Amino Acids (10)

These amino acids are not synthesized by the body but must be supplied in the diet. It can be divided into two subtypes:

A. *Fully essential amino acids:*
  - Valine
  - Leucine
  - Isoleucine
  - Threonine
  - Lysine
  - Methionine
  - Phenylalanine
  - Tryptophan

Note
To recall, use the code PVT TIM HALL.

B. *Semi-essential amino acids:* These amino acids are not synthesized in the body in adequate amount during growth especially in children and also in pregnancy and lactation, e.g.,
  - Histidine
  - Arginine

Biomedical Importance

❑ For the optimal growth of the young
❑ For maintenance of nitrogen equilibrium in adult
❑ Omission of any essential amino acid results in decrease in growth and negative nitrogen balance.

Nonessential Amino Acids (10)

These amino acids can be synthesized in the body. They need not be supplied in the diet, e.g.,
- Glycine
- Serine
- Alanine
- Aspartic acid
- Asparagine
- Glutamic acid
- Glutamine
- Proline
- Cysteine
- Tyrosine

■ PROPERTIES

Physical Properties

- *State:* Colorless, crystalline substances
- *Taste:* May be tasteless, sweet or bitter
- Monosodium glutamate (MSG— ajinomoto) is used as a flavoring agent in foods.
- *Solubility:* More soluble in water than in polar solvents.
- *Isomerism:* All amino acids, except glycine exist as D and L isomers and are optically active:

$$\begin{array}{cc} \text{COOH} & \text{COOH} \\ | & | \\ \text{H—C—NH}_2 & \text{H}_2\text{N—C—H} \\ | & | \\ \text{R} & \text{R} \\ \text{D-Amino acid} & \text{L-Amino acid} \end{array}$$

Amino acids present in biological proteins contain L-α amino acids.

Ampholytes

Definition

Amino acids can act as acids and bases. So they are called as ampholytes.

Ionic State

Each amino acid has at least two ionizable groups namely —NH_2 group and COOH group. In strongly acidic pH medium, the amino acid will be in cationic form. In strongly alkaline pH medium, it will be in anionic form. In aqueous solution (neutral pH) it will behave both as cationic form and anionic form. At this point, each amino acid carries both charges (+ and −) in equal number and hence the net charge is zero (zwitterion/dipolar ion).

$$\begin{array}{ccc} \text{R—CH—COOH} & \text{R—CH—COO}^- & \text{R—CH—COO}^- \\ | & | & | \\ \text{NH}_3^+ & \text{NH}_3^+ & \text{NH}_2 \\ \text{Cation} & \text{Zwitterion} & \text{Anion} \end{array}$$

Depending on the pH of the solution, each amino acid can behave as an acid or a base. This property is called as amphoteric. So amino acids are called as ampholytes.

Isoelectric pH (or) Isoelectric Point (pI)

Definition

It is the pH at which the amino acid does not migrate to any electrode in an electric field. At this pH, the amino acid molecule exits in the form of zwitterion, i.e., it carries equal number of positive charge and equal number of negative charge and the net charge is zero (electrically neutral).

Application

- The isoelectric point characteristic of the amino acids forms the basis of electrophoresis.
- Proteins act as buffers on both the sides of isoelectric pH.

Chemical Properties

- *Reactions due to carboxyl group (—COOH):*
  - *Formation of esters:* Amino acids can form ester with alcohols

$$\begin{array}{c} \text{CH}_2\text{—COOH} + \text{C}_2\text{H}_5\text{OH} \xrightarrow{-\text{H}_2\text{O}} \text{CH}_2\text{—COOC}_2\text{H}_5 \\ | \qquad\qquad\qquad\qquad\qquad\qquad | \\ \text{NH}_2 \qquad\qquad\qquad\qquad\qquad\qquad \text{NH}_2 \\ \text{Glycine} \qquad\qquad\qquad\qquad\qquad \text{Glycine ester} \end{array}$$

α-amino acids which do no occur in proteins but perform important functions in mammalian body.		
Ornithine	Citrulline	Homocysteine
Nonamino acids		
β-alanine	γ-aminobutyric acid	Taurine
Amino acids which are formed from post-translational modifications		
4-hydroxyproline	5-hydroxylysine	γ-carboxyglutamic acid
21st amino acid = selenocysteine—present in glutathione peroxidase		

- *Formation of amines:* Amino acids can be converted to their respective amines by heating with barium hydroxide. Important amines are formed from amino acids in the body.

$$R-CH(NH_2)-COOH \xrightarrow{-CO_2} R-CH_2-NH_2$$

Histidine $\xrightarrow{-CO_2}$ Histamine

Tryptophan $\xrightarrow{-CO_2}$ Tryptamine

- *Formation of amides:* With ammonia, they form the corresponding amides. Asparagine (amide of aspartic acid) and glutamine (amide of glutamic acid).
- Glutamine is involved in transport of ammonia in the body.
  Aspartic acid + NH_3 → Asparagine
  Glutamic acid + NH_3 → Glutamine
☐ *Reactions due to amino (–NH_2) group:*
  - *Salt formation:* The amino group reacts with mineral acids, such as HCl to form salts.

$$CH_2(NH_2)-COOH \xrightarrow{+HCl} CH_2(NH_3Cl)-COOH$$

Glycine → Glycine hydrochloride

- *Transamination:* Amino group of amino acid is transferred to a keto acid to form the corresponding new amino acid and new keto acid.

  Glutamate + Pyruvate → α-ketoglutarate acid + Alanine

  This reaction is important in interconversion of amino acids and also in synthesis of non-essential amino acids.
- *Formation of acyl derivatives:* Amino group reacts with acyl anhydride or acyl halide, such as benzoyl chloride and produces acyl amino acids, such as benzoyl glycine (hippuric acid). This is one of the mechanisms of detoxification and also a liver function test.
  Benzoyl + Glycine → Benzoyl glycine
  chloride   (hippuric acid)
☐ *Reaction due to both amino and carboxyl groups:*
  - Formation of chelated complex: Amino acids form chelated coordination complexes with certain heavy metals.
    Glycine + Calcium → Calcium diglycinate

Amino acids resulting from breakdown of enamel and dentine form soluble calcium complexes resulting in loss of calcium and development of caries.

☐ *Reactions to identify N-terminal amino acid:*
  - *Reaction with Sanger's reagent:* Sanger's reagent (1 Fluoro, 2, 4, dinitrobenzene FDNB) condenses with the free amino group in an alkaline medium. The compound formed enables the identification of N-terminal amino acid.
  - *Reaction with Edman's reagent:* Reaction between Edman's reagent (Phenyl isothiocyanate) and the amino acid also enables the identification of N-terminal amino acid.
☐ *Reactions to identify C-terminal amino acid:*
  - *Enzymatic cleavage:* Carboxypeptidase attacks only peptide bond joining the last residue with a free α-carboxyl group of the peptide chain. Amino acids released are identified by chromatography.
  - *Sorenson's formal titration:* This method is also used to estimate the free carboxyl group in amino acid.
  - *Color reactions*: Refer page 57.
  - *Technique for separation of amino acids*: Chromatography (*refer* Chapter 28).

PROTEINS

■ DEFINITION

Proteins are high molecular weight organic compounds. They are formed from amino acids which are linked together through peptide bonds.

■ MEANING

The term protein is derived from Greek word 'proteios' meaning 'Primary or Holding first place'.

■ COMPOSITION

Proteins are polymers of amino acids. Only 20 different amino acids occur in mammalian proteins though more than 300 amino acids are present in nature.

■ OCCURRENCE

They are present in all forms of life.

BIOMEDICAL IMPORTANCE/FUNCTIONS

- *Energy:* Proteins supply energy to a minor extent (12–15%).
- *Structural elements:* Proteins are the main structural components of the cytoskeleton, e.g., collagen, elastin.
- *Enzymes:* All enzymes except ribozymes are proteins. They act as biocatalysts.
- *Transport:* Some proteins are involved in the transport of specific substances across the membrane or in the body fluids, e.g., albumin, transferrin, hemoglobin.
- *Blood clotting:* They are involved in blood clotting through thrombin, fibrinogen and other protein factors.
- *Hormones:* Some hormones are proteins, e.g., Insulin, GH.
- *Immunity:* They provide defense against infection by means of protein antibodies, e.g., Immunoglobulins.
- *Homeostasis:*
  - *Water and electrolyte balance:* Proteins by exerting osmotic pressure help in maintenance of water and electrolyte balance in the body.
  - *Acid-base balance:* Protein buffers play an important role in maintenance of acid-base balance of blood.
- *Miscellaneous:*
  - *Storage:* Ferritin
  - *Contractile elements:* Actin
- *Regulatory role:* Calmodulin, G-proteins
- *Pharmacopeial products:* Human immunoglobulins.

Clinical Importance

- Analysis of certain proteins in blood is widely used for diagnostic purpose, e.g., liver disease
- Analysis of plasma immunoglobulins has diagnostic use in immune disorders
- Many genetic diseases arise due to deficiency of proteins
- Altered structure of protein leads to prion disease.

CLASSIFICATION

Proteins are classified in different ways as follows:

A. Classification (Fig. 4.2)

Classification of proteins is mainly based on composition and physical properties, such as solubility, heat coagulation. This is the most commonly employed classification. According to this classification, proteins are classified into three major classes with many subclasses.
1. Simple proteins (**Table 4.1**)
2. Conjugated proteins (**Table 4.2**)
3. Derived proteins (**Table 4.3**)

B. Classification

It is based on shape of proteins:
- *Globular proteins:* They are oval or spherical in shape. They have axial ratio less than 10

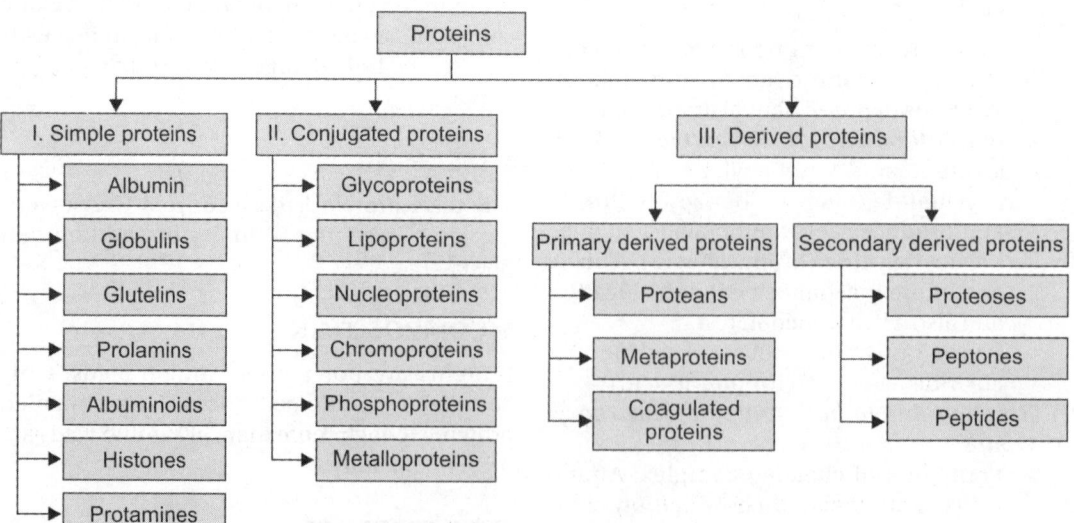

Fig. 4.2: Classification of proteins.

(ratio of length to breadth), e.g., albumin, globulins.
- *Fibrous proteins:* They are elongated or needle shaped. They have axial ratio greater than 10, e.g., collagen, keratin, elastin.

C. Classification

It is based on functions of proteins:
- *Structural proteins:* Proteoglycans
- *Storage proteins:* Ferritin, myoglobin
- *Enzymes:* Dehydrogenases, kinases
- *Transport proteins:* Hemoglobin, lipoproteins
- *Protective proteins:* Immunoglobulins, blood clotting factors
- *Contractile proteins:* Actin, tubulin
- *Hormones:* Insulin, GH

D. Classification: Based on Nutritional Value (*refer* Chapter 21)

- Complete proteins
- Incomplete proteins

Simple Proteins

These proteins yield amino acids on hydrolysis. They are further classified as in **Table 4.1**.

Conjugated Proteins

- These are simple proteins combined with a nonprotein group.
- Protein part + Nonprotein part (prosthetic group) = Conjugated protein
- Depending on the nature of prosthetic group, they are subclassified in **Table 4.2**.

Derived Proteins (Table 4.3)

This class of proteins includes those proteins formed from simple and conjugated proteins by various physical and chemical factors. These are subdivided on the basis of their progressive cleavage into two subclasses which may again be of several types **(Table 4.3)**.

Table 4.1: Simple proteins.

Sl. No.	Subclass	Properties	Examples
1.	Albumin	Soluble in water and dilute salt solutions. Coagulable by heat, precipitated by full saturated salt (ammonium sulfate) solution	Albumin in blood, ovalbumin in egg, lactalbumin in milk, myogen in muscle, legumelin in soya beans, leucosin in wheat
2.	Globulins	Sparingly soluble in water. Soluble in dilute salt solution. Heat coagulable. Precipitated by half saturated salt (ammonium sulfate) solution	Globulins in blood, ovoglobulin in egg yolk, lactoglobulin in milk, myosinogen in muscle, tuberin in potato, legumin in peas
3.	Glutelins	Insoluble in water and salt solutions. Soluble in dilute acids and alkalis. Coagulated by heat	Plant proteins, glutenin in wheat, oryzenin in rice
4.	Prolamines	Soluble in alcohol (60–70%). Insoluble in water and salt solution and absolute alcohol. Not coagulated by heat	Plant proteins, gliadin in wheat, zein in maize
5.	Albuminoids (Scleroproteins)	Insoluble in water, dilute salt solutions, acids and alkalis. Not heat coagulated	• Keratin (in hair, horn, nail, wool, feather) • Collagen (in bone, cartilage and tendons) • Elastin (in connective tissue and ligaments)
6.	Histones	Slight basic proteins. Soluble in water, dilute acids and salt solutions. Not coagulated by heat	Globin in hemoglobin, histones in nucleoproteins
7.	Protamines	Strong basic proteins soluble in water, dilute acids and alkalis. Not heat coagulable	Salmine Present in nucleoproteins

Section 2: Chemistry of Biomolecules

Table 4.2: Conjugated proteins.

Sl. No.	Subclass	Composition	Examples
1.	Glycoproteins	Protein + Carbohydrate	Mucin in saliva, ovomucoid in egg white, present in tendon, bones
2.	Lipoproteins	Protein + Lipid	Present in egg yolk, milk, cell membranes
3.	Nucleoproteins	Simple basic proteins (protamine, or histone) + Nucleic acids	Present in nucleus, cytoplasm
4.	Chromoproteins	Protein + Colored substance	Hemoproteins: (Protein + Heme) • Hemoglobin: Cytochromes • Others: Flavoprotein (Protein + Riboflavin)
5.	Phosphoproteins	Protein + Phosphorus	Casein in milk, ovovitellin in egg yolk
6.	Metalloproteins	Protein + Metal ion	Ferritin (Protein + Fe), Ceruloplasmin (Protein + Cu)

Table 4.3: Derived proteins.

Sl. No.	Subclass	Characteristics	Examples
A. *Primary derived proteins:* These are the derivatives of proteins formed during early stages of hydrolysis by dilute acids, alkalis or enzymes.			
1.	Proteans	Insoluble in water	Fibrin from fibrinogen
2.	Metaproteins	Insoluble in water	Acid and alkali metaproteins
3.	Coagulated proteins	These are insoluble products formed by the action of heat or alcohol or other factors, such as high pressure	Cooked meat, cooked egg albumin
B. *Secondary derived proteins:* These are the derivatives of proteins formed by the progressive hydrolysis of proteins at their peptide linkages.			
1.	Proteoses	• Formed at the next stage of hydrolysis of metaproteins • Soluble in water. Not coagulated by heat Precipitated by full saturated ammonium sulfate	• Albumose from albumin • Globulose from globulin • Gelatin from collagen
2.	Peptones	Soluble in water. Not coagulable by heat. Not precipitated by saturated ammonium sulfate	Proteins formed by the enzymatic digestion by proteases
3.	Peptides	Combination of two or more amino acids linked by peptide bonds	Glutathione Angiotensins, etc.

STRUCTURAL ORGANIZATION OF PROTEINS

Proteins are macromolecules. The biological functions of proteins are based on their conformation (structural arrangement).

They have four levels of structure:
1. Primary structure
2. Secondary structure
3. Tertiary structure
4. Quaternary structure

Primary Structure

It is the linear sequence of amino acids joined together by peptide bonds in their peptide chains.

$$H_2N-CH_2-CO-NH-CH_2-COOH$$
Glycylglycine
(Glycine + Glycine)

The free NH_2 group of terminal amino acid is called *N*-terminal end. The free COOH group is called *C*-terminal end.

Primary structure of insulin was described by Sanger in 1955.

Secondary Structure (Fig. 4.3)

The peptide chain thus formed assumes secondary structure by folding or coiling through hydrogen bonds and disulfide bonds.
- *Hydrogen bonds:* These are weak low-energy noncovalent bonds. They are formed by sharing H-atoms between oxygen of CO and nitrogen of $-NH_2$.
- *Disulfide bonds:* These are strong, high-energy covalent bonds. They are formed between two cysteine residues.

Hydrogen bonding in secondary structure produces either α helix or β pleated sheet structure as proposed by Pauling and Corey.

α-helix: A peptide chain forming regular helical coils is called α-helix. These coils are stabilized by hydrogen bonds between carbonyl 0 of 1st amino acid and amide N of 4th amino acid residues. Hydrogen bond is intrachain. α helices can be right handed or left handed. The proteins of hair nail, skin contain a group of proteins called keratins which have a helical structure. Collagen forms a triple helical structure.

β pleated sheet: This type of structure is formed when hydrogen bonds are formed between the carbonyl oxygens and amide nitrogens of two or more adjacent extended polypeptide chains. Hydrogen bonding in β pleated sheet is interchain. Polypeptide chain in this structure is fully extended. The adjacent chains may be parallel or antiparallel. Silk fibroin, a protein of silk worm, is rich in β pleated sheet.

(Some proteins may have nonhelical non-pleated structure called random coil in addition to the above).

Tertiary Structure (Fig. 4.4)

The polypeptide chain with secondary structure may be further folded or twisted forming many sizes. Such a structural conformation is called as tertiary structure. It refers to three-dimensional structure. Protein in this conformation is called as a native protein which is biologically active. The bonds responsible for interaction between groups of amino acids are:
- Hydrophobic bonds
- Hydrogen bonds
- Ionic or electrostatic interactions
- Van der Waals forces
- Disulfide bonds

Quaternary Structure (Fig. 4.5)

All the polypeptide chains with primary, secondary and tertiary structures (monomers/subunits) may be held together by noncovalent interactions or covalent crosslinks to form quaternary structure of proteins (oligomeric protein).

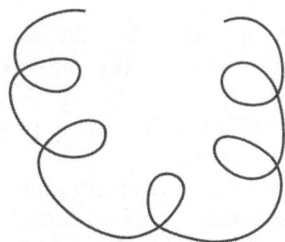

Fig. 4.4: Tertiary structure.

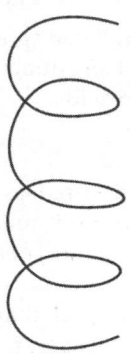

Fig. 4.3: Secondary structure.

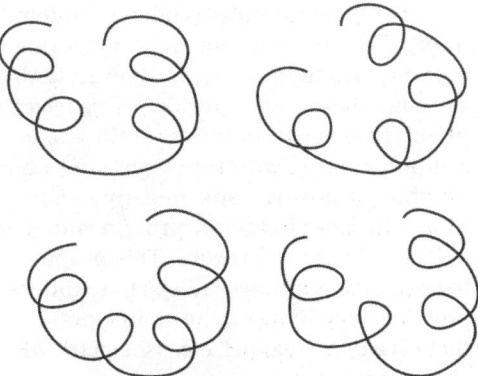

Fig. 4.5: Quaternary structure.

For example,

Creatine phosphokinase (CPK)	= Dimer (2 monomers)
Lactate dehydrogenase (LDH)	= Tetramer (4 monomers)
Hemoglobin	= Tetramer (4 monomers)

These proteins are involved in metabolism and cellular function.

> **Clinical Importance**
>
> Some diseases occur due to altered structure of patient.
> ❖ *Prion disease:* It occurs due to misfolding of three dimensional structure of proteins, e.g., Transmissible spongiform encephalopathies in humans; mad cow disease in cattle.
> ❖ *Amyloidosis:* It occurs due to altered protein structure of β pleated sheets (amyloid proteins), e.g., Alzheimer's disease (neuroregnerative disorder).

■ PROPERTIES

Physical Properties

- *Taste:* Pure proteins are generally tasteless. But their hydrolytic products are bitter in taste.
- *Odor:* Pure proteins are odorless but when heated they give off the odor of burning feather.
- *State:* Aqueous solution of proteins are colloidal in nature.
- *Molecular weight:* They are high molecular weight compounds. For example, mol. wt. of Albumin: 69,000, Globulin: 1,76,000
- *Viscosity:* It is related to molecular size. Long molecules (fibrous proteins) are more viscous than globular molecules (globular proteins).
- *Ampholytes:* Proteins are ampholytes due to presence of amino acids, i.e., they act both as acids and bases. At a specific pH (isoelectric pH or isoelectric point) protein exists as a dipolar ion (Zwitterion) carrying equal number of positive and negative charges. Thus, the net charge on protein molecule at its isoelectric pH is zero. This property is used in electrophoresis to separate different proteins depending on the charge present in them at a particular pH, e.g., isoelectric pH of albumin is 4.7, casein 4.6.

Chemical Properties

Precipitation

- *By electrolytes or alcohol:* Polar groups of proteins, such as NH_2 and COOH groups become hydrated and swell up when electrolytes or alcohol is added to it. Finally these agents dehydrate proteins and precipitate them from solution.
- *By positive (+) ions:* The commonly used positive (+) ions are the heavy metals of Hg^{++}, Pb^{++}, etc. The metals precipitate proteins at the pH alkaline to its isoelectric pH.
  - Clinical application
    - Proteins are used as antidotes to metallic poisons
    - $AgNO_3$ is used in cauteries.
- *By negative (–) ions:* The commonly used negative (–) ions are tungstic acid, trichloroacetic acid, etc. These agents precipitate proteins when pH of the medium is on the acidic side of its isoelectric pH.
  - Clinical application
    - To prepare protein free filtrate of blood and other biological fluids prior to analysis of some constituents, such as sugar and urea.
    - Proteins can combine with acidic dyes (–) or basic dyes (+) forming protein dye-complex. This property is applied in staining the tissue in histopathological specimens.

Hydrolysis

The sequence of reactions and various products obtained during hydrolysis of proteins are:

Proteins → Proteans → Metaproteins
↓
Amino acids ← Peptides ← Peptones ← Proteoses

It can be brought out by proteolytic enzymes. The ultimate end products of hydrolysis of proteins are amino acids.

Denaturation

Definition: It is defined as a disruption of secondary, tertiary and quaternary structure (except primary structure) of the native protein. It results in the alterations of the physical, chemical and biological characteristics of the protein by a variety of agents.

Causative Agents

- *Physical agents:* Heat, violent shaking, UV light, high pressure.
- *Chemical agents:* Acids, alkalis, enzymes, heavy metal salts, detergents, organic solvents, urea, salicylate.

Changes in Denatured Proteins

- *Physical*
  - Denatured proteins cannot be crystallized
  - Viscosity is increased
  - Solubility is decreased
- *Chemical*
  - Many chemical groups which were rather inactive become exposed, e.g., SH group
  - Enzymatic and hormonal activity is destroyed
- *Biological*
  - Increased digestibility by proteolytic enzymes
  - Becomes inactive

Importance: This process is utilized in clinical laboratory for analyzing constituents of blood.

Denaturation and renaturation of proteins: Denatured proteins can be reversed in some cases and cannot be reversed in other cases.

Reversibility: Protein ribonuclease becomes denatured when treated with urea and β-mercaptoethanol. Denatured protein ribonuclease when freed from urea and β-mercaptoethanol is converted to native protein and gain enzymatic activity.

Irreversibility: When egg albumin (native protein) is heated, it is coagulated and then denatured protein becomes irreversible **(Fig. 4.6)**.

Color Reactions of Proteins (Table 4.4)

Proteins produce color in certain reactions, which is due to characteristic group of particular amino acid(s) present in them. Color reactions are used to identify amino acids and hence proteins.

Table 4.4: Color reactions of proteins.

	Name of the test	To detect
1.	Biuret test (general test)	Proteins
2.	Ninhydrin test	α amino acids
3.	Xanthoproteic test	Aromatic amino acids
4.	Million's test	Tryptophan, tyrosine
5.	Hopkins–Cole test	Tryptophan
6.	Sakaguchi test	Arginine
7.	Sulfur test	Sulfur containing amino acids (except methionine)
8.	Pauly's test	Histidine
9.	Molisch test	Glycoproteins

ESTIMATION OF PROTEINS (IN BLOOD)

- Biuret method
- Kjeldahl method

CRITERIA FOR PURITY OF PROTEINS

Purity of proteins can be tested by the following methods:
- Molecular weight
- Solubility curves
- Immunoreactivity

METHODS OF SEPARATION OF PROTEINS

- Ultracentrifugation
- Salting out methods
- Electrophoresis

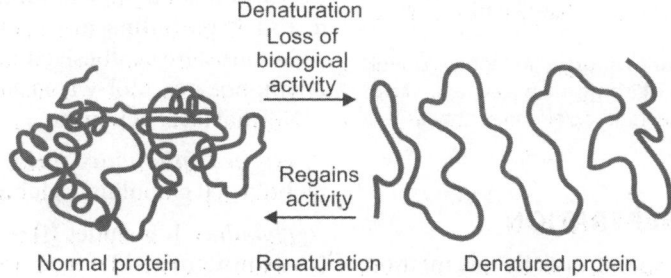

Fig. 4.6: Protein denaturation.

PLASMA PROTEINS

The human plasma proteins consist of a mixture of simple proteins, such as albumin, globulins and conjugated proteins, such as lipoproteins, glycoproteins, etc.

BIOMEDICAL IMPORTANCE/FUNCTIONS

- *Tissue building:* The amino acids from plasma proteins can be used for building up new tissue proteins and vice versa.
- *Nutrition:* Plasma simple proteins are useful in hypoproteinemic state.
- *Fluid exchange:* The colloid osmotic pressure of plasma proteins maintains the distribution of water (fluid) between the blood and tissues.
- *Viscosity of blood:* Due to presence of proteins, the viscosity of blood maintains blood pressure within normal range.
- *Blood coagulation and fibrinolysis:*
  - *Blood clotting:* Plasma contains a number of components, several enzymes and clotting factors which participate in the process of coagulation of blood.
  - *Fibrinolysis:* Thrombus (intravascular clot) is digested by enzymes of fibrinolytic system in the plasma, thus avoiding thrombosis.
- *Transport:* Some proteins are involved in the transport of specific substances either across the membrane or in the body fluids.
  - *Transferrin:* Transports iron
  - *Lipoproteins:* Transport lipids
- *Immunity:* γ globulins present in plasma are antibodies. They protect the body against infections.
- *Buffers:* The protein buffers constitute relatively a small fraction of total blood buffers which maintain acid-base balance of blood.

Clinical Importance

- Analysis of certain proteins has diagnostic value, e.g., liver disease
- Estimation of enzymes (protein) in blood is useful in the diagnosis of some diseases, e.g., Acid phosphatase—prostatic carcinoma. Amylase—acute pancreatitis.

METHOD OF SEPARATION

- *Precipitation by 'salting out':* By this method, different concentrations of salt solutions are used to precipitate the various fractions of proteins, which are then separated.
- Electrophoresis (*refer* Chapter 28).

INDIVIDUAL PLASMA PROTEINS

The plasma proteins are divided into three major types:
1. Albumin
2. Globulins
3. Fibrinogen

Albumin

It is a simple protein. 50–60% of the total proteins of plasma is albumin. It is synthesized in liver. Mol. wt. is 69000.

Functions

- Involved in the transport of several substances, e.g., free fatty acids, unconjugated bilirubin, calcium and steroid hormones and some drugs.
- Maintains osmotic pressure and plays an important role in exchange of water between tissue fluid and blood.
- Nutritionally important constituent.

Normal Level in Plasma

3.5–5 g/100 mL.

Clinical Importance

It is decreased (hypoalbuminemia):
- Severe protein calorie malnutrition
- Liver disease, such as liver cirrhosis
- Nephrotic syndrome

Increased (hyperalbuminemia): Dehydration

Globulins

Constitute about 40% of total plasma proteins. α and β globulins are synthesized in liver. γ globulins are synthesized in plasma cells and B lymphocytes. Mol. wt. 90,000–13,00000.

Normal level in plasma = 2.5–3.5 g/100 mL.

These are subdivided into: α_1 globulins, α_2 globulins, β globulins, γ globulins.

α_1 *globulins:* It includes (i) α_1 acid glycoprotein (orosomucoid)—It is a reliable indicator of acute inflammation (ii) α_1-fetoglobulin

(α_1 fetoprotein)—It is useful diagnostically in determining the presence of hepatocellular carcinoma. (iii) α_1 - antitrypsin—It is principal protease inhibitor of plasma. It is decreased in emphysema of lungs.

α_2 *globulins:* It includes (i) Ceruloplasmin—is a copper-containing protein. It mainly functions as the enzyme ferroxidase which is involved in the conversion of Fe^{++} to Fe^{+++} to be incorporated into transferrin. It is decreased in Wilson's disease. (ii) Haptoglobulin—is used to evaluate rheumatic disease. It is increased in inflammatory conditions.

β_1 *globulins:* It includes (i) Transferrin (siderophilin)—is an iron containing protein. Its sole function is the transport of iron between intestine and site of synthesis of hemoglobin and other heme containing proteins. (ii) C-reactive protein—is indicator of early phase of inflammatory process. (iii) β lipoprotein (LDL)—transports cholesterol esters throughout the body.

γ *globulins:* These are immunoglobulins which have antibody activity (refer to immunoglobulins).

Fibrinogen

It is a clotting factor I. It is a soluble glycoprotein. It is the precursor of fibrin the substance required for clotting of blood. It constitutes 4–6% of total proteins of blood. It is synthesized in liver.

Normal level in plasma = 200 – 400 mg/100 mL.

ABNORMALITIES IN PLASMA PROTEINS (CLINICAL IMPORTANCE)

- *Hyperproteinemia* (increase in plasma total protein):
  - Hemoconcentration due to dehydration
  - Hypergammaglobulinemia, e.g., chronic liver disease, multiple myeloma
- *Hypoproteinemia* (decrease in plasma total protein):
  - Hemodilution due to water intoxication
  - Hypoalbuminemia
    - Loss from the body as in nephrotic syndrome
    - Decreased synthesis of albumin
  - Hypogammaglobulinemia

IMMUNOGLOBULINS

DEFINITION

The immunoglobulins (Ig) constitute a heterogeneous family of plasma proteins. They occupy γ globulin fraction of plasma proteins in electrophoresis.

GENERAL FUNCTION

They act as antibodies against infections.

Synthesis: They are produced by plasma cells.

CLASSIFICATION

They are divided into five major classes based on their molecular weight, electrophoretic mobility, ultracentrifugal sedimentation and other properties.

1. IgG
2. IgM
3. IgA
4. IgD
5. IgE

- *IgG:* It comprises 70–80% of total immunoglobulins in an adult. Its mol. wt. is 1,45,000 (approx). It can cross the placenta freely. It is the major protective antibody in new-borns. It represents the most of antibacterial and antiviral antibodies, e.g., immune anti-A and anti-B, anti-Rh antibodies, anti-toxins (diphtheria, tetanus, streptococcal), antiviral antibodies, complement fixing antibodies, autoantibodies to thyroid.
- *IgM:* It constitutes approximately 7% of total immunoglobulins in the normal adult. It is the larger Ig molecule, mol. wt. is 9,00,000 to 10,00,000. IgM antibodies are prominent in early immune response to most antigens. It predominates in certain antibody responses such as natural blood group antibodies. Excessive production of IgM occurs in Waldenstrom's macroglobulinemia.
- *IgA:* It constitutes 10–20% of total Ig in the normal adult. Its molecular weight varies from 1,50,000 to 5,00,000. It provides the primary defense mechanism against some local infections due to its presence in saliva, tears, bronchial secretions, nasal mucosa, prostatic fluid, vaginal secretions and mucus secretions of small intestine.

- *IgD:* It is present in serum in trace amount, i.e., 0.2% of total immunoglobulin. Its molecular weight is approximately 1,80,000. It is supposed to have antibody activity towards certain antigens such as diphtheria toxoid, certain thyroid antigens.
- *IgE:* It comprises only 0.04% of the total serum immunoglobulins. Its mol. wt. is 1,90,000 to 2,00,000. It has antibody function and antiallergic function.

STRUCTURE OF IMMUNOGLOBULINS (FIG. 4.7)

Each immunoglobulin molecule is a Y-shaped tetramer. Each molecule has equal member of two heavy polypeptide chains (H-chains) and two light polypeptide chains (L-chains). Hence, each molecule can be represented as H_2L_2. The major bond between H and L chains, and also between the two halves of the molecule are connected by disulfide linkages between cysteine residues and also by noncovalent forces.

Each heavy chain (mol. wt. 53,000 to 75,000) consist of approximately 450 amino acids and each ligh chain (mol. wt. 23,000) consist of 212 amino acids. As heavy chains of Ig are linked to carbohydrates, immunoglobulins are called as glycoproteins.

Each chain (L or H) has two regions. The amino terminal half of the light chain is the variable region (V_L), While the carboxy terminal half is the constant region (CL). In the heavy chain, approximately one-quarter of the amino terminal region is variable (V_H) and the remaining three quarters is constant regions.

Amino acid sequence of variable regions of light and heavy chains is responsible for the specific binding of Ig (antibody) with antigen.

Type of heavy chain determines the class of immunoglobulins.

	IgG	IgA	IgM	IgD	IgE
Heavy chain types	γ	α	μ	S	Σ
No. of peptide chains	1	2	5	1	1
Light chains	κ (Kappa) or λ (Lambda) in all classes				

Clinical Importance

- Increased in chronic infections, paraproteinemias (multiple myeloma)
- Decreased in some congenital disorders

PEPTIDES

Peptides are the hydrolytic products of proteins.

$$\text{Protein} \xrightarrow{\text{Hydrolysis}} \text{Peptides}$$

DEFINITION

They are formed from two or more amino acids linked through peptide bonds. These are named according to the number of amino acids present in them.

$$\text{Amino acids} \xrightarrow{\text{Linkage}} \text{Peptides}$$

COMPOSITION

- *Dipeptide:* Made up of two amino acids, e.g., glycylglycine

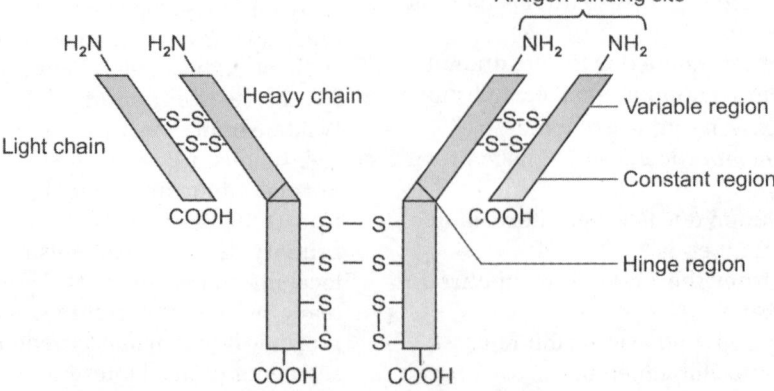

Fig. 4.7: Structure of immunoglobulin.

NH$_2$-CH$_2$-CO — NH-CH$_2$-COOH
(glycine)　　　　　(glycine)

- *Tripeptide:* Made up of three amino acids, e.g., glutathione
  Glycine + Cysteine + Glutamic acid

The linking together of more than two amino acids by peptide bonds produces polypeptide chains. Many polypeptide chains combine together to form proteins. Total number of amino acids present in peptides may vary from 2–50.

■ FORMATION

A peptide is formed by linking the carboxyl group of one amino acid and the amino group of next amino acid by the removal of water.

■ STRUCTURE

Peptides are written with N-terminal residue (the residue with a free amino group) at the left and with the C-terminal residue (the residue with a free carboxyl group) at the right. The linear sequence of amino acids in a polypeptide constitutes its primary structure.
Example: (Table 4.5)

■ PROPERTIES

Peptides are soluble in water. They are not coagulated by heat.

■ BIOMEDICAL IMPORTANCE/ FUNCTIONS

The following are the physiologically important peptides used in various fields of medicine.

■ MISCELLANEOUS PROTEINS/ PEPTIDE

Glycoproteins

Glycoproteins are conjugated proteins.
- *Composition:* They are complex of proteins and oligosaccharides.
  Proteins + Oligosaccharides = Glycoproteins
- *Occurrence:* They are widely distributed in almost all tissues and cell membranes.

Examples
- Plasma proteins, e.g., albumin
- Structural proteins, e.g., collagen
- Enzymes, e.g., alkaline phosphatase
- Hormones, e.g., thyroglobulin
- Transport proteins, e.g., transferrin
- Immunoproteins, e.g., immunoglobulin

Functions
- They form viscous solutions which act as lubricants and protection covers in the body
  • Intestinal mucus protects intestinal cell against mechanical damage.
  • Respiratory tract mucus protects against invasion by bacteria.
  • Uterus is protected from vaginal microbial flora by the cervical mucus.
- They play key role in fertilization and inflammation.
- Glycoproteins are involved in many diseases, e.g., AIDS, cystic fibrosis, influenza, peptic ulcer and rheumatoid arthritis.

$$H_2N\text{-}CH_2\text{-}COOH + H_2N\text{-}CH_2\text{-}COOH \xrightarrow{-H_2O} H_2N\text{-}CH_2\text{-}CO\text{-}NH\text{-}CH_2\text{-}COOH$$
Amino acid 1　　Amino acid 2　　　　　　　Peptide

Table 4.5: Physiologically active peptides.

Sl. No.	Examples	Importance
1.	Glutathione	It is a tripeptide. It is required for the action of several enzymes and also insulin. It functions in oxidation and reduction systems (*refer* page 62)
2.	Bradykinin and kallidin	Smooth muscle hypotensive agents
3.	Angiotensins	Role in hypertension
4.	Hormones	Oxytocin and vasopressin, ACTH, gastrin
5.	Antibiotics	Penicillin, actinomycin
6.	Brain peptides	Enkephalins: Reduces intestinal motility
7.	Carnosine, anserine	Present in muscles, histidine derivatives, dipeptide

Proteoglycans

Proteoglycans are conjugated proteins which contain covalently linked glycosaminoglycans (GAG).

    Protein + Glycosaminoglycans (Mucopolysaccharides) = Proteoglycans

They are also called as mucoproteins.

Occurrence: They are found in all the tissues of the body mainly extracellular matrix (ground substance).

Functions

- Proteoglycans are associated with the major structural components of the extracellular matrix (collagen, elastin).
- They are components of plasma membrane.
- They play a role in corneal transparency.

Apolipoproteins (Apoproteins)

Definition: The protein components of the lipoproteins are known as apolipoproteins.

Functions

- They act as structural components of lipoproteins.
- They may act as activator or inhibitor of some enzymes
- They act as lipid transfer proteins.
- They recognize the cell membrane receptors.

Types: Different types of apolipoproteins are present in lipoproteins.

Lipoproteins	Major apolipoproteins
Chylomicron	B-48
VLDL	B-100, C-I, C-II, C-III
LDL	B-100
HDL	A-I, A-II

Collagen

It is major protein of connective tissue in animals and humans. It is a structural protein and constitutes about 25% of the total body protein.

Functions

- It provides an extracellular matrix (ECM) in the tissues.
- It provides strength, support and shape to the tissues.
- It helps in cell proliferation and differentiation.
- It may contribute to thrombus formation.

Types

Approximately 28 different types of collagens have been identified in human tissue. They are triple helix in structure.

> **Clinical Importance**
> A number of genetic diseases occur due to abnormalities in the synthesis of collagen, e.g., osteogenesis imperfecta, Ehler's–Danlos syndrome.

> **Note**
> Contractile proteins (myosin, actin, and troponins) are involved in the movement of body organs (muscle, heart, gut and cells).

Glutathione (Peptide)

- *Composition:* It is a tripeptide consisting of three amino acids, namely—glutamic acid, cysteine and glycine. Its chemical name is γ-glutamyl cysteinyl glycine. It is a pseudopeptide.
- *Occurrence:* It is widely present in nature.

Functions

- It is an important reducing agent in the tissues.
  - It is required as coenzyme for activation of methionine to form S-adenosyl methionine (active methionine).
  - It also acts as coenzyme for PG synthetase.
  - It takes part in glutamyl cycle for absorption of amino acids from the intestine.
- Glutathione peroxide containing selenium as cofactor helps to destroy H_2O_2 and free radicals in cells.
- It maintains structure and integrity of RBC membrane.
- It prevents oxidation of S-H groups of proteins and enzymes to S-S groups to protect their functions.
- It is involved in the detoxification of certain toxic compounds, such as organophosphate and nitro compounds.

5. Chemistry of Nucleic Acids

Chapter Outline

- Definition
- Discovery
- Types
- Occurrence
- Biomedical Importance/Functions
- Composition
- Nucleosides
- Nucleotides
- Nucleic Acids
- Biologically Important Nucleotides
- Nucleoproteins
- Additional Information

DEFINITION

Nucleic acids are macromolecules. They are polynucleotides. They are hereditary determinants of living organisms.

DISCOVERY

Miescher (1871) isolated nucleic acid from pus cells and named it as nuclein. Altmann in 1899 introduced the term nucleic acid to replace nuclein. Avery, MacLeod and McCarty in 1944 demonstrated that DNA contained genetic information.

TYPES

There are two types of nucleic acids in the cells (**Fig. 5.1**):

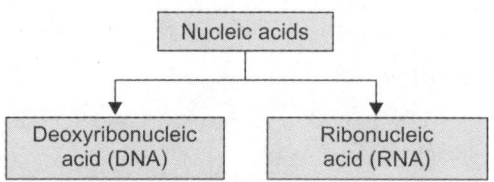

Fig. 5.1: Type of nucleic acids.

OCCURRENCE

Both nucleic acids are present in all animals, plants, bacteria and viruses. They may be present in free state or in combination with proteins as nucleoproteins.

BIOMEDICAL IMPORTANCE/FUNCTIONS

- Study of the chemistry and functions of nucleic acids is essential to understand normal cellular physiology and disease at molecular level.
- DNA is the fundamental unit of genetic information. It stores and transmits the genetic properties of an organism.
- RNA is involved in the synthesis of proteins after receiving genetic information from DNA.

$$DNA \xrightarrow{Transcription} RNA \xrightarrow{Translation} Protein$$

Clinical Importance

Defect in DNA may lead to inherited disorders: Xeroderma pigmentosum.

COMPOSITION

Nucleic acids are made up of several mononucleotides. Each mononucleotide contains nitrogenous base, sugar and phosphoric acid.

Nitrogenous Bases

Two types of nitrogenous bases are found in nucleic acids (**Fig. 5.2**). They are heterocyclic (ring) compounds.

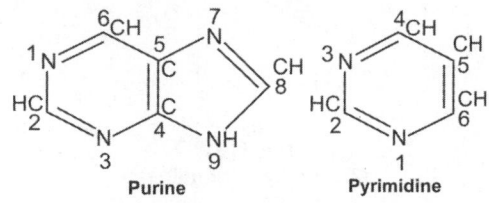

Fig. 5.2: Nitrogenous bases.

a. *Purine:* It is a two-ring nitrogenous base. It contains a six-membered pyrimidine ring fused with a five membered imidazole ring.
Purine bases present in nucleic acids are **(Fig. 5.3)**:
- Adenine (A)
- Guanine (G)

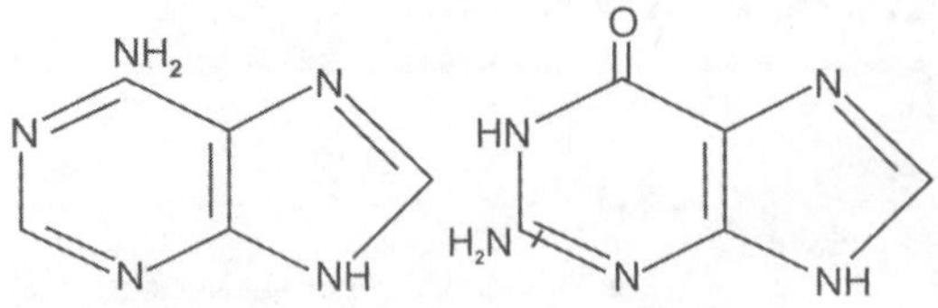

Adenine (A)
(6-aminopurine)

Guanine (G)
(2-amino 6-oxypurine)

Fig. 5.3: Purine bases.

b. *Pyrimidine:* It is a single ring nitrogenous base. It contains a heterocyclic nucleus with two nitrogen atoms at 1 and 3 positions.
Pyrimidine bases present in nucleic acids are **(Fig. 5.4)**:

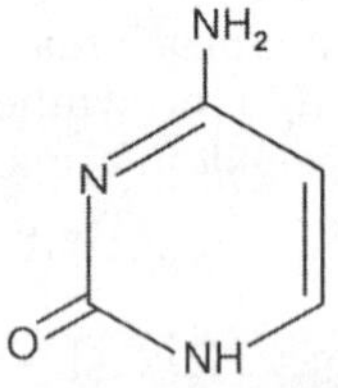

Cytosine (C)
(2-oxy-4-aminopyrimidine)

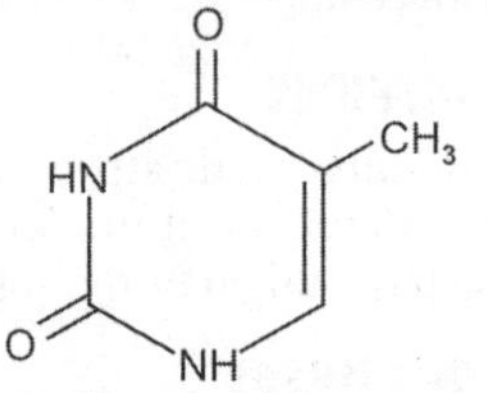

Thymine (T)
(2, 4-dioxy-5-methylpyrimidine)

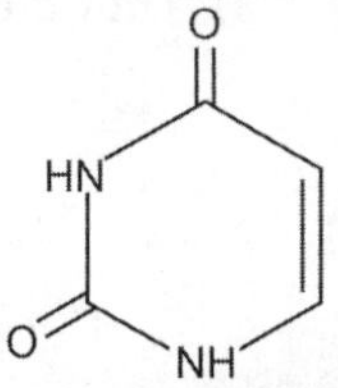

Uracil (U)
(2, 4-dioxy pyrimidine)

Fig. 5.4: Pyrimidine base.

Sugars

Ribose and deoxyribose are pentose sugars present in nucleic acids. Ribose is a 5-carbon aldose sugar present in ribonucleic acid (RNA). D-2 deoxyribose is present in deoxyribonucleic acid (DNA). Both sugars are present in nucleic acids in β-furanose forms **(Fig. 5.5)**.

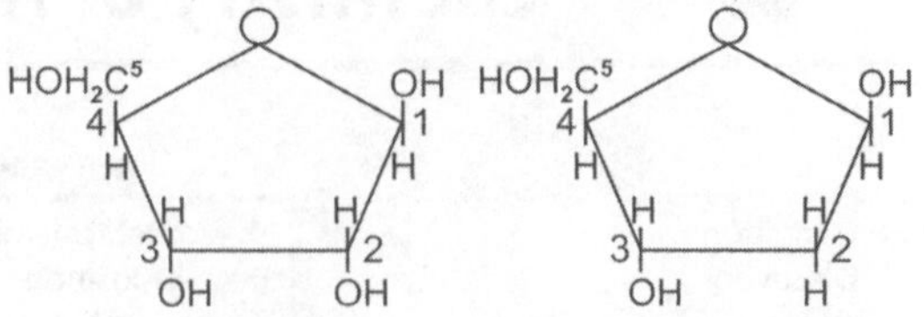

D-ribose

D-2-deoxyribose

Fig. 5.5: Pentose sugars.

Phosphoric Acid (Phosphate)

It is present both in DNA and RNA as phosphate:

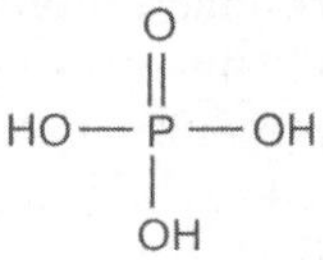

■ NUCLEOSIDES

Nucleosides are compounds in which nitrogenous bases are attached to sugars through glycosidic linkage.

Nucleoside = Base + Sugar

First carbon of the sugar (Ribose or Deoxyribose) is attached to nitrogen at 9th position of purine base or 1st position of pyrimidine base **(Fig. 5.6)**.

Purine
9 N
|
1 C
Sugar

Pyrimidine
1 N
|
1 C
Sugar

Examples

Nucleosides	Base	Sugar
1. Ribonucleosides		
• Adenosine	Adenine	Ribose
• Guanosine	Guanine	Ribose
• Cytidine	Cytosine	Ribose
• Uridine	Uracil	Ribose
2. Deoxyribonucleosides		
• Deoxyadenosine	Adenine	Deoxyribose
• Deoxyguanosine	Guanine	Deoxyribose
• Deoxycytidine	Cytosine	Deoxyribose
• Deoxythymidine	Thymine	Deoxyribose

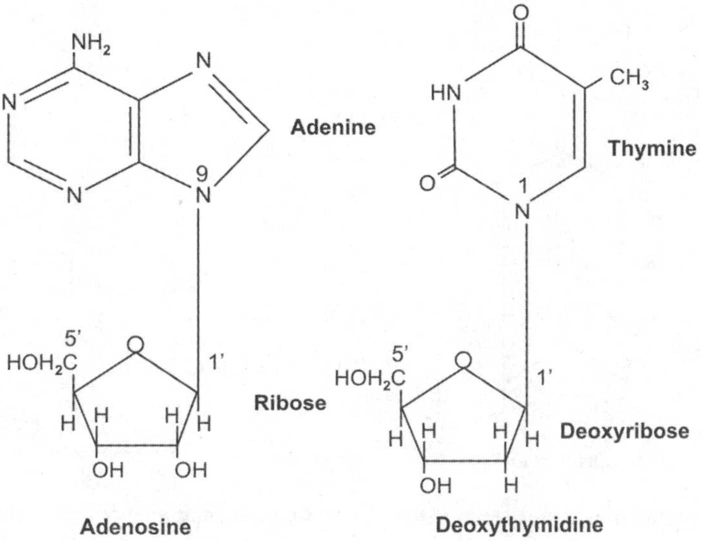

Fig. 5.6: Structure of nucleosides.

■ NUCLEOTIDES (TABLE 5.1)

They are phosphoric acid esters of nucleosides. A nucleotide is a combination of nitrogenous base, sugar and phosphate **(Fig. 5.7)**.

Nucleotide = $\underbrace{\text{Base + Sugar}}_{\text{Nucleoside}}$ + Phosphate

[A nucleotide is a nucleoside with phosphate. Phosphate group may be attached on one or more of hydroxyl groups of the sugar (3' or 5' position of carbon by ester linkage)].

Polynucleotide: It is formed by linking together two or more nucleotides **(Fig. 5.8)**.

Table 5.1: Nucleotides.

Nucleotides	Base	Sugar	Acid
1. Ribonucleotides (Present in RNA)			
▪ Adenylate [Adenylic acid/adenosine monophosphate (AMP)]	Adenine	Ribose	Phosphoric acid (as phosphate)
▪ Guanylate [Guanylic acid/guanosine monophosphate (GMP)]	Guanine	Ribose	Phosphoric acid (as phosphate)
▪ Cytidylate [Cytidylic acid/cytidine monophosphate (CMP)]	Cytosine	Ribose	Phosphoric acid (as phosphate)
▪ Uridylate [Uridylic acid/uridine monophosphate (UMP)]	Uracil	Ribose	Phosphoric acid (as phosphate)
2. Deoxyribonucleotides (Present in DNA)			
▪ Deoxyadenylate (Deoxyadenylic acid/deoxyadenosine monophosphate (d-AMP)	Adenine	Deoxyribose	Phosphoric acid (as phosphate)
▪ Deoxyguanylate (Deoxyguanylic acid/deoxyguanosine monophosphate (d-GMP)	Guanine	Deoxyribose	Phosphoric acid (as phosphate)
▪ Deoxycytidylate (Deoxycytidylic acid/deoxycytidine monophosphate (d-CMP)	Cytosine	Deoxyribose	Phosphoric acid (as phosphate)
▪ Deoxythymidylate (Deoxythymidylic acid/(deoxy) thymidine monophosphate (d-TMP)/thymidylate	Thymine	Deoxyribose	Phosphoric acid (as phosphate)

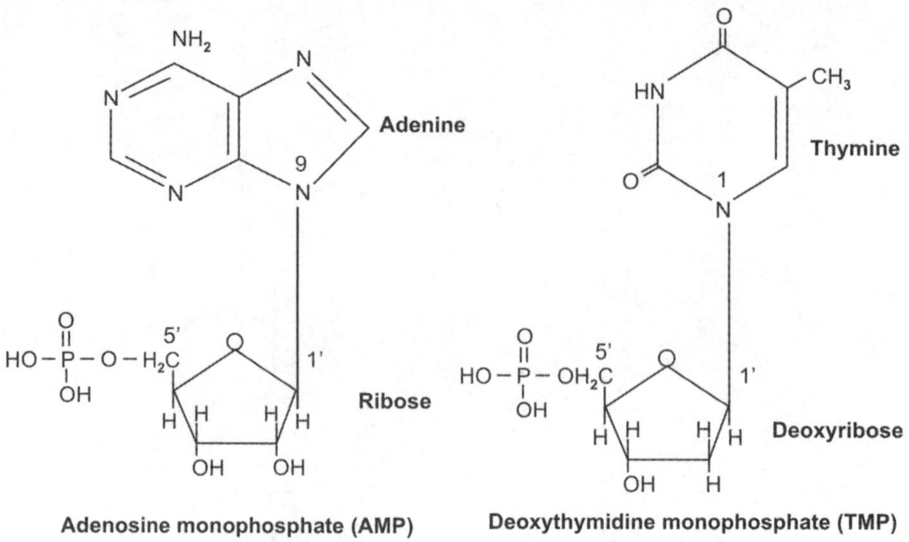

Section 2: Chemistry of Biomolecules

Fig. 5.7: Structure of nucleotides.

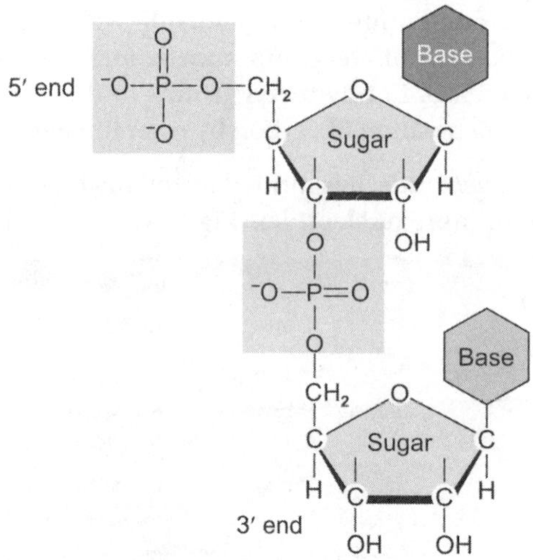

Fig. 5.8: Polynucleotide.

NUCLEIC ACIDS

Two types of nucleic acids are present in living systems:
1. Deoxyribonucleic acid
2. Ribonucleic acid

Deoxyribonucleic Acid

Location

DNA is present mainly in the nucleus of cells (a very small amount is also present in mitochondria).

Structure

It is a polymer of four types of deoxyribonucleotides. It contains 10^{10} nucleotides (**Table 5.2**).

All these deoxyribonucleotides have D-2 deoxyribose as sugar moiety. Each nucleotide contains one of the nitrogenous bases: adenine/guanine (purine bases)/cytosine/thymine (pyrimidine bases). Each one has phosphate group. Purine and pyrimidine bases carry genetic information. Sugar and phosphate groups perform a structural role.

Mononucleotides are linked to one another by phosphodiester bridges at 3'–5' position of deoxyribose constituting a single polynucleotide strand.

Table 5.2: Structure of deoxyribonucleotide.

Deoxyribonucleotides	Base	Sugar	Acid
Deoxyadenylate	Adenine	Deoxyribose	Phosphoric acid
Deoxyguanylate	Guanine	Deoxyribose	Phosphoric acid
Deoxycytidylate	Cytosine	Deoxyribose	Phosphoric acid
(Deoxy) thymidylate	Thymine	Deoxyribose	Phosphoric acid

DNA Double Helix

Watson and Crick (1953) proposed *double helical structure* of DNA **(Fig. 5.9)** (N.P 1962).

DNA molecule consists of two right-handed strands coiled around the common axis. It looks like a twisted/spiral staircase. The two strands are held together by hydrogen bonds between purine and pyrimidine bases of the respective strands.

A with T (two hydrogen bonds); G with C (Three hydrogen bonds).

This union of bases is known as base complementary rule (Chargaff rule). In DNA molecule content of (purine to pyrimidine is equal) A = T; G = C:

Sugar-phosphates are seen on the outer side and bases are on the inner side of the strands. The two strands run in opposite directions and antiparallel, i.e., one strand runs in 5′ to 3′ direction and the other in opposite directions. The terminal phosphate groups are at opposite ends of the double helix. Each strand acts as a template for synthesis of opposite strand during replication. The double helix has also alternating major and minor grooves along its long axis. The width (diameter) of a double helix is 20Å (2 mm). Each turn of the helix is 34Å (3.4 nm) with 10 pairs of nucleotides. Proteins interact with DNA molecules at these grooves.

Types

DNA may exist in different double helix forms: A, B, C, D, E and Z. B form of DNA double helix described above is the most predominant form under physiological conditions. It is right handed double helix.

Formation

It is formed from already existing DNA through replication in the nucleus.

$$DNA \xrightarrow{Replication} DNA$$

Properties

State

DNA is viscous in nature. It has the property of fiber.

Denaturation

Acid, alkali and heat can denature DNA. When hydrogen bonds between bases break, two strands of DNA double helix can separate or unwind during this process. It occurs during DNA synthesis (replication), RNA synthesis (transcription) and genetic recombination. The temperature at which DNA is half denatured is melting temperature (Tm).

Renaturation

Separated strands of DNA can also be reunited. It is known as annealing.

Biomedical Importance/Functions

- *Genetic carrier*: A chromosome is a long DNA molecule. A segment of DNA is gene. It carries genetic information.
- *Inheritance*: It provides the information inherited by daughter cells and offsprings.
- *Synthesis of DNA*: New DNA is formed from existing DNA.

$$(DNA \xrightarrow{Replication} DNA)$$

- *Synthesis of RNA and protein*: It is the source of genetic information for synthesis of:

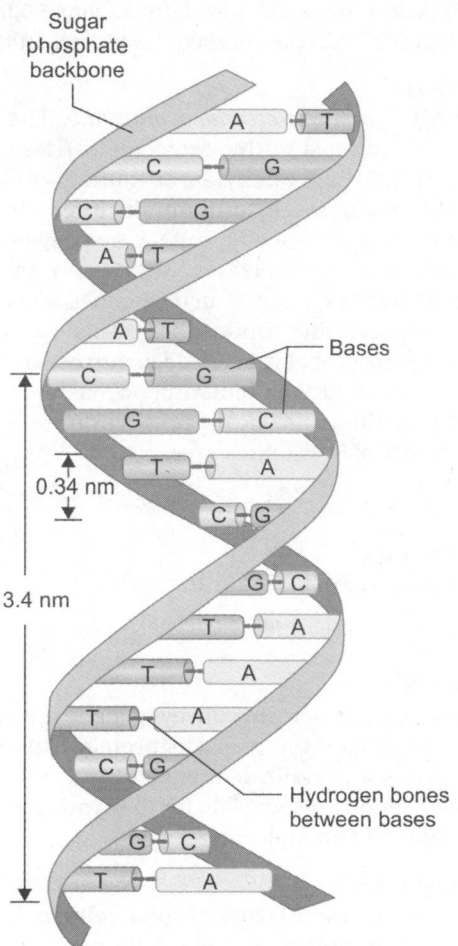

Fig. 5.9: DNA double helix.
(For color version, see Plate 1)

- All types of RNA:

  (DNA $\xrightarrow{\text{Transcription}}$ RNA)

- Proteins:

  (RNA $\xrightarrow{\text{Translation}}$ Protein)

Organization of DNA in the Cell

- *Prokaryotes (Bacteria):* No distinct nucleus is present DNA is loosely packed.
- *Eukaryotes:* DNA is present in association with basic proteins namely histones to form nucleosomes (*refer* Chapter 26).

Ribonucleic Acid

Location

RNA is found mainly in the cytoplasm.

Structure

It is a polynucleotide containing four types of ribonucleotides. It contains 60–6,000 ribonucleotides.

Ribonucleotides	Base	Sugar	Acid
Adenylate	Adenine	Ribose	Phosphoric acid
Guanylate	Guanine	Ribose	Phosphoric acid
Cytidylate	Cytosine	Ribose	Phosphoric acid
Uridylate	Uracil	Ribose	Phosphoric acid

Ribonucleotides are linked together by 3′, 5′ phosphodiester bonds to form RNA.

RNA molecule usually exists as a single stranded molecule. Hence its guanine content does not necessarily equal its cytosine content and its adenine content does not necessarily equal to its uracil content.

Bases present in RNA are:
- Adenine, guanine (Purine bases)
- Cytosine, uracil (Pyrimidine bases)

The sugar moiety in RNA is: D-ribose. Each ribonucleotide contains a phosphate group.

Formation

It is formed from DNA in the nucleus by transcription.

DNA $\xrightarrow{\text{Transcription}}$ RNA

Biomedical Importance/Functions

- RNA is involved in protein synthesis by translation after receiving genetic information from DNA

RNA $\xrightarrow{\text{Translation}}$ Protein

- Some RNAs act as catalysts (ribozymes).
- Some RNAs are genetic material of viruses.

Types of RNA

There are three major types of RNA. They differ from each other by size, structure, stability and functions.
1. Messenger RNA (mRNA)
2. Transfer RNA (tRNA)
3. Ribosomal RNA (rRNA)

> **Note**
> All RNAs are formed from DNA in the nucleus. They are single stranded.

Messenger RNA

mRNA accounts for 5–10% of total cellular RNA. It has low molecular weight 30,000–50,000. mRNA of *E.coli* contains 900–1,540 nucleotides.

Structure

mRNA is a single stranded molecule: The 3′-OH end of most mRNA molecule carries poly A tail (20–250 adenylate ribonucleotides) which is supposed to maintain intercellular stability of the specific mRNA by preventing attack of 3′-exonucleases. The 5′-OH end of mRNA carries a cap structure consisting of 7 methylguanosine triphosphate. This cap mini structure is probably involved in the recognition of mRNA by protein biosynthetic machinery. It also helps in stabilizing the mRNA by preventing the attack of 5′-exonucleases.

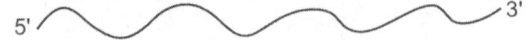

Formation

It is formed from DNA by transcription:

DNA $\xrightarrow{\text{Transcription}}$ mRNA

Function

It acts as a messenger, conveys genetic message from nucleus to cytoplasm for protein synthesis. It carries a specific sequence of nucleotides, called codons responsible for the synthesis of a specific protein molecule.

Transfer RNA

It accounts for 10–20% of total cellular RNA. It has low molecular weight about 25,000. It is the smallest form of RNA. It contains about 75 nucleotides.

Structure (Fig. 5.10)

tRNA is also a single stranded molecule. It undergoes folding to form a *clover leaf structure*. These folds are stabilized by hydrogen bonds between complementary bases in different positions of the same strand. These structures are called as arms. Each arm contains a base paired stem.

All tRNA molecules contain four main arms:
1. *Acceptor arm:* It consists of paired sequence of Cytosine-Cytosine-Adenine. Amino acid is attached to acceptor arm.
2. *Anticodon arm:* It has paired and nonbonded loop carrying sequence of three bases forming anticodon.
3. *D arm:* It contains dihydrouridine.
4. *TΨC arm:* It contains thymine, pseudo-uridine and cytosine.
  Long tRNAs have also fifth (extra/variable) arm.

Formation
They are formed from DNA by transcription:

$$DNA \xrightarrow{Transcription} tRNA$$

Functions
- They transfer amino acid from amino acid pool to the site of protein synthesis, i.e., ribosomes.
- They serve as adapters for the translation of the information present in the sequence of nucleotides of mRNA into specific amino acids.

Ribosomal RNA
It forms 80% of total cellular RNA. It has high molecular weight of 4.2×10^6.

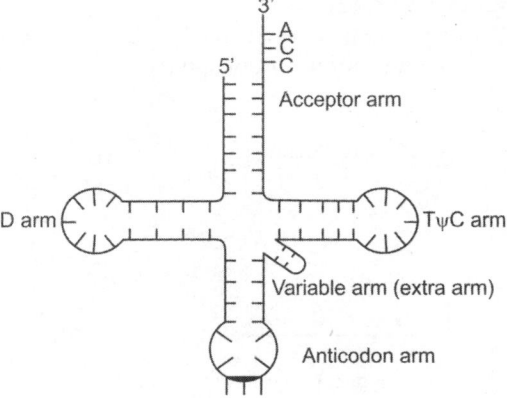

Fig. 5.10: Structure of tRNA.

Location
It is present in ribosomes.

Structure
There are different types of rRNAs, and are single stranded. Mammalian 5s, 18s, and 28s, rRNAs are made up of 120, 1900 and 4750 nucleotides respectively.

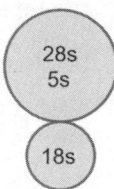

Formation
rRNAs are also formed from DNA by transcription in the nucleus.

$$DNA \xrightarrow{Transcription} rRNA$$

Functions
- Maintains structural integrity of ribosomes
- Binds mRNA with ribosomes for protein synthesis (translation)

Different between DNA and RNA is shown in **Table 5.3**.

BIOLOGICALLY IMPORTANT NUCLEOTIDES

Some nucleotides are not present in DNA or RNA but they are biologically important.

General functions:
- Energy metabolism
- Protein synthesis
- Coenzymes of B complex vitamins
- Control of enzyme activity
- Synthesis of glycogen
- Lipid biosynthesis
- Second messengers

They are of two types:
1. Naturally occurring nucleotides
2. Synthetic nucleotides

Naturally Occurring Nucleotides

Free nucleotides are also present in the cells. They serve several physiological functions in the body:

They are subdivided into:
- Purine nucleotides
- Pyrimidine nucleotides
- Miscellaneous nucleotides

Table 5.3: Differences between DNA and RNA.

Features	DNA	RNA
• Location	Mainly in nucleus	Mostly in cytoplasm
• Structure	Double stranded helix	Single stranded
• Components: ▪ Sugar ▪ Base	Deoxyribose Thymine present Uracil absent	Ribose Thymine absent Uracil present
• Base pairing	Adenine to thymine Guanine to cytosine	No such base pairing
• Stability	It is alkali stable	It is alkali labile
• No. of nucleotides	It consists of a large number of nucleotides	It consists of fewer nucleotides
• Genetic material	It is the genetic material of all organisms	It is the genetic material of some viruses only

Purine Nucleotides

(Purine + Sugar + Phosphate)

Examples

Adenine nucleotides
Adenosine monophosphate (AMP)
Composition: Adenine + Ribose + Phosphate

Importance
- It is a low energy compound.
- It acts as an activator of several enzymes in the body.
- It acts as inhibitor of certain enzymes, such as fructose 1, 6 diphosphatase in glycolysis.

Adenosine diphosphate (ADP)
Composition: Adenine + Ribose + Phosphate + Phosphate.

Importance
- It is a low-energy compound.
- It is primary phosphate acceptor in oxidative phosphorylation.
- It has control on cellular respiration, muscular contraction.
- It is an activator of enzyme glutamate dehydrogenase.

Adenosine triphosphate (ATP)
Composition: Adenine + Ribose + Phosphate + Phosphate + Phosphate

Formation: It is formed in electron transport chain through oxidative phosphorylation in mitochondria and also by substrate level phosphorylation during oxidation in metabolic pathway (e.g., Glycolysis, TCA cycle).

Importance:
- It is a high-energy compound. It is known as energy currency of the cell.
- It is an important source of energy for muscle contraction, transmission of nerve impulse, transport of nutrients across cell membrane, spermatozoa, etc.
- It is required for the synthesis of various important compounds in the body, e.g., glucose, fatty acids, phosphocreatine, S adenosyl methionine, etc.
- It denotes phosphate for a variety of phosphotranferase reactions.

Cyclic AMP (cAMP) or 3′, 5′ adenosine monosphosphate (Fig. 5.11)
Composition: It is a cyclic nucleotide.
Adenine + Ribose + Phosphate

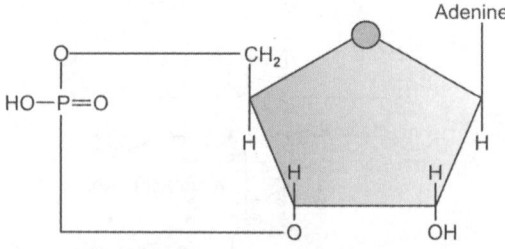

Fig. 5.11: Structure of cAMP.

Synthesis: It is formed from ATP by the enzyme adenylate cyclase.

$$ATP \xrightarrow{E} cAMP$$

Degradation: It is destroyed in tissues by conversion to AMP by the enzyme cAMP phosphodiesterase.

$$cAMP \xrightarrow{E} AMP$$

Importance
- It acts as a second messenger for hormone action, e.g., glucagon, ADH, etc.
- It plays an important role in:
  - Glycogenolysis
  - Lipolysis
  - Steroid synthesis
- It modulates transcription and translation in protein biosynthesis.
- It regulates permeability of cell membranes.
- Measurement of cAMP levels in blood is useful in the diagnosis of liver disease, thyroid disorder, etc.
- Plays an importance role in cell differentiation.

Guanine nucleotides
Composition
Guanine + Sugar + Phosphate (s)
- *Guanosine monophosphate (GMP)*
- *Guanosine diphosphate (GDP)*: It is a low-energy compound.
- *Guanosine triphosphate (GTP)*:
  - It is a high-energy compound.
  - Required for synthesis of proteins.
  - Involved in oxidation of succinyl CoA in citric acid cycle.
- *Cyclic GMP*: It is formed from GTP by the enzyme guanylate cyclase. It is involved in phosphorylation of protein hormones. It acts as second messenger for hormone action, e.g., atrial natriuretic factor.

Pyrimidine Nucleotides
(Pyrimidine + Sugar + Phosphate)

Uridine nucleotides
Composition
Uracil + Sugar + Phosphate

Uridine monophosphate (UMP): It is formed in the biosynthetic pathway of pyrimidine nucleotide. UDP glucose is involved in glycogen synthesis and formation of lactose in mammary gland. UDP glucuronic acid is used for detoxification of toxic compounds such as bilirubin.

Cytidine nucleotides
Composition
Cytosine + Sugar + Phosphate
- *CTP:* It is required for the synthesis of phosphoglycerides.
- *CDP choline:* It is involved in biosynthesis of phospholipids.

Thymine nucleotide
Composition: Thymine + Sugar + Phosphate

Miscellaneous Nucleotides
- *Coenzyme nucleotides:* B-complex vitamins act as coenzymes, e.g.,
  - Nicotinamide adenine dinucleotide (NAD)
  - Nicotinamide adenine dinucleotide phosphate (NADP)
  - Flavin mononucleotide (FMN)
  - Flavin adenine dinucleotide (FAD)
  - *Coenzyme A* (adenosyl nucleotide)
- *Component of S-adenosyl methionine (SAM)*: It is involved in one carbon metabolism (*refer* methionine metabolism).

Synthetic Nucleotides
Definition
Nucleotides can be prepared synthetically by altering heterocyclic ring or sugar moiety in nucleotides.

Mechanism of Action
- Inhibits specific enzymes essential for nucleic acid synthesis
- Affects base pairing in DNA

Examples
Synthetic nucleosides/nucleotides/nucleobases
- *Cytarabine:* Used in the chemotherapy of cancer
- *5-Iododeoxyuridine:* Used to treat hepatic keratitis
- *Allopurinol:* Used in the treatment of gout.
- *Azathioprine:* Used during organ transplantation.

■ NUCLEOPROTEINS

Location

These are essential constituents of nuclei of animal and plant cells. They are also found in the cytoplasm particularly associated with ribosomes.

Composition

They are conjugated proteins:

Nucleoprotein = Nucleic acid + Protein

Protein present in nucleic acid is a basic protein like histone or protamine. In cells, nucleic acids are present as nucleoproteins. They are ribonucleoproteins and deoxy-ribonucleoproteins according to sugar unit present. Bacteriophages and viruses are nucleoproteins containing either DNA and RNA.

Functions

They may be considered as the sites for the synthesis of proteins and enzymes.

■ ADDITIONAL INFORMATION

- γRNA may function as ribozymes (*refer* Chapter 7)
- Minor type RNAs: hnRNAs, snRNAs
- Unusual nuclear bases—dihydrouridine, pseudouridine.

6 Chemistry of Hemoglobin

Chapter Outline

- Definition
- Biomedical Importance/Functions
- Composition
- Porphyrin
- Normal Human Hemoglobins
- Spectroscopic Analysis of Hemoglobin and its Derivatives
- Hemoglobinopathies
- Technique for Identification (Separation) of Hemoglobins
- Estimation of Hemoglobin in Blood
- Test for Hemoglobin in Abnormal Urine

Other Hemoproteins
- Myoglobin

■ DEFINITION

Hemoglobin (Hb) is an important hemoprotein (conjugated protein). It is present in red blood cells and is responsible for red coloration of blood.

■ BIOMEDICAL IMPORTANCE/FUNCTIONS

Transport of Gases

- It transports oxygen from lungs to the capillaries of peripheral tissues.
- It transports carbon dioxide from capillaries of peripheral tissues to lungs for subsequent excretion.

Blood Buffer

It is an important blood buffer and helps to maintain pH of blood (acid base balance).

Pigments

Various pigments of bile, blood, stool, urine, etc. are derived from it, e.g., bilirubin.

Clinical Importance

- Study of hemoglobin chemistry explains the molecular basis of genetic diseases such as hemoglobinopathies.
- Poisoning by cyanide and carbon monoxide is fatal because they disturb the physiological functions of hemoglobin.

■ COMPOSITION

Hemoglobin is a macromolecule. It has four levels of structure of a protein (tetramer). It is a conjugated protein. It consists of protein globin and nonprotein heme.

Hemoglobin = Heme + Globin
(cojugated protein) (nonprotein) (protein)

Heme

It is the prosthetic group (nonprotein part) of hemoglobin. It is the colored component of hemoglobin.

Composition

Heme is a porphyrin containing iron in ferrous (reduced) state (Fe^{++}), i.e., iron porphyrin is called as heme.

Heme = Porphyrin + Iron

■ PORPHYRIN

Porphyrin is a heterocyclic compound. It is derived from prophin which is formed by linkage of four pyrrole rings through methyne (= CH –) bridges **(Fig. 6.1)**.

Pyrrole → Porphin → Porphyrin

[Porphobilinogen is substituted pyrrole ring. Porphyrinogens are similar to porphyrins but pyrrole rings are linked through methylene bridges ($-CH_2$)].

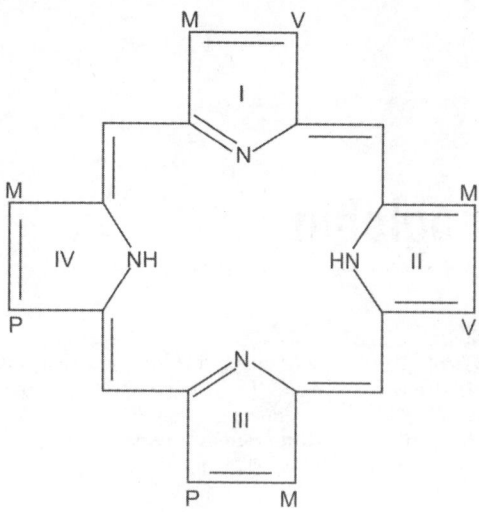

Fig. 6.1: Structure of porphyrin.

Structure (Fig. 6.1)

Porphyrins in nature are compounds in which various side chains are substituted for 8 hydrogen atoms in the porphyrin ring. According to Hans Fischer, simplified structural formula for porphyrin is represented as follows:

The side chains may be:

–CH$_2$COOH	(Acetate group)	–	Represented as A
–CH$_2$CH$_2$COOH	(Propionate group)	–	Represented as P
–CH$_3$	(Methyl group)	–	Represented as M
–CH = CH$_2$	(Vinyl group)	–	Represented as V
–CH$_2$CH$_2$	(Ethyl group)	–	Represented as E

Depending on the type of arrangements of substituents, two main types of porphyrins occur in nature.
1. Type I porphyrin
2. Type III porphyrin

Among these, type III porphyrin is abundant in nature.

Porphyrin present in heme is *type III porphyrin*, i.e., protoporphyrin III (it is also called as type IX porphyrin or protoporphyrin IX).

Occurrence

Porphyrins are found in urine, feces, bile, blood and bone marrow.

Properties

Physical properties

- *Solubility:* They are readily soluble in organic solvents.
- *Fluorescence:* Solutions of porphyrins in organic solvents or mineral acids emit red fluorescence under ultraviolet light. This property is used in the detection of porphyrins in urine.
- *Absorption spectrum:* Porphyrins are colored compounds. Porphyrins exhibit characteristic absorption spectrum, (e.g., Soret band) in visible and ultraviolet regions. This property is used in spectroscopic analysis of hemoglobin and its derivatives in blood.

Chemical properties

- *Amphoteric nature:* Porphyrins behave as weak bases, due to presence of two tertiary nitrogen atoms in the molecule. Porphyrins also behave as acids if they have carboxyl groups in the side chain. Thus natural porphyrins are amphoteric compounds.
- *Formation of metal complex:* Nitrogen atoms of pyrrole nucleus will form complexes with certain metals, such as iron, copper, zinc or magnesium. Metal will occupy in the central position of porphyrin ring. This metal complex is called as metalloporphyrin, e.g., heme is metalloporphyrin because iron is attached to porphyrin.

Iron

Iron present in heme is ferrous (reduced) form (Fe^{++}). It is attached to porphyrin through nitrogen atoms of the pyrrole rings by coordinate linkages.

Iron + Porphyrin → Iron porphyrin (heme)

Iron porphyrin is a metalloporphyrin. It is the prosthetic group of hemoglobin **(Fig. 6.2)**.

Globin

The protein part of hemoglobin is globin. Globin is an example of simple protein (histone group).

Functions

- It helps iron to remain at ferrous state.
- It helps to combine loosely and reversely.

Structure

It consists of four parallel layers of closely packed polypeptide chains, arranged in the

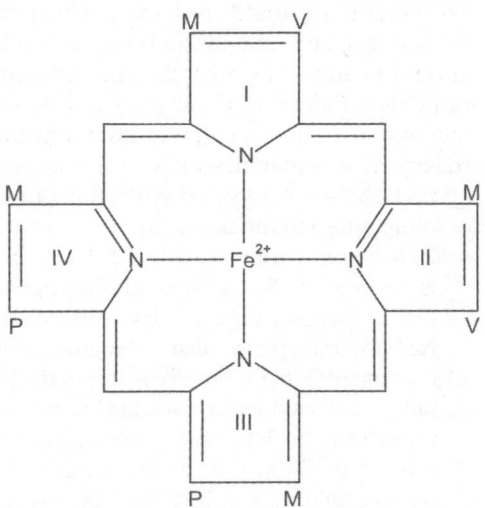

Fig. 6.2: Structure of heme.

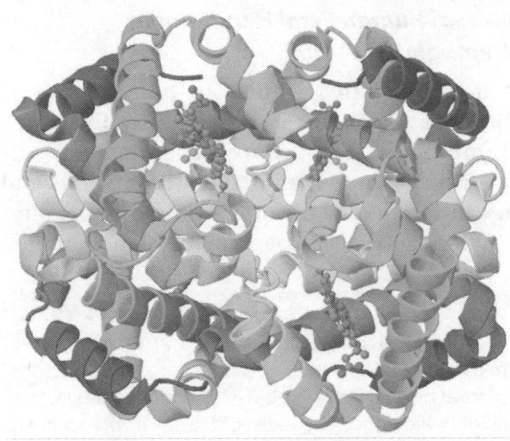

Fig. 6.3: Hemoglobin structure.
(For color version, see Plate 1)

configuration of a tetrahedron. The four polypeptide chains form 2 pairs of chains. One pair of chains possessing valine - leucine - serine as N terminal residue and lysine - tyrosine - arginine as C-terminal residue are called as α-chains. Each chain has identical amino acid composition of 141 amino acids. The other pair is designated as β-chains. Each of the β-chains has 146 amino acids and differs in N-terminal amino acids and C-terminal amino acids.

Name of the chain	N-terminal	C-terminal
α-chain	Valine - Leucine - Serine	Lysine - Tyrosine - Arginine
β-chain	Valine - Histidine - Leucine	Lysine - Tyrosine - Histidine

Linkage of Globin to Heme (Fig. 6.3)

As already stated, globin has four polypeptide chains. One heme molecule is attached to each polypeptide chain of globin molecule through linkage of Fe^{++} in heme and imidazole nitrogen of histidine in globin. Thus each globin molecule containing four polypeptide chains possesses four heme molecules to form hemoglobin.

Heme + Globin = Hemoglobin

$HbA \longrightarrow$ 4 Heme
$ \longrightarrow$ 1 Globin $\begin{cases} 2\alpha \\ 2\beta \end{cases}$

NORMAL HUMAN HEMOGLOBINS

Red blood cells (RBCs) contain same or different types of normal hemoglobin. The differences in various hemoglobins lie in globin (protein) part only. Heme part is same in any hemoglobin. The different globins differ in the amino acid composition of polypeptide chains in other than α chains, i.e, α-chains are identical in all hemoglobins, but β-chains will differ.

Normal human adult blood contains:
❑ Hemoglobin A (A_1): 98% (major form)
❑ Hemoglobin A_2: 2% (minor form)

Major Form

Normal Human Adult Hemoglobin: Hemoglobin A or A_1/HbA or HbA_1

Hemoglobin A contains 2α chains and 2β chains. It is represented as $\alpha_2\beta_2$. Each α chain has 141 amino acids and each β chain has 146 amino acids. Hence total number of amino acids present in hemoglobin A:

α. 2 × 141 = 282
β. 2 × 146 = 292
Total 574

Minor Forms

Normal Human Adult Hemoglobin: Hemoglobin A_2

Hemoglobin A_2 contains two α-chains similar to hemoglobin A. But it has two –δ chains in place of two β chains. It is represented as $\alpha_2\delta_2$.

Normal Human Fetal Hemoglobin (Hemoglobin F)/HbF

It has 2α chains similar to hemoglobin A. But it has 2γ chains in place of two β-chains. Hemoglobin F is represented as $\alpha_2\gamma_2$. It contributes more than half in human fetus and newborn child. It disappears six months after birth and its place is taken up by hemoglobin A.

Glycosylated Hemoglobin (HbA_{1C})

Glycosylated hemoglobin (HbA_{1C}) is glucose + hemoglobin. In normal adult, it is present up to 5% of total normal hemoglobin. In diabetic patients, this level is elevated. The level of HbA_{1C} in blood is an index of diabetic control (*refer* Chapter 11).

Properties

Physical Properties

- *State:* It is a crystalline compound. Its shape resembles a spheroid.
- *Molecular weight:* Its molecular weight is 65,000 approx.
- *Color:* It is red colored.
- *Isoelectric point:* Its isoelectric point is 6.8.
- *Absorption band:* It can exhibit characteristic absorption bands.

Chemical Properties

- *Transport of oxygen (formation of oxyhemoglobin)* **(Fig. 6.4)***:* The relationship between pO_2 and the binding capacity of hemoglobin with oxygen may be expressed graphically as oxygen dissociation curve of hemoglobin.

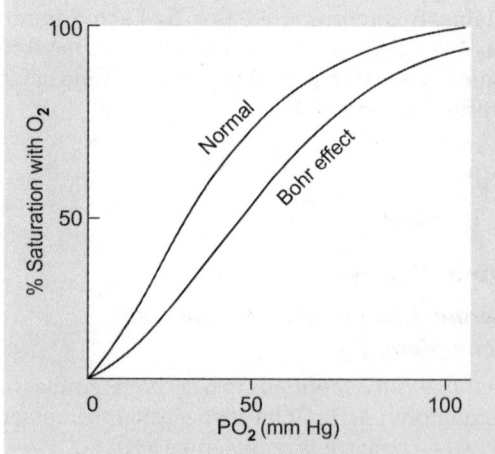

Fig. 6.4: Oxygen dissociation curves of hemoglobin.

The latter is sigmoidal in shape. It illustrates oxygen uptake and release. It is affected by several factors. CO_2 *and pH:* The influence of pCO_2 (High pCO_2) and pH (high H^+) to facilitate uptake of oxygen in the lungs and release of oxygen in tissues is known as *Bohr effect*. It shifts the oxygen dissociation curves of hemoglobin to the right.

- *2, 3-bisphosphoglycerate (2,3-BPG):* It is formed in RBCs through Rapoport-Luebering cycle (glycolysis) in carbohydrate metabolism. It regulates the binding of O_2 to hemoglobin. It specifically binds to deoxyhemoglobin and decreases O_2 affinity to Hb, which facilitates the release of O_2 at partial pressure in the tissues. Thus 2,3 BPG shifts oxygen dissociation curve to the right.

$$HbO_2 + 2,3\ BPG \rightarrow Hb\text{-}2,3\ BPG + O_2$$

Clinical Importance

2,3 BPG has a lot of biomedical significance:
- *In hypoxia:* It is elevated in chronic hypoxia (high attitude, obstructive pulmonary emphysema) associated with difficulty in O_2 supply.
- *In anemia:* It is increased in severe anemia in order to maintain the oxygen demands of the body.

- *Transport of carbon dioxide (formation of carbaminohemoglobin):* Hemoglobin can combine with carbon dioxide through free amino group present in globin to form carbaminohemoglobin. It is a reversible process. About 10% of carbon dioxide is carried towards lungs by hemoglobin through this route.

$$HbNH_2 + CO_2 \rightleftharpoons HbNHCOOH$$

- *As buffer:* As hemoglobin is a protein, it can act as a buffer. Thus reduced hemoglobin and oxyhemoglobin is a buffer $\left(\dfrac{Hb}{HHb}\right)$. Hemoglobin exerts its buffer action through its ionizable imidazole ring of histidine.

- *Formation of carboxyhemoglobin:* Hemoglobin combines more readily with carbon monoxide to form carboxyhemoglobin, which is very poisonous in nature.

$$Hb + CO \rightarrow CO\text{-}Hb$$

We inhale carbon monoxide through coal gas, artificial illuminator lamps, tobacco smoking and automobile gases. It deprives blood of its ability to transport oxygen. The tissues may not receive oxygen and patient may die of anoxia. The condition is called as carboxyhemoglobinemia. Its symptoms are breathlessness and headache. Blood shows cherry red color when treated with NaOH. It shows two absorption bands. Patient should be treated by exposing him to high pressure of oxygen.

- *Formation of methemoglobin (met Hb):* When hemoglobin is treated with mild oxidizing agents (potassium ferricyanide or potassium chlorate), it is oxidized to methemoglobin. Methemoglobin is a stable inactive form of hemoglobin. So it cannot transport oxygen.

Methemoglobinemia

Hemoglobin → Methemoglobin
(Fe^{++})   (Fe^{+++})

Definition: In normal condition, only trace of methemoglobin exists. Increased amount of methemoglobin in blood is known as methemoglobinemia.

Causes: It is due to ingestion or exposure of nitrites (baby food, chlorates, potassium ferricyanide and free radicals). It is also present in hereditary methemoglobinemias and in individuals with abnormal hemoglobin Hb-M.

Symptoms: Cyanosis, dyspnea, loss of consciousness, and death.

Test: It shows characteristic absorption bands. It can be detected by Schumm's test.

Treatment: Vitamin C is used to reduce methemoglobin to hemoglobin in these patients.

- *Formation of cyanmethemoglobin:* Methemoglobin cannot combine with oxygen or carbon dioxide. But it can combine with several anions. During cyanide poisoning a small amount of hemoglobin is converted to methemoglobin by giving nitrite. Methemoglobin will combine with cyanide to form nontoxic cyanmethemoglobin.

Methemoglobin → Cyanmethemoglobin

- *Formation of sulfhemoglobin:* It is formed by action of H_2S on oxyhemoglobin. It is found in blood after administration of sulfonamide drugs or during constipation. The condition is *sulfhemoglobinemia.*

Hemoglobin $\xrightarrow{H_2S}$ Sulfhemoglobin

- *Action of acids:* When Hb (of blood) is treated with glacial acetic acid, acid hematin is formed.

Hemoglobin + Acid → Acid hematin

- *Action of alkalis:* Hb (of blood) is boiled with ammonia, cooled and a little alcohol is added, alkali hematin is formed.

Hemoglobin + Alkali → Alkali hematin

- *Formation of hemin:* When Hb (of blood) is heated gently with Nippe's fluid (KCl + KBr + KI in acetic acid), hemin is formed. It appears as characteristic brown crystals, when observed under microscope. These crystals can be prepared from aged samples of blood or blood stains in clothes. Hence, this test has medicolegal significance **(Fig. 6.5)**.

Hemoglobin $\xrightarrow{\text{Nippe's fluid}}$ Hemin

- *Formation of hematoporphyrin:* Centration H_2SO_4 converts hemoglobin to hematoporphyrin. It is found in the blood and urine in sulfonal poisoning.

Hemoglobin $\xrightarrow{\text{Concentration } H_2SO_4}$ Hematoporphyrin

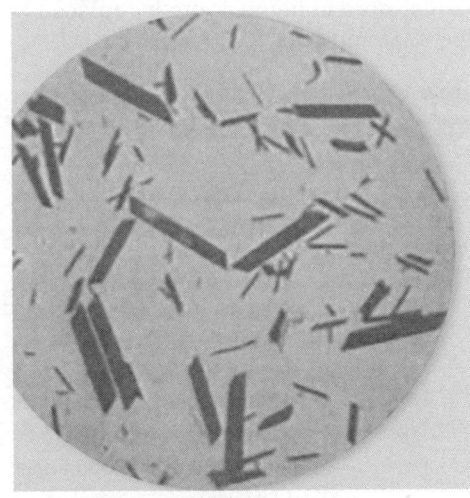

Fig. 6.5: Hemin crystals.
(For color version, see Plate 2)

SPECTROSCOPIC ANALYSIS OF HEMOGLOBIN AND ITS DERIVATIVES

Hemoglobin and its derivatives can absorb solar light. The absorbed portion of spectrum appears as dark bands when seen through spectroscope. These bands are called as absorption bands. Each derivative has its characteristic band (s). Hence this property is used to identify different Hb derivatives.

- *Oxyhemoglobin:* One narrow band, one wide band in green region of spectrum.
- *Reduced hemoglobin:* One broadband of spectrum in green region.
- *Carboxyhemoglobin:* Two bands in green region
- *Methemoglobin:* One band of spectrum in red region, two bands in green portion.

HEMOGLOBINOPATHIES

Definition

These are genetic disorders caused by:
- Production of structurally different abnormal hemoglobins, or
- Synthesis of insufficient quantities of normal hemoglobin (thalassemia).

Abnormal Hemoglobins (Table 6.1)

Abnormal hemoglobins differ in the globin part only and not in heme part. One amino acid of globin of normal hemoglobin is replaced by a different amino acid.

Sickle Cell Disease (Sickle Cell Anemia/Sickle Cell Hemoglobin Hbs)

It is a hereditary blood disorder in which erythrocytes (RBCs) assume an abnormal rigid, sickle shape (**Fig. 6.6**).

Cause

It occurs due to missense mutation in the β globin gene. It causes an abnormal hemoglobin namely Hbs, in erythrocytes.

It is the most common type of abnormal hemoglobin. It is also called as sickle cell hemoglobin (Hbs).

Changes

- Glutamic acid present at 6th position of both β chains of normal hemoglobin is replaced

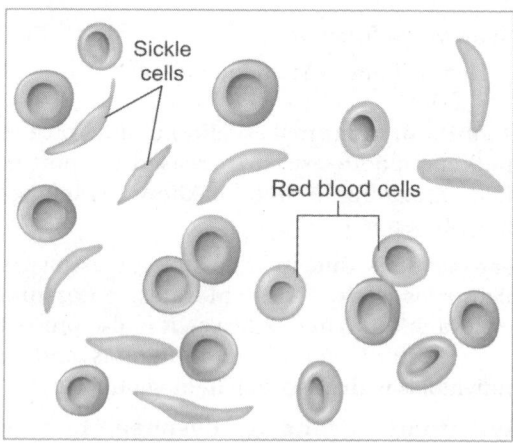

Fig. 6.6: Sickle cell disease.

Table 6.1: Examples of abnormal hemoglobins.

Sl. No.	Type of abnormal hemoglobin	Replacement of position of amino acid	Amino acid presenting normal hemoglobin at that position	Replaced by	Features
1.	Hb-S	6th position of β chain	Glutamic acid	Valine	Sickle cell anemia (**Fig. 6.6**)
2.	Hb-C	6th position of β chain	Glutamic acid	Lysine	Present in blood of Negroes. Leads to mild hemolytic anemia. It also produces sickling
3.	Hb-D (Punjab)	121st position of β chain	Glutamic acid	Glutamine	It does not produce sickling; common in Punjab population
4.	Hb-E	26th position of β chain	Glutamic acid	Lysine	Seen in South East Asia. RBC may have increased fragility.
5.	Hb-M (Boston)	58th position of α chain	Histidine	Tyrosine	Fe^{++} in hemoglobin is oxidized to Fe^{+++} thus producing methemoglobin

by valine (Glutamic acid → valine). It leads to polymerization of hemoglobin molecules inside RBCs.
- Amino acid substitution causes distortion of RBCs into sickle. The sickle cells may lead to infarction in organs, such as spleen.

Incidence
1 in 500 newborns.

Occurrence
Common in central and West Africa (mostly tropical areas)

Effects
- Hemolytic anemia
- More incidence to *Salmonella* infections
- More resistant to malaria
- Tissue damage and pain
- Premature death

Detection
- Sickling test
- Electrophoresis
- Finger—printing technique

Treatment
- Blood transfusion
- Antisickling agents such as urea and aspirin.

Thalassemias

Thalassemias are a group of genetic blood disorders due to defective synthesis of α or β chains of Hb **(Fig. 6.7)**.

Incidence
1 in 100.

Occurrence
More common in Mediterranean countries. Also prevalent in South East Asia.

Meaning
Thalassea (Greek—sea)

Cause
They occur due to defect in the synthesis of α or β globin chain of hemoglobin due to mutation.

Types
Two types depending upon whether the genetic defect lies in the synthesis of α or β globin chains of Hb.
1. α-thalassemias: These disorders occur due to decreased synthesis or total absence of α-globin chains of Hb.
   Symptoms:
   - Fatigue
   - Jaundice
   - Slow growth
   - Swollen abdomen
   - Irritability
   - Dark urine
2. β-thalassemias: These disorders occur due to decreased synthesis or total absence of β globin chains. There are two subtypes of β-thalassemias.
   - β-thalassemia minor: It is a heterozygous state with defect in only one of the two β globin chains. It is mostly asymptomatic and less serious.
   - β-thalassemia major: It is a homozygous state in which both genes responsible for β globin synthesis is defective.

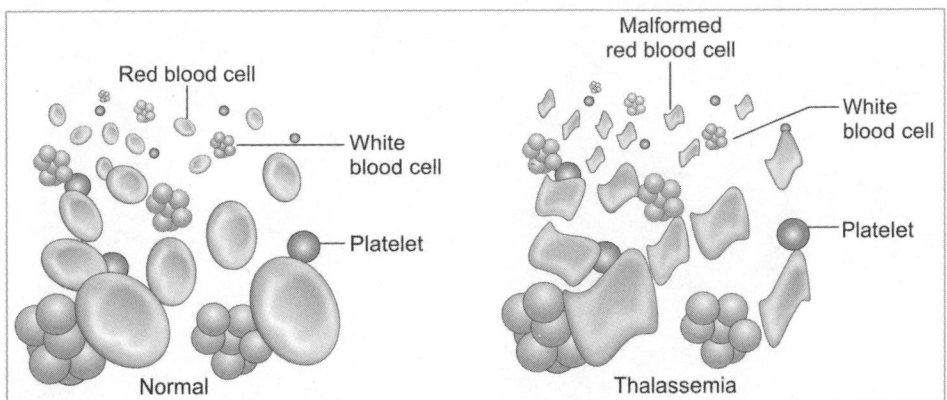

Fig. 6.7: Thalassemia.

It is associated with severe anemia of infancy described by Cooley, hence called as Cooley's anemia. In this condition, infants have mongoloid features and stunted growth and suffer from severe hemolytic anemia. It is more serious than minor type.

Diagnosis
Complete blood count (CBC), electrophoresis, gene analysis.

Treatment
Blood transfusion.

TECHNIQUE FOR IDENTIFICATION (SEPARATION) OF HEMOGLOBINS

Various hemoglobins can be identified by:
- Electrophoresis
- Finger printing

ESTIMATION OF HEMOGLOBIN IN BLOOD

- Sahli's method
- Colorimetric method

Normal Level of Hemoglobin in Blood
- *Men:* 13–17 g/100 mL blood
- *Women:* 12–15 g/100 mL blood

TEST FOR HEMOGLOBIN IN ABNORMAL URINE

It occurs in hematuria and hemoglobinuria. It can be detected by benzidine test.

OTHER HEMOPROTEINS

There are other hemoproteins in the body which have specific functions.

MYOGLOBIN

It is located primarily in capillaries of red muscles. It contains heme and globin with one polypeptide chain. It differs from blood hemoglobin in its absorption spectrum. Molecular weight is 17,000. It is mainly involved in the transport of oxygen within muscle. Rate of combination with gases also differs from Hb. It has little affinity for carbon dioxide. It can be detected in blood following myocardial infarction.

Cytochromes
They function as heme enzymes in electron transport chain present in mitochondria.

Catalases
They are also heme containing enzymes. They are found in blood, bone marrow, mucous membrane, liver and kidney. They destroy H_2O_2 formed in tissues.

Peroxidases
They are found in erythrocytes, leukocytes, and lens fibers. For example, glutathione peroxidase is an important enzyme of this group. It catalyzes destruction of H_2O_2.

7 Enzymes

Chapter Outline

- Definition
- Discovery
- Meaning
- Biomedical Importance/Functions
- Commercial Uses
- Composition
- Properties
- Substrate
- Naming Enzymes
- Classification of Enzymes
- Numbering Enzymes
- Enzyme Specificity
- Cofactors
- Mechanism of Enzyme Action
- Factors Affecting Activity of Enzymes or Velocity of Enzymatic Reaction (Enzyme Kinetics)
- Regulation of Enzyme Activity
- Expression of Enzyme Activity
- Application of Enzymes in Medicine
- Isoenzymes
- Additional Information

■ DEFINITION

Enzymes are biocatalysts produced by living organisms. They accelerate the rate of reactions occurring in the cells. They are proteins, except ribozymes.

■ DISCOVERY

Discovery and characterization of enzymes are based on the research work of several scientists like Berzelius, Pasteur, Buchner, Sumner, etc. The name "Enzyme" was first proposed by Kunhe in 1878.

■ MEANING

Enzyme means 'in yeast'.

■ BIOMEDICAL IMPORTANCE/ FUNCTIONS

- As biocatalysts, they regulate all physiological processes, thus maintaining homeostasis.
- Homeostasis will be disturbed in pathological states resulting in changes in the enzyme levels.
- All enzymes in biological systems are under genetic control. Enzyme deficiency will lead to inborn errors of metabolism (genetic disorders), e.g., phenylketonuria, albinism, etc.

Clinical Importance

- Measurement of some intracellular enzymes in blood provides physicians with diagnostic and prognostic information (clinically important enzymes/diagnostic enzymes), e.g., serum amylase, serum glutamate oxaloacetate transaminase (SGOT), serum glutamate pyruvate transaminase (SGPT), etc.
- They are used as therapeutic agents, e.g., streptokinase, pepsin, etc.

■ COMMERCIAL USES

They have wider applications in industries related to:
- Pharmaceuticals
- Biotechnology
- Textiles
- Agriculture and food
- Veterinary
- Laboratory reagents

■ COMPOSITION (FIG. 7.1)

Enzymes, except ribozymes, are proteins in nature. Many enzymes contain nonprotein called cofactors that are essential for the functions of the enzymes.

Base on composition, enzymes are of three types:

Section 2: Chemistry of Biomolecules

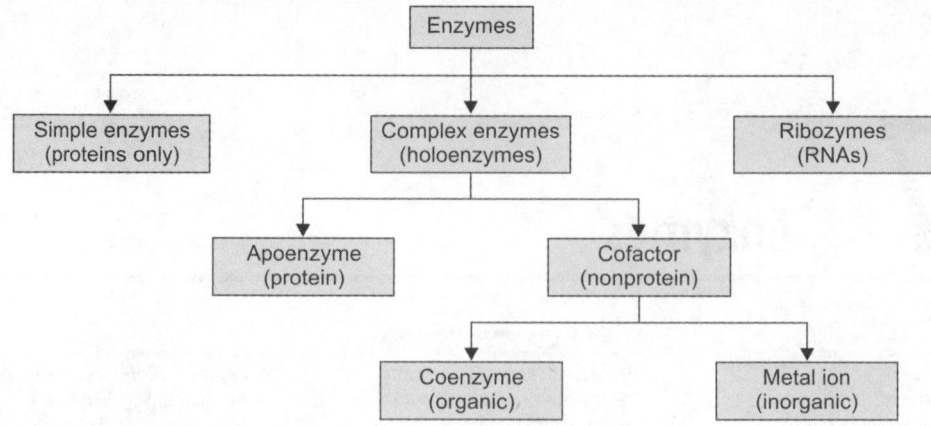

Fig. 7.1: Composition of enzymes.

1. Simple enzymes (proteins only)
2. Complex enzyme (holoenzyme)
   = Apoenzyme + Cofactor (coenzyme/metal ion)
      (protein)   (nonprotein)
3. Ribozymes (RNAs)

■ PROPERTIES

Enzymes resemble proteins in their properties:

Physical Properties

- Higher molecular weight compounds
- Soluble in water or salt solution
- Amphoteric colloidal electrolytes

Chemical Properties

- They are organic compounds.
- They have enormous catalytic activity.
- Enzymes accelerate the rate of reaction by lowering the energy of activation.
- Velocity (rate) of enzyme catalyzed reactions may be altered by substrate concentration, enzyme concentration, pH, temperature, physical and chemical agents.
- They are highly specific in reaction catalyzed.
- Some enzymes may exist in different forms (isoenzymes). They show different electrophoretic mobilities.

Important Definitions

- *Intracellular enzymes or endoenzymes:* These enzymes act in the cells which produce them, e.g., metabolic enzymes.
- *Extracellular enzymes or exoenzymes:* These enzymes are produced by some cells and are secreted into other parts of the body where they catalyze the reaction, e.g., digestive enzymes.
- *Zymase (active form of enzyme):* An extracellular enzyme which is secreted ready for action is called as zymase, e.g., amylase in saliva.
- *Zymogen (proenzyme):* An enzyme which is secreted in inactive form and ultimately activated by an agent (kinase) is a zymogen, e.g., trypsinogen (in pancreatic juice) is a zymogen. It is activated by enterokinase (in intestinal mucosa) to form trypsin.

$$\text{Zymogen (inactive)} \xrightarrow{\text{Kinase}} \text{Zymase (active)}$$

$$\text{Trypsinogen (zymogen)} \xrightarrow{\text{Enterokinase}} \text{Trypsin (zymase)}$$

■ SUBSTRATE

The substance on which an enzyme acts is called the substrate, e.g., maltose is the substrate for the enzyme maltase.

$$\text{Maltose (substrate)} \xrightarrow{\text{Maltase (enzyme)}} \text{Glucose (product)} + \text{Glucose (product)}$$

Location of enzymes in the cell is discussed in **Table 7.1**.

■ NAMING ENZYMES

- Enzymes are usually named by adding suffix - "ase" to the main part of the substrate on which they act, e.g., maltase is named after maltose.
- Some enzymes are named by their function, e.g., dipeptidase, decarboxylase, deaminase, dehydrogenase.
- Some enzymes are named according to their source, e.g., salivary amylase, pancreatic amylase.

Chapter 7: Enzymes

Table 7.1: Location of enzymes in the cell.	
Subcellular organelles	**Enzymes present for**
Cytosol	• Glycolysis • Glycogenolysis • Glycogenesis • Synthesis of fatty acids
Mitochondria	• Electron transport chain • Citric acid cycle, β-oxidation, urea cycle
Ribosomes	Protein synthesis
Lysosomes	Hydrolytic processes
Endoplasmic reticulum	Synthesis of various lipids, protein synthesis
Golgi apparatus (Golgi bodies)	Sorting of proteins, glycosylation reactions
Nucleus	Synthesis of DNA, RNA

■ CLASSIFICATION OF ENZYMES

According to International Union of Biochemistry (IUB) Nomenclature System in 1961, enzymes are classified into six major classes, based on the type of chemical reactions catalyzed and reaction mechanism. Each major class has many subclasses (**Fig. 7.2**).

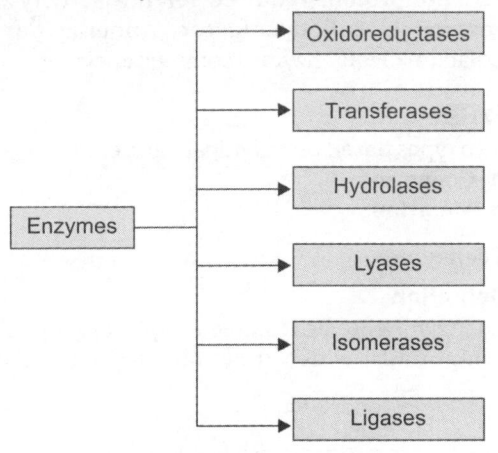

Fig. 7.2: Classification of enzymes.

Oxidoreductases

Catalyze oxidoreductions between two substrates involving transfer of hydrogen or electrons.
- *Dehydrogenases*, e.g., lactate dehydrogenase (LDH)

$$CH_3-CH(OH)-COOH \rightleftharpoons CH_3-CO-COOH$$
Lactic acid → Pyruvic acid

- *Oxidases*, e.g., cytochrome oxidases
- *Oxygenases*, e.g., typtophan oxygenase
- *Hydroperoxidases*, e.g., peroxidase, catalase

Transferases

Catalyze transfer of groups (other than hydrogen) between two substrates.
- Transaminases (aminotransferases) *(Transfer of amino group):* SGOT (AST), SGPT (ALT)—they require pyridoxal phosphate as coenzyme.

Aspartate + α ketoglutarate $\underset{}{\overset{SGOT}{\rightleftharpoons}}$ Oxaloacetate + Glutamate

Alanine + α ketoglutarate $\underset{}{\overset{SGPT}{\rightleftharpoons}}$ Pyruvate + Glutamate

- Methyltransferases
- Transphosphorylases
- Transaldolase
- Transketolase

Hydrolases

Catalyze hydrolysis of ester, ether, peptide, glycosyl groups with addition of water.
- Esterases, e.g., choline esterase

$$CH_3CO\text{-choline} + H_2O \rightarrow CH_3COOH + Choline$$
Acetylcholine   Acetic acid

- Peptidases
- Glycosidases
- Phosphatases
- Thiolases
- Ribonucleases
- Deaminases

Lyases

Catalyze removal of groups from substrates by mechanism other than hydrolysis.
- *Decarboxylases*

$$CH_3\text{-}CO\text{-}COOH \xrightarrow[\text{Decarboxylase}]{\text{Pyruvate}} CH_3\text{-}CHO + CO_2$$
Pyruvic acid   Acetaldehyde

- *Synthases*, e.g., glycogen synthase (they do not require ATP).

Isomerases

Catalyze isomerization (interconversion of optical or geometric isomers).
- Racemases

L-alanine $\xrightarrow[\text{racemase}]{\text{Alanine}}$ D-alanine

- Isomerases
- Epimerases
- Mutases

Ligases

Catalyze linking together of two compounds coupled with the breaking of a pyrophosphate bond of high energy phosphates (ATP, GTP, etc.).

- *Synthetases*, e.g., glutamine synthetase
  Glutamic acid + NH_3 → Glutamine
- *Carboxylases*

■ NUMBERING ENZYME

Each enzyme is given a systematic code number called Enzyme Commission (EC) Number. It is a four-digit number. Thus enzyme lactate dehydrogenase is EC 1.1.1.27.

Where,
- EC = Enzyme commission
- First digit 1 = Class (oxidoreductase)
- Second digit 1 = Subclass (CHOH is oxidized)
- Third digit 1 = Sub sub class (NAD^+ as cofactor)
- Fourth digit 27 = Serial number (specific enzyme), e.g., lactate dehydrogenase

■ ENZYME SPECIFICITY

Enzymes are specific in their action. Enzymes (organic catalysts) differ from inorganic catalysts in their extraordinary specificity. Different types of enzyme specificity have been recognized.

Substrate Specificity

Some enzymes are capable of acting on only one substrate, e.g., urease acts only on urea to produce ammonia and carbon dioxide.

$$NH_2-CO-NH_2 \xrightarrow[\text{Urease}]{\text{HOH}} 2NH_3 + CO_2$$

Group Specificity

Some enzymes act only on particular groups, e.g., Glycosidases act on glycoside linkages. Proteases act on peptide linkages.

Stereo Specificity

- *Optical specificity:* Some enzymes will react with only one of the two optical isomers, e.g., Most of the mammalian enzymes act on L-amino acids.
- *Geometrical specificity:* Some enzymes show specificity towards cis or trans isomer, e.g., fumarase acts on transisomer (fumaric acid) only and not on cis isomer (maleic acid).

■ COFACTORS (FIG. 7.3)

Definition

Any nonprotein required for the activity of enzyme is called cofactor. Apoenzyme + Cofactor = Holoenzyme (complex enzyme).

Type

Two types based on chemical nature:
- Coenzymes
- Metal ions

Coenzymes

Definition

Coenzymes are heat stable nonprotein organic compounds, which function as cofactors in

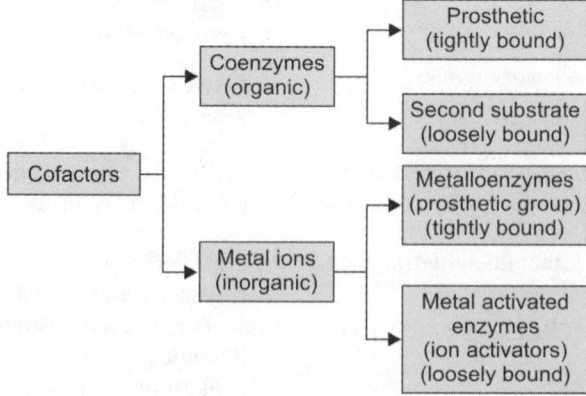

Fig. 7.3: Cofactors.

enzymatic catalysis. They are mostly vitamin derivatives and nucleotides.

Apoenzyme + Coenzyme → Holoenzyme
                (cofactor)

e.g., Protein + Thiamine → Transketolase
              Pyrophosphate

Functions
- Accept atoms or groups from a substance and transfer to other molecule
- Less specific
- Cannot function individually as enzymes
- May function as cosubstrates
- Required for oxidation reduction, group transfer, isomerization reactions, etc.

Types
Two types according to the group transferred:

Group transferring coenzymes
- *Thiamine pyrophosphate:* Decarboxylation
- *Pyridoxal phosphate:* Transamination
- *Biotin:* CO_2 fixation
- *Coenzyme A (CoA):* Acetylation
- *Folate coenzymes:* One carbon transfer
- *Cobamide coenzymes:* Carbon chain isomerism
- *Lipoic acid:* Oxidative decarboxylation
- *ATP and related compounds:* Donate phosphate.

Hydrogen transferring coenzymes
- NAD+
- NADP+
- FMN
- FAD
- Coenzyme Q

Metal Ions (Fig. 7.4)

Definition
Metal ions function as cofactors for some enzymes during catalysis.

Apoenzyme + Metal ion → Holoenzyme
                (cofactor)

For example,
Protein + Zinc → Carbonic anhydrase

Types
Two types depending on the affinity of a particular enzyme for its metal ion.
- Metalloenzymes, e.g., xanthine oxidase
- Metal activated enzymes, e.g., ATPase enolase.

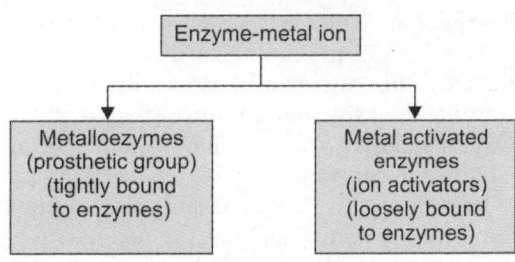

Fig. 7.4: Enzyme-metal ion.

Mode of action/function
Almost similar in both types
- Facilitates substrate binding and catalysis by forming bridge complexes of enzyme, metal and substrate
- Function as general acid-base catalysis
- Induce structural changes in enzyme or substrate molecules.

Ribozymes
These are a class of non-protein enzymes. They are RNA enzymes (also known as catalytic RNAs). They catalyze the specific reactions like protein enzymes. They are found in ribosomes. They were discovered in 1980 by Sidney Altman and Thomas Cech (N.P. 1989).

For example,
- Peptidyl transferase: It catalyzes the formation of peptide bond in protein synthesis (translation).
- Ribonuclease: It cleaves tRNA precursors to produce mature tRNA.

MECHANISM OF ENZYME ACTION (FIG. 7.5)
Catalysis is the primary function of enzymes. The energy needed by the reactants to undergo

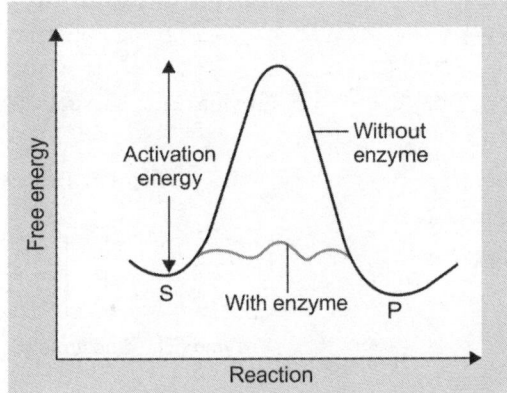

Fig. 7.5: Enzyme mechanism.

the reaction is known as activation energy. The enzyme in the biological system reduces the activation energy and causes the reaction to proceed at low temperature (below 40°C). Enzymes speed up the reaction without altering equilibrium constant.

During enzyme catalysis substrate(s) must combine with enzyme(E) at the active site to form enzyme substrate (ES) complex which finally results in production of product (P). This concept has been explained by the following theories.

$$E + S \rightarrow ES\ complex \rightarrow E + P$$

Active Site (Catalytic Site)

Substrate molecules are comparatively much smaller than enzyme molecules. There are some specific regions or sites on the enzymes for binding with the substrate. Such sites of attachment are called as active sites or catalytic sites. The active sites in the enzymes are like grooves and look like three-dimensional structure. They form a small part of the total portion of the enzyme. They are made up of different amino acids and serine is the predominant amino acid.

Allosteric Site

Some enzymes have also other sites to which substrates can bind. These sites are called as allosteric sites.

Theories of Mechanism of Enzyme Action

- *Emil Fischer's lock and key model:* According to this theory, substrate units with active site of an enzyme like a key fitting into a lock. Thus enzyme substrate complex (E-S complex) is formed. This complex is unstable and immediately decomposes to produce reaction products and free enzyme **(Fig. 7.6)**. This model is rigid (not flexible) and does not explain the effect of allosteric modulators.
- *Koshland's induced fit model:* This theory states that the substrate induces some configurational or geometrical changes in the active site of the enzyme molecule. Consequently, the enzyme molecule is made to fit completely with the substrate **(Fig. 7.7)**. This model explains the action of allosteric modulators and competitive inhibition of enzyme activity.
- *Substrate strain theory (recent theory):* The enzyme induces a strain to the substrate and leads to the formation of product.

FACTORS AFFECTING ACTIVITY OF ENZYMES OR VELOCITY OF ENZYMATIC REACTION (ENZYME KINETICS)

Various factors affect the activity of enzymes or the velocity of reactions.

1. Effect of substrate concentration
2. Effect of enzyme concentration
3. Effect of pH
4. Effect of temperature
5. Oxidation
6. Physical agents
7. Enzyme activators
8. Enzyme inhibitors

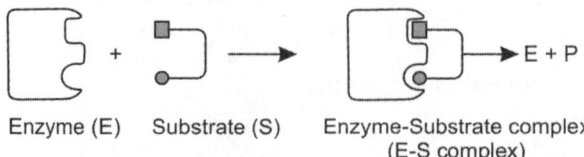

Fig. 7.6: Fisher's lock and key model.

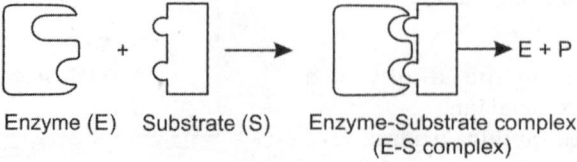

Fig. 7.7: Koshland's induced fit model.

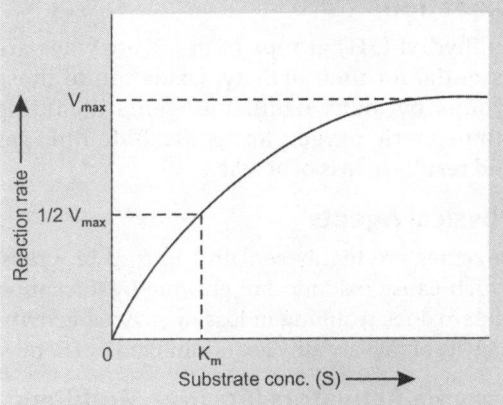

Fig. 7.8: Effect of substrate concentration on enzyme activity.

Effect of Substrate Concentration

According to Michaelis and Menten hypothesis, the enzyme forms a weakly bonded complex with the substrate. This unstable complex decomposes to yield free enzyme and reaction products (**Fig. 7.8**).

$$E + S \rightarrow ES \rightarrow E + P$$

The velocity of an enzymatic reaction increases first in a linear fashion, as the concentration of the substrate increases but later on the curve flattens and remains constant because enzyme is saturated with the substrate.

The effect of substrate concentration on velocity of reaction is graphically represented as Michaelis curve. It has rectangular hyperbola. The velocity of the reaction at high substrate concentration is called as maximum velocity (V). The substrate concentration mol/L that produces half-maximum velocity (V/2) is called as Michaelis constant or K_m.

The kinetic equation can be expressed mathematically by Michaelis Menten equation.

$$V/2 = \frac{V(S)}{Km + (S)}$$

Use of K_m

- It is a measure of affinity of an enzyme for its substrate.
- High K_m indicates weak binding. Low K_m indicates strong binding.
- It indicates a number of active sites filled.
- It gives an idea of type of inhibition of an enzyme by the inhibitor.

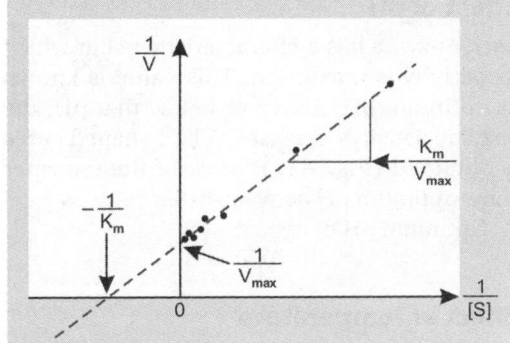

Fig. 7.9: Lineweaver–Burk plot.

Lineweaver–Burk Plot (Double Reciprocal Plot) (Fig. 7.9)

It is graphical representation of effect of substrate concentration on enzyme activity described by Lineweaver and Burk in 1934. It is widely used to determine accurately V_{max} and K_m in enzyme kinetics. By taking the reciprocals of the equation straight-line graph is obtained. It is useful to understand the effect of various enzyme inhibitors.

$$\frac{1}{V_a} = \frac{K_m}{V_{max}} \frac{1}{[s]} + \frac{1}{V_{max}}$$

Effect of Enzyme Concentration

The rate of an enzyme catalyzed reaction is directly proportional to the concentration of enzyme. The greater the concentration of enzyme, the faster will be the reaction (**Fig. 7.10**).

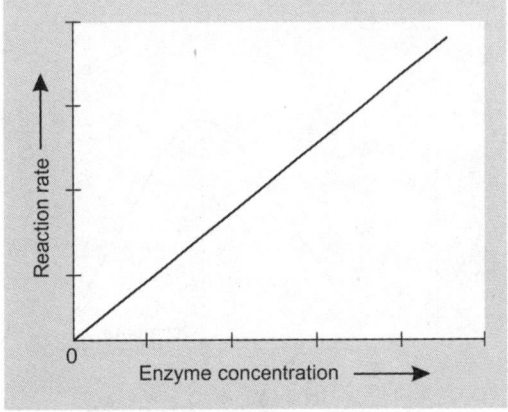

Fig. 7.10: Effect of enzyme concentration on enzyme activity.

Effect of pH

Each enzyme has a characteristic pH at which its activity is maximum. This value is known as optimum pH. Above or below that pH, the enzyme activity decreases. A bell-shaped curve is obtained **(Fig. 7.11)**. Most of the enzymes show optimum pH between 6–8.

Optimum pH of trypsin = 8
ACP = 5

Effect of Temperature

Enzyme catalyzed reactions have an optimum temperature at which the reaction is most rapid. Above this temperature, reaction rate decreases due to denaturation of enzyme protein. Below this temperature, enzyme reaction is slow (At 0°C most enzymes are inactive). The curve is bell shaped **(Fig. 7.12)**. Most of the enzymes show maximum activity between 37–40°C.

Oxidation

Sulfhydryl (SH) groups of many enzymes are essential for their activity. Oxidation of these groups by many oxidizing agents including atmospheric oxygen forms disulfide linkages and results in loss of activity.

Physical Agents

Enzymes are highly sensitive to α, β or γ rays, which cause oxidation of enzyme by formation of peroxides resulting in loss of enzyme activity. Activity of salivary amylase is inhibited by UV rays.

Enzyme Activators (Positive Modifiers)

Those molecules which increase enzyme activity are called activators, e.g., metal ion, kinases, etc. (*refer* page 85).

Enzyme Inhibitors (Negative Modifiers)

Definition

Compounds which convert the enzymes into inactive substances, thus affecting enzyme catalyzed reactions are called as *enzyme inhibitors*. The phenomenon is *enzyme inhibition*.

Types

It can be classified into two types, depending on whether the reaction is reversible or irreversible **(Fig. 7.13)**.

- *Reversible inhibition:* Inhibitor can dissociate from target enzyme because it is loosely bound with it. It is of three types:
  - *Competitive inhibition:* Certain inhibitors are structurally similar to substrates. These compete with the substrate for the enzyme. These so called competitive inhibitors occupy the available active site of the enzyme, thus decreasing the rate of formation of E-S complex. Thus they inhibit enzyme reaction **(Fig. 7.14)**.

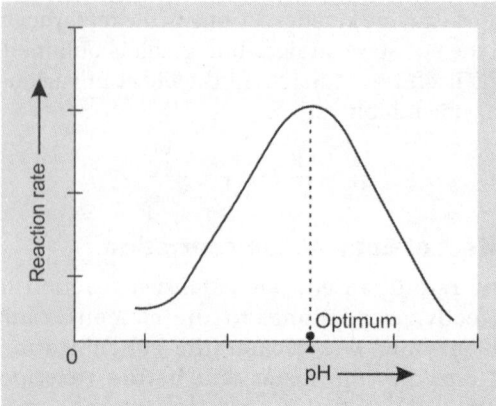

Fig. 7.11: Effect of pH on enzyme activity.

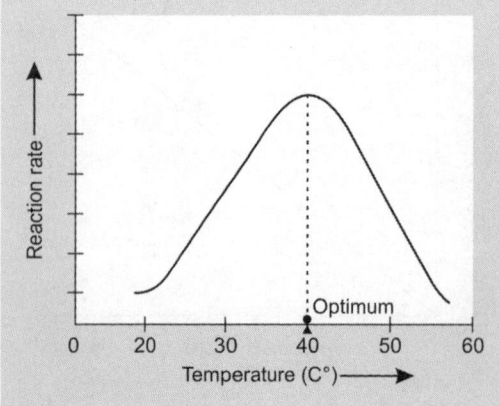

Fig. 7.12: Effect of temperature on enzyme activity.

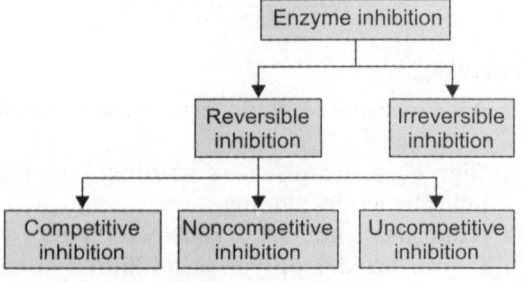

Fig. 7.13: Enzyme inhibition.

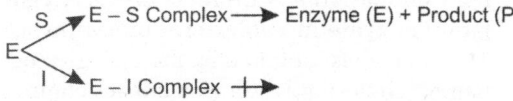

Fig. 7.14: Competitive inhibition.

For example:

1. Succinic acid $\xrightarrow{\text{Succinate dehydrogenase}}$ Fumaric acid
(malonic acid is competitive inhibitor)

2. Xanthine $\xrightarrow{\text{Xanthine oxidase}}$ Uric acid
(allopurinol is competitive inhibitor)

3. p-aminobenzoic acid $\xrightarrow{\text{Enzyme in bacteria}}$ Folic acid
(sulfonamide is competitive inhibitor)

4. Vitamin K $\xrightarrow[\text{Discoumarol}]{\text{Vitamin K epoxide}}$ glutamate

5. HMG-CoA $\xrightarrow{\text{HMG-CoA reductase}}$ Cholesterol
(lovastatin is competitive inhibitor)

Note
Pharmacological action of several drugs can be explained by the principle of competitive inhibitors.

- *Noncompetitive inhibition:* No structural resemblance between substrate and inhibitor. They do not compete for active sites. These inhibitors react with functional groups, (e.g., SH) of the enzyme and make them inactive.
  For example, $ESH + Hg^{++} \rightarrow E\text{-}S\text{-}Hg^{++} + H^+$
- *Uncompetitive inhibition:* It occurs when the inhibitor binds after the substrate has bound to the enzyme and then stops the reaction occurring, i.e., it combines with ES complex, e.g., inhibition of placental alkaline phosphatase (Regan isoenzyme) by phenylalanine.
- *Irreversible inhibition:* Inhibitor binds at the active site of the enzyme through covalent modification. It involves chemical modification of the enzyme molecule.
  For example:
  - E + p-chloromercuribenzoate → E-mercuri-benzoate
  - Organophosphorus insecticides
  - Di-isopropyl fluorophosphate (DFP)- Nerve gas

Importance of Enzyme Inhibitors
❏ Used to study the mechanism of enzyme action.
❏ Used to follow the course of reaction in metabolic pathways.
❏ Some enzyme inhibitors function as drugs:
  - Sulfonamide—acts as an antimetabolite
  - Allopurinol—used to treat gout
  - Monoamine oxidase inhibitors—used to treat depression
❏ Statin drugs—to treat hypercholesterolemia

REGULATION OF ENZYME ACTIVITY

Regulation of enzyme activity contributes in a major way in preserving homeostasis of the body. To achieve this, biochemical reactions (metabolic processes) are regulated in the following ways in response to the physiological needs.

❏ *Compartmentation of metabolic pathways:* The enzymes of anabolism (synthesis) and catabolism (breakdown) are operative in different cellular organelles to achieve maximum economy, e.g., enzymes of fatty acid synthesis are found in cytosol. Enzymes of fatty acid oxidation are found in mitochondria.
❏ *Activation of latent enzyme:* Certain enzymes exist in the active (zymase) and inactive (zymogen) forms which are interconvertible depending on the needs of the body, e.g., glycogen phosphorylase.
❏ *Enzyme degradation:* Some enzymes are most rapidly degraded if not needed; they are synthesized when they are required.
❏ *Stimulation/inhibition by control proteins:* Some enzymes are regulated by control proteins, e.g., calmodulin.
❏ *Control of enzyme synthesis:*
  - *Adaptive enzymes:* Syntheses of these enzymes are controlled by genes. Their concentration decreases (repression) or increases (induction) as per the body needs.
  - *Constitutional enzymes:* These enzymes are not controlled and remain constant.

Section 2: Chemistry of Biomolecules

☐ *Allosteric regulation (allosteric enzymes):* Oligomeric enzymes (having two or more subunits) have two different sites.
- Active site (substrate binding site)
- Allosteric site (regulatory site)

Enzymes having allosteric site in addition to active site are known as *allosteric enzymes*. Both are located at different sites (peptide units) in the enzyme molecule. Allosteric enzymes frequently catalyze the committed step present in the beginning of the pathway (*see* below). These enzymes are known as regulatory enzymes or rate limiting enzymes or key enzymes.

For example, hexokinase, phosphofructokinase. Certain substances referred to as allosteric modulators bind at the allosteric site and regulate the enzyme activity.

☐ *Feedback inhibition (end-product inhibition):* It is a specialized type of allosteric inhibition, necessary to control metabolic pathways for efficient cellular function. The process of initiating the first step by the final product in a series of enzyme catalyzed reactions of a metabolic pathway is known as feedback inhibition.

$$A \xrightarrow{E_1} B \xrightarrow{E_2} C \xrightarrow{E_3} D$$

For example, HMG CoA reductase is a regulatory enzyme in cholesterol biosynthesis. The enzyme is inhibited by the end-product namely cholesterol through feedback control.

■ EXPRESSION OF ENZYME ACTIVITY

Various expressions are used to denote enzyme activity in serum/plasma.

For example, IU/L, King Armstrong Units, Somogyi Units, etc.

It is preferable to express enzyme activity in serum/plasma as IU/L.

Definition [Enzyme Unit (IU/L)]

It is the quantity of enzyme which transforms one micromole of substrate per minute under the defined conditions.

Measurement of enzymes in serum/plasma-spectrophotometric methods.

■ APPLICATION OF ENZYMES IN MEDICINE

Diagnostic Significance of Enzymes (Clinically Important Enzymes)

Diagnosis and prognosis of several diseases can be arrived at by estimating the levels of specific enzymes in serum/plasma (**Table 7.2**).

Table 7.2: Clinically important enzymes.

Sl. No.	Name of enzyme	Normal level in plasma/serum	Increased in (diagnosis)
1.	Acid phosphatase	2–12 IU/L	Metastatic prostatic carcinoma
2.	Alkaline phosphatase	40–125 IU/L	Rickets, Paget disease, hyperparathyroidism, obstructive jaundice
3.	Amylase	25–85 IU/L	Acute pancreatitis
4.	Lipase	50–175 IU/L	Acute pancreatitis
5.	Creatine phosphokinase (CPK) or creatine kinase (CK)	10–50 IU/L	Muscular dystrophy, myocardial infarction, trauma
6.	Gamma glutamyl transferase (γGT)	10–50 IU/L (M) 7–30 IU/L (F)	Various liver diseases, alcoholism
7.	Lactate dehydrogenase (LDH)	90–200 IU/L	Myocardial infarction, hepatitis, carcinoma
8.	SGOT (AST)[Serum glutamate oxaloacetate transaminase]	5–45 IU/L	• Highly increased in myocardial infarction. • Slightly increased in liver diseases
9.	SGPT (ALT)[Serum glutamate pyruvate transaminase]	3–40 IU/L	Highly increased in liver diseases. Slightly increased in myocardial infarction
10.	Cholinesterase	5–10 IU/L	Increased in organophosphorus poisoning, nephrotic syndrome

(AST: aspartate transaminase; ALT: alanine transferase)

Therapeutic Uses

Some enzymes are used to treat diseases:
- *Penicillinase:* To treat allergy to antibiotic penicillin
- *Lysozyme:* Present in tears, used as an antibiotic in the treatment of eye infections
- *Asparaginase:* For treatment of some types of leukemia
- *Urokinase, streptokinase:* To dissolve blood clot
- *Pepsin, amylase and pancreatic enzymes:* To correct indigestion
- *Trypsin:* Used in cataract surgery.

ISOENZYMES

Some enzymes exist in different form and are called as isoenzymes.

Definition

Isoenzymes are the physically distinct forms of the same enzyme. They catalyze the same chemical reaction though at different rates.

Alternative Name

Isozymes.

Characteristics

Each isoenzyme shows different electrophoretic mobility during electrophoresis. They have different pH optima and K_m value. They have immunological differences. Each isoenzyme is made up of same or different peptide subunits.

Occurrence

Isoenzymes are present in serum and tissues of all living organisms.

Method of Separation

Polyacrylamide gel electrophoresis (PAGE).

Examples and Clinical Importance

Lactate Dehydrogenase (LDH)

It is a glycolytic enzyme involved in the conversion of lactic acid to pyruvic acid and vice versa using coenzyme NAD^+.

$$CH_3CHOHCOOH \underset{NADH+H^+}{\overset{NAD+}{\rightleftharpoons}} CH_3COCOOH$$
Lactic acid Pyruvic acid

LDH occurs as five different isoenzymes. Each isoenzyme is a tetramer, i.e., having same or two different subunits (H and M units).

Name	Subunits	Normal %
LDH_5	MMMM	5%
LDH_4	HMMM	10%
LDH_3	HHMM	20%
LDH_2	HHHM	35%
LDH_1	HHHH	30%

Estimation of LDH in serum will not reveal precisely whether the disease is that of heart (myocardial infarction) or liver (hepatitis). Study of isoenzymes of LDH are useful in the differential diagnosis of heart and liver diseases. LDH_1 and LDH_2 are increased in heart disease. But in liver diseases, LDH_4 and LDH_5 are increased.

Creatine Phosphokinase (CPK)/Creatine Kinase (CK)

This enzyme is involved in the formation of phosphocreatine from creatine and ATP.

$$Creatine + ATP \rightarrow Phosphocreatine$$

It has three isoenzymes:

Name	Location	Normal %	Diagnosis (increased in)
CPK1 (CPK-BB)	Brain	1%	Brain trauma
CPK2 (CPK-MB)	Heart muscle	5%	Myocardial infarction
CPK3 (CPK-MM)	Skeletal muscles	94%	Muscular dystrophy

Type of Enzymes Present in Blood

1. *Plasma specific enzymes (plasma functional enzymes):* These enzymes are normally present in the plasma and they have specific function to perform, e.g., lipoprotein lipase, coagulation factors.
2. *Plasma nonspecific enzymes (plasma nonfunctional enzymes):* These enzymes may be absent or present at low concentration in plasma. They enter into circulation due to increased cell turn over, cellular damage, diseases, etc. They are clinically important enzymes (diagnostic enzymes), e.g., LDH, CPK, etc., **(Table 7.2)**.

Analytical uses: Enzymes used as laboratory reagents:
- Glucose oxidase and peroxidase: To estimate glucose in blood.
- Urease: To estimate urea in blood.
- Cholesterol oxidase: To estimate cholesterol in blood.

■ ADDITIONAL INFORMATION

Enzyme Pattern in Diseases

Measurement of a single enzyme or a group of enzymes helps in the diagnosis of various diseases **(Table 7.3)**.

Enzymes in Myocardial Infarction

The following three enzymes are used for the diagnosis of myocardial infarction (MI):
- Creatine kinase (CK)/creatine phosphokinase (CPK)
- SGOT (AST)
- Lactate dehydrogenase (LDH)

These enzymes are elevated in myocardial infarction but the time of their increase and decrease differ **(Fig. 7.15)**.

CPK: It increases first within 3 hours after MI, reaches peak value within 24–30 hours and returns to normal within 2–4 days.

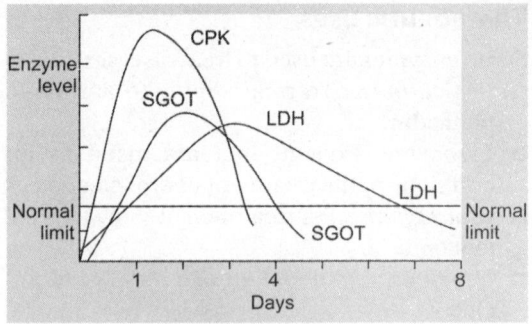

Fig. 7.15: Enzymes in MI.
(SGOT: Serum glutamic oxaloacetic transaminase; CPK: creatine phosphokinase; LDH: Lactate dehydrogenase)

SGOT (AST): It rises after CPK and reaches a peak within 48 hours after MI and returns to normal level within 4–5 days.

LDH: It rises from 8–16 hours, reaches peak on 3rd or 4th day returns to normal level within 9–12 days.

> **Note**
> Some nonenzymatic biomarkers are also used in clinical practice, e.g., troponins I, lipid profile, etc.

Table 7.3: Enzyme pattern in diseases.

Sl. No.	Enzyme (s)	Diagnosis
1.	Liver diseases: • SGPT (ALT) • SGOT (AST)	Both enzymes are increased in liver diseases. But SGPT is increased more than SGOT
	• LDH	Also increased in liver disease (LDH$_5$)
	• Alkaline phosphatase	Highly increased in obstructive jaundice
	• γ glutamyl transferase (γGT)	Highly increased in alcoholic liver disease
2.	Heart diseases (myocardial infarction):	**Fig. 7.14**
	• CPK (CK)	Highly increased in MI especially CPK-MB
	• SGOT (AST) • LDH (LDH$_2$)	Also highly increased in MI
3.	Muscle disease: CPK (CK)	Marked increase in muscle wasting disease (muscular dystrophy), especially CPK-MM
4.	Bone diseases: Alkaline phosphatase (ALP)	Highly increased in bone diseases, such as rickets, osteomalacia, Paget disease
5.	Pancreatic disease: • Amylase • Lipase	Both enzymes are increased in acute pancreatitis
6.	Cancer: Acid phosphatase (ACP)	Increased in prostate cancer

8 Vitamins

Chapter Outline

- Definition
- Alternative Name
- Discovery
- Biomedical Importance/ Functions
- Classification

Fat-Soluble Vitamins (Lipid-Soluble Vitamins)
- Vitamin A
- Vitamin D
- Vitamin E
- Vitamin K

Water-Soluble Vitamins
- B-Complex Vitamins
- Non B-Complex Vitamin
- Vitamin-like Compounds
- Antivitamins
- Vitamins-Table

■ DEFINITION

Vitamins are defined as organic compounds occurring in natural foods either as such or as precursors. They are required in small quantities in the diet for the vital functions of the body.

■ ALTERNATIVE NAME

Accessory food factors.

■ DISCOVERY

Normal nutrition and health cannot be maintained in humans by diets containing only carbohydrate, lipids, proteins, and minerals. This fact was recognized by demonstration of deficiency diseases due to absence or deficiency of some substances in the diet which are known as vitamins. Scientists who tried to find out the existence of these substances are Takaki (1880), Lunin (1881), Eijkman (1897), Hopkins (1912), McCollum (1915), etc. Funk (1913) named a factor in rice polishings as vitamins as it was found to be an amine and vital for life. Later it was known that only few vitamins were amines. Hence, the term vitamin was used.

■ BIOMEDICAL IMPORTANCE/ FUNCTIONS

- They are required for growth, maintenance and reproduction.
- Most of the vitamins cannot be synthesized by the body and hence must be supplied in the diet.
- They are necessary for several biochemical functions, (e.g., visual cycle, coenzymes in metabolic reactions).

Clinical Importance

- They are used as pharmacological/therapeutic agents (e.g., vitamin C, niacin).
- They may produce deficiency and/or toxicity symptoms, e.g., xerophthalmia, hypervitaminosis.

■ CLASSIFICATION (FIG. 8.1)

Vitamins are broadly divided into two groups depending on their solubility.
1. Fat-soluble vitamins
2. Water-soluble vitamins

FAT-SOLUBLE VITAMINS (LIPID- SOLUBLE VITAMINS)

This group consists of the following vitamins:
1. Vitamin A
2. Vitamin D
3. Vitamin E
4. Vitamin K

■ VITAMIN A

Alternative Names

- Antixerophthalmic factor
- Anti-nightblindness factor

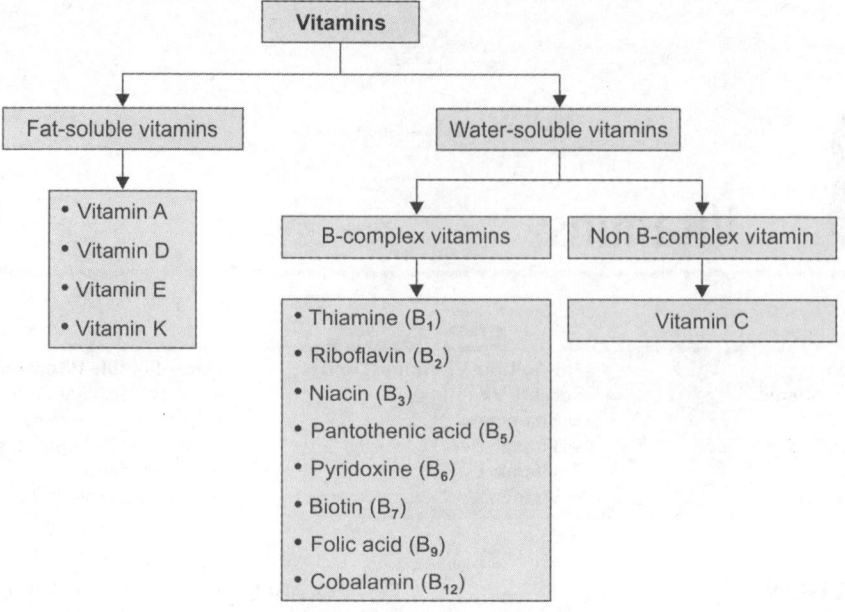

Fig. 8.1: Classification of vitamins.

Chemistry

Structure (Fig. 8.2)

Vitamin A refers to all compounds having the biological activity of vitamin A (vitamers).

Three important forms of vitamin A are:
1. *Retinol (vitamin A alcohol):*
   - It is usually called as vitamin A (or) vitamin A_1
   - Vitamin A_2 is 3 dehydroretinol
2. *Retinal (vitamin A aldehyde):* It is also known as retinene.
3. *Retinoic acid (vitamin A acid)*

All the three compounds contain the following common structural unit. They consist of a β ionone ring and an isoprenoid side chain. All these three forms are referred to as retinoids.

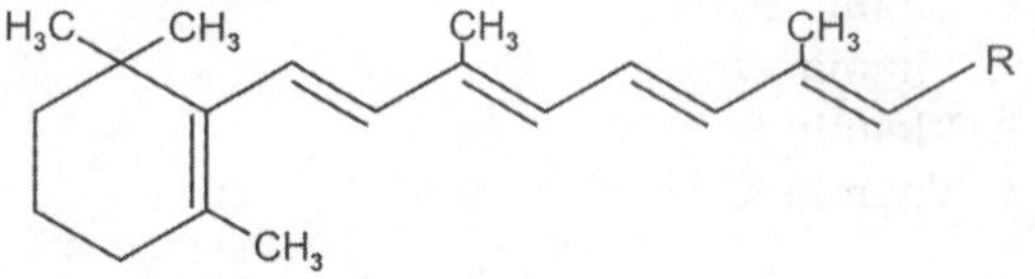

R = CH$_2$OH (retinol)
R = CHO (retinal)
R = COOH (retinoic acid)

Fig. 8.2: Structure of vitamin A.

Provitamins A

A number of plant pigments can be converted into vitamin A by animal tissues. These pigments are known as carotenes. They are precursors of vitamin A (provitamins A).

There are many types of carotenes, such as α-carotenes; β-carotenes; γ-carotenes, etc.

All these compounds are known as carotenoids. Of these, the yellow pigment β-carotene is the most important provitamin A. It contains two terminal β-ionine rings linked by a hydrocarbon chain.

Conversion of provitamin A into vitamin A:

β-carotene → Vitamin A
(one molecule) (two molecules)

Properties

- It is a crystalline substance.
- It is soluble in fat solvents but insoluble in water.
- It is not destroyed during cooking.

Sources

- *Animal (in the form of vitamin A):* Fish liver oil, milk, butter, cheese, egg yolk
- *Plant (in the form of provitamin A):* Carrots, tomatoes, and green leafy vegetables, mangoes, papayas.

Metabolism

Biosynthesis
Refer above.

Absorption
Dietary vitamin A is present as fatty acid ester form which is hydrolyzed by esterase in the intestinal lumen into free vitamin A and fatty acid. Free vitamin A is absorbed and undergoes re-esterification in the intestinal epithelial cells and finally absorbed into lymphatics.

Storage
About 95% of vitamin A is stored as its ester retinol palmitate in the liver. The rest is stored in other tissues, such as lactating breast, adrenals, lung, and intestine.

Transport
In man, liver is the major site for conversion of provitamin A to vitamin A and also for storage. From the liver, vitamin A is transported to various organs through blood in association with retinol binding protein (RBP).

Excretion
Under normal conditions, only very small amounts of vitamin A is excreted in the urine.

Functions

Biochemical
- *Wald's visual cycle (rhodopsin cycle):* It describes the role of vitamin A in visual process. It was proposed by George Wald (1966) **(Fig. 8.3)**.

  The retina of the eye contains two types of receptor cells: (1) Rods (2) Cones.
  1. *Rods:* The rods are concerned with vision at dim light (night vision).
     - The rods contain a photosensitive visual pigment called rhodopsin (conjugated protein). When light strikes retina, rhodopsin splits into opsin (protein) and all-trans-retinal. This reaction triggers a nerve impulse to be perceived by the brain.
     - The all-trans-retinal is immediately isomerized to 11-cis-retinal in the dark by retinal isomerase. 11-cis-retinal recombines with opsin to generate rhodopsin and complete the visual cycle.
     - But conversion of all trans-retinal to 11-cis-retinal is incomplete. Hence most of all trans retinal is transported through blood to the liver where it is converted to all trans retinol by alcohol dehydrogenase.

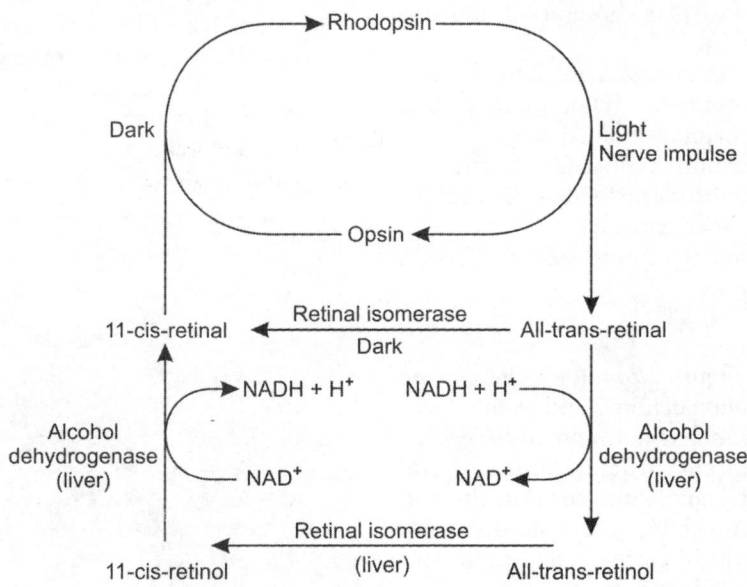

Fig. 8.3: Wald's visual cycle.

The all-trans-retinol is isomerized to 11-cis-retinol which is then transported to retina via blood after oxidized to 11-cis-retinal to take part in the visual cycle.

Dark adaptation time: When a person enters from an area of bright light to dim light rhodopsin stores are depleted impairing the vision. But within the few minutes (dark adaptation time) rhodopsin is resynthesized improving the vision.

2. *Cones:* These are responsible for vision at bright light. Cones contain 3-photosensitive pigments (conjugated proteins)
   - Cyanopsin
   - Iodopsin
   - Porphyropsin

   All three pigments are sensitive to blue, green, and red colors respectively. When light strikes the retina a particular pigment is bleached depending on the color of the light. It results in generation of nerve impulse and perception by the brain. Reduction in the number of cones will lead to color blindness.

- *Glycoprotein synthesis:* Retinoic acid has an important role in glycoprotein synthesis. Thus it is responsible for the development and maintenance of the ground substance in collagenous tissues.
- *Mucopolysaccharide synthesis:* Retinoic acid is involved in synthesis of chondroitin sulfate, a constituent of ground substance.
- *Antioxidants:* Both retinoids and carotinoids act as antioxidants which account for their anticancer activity.
- *Gene expression:* Retinol may be involved in protein synthesis.

Others

- *Bone and teeth formation:* It accelerates the normal formation of bones and teeth.
- *Epithelialization:* It is found to be essential for the normal structural integrity and behavior of the epithelium covering the skin and forming the lining of the nasal sinuses, mouth, pharynx, digestive tract, respiratory tract, and genitourinary tract.
- *Growth:* It has a role in growth especially in children.
- *Reproduction:* It is necessary for the normal development of testis and sperm maturation in male and pregnancy in female.
- *Immunity:* It is essential for combating infection due to its immune response.

Daily Requirements (RDA)

- *Adults:* 5,000 IU/day
- *Children:* 3,000 IU/day

Deficiency

Causes

- Low dietary intake
- Defective absorption

Symptoms

Changes in eyes

- *Nightblindness (nyctalopia):* Visual acuity is decreased. Dark adaptation time is increased. The affected persons have difficulty to see in dim light. It is one of the earliest symptoms of vitamin A deficiency.
- *Xerophthalmia:* Dryness of conjunctiva and cornea **(Fig. 8.4)**.
- *Bitot's spots:* White opaque spots appear in conjunctiva.
- *Keratomalacia:* Corneal epithelium becomes keratinized softened and ulcerated.

Changes in other parts of the body

- It may result in keratinization in which:
  - Skin becomes dry, scaly, and rough
  - Epithelium of respiratory tract shows increased susceptibility to infection
  - Reduced mucous secretion occurs in GI tract epithelium
  - Urolithiasis occurs in urinary tract.

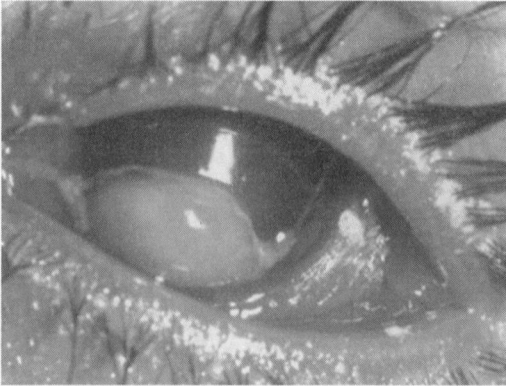

Fig. 8.4: Xerophthalmia.
(For color version, see Plate 2)

- Defective teeth and bone formation is seen due to lowered osteoblastic activity
- Therapeutic uses:
  - Antioxidant against cancer
  - Protect against xerophthalmia, night blindness
  - Role in vision

Toxicity (Hypervitaminosis A)

Excess of vitamin produces a series of toxic effects known as hypervitaminosis A. Its symptoms include: Headache, nausea, vomiting, and drowsiness, peeling of the skin, painful bones, anorexia, loss of weight.
Assay: Based on Carr-Price reaction.

■ VITAMIN D

Alternative Names

Antirachitic factor; Calciferols, sunshine vitamin.

Chemistry

Structure (Figs. 8.5A and B)

Vitamin D refers to a group of steroid compounds having vitamin D activity. They are also called as calciferols.

The most important vitamin D compounds are:
- Vitamin D_2 (ergocalciferol)
- Vitamin D_3 (cholecalciferol)

Both compounds are similar in structure, except that ergocalciferol has an additional methyl group and a double bond.

Provitamins D

Many precursors of vitamin D (provitamins D) are known, but only two of them are found in nature.
1. *Ergosterol:* It is the provitamin D_2. It is present in plants.
2. *7-dehydrocholesterol:* It is the provitamin D_3. It is found in animals and humans.

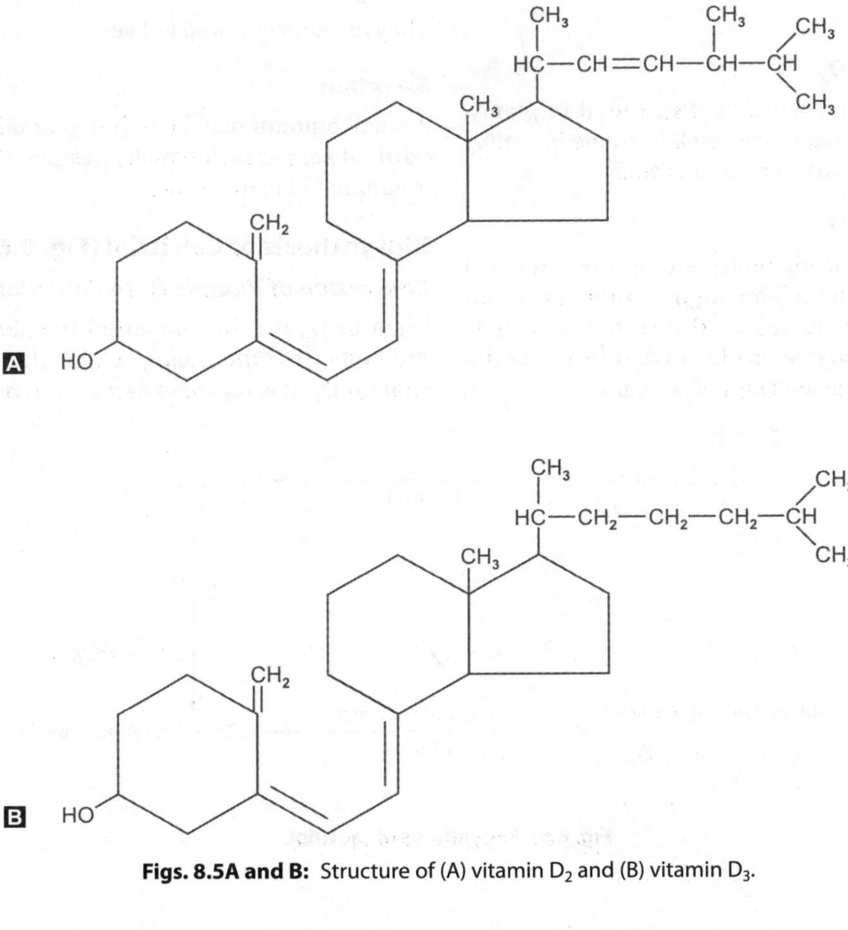

Figs. 8.5A and B: Structure of (A) vitamin D_2 and (B) vitamin D_3.

Conversion of provitamins D to vitamins D

Formation of vitamin D_2

Ergosterol (provitamin D_2) can be commercially converted to ergocalciferol (vitamin D_2) in plants.

$$\text{Ergosterol (provitamin } D_2) \xrightarrow[\text{(commercial)}]{\text{Photolysis}} \text{Ergocalciferol (vitamin } D_2)$$

Formation of vitamin D_3

7-dehydrocholesterol (provitamin D_3) is converted to cholecalciferol (vitamin D_3) in exposed skin of humans and animals due to sunlight.

$$\text{7-dehydrocholesterol (provitamin } D_3) \xrightarrow[\text{Photolysis}]{\text{Sunlight}} \text{Cholecalciferol (vitamin } D_3)$$

Properties

- It is a white crystalline substance.
- It is soluble in fat solvents.
- It is resistant to heat and oxidation.
- It is not affected by acids and alkalis.

Sources

Provitamin D_2

Provitamin D_2 is widely distributed in plants. Since it is not absorbed well from the intestine, it is of no dietary nutritional value.

Provitamin D_3

It is formed from cholesterol in the intestinal mucosa of men and higher animals. From intestine, it passes to the skin where it is converted (activated) into vitamin D_3 by the action of ultraviolet rays of sunlight.

Vitamin D_2

Plants (ergot, yeast)

Vitamin D_3

- *Rich:* Liver and viscera of fish
- *Good:* Egg yolk, butter
- *Poor:* Milk, plant foods
- *Cheaper source:* Sunlight (as activator)

Metabolism

Biosynthesis

Refer above.

Absorption

Provitamins D are poorly absorbed from small intestine. But vitamin D is readily absorbed from the small intestine and from the skin surface. Its absorption from the small intestine is enhanced by factors, such as bile salts.

Storage

They are largely stored in liver.

Excretion

A small amount may be excreted in bile, but is partly absorbed in the small intestine. None of it is eliminated in the urine.

Biosynthesis of Calcitriol (Fig. 8.6)

Conversion of Vitamin D_3 to Calcitriol

Vitamin D_3 can be converted to calcitriol in the body. It is the biologically active form of vitamin D_3. It is regarded as a steroid hormone.

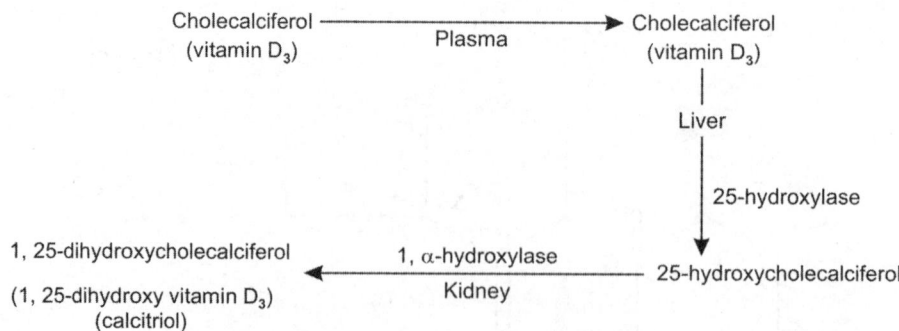

Fig. 8.6: Biosynthesis of calcitriol.

It is synthesized in kidney and acts on bone, intestine, kidney (target organs).

Site
Liver, kidney.

Steps
- Cholecalciferol (vitamin D_3) after absorption from the intestine circulates in the blood bound to a specific globulin and transported to the liver.
- In the liver, it is hydroxylated at 25th position to form 25-hydroxycholecalciferol by the enzyme 25-hydroxylase.
- A specific vitamin D binding protein carries 25-hydroxycholecalciferol to the kidneys, where it undergoes further hydroxylation at position 1 to form 1, 25-dihydroxycholecalciferol (calcitriol) by the enzyme 1-α-hydroxylase.

Functions
Vitamin D_3 (as calcitriol) is involved in the following functions:

Biochemical
- *Calcium and phosphate metabolism:* Vitamin D acts on target organs, such as bones, kidneys, intestinal mucosa to regulate calcium and phosphate metabolism in association with parathyroid hormone (PTH) and calcitonin.
  - Intestinal absorption of calcium and phosphate
    - Vitamin D directly stimulates the intestinal absorption of calcium and indirectly that of phosphate. It decreases pH in the lower intestinal tract which helps in increasing the absorption of calcium and phosphate.
  - It stimulates transcription of mRNA for the synthesis of a calcium binding protein by the intestinal epithelium. This protein, in turn, participates in transport of calcium across the intestinal mucosa.
  - *Mineralization of bone:* It is necessary for the normal development of bones. It stimulates the calcification of bones in both adults and growing children.
- It increases the citrate level of blood, bone, kidney and heart tissues and also its excretion in urine.
- It induces phytase which catalyzes hydrolysis of phytate in the intestine.

Others
It is involved in cell differentiation and immune function.

Therapeutic Uses
- Maintains healthy bones and teeth, protects against osteomalacia **(Fig. 8.7)** and rickets **(Fig. 8.8)**.
- Protection against DM type-I, cancer, multiple sclerosis.
- Reduces depression, heart disease, and anxiety.

Daily Requirements (RDA)
- *Adult:* 200 IU/day
- *Children:* 400 IU/day

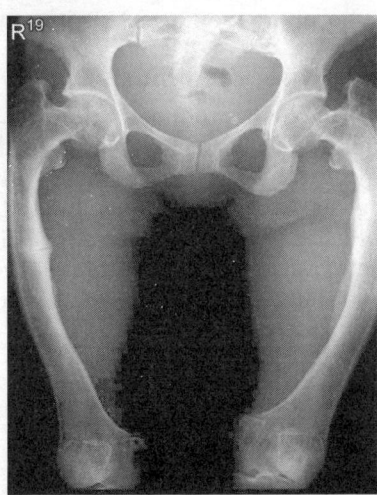

Fig. 8.7: Osteomalacia.

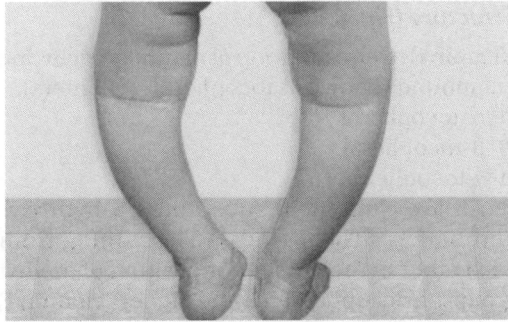

Fig. 8.8: Rickets.
(For color version, see Plate 2)

Deficiency

Causes
- Low intake of vitamin D
- Insufficient exposure to sunlight
- Defective absorption

Symptoms
- *Rickets:* It occurs in growing children. It is characterized by defective vascularization and mineralization of bones. Ends of long bones become bulky and soft. Bow legs, knock knees, rickety rosary, pigeon chest, occur. Plasma level of vitamin D is decreased and that of alkaline phosphatase is increased.
- *Osteomalacia:* It is seen in adults. It may occur in women who are not exposed to sunlight. Mineralization of osteoid to form bone is affected and thus bones become soft. It affects mostly pelvic bones. Delay in teeth formation may occur. Low serum calcium and phosphorus and high ALP present.

Toxicity (Hypervitaminosis D)

Vitamin D toxicity produces, anorexia, thirst, constipation, polyuria followed by: nausea, vomiting, and diarrhea; urinary lithiasis. Hypercalcemia and hyperphosphatemia may occur which may lead to metastatic calcification in kidneys, muscles, gastric mucosa, bronchi, etc. Renal failure leading to death may also occur.

■ VITAMIN E

Alternative Names
Tocopherol, antisterility factor.

Chemistry

Structure (Fig. 8.9)

Vitamin E refers to a group of naturally occurring compounds known as tocopherols (vitamers).
- α-tocopherol
- β-tocopherol
- γ-tocopherol, etc.

All are isoprenoid substituted 6-hydroxy-chromanes (Tocol rings). They differ from each other in the number or position of methyl groups. α-tocopherol has the highest vitamin E activity.

Properties
- It is a light yellow oil.
- It is insoluble in water but soluble in fat solvents.
- It is destroyed by alkali and also by food processing and cooking.
- Oxidation and UV light destroy vitamin E activity.

Sources
- *Plant:* Wheat germ oil, sunflower seed oil, safflower seed oil, corn, and soya bean oil.
- *Animal:* Meat, fish, liver, eggs.

Metabolism

Biosynthesis, Absorption, Storage and Excretion

It is not synthesized in the body. It is dissolved in the fat of the diet and absorbed in the small intestine. It is stored in adipose tissue. Under normal conditions, there is no significant excretion of tocopherol in urine or feces. However, milk contains small amount.

Functions

Biochemical

Antioxidant

Vitamin E acts as an antioxidant to prevent many undesirable peroxidations in the body through removal of free radicals (O_2^-, H_2O_2).
- It preserves the integrities of membrane bound organelles and thereby prevents muscular hepatic necrosis, and increased erythrocyte fragility.
- It prevents damage to lung tissues.
- It protects selenide at the active site of membrane selenoproteins.
- It increases the rate of oxidative phosphorylation.

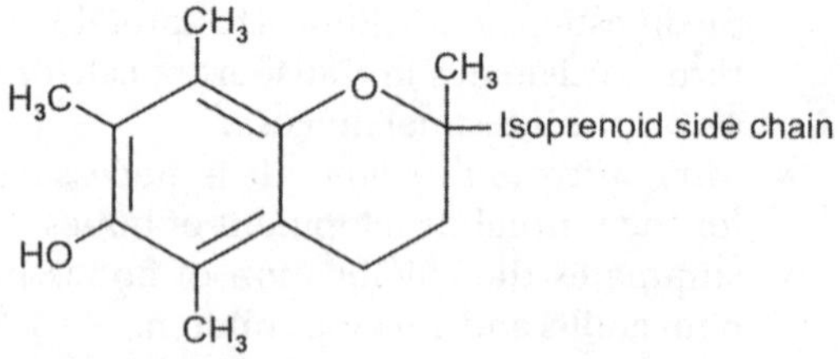

Fig. 8.9: Structure of vitamin E.

- It prevents oxidation of vitamin A and carotenes thereby reducing their wastage.
- It prevents ageing, cancer, etc.

Synthesis of Biologically Important Compounds

It may be involved in the synthesis of heme, coenzyme Q and nucleic acids.

Others

- It helps in maintaining seminiferous epithelium. It prevents sterility.
- It is used in the treatment of nocturnal muscle cramps, fibrocystic breast disease, atherosclerosis (therapeutic use).

Daily Requirements (RDA)

- *Adults:* 20–25 IU/day
- *Children:* 10–15 IU/day

Deficiency

In humans.

Symptoms

- Muscular dystrophy
- Anemia in newborn infants and pregnant and/lactating women
- Hepatic necrosis
- Neurological disorders

In rats
Permanent sterility
Toxicity: Not reported

■ VITAMIN K

Alternative Name

Antihemorrhagic factor.

Chemistry

Structures (Fig. 8.10)

Vitamin K exists in three forms which are naphthaquinone derivatives.

Vitamin K_1 (phylloquinone), vitamin K_2 (menaquinone), vitamin K_3 (menadione).

Properties

- Vitamin K_1 is yellowish oil, vitamin K_2 is yellowish crystalline solid. They are soluble in fat solvents, but insoluble in water. They are stable to heat but their activity is lost by strong acids and alkalis.
- But vitamin K_3 is soluble in water and can be given parenterally.

Sources

Vitamin K_1	Vitamin K_2	Vitamin K_3
Green leafy vegetables	Putrid fish meal	Synthetic
(Cauliflower, cabbage, tomatoes, etc.)	(Intestinal bacteria)	
Meat, egg yolk, dairy products		

Metabolism

Biosynthesis, Absorption, Storage, and Excretion

It is not synthesized in the body, but is adequately synthesized by the intestinal bacteria. It is readily absorbed from the small intestine in the presence of bile salts (vitamin K_3 is absorbed even in the absence of bile salts). It is not stored to any appreciable amount. It is not excreted in the urine or bile. Large amounts may be excreted in the feces. Women may excrete in milk.

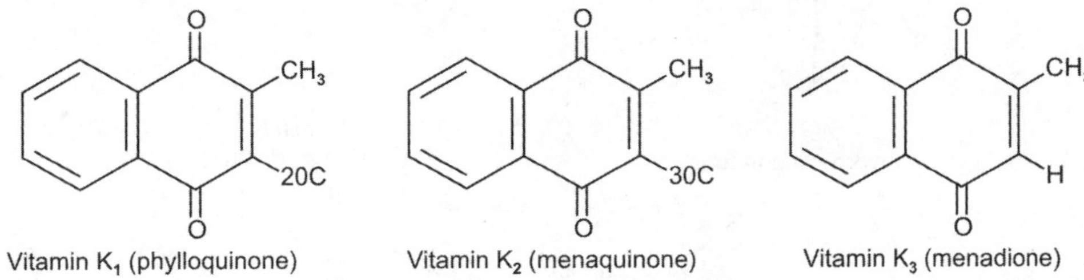

Vitamin K_1 (phylloquinone)   Vitamin K_2 (menaquinone)   Vitamin K_3 (menadione)

Fig. 8.10: Structures of vitamin K.

Functions

Biochemical

Blood coagulation/vitamin K-cycle (Fig. 8.11)
Vitamin K is necessary for blood coagulation. It brings about the post-translational modification of certain blood clotting factors (proteins). In the liver, the clotting factors namely factor II (prothrombin) VII, IX, and X are synthesized as inactive precursors. Vitamin K acts as a coenzyme for the enzyme carboxylase which catalyzes carboxylation of glutamic acid residues in the protein (clotting factors). γ-Carboxylation generates calcium binding sites essential for blood clotting. This process can be represented as a cycle called *vitamin K-cycle*. Dicumarol is an inhibitor of this cycle.

Calcium-binding proteins
It is required for carboxylation of specific glutamate residues of calcium binding proteins of bones.

Electron transport chain
It is involved in the respiratory chain mechanism and oxidative phosphorylation.

Others
It is used as an antidote to poisoning by dicumarol type drugs (therapeutic use).

Daily Requirements (RDA)
- *Adults:* 50–100 µg/day
- *Children:* 1 µg/kg body weight/day

Deficiency

Causes
- Fat malabsorption
- Sterilization of large intestines by antibiotics

Symptoms

Hemorrhagic disease
This occurs due to lowered prothrombin level and increased clotting time of blood and hence bleeding tendency. This may lead to mucous membrane bleeding, post-traumatic bleeding, and internal bleeding.
Toxicity: Hemolytic anemia, jaundice.

Antivitamins/Antagonists
Dicoumarol type drugs, e.g., warfarin.
Anticoagulants, e.g., heparin

WATER-SOLUBLE VITAMINS

Water-soluble vitamins are divided into two subgroups:
1. B-complex vitamins
    - Thiamine (B_1)
    - Riboflavin (B_2)
    - Niacin (B_3)
    - Pantothenic acid (B_5)
    - Pyridoxine (B_6)
    - Biotin (B_7)
    - Folic acid (B_9)
    - Cobalamin (B_{12})
2. Non B-complex vitamin
    - Vitamin C (ascorbic acid)

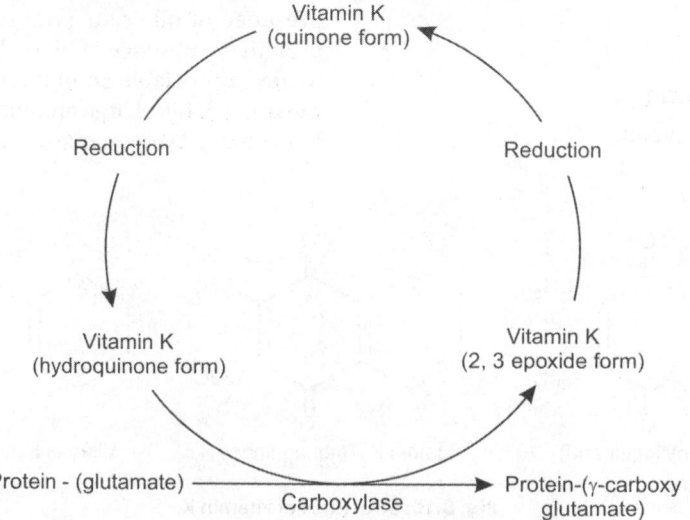

Fig. 8.11: Vitamin K-cycle.

B-COMPLEX VITAMINS

Thiamine (Vitamin B_1)

Alternative Names
Antiberiberi factor, antineuritic factor, aneurin.

Chemistry
Structure (Fig. 8.12)
It contains a pyrimidine ring and a thiazole ring linked by a methylene bridge. It is a sulfur containing vitamin.

Properties
- It is a white crystalline basic substance.
- It is readily soluble in water.
- It is destroyed at high temperature.
- It is oxidized to thiochrome which exhibits fluorescence.

Sources
- *Plant:* Rice polishings, peas, beans, whole cereal grains, nuts, etc.
- *Animal:* Ham/pork meats, liver, mutton, beef, eggs.

Metabolism
Biosynthesis, absorption, storage, and excretion
It is not synthesized by human beings. It is readily absorbed from the small intestine. Heart has the highest concentration of thiamine followed by brain, liver, kidney. About 10% is excreted in urine. It is also secreted in milk as thiamine protein complex.

Coenzyme
Thiamine pyrophosphate (TPP) is the coenzyme form of thiamine.
Thiamine – p – p
(Alternate name: Cocarboxylase)

Functions
Biochemical
Oxidative decarboxylation
- *Carbohydrate metabolism:* It acts as a coenzyme with pyruvate dehydrogenase complex which converts pyruvate to acetyl-CoA.

    Pyruvate → Acetyl-CoA
- It acts as a coenzyme with α-ketoglutarate dehydrogenase complex which converts α ketoglutarate to succinyl-CoA in the citric acid cycle.

    α-ketoglutarate → Succinyl-CoA
- *Protein metabolism:* It acts as a coenzyme for α-keto acid decarboxylase which catalyzes α-keto acids formed in the catabolism of branched chain amino acids (valine, leucine and isoleucine).

Transketolase reaction
Carbohydrate metabolism
It acts as a coenzyme for transketolase in hexose monophosphate (HMP) shunt.

Ribose - 5 - p + Xylulose 5 - p → Sedoheptulose 7 - p + Glyceraldehyde - 3 - p.

Others
It plays an important role in the transmission of nerve impulse as TPP is required for synthesis of acetylcholine.

Daily Requirements (RDA)
- *Adults:* 1–1.5 mg/day
- *Children:* 0.7–1.2 mg/day

Deficiency
Beriberi (Fig. 8.13)
It is a nutritional disorder caused by deficiency of thiamin (vitamin B_1). It is characterized by impairment of heart and nerves.

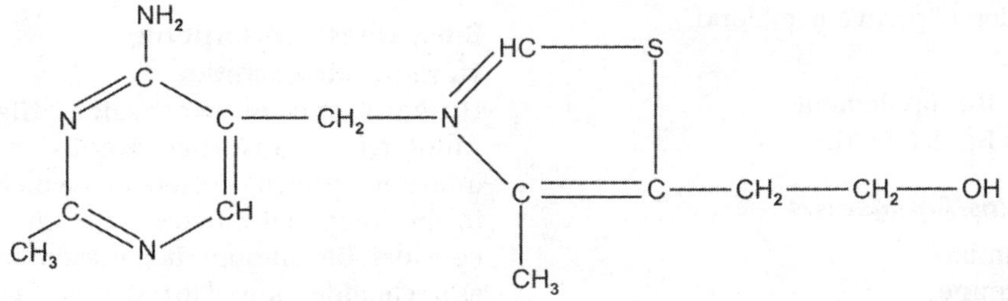

Fig. 8.12: Structure of thiamine.

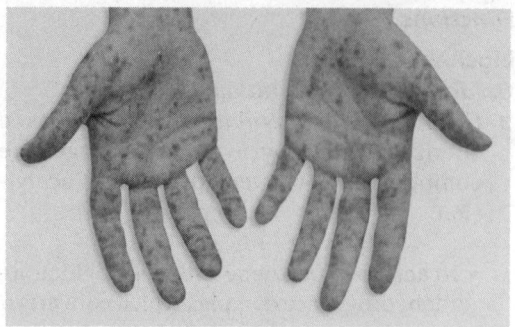

Fig. 8.13: Beriberi.
(For color version, see Plate 2)

Causes:
- Thiamin deficiency in the diet
- Diet with polished rice
- Alcoholism

Types: Two types of beriberi occur.
1. Wet beriberi (cardiovascular beriberi): It affects the heart and circulatory system, and may cause heart failure. It causes edema of face, legs, trunk, and serous cavities. Dyspnea is present.
2. Dry beriberi (neurological beriberi): It occurs when poor calorie intake and physical inactivity are present. The neurological findings may be peripheral neuropathy, loss of sensation in hands and feet, paralysis of lower eggs, mental confusion, etc.

Wernicke encephalopathy in alcoholics and Korsakoff syndrome are two forms of dry beriberi.

Note
Other types of beriberi are also known in clinical practice:
- Infantile beriberi
- Cerebral beriberi
- Mixed beriberi

Diagnosis:
- Estimation of transketolase in erythrocytes
- Estimation of pyruvate in blood

Treatment:
- Vitamin B_1, supplement
- Vitamin B_1, rich foods

Antivitamins/Antagonists
- Pyrithiamine
- Oxythiamine

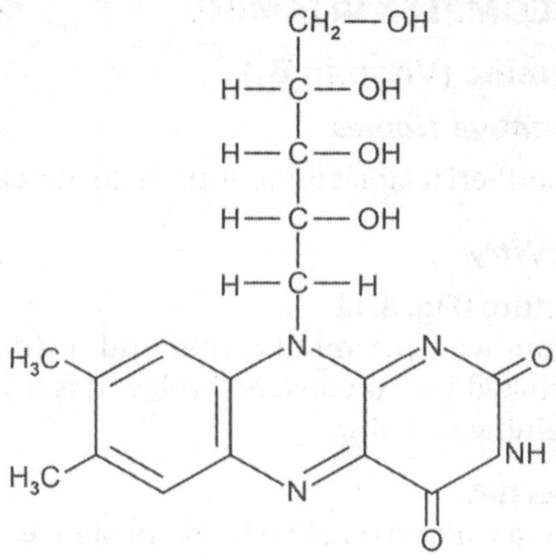

Fig. 8.14: Structure of riboflavin.

Riboflavin (Vitamin B_2)

Alternative Name
Lactoflavin

Chemistry

Structure (Fig. 8.14)
It contains D-ribitol (a ribose alcohol) attached to flavin nucleus (a heterocyclic ring isoalloxazine).

Properties
- It is an orange-yellow compound.
- It is water-soluble, heat-stable in acid and neutral medium but not in alkaline solution.
- On exposure to UV rays, it is converted to lumiflavin which exhibits greenish-yellow fluorescence.
- It undergoes reversible reduction to form a colorless substance leukoriboflavin.

Sources
- *Plant:* Germinating seeds, vegetables, fruits
- *Animal:* Liver, kidney, milk, meat, eggs

Metabolism

Biosynthesis, absorption, storage, and excretion
Humans cannot synthesize this vitamin. Riboflavin is absorbed readily in the small intestine as flavin nucleotides which is formed in the intestinal mucosa. It is not stored to a considerably amount. It is present in all tissues as nucleotides bound to proteins (flavoproteins).

It is excreted mainly in the urine (50%) as nucleotides. Minor part in feces. It is also secreted in milk.

Coenzymes

Riboflavin is a component of two coenzymes.

Flavin mononucleotide (FMN)
Riboflavin – P

Flavin adenine dinucleotide (FAD)
Riboflavin – P – P – Ribose - Adenine

Functions

Biochemical

FMN and FAD function as coenzymes of flavoprotein enzymes (oxidoreductases) in metabolism. They are involved in oxidation reduction reactions. In this role, they undergo reversible oxidation reductions, and reduced forms $FMNH_2$ and $FADH_2$ are formed.

- Reactions in which FMN is involved as a coenzyme, are:
  - It is a constituent of electron transport chain.
  - Amino acid metabolism

    Amino acid $\xrightarrow{\text{L-amino acid oxidase}}$ α-keto acid + NH_3

- Reactions in which FAD is involved as a coenzyme, are:
  - Carbohydrate metabolism

    Pyruvate $\xrightarrow{\text{PDH}}$ Acetyl-CoA

    Succinate $\xrightarrow{\text{Succinate dehydrogenase}}$ Fumarate

    α ketoglutarate $\xrightarrow{\text{KDH}}$ Succinyl-CoA

  - Lipid metabolism

    Acyl-CoA $\xrightarrow{\text{Acyl-CoA dehydrogenase}}$ α, β-unsaturated acyl-CoA

  - Amino acid metabolism

    Glycine $\xrightarrow{\text{Glycine oxidase}}$ Glyoxylate + NH_3

Others

- Riboflavin is involved in the regulatory functions of some hormones in carbohydrate metabolism.
- Riboflavin present in retina is converted by light to a compound involved in stimulation of the optic nerve.

Daily Requirements (RDA)

- *Adults:* 1.5–1.8 mg/day
- *Children:* 0.8–1.2 mg/day

Deficiency

Causes
- Defective absorption
- Alcoholism

Symptoms
- *Lips:*
  - Pink parts of lips become bright, red, swollen, and cracked (cheilosis).
  - The tissues at the corners of the lips are swollen and fissured (angular stomatitis).
- *Tongue:* Becomes enlarged, tender, and red purple (magenta) in color (glossitis).
- *Skin:* Skin becomes rough and scaly. (seborrhea).
- *Eyes:* Corneal vascularization, inflammation, photophobia.

Antivitamins/Antagonists
- Dichlororiboflavin
- Isoriboflavin
- Galactoflavin

Niacin (Vitamin B_3)

Alternative Names
Nicotinic acid/nicotinamide; pellagra preventive factor of Goldberger.

Chemistry
Niacin is the generic name for nicotinic acid and nicotinamide (niacinamide).

Structure (Fig. 8.15)
Nicotinic acid is a pyridine derivative (Pyridine-3-carboxylic acid). Nicotinamide is the amide of nicotinic acid.

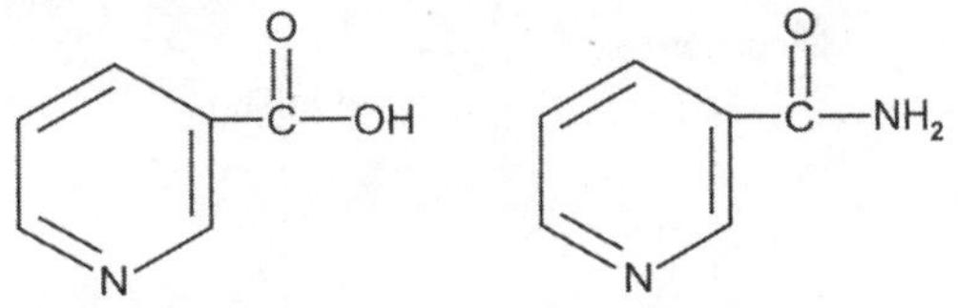

Fig. 8.15: Structure of niacin.

Properties
- It is a white crystalline substance.
- It is soluble in water, alcohol, and alkali.
- It forms salts with hydrochloride and metals.

Sources
- *Animal:* Liver, kidney, meat, fish
- *Plant:* Legumes, nuts, green vegetables, coffee, tea.

Metabolism
Biosynthesis, absorption, storage, and excretion
Niacin can be synthesized from the amino acid tryptophan in humans. 60 mg tryptophan produces 1 mg of niacin. It is also synthesized by intestinal bacteria. It is absorbed from the small intestine. It is not stored in the body. It is mainly excreted in urine as follows:
- N'-methyl nicotinamide and its oxidation products.
  Glycine conjugates of methyl derivatives.
- Traces of nicotinamide are also eliminated in sweat and milk.

Coenzymes
Niacin is a component of two coenzymes for oxidoreductase enzymes.

Nicotinamide adenine dinucleotide (NAD$^+$): Oxidized form

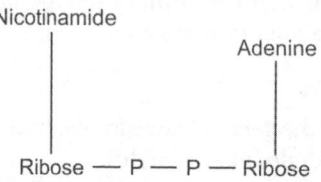

Reduced form of this coenzyme is dihydro-nicotinamide adenine dinucleotide (**NADH + H$^+$**).

Nicotinamide Adenine Dinucleotide Phosphate (NADP$^+$): Oxidized form

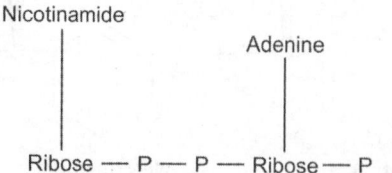

Reduced form of this coenzyme is dihydro-nicotinamide adenine dinucleotide phosphate (**NADPH+ H$^+$**).

Functions
Biochemical
NAD$^+$ and NADP$^+$ function as coenzymes for oxidoreductases by acting as hydrogen and electron transfer agents.

Reactions in which NAD$^+$ acts as coenzyme
Carbohydrate metabolism
- Lactate $\xrightarrow{\text{Lactate dehydrogenase}}$ Pyruvate
- Pyruvate $\xrightarrow{\text{Pyruvate dehydrogenase complex}}$ Acetyl-CoA
- α-ketoglutarate $\xrightarrow{\text{α-ketoglutarate dehydrogenase complex}}$ Succinyl-CoA

Lipid Metabolism
- β-hydroxy acyl-CoA $\xrightarrow{\text{β-hydroxy acyl-CoA dehydrogenase}}$ β-ketoacyl-CoA
- β-hydroxy - butyrate $\xrightarrow{\text{β-hydroxy butyrate dehydrogenase}}$ Acetoacetate

Protein Metabolism
- α-keto acids of branched chain amino acids $\xrightarrow{\text{Branched chain α-keto acid dehydrogenase}}$ Corresponding acyl-CoA thioesters

Reactions in which NADP$^+$ acts as a coenzyme
Carbohydrate metabolism
Glucose 6-P $\xrightarrow{\text{Glucose 6-P dehydrogenase}}$ 6-Phospho-gluconolactone

Malate $\xrightarrow{\text{Malic enzyme}}$ Pyruvate

NADPH dependent reactions
Lipid metabolism
HMG-CoA $\xrightarrow{\text{HMG-CoA reductase}}$ Mevalonate

Protein metabolism
Phenylalanine $\xrightarrow{\text{Phenylalanine hydroxylase}}$ Tyrosine

Reactions in which NAD$^+$ or NADP$^+$ Acts as a coenzyme
Glutamate $\xrightarrow{\text{Glutamate dehydrogenase}}$ α-ketoglutarate +NH$_3$

Others
- Essential for the normal functioning of skin, intestinal tract and nervous system
- Used for lowering cholesterol (therapeutic use).

Daily Requirements (RDA)
- *Adults:* 16–20 mg/day
- *Children:* 9–16 mg/day

Deficiency
Causes
- Low intake of niacin and tryptophan
- Carcinoid syndrome

Symptoms
Deficiency of niacin in human leads to a syndrome known as pellagra **(Fig. 8.16)**. It is a special type of dermatitis followed by malfunction of digestive and nervous systems which may eventually lead to death. The chief clinical symptoms of this disease have been referred to as 3 Ds, i.e., dermatitis, diarrhea, dementia [It may lead to death (4th D) if not treated].

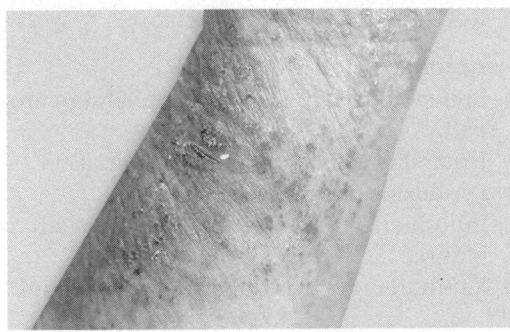

Fig. 8.16: Pellagra.
(For color version, see Plate 2)

Skin symptoms
Skin of those parts of the body exposed to sunlight or heat becomes red, later brown, rough, and scaly (dermatitis).

Gastrointestinal symptoms
Anorexia, nausea, vomiting, abdominal pain with alternating constipation/*diarrhea*, gingivitis, stomatitis; thickening and inflammation of the colon.

Cerebral symptoms
Headache, insomnia, depression, and dementia.

Antivitamins/Antagonists
- Pyridine 3-sulfonic acid
- 3-acetyl pyridine

Pyridoxine (Vitamin B_6)

Alternative Name
Rat antidermatitis factor.

Chemistry
Structure (Fig. 8.17)
Vitamin B_6 refers to a group of three compounds namely (vitamers):
1. Pyridoxine (Alcohol)
2. Pyridoxal (Aldehyde)
3. Pyridoxamine (Amine)

All are derivatives of pyridine. As the pyridoxine is the first member of this group, it is usually known as vitamin B_6.

Properties
- It is a white crystalline substance.
- It is soluble in water and alcohol.
- It is resistant to heat but destroyed at high temperature.

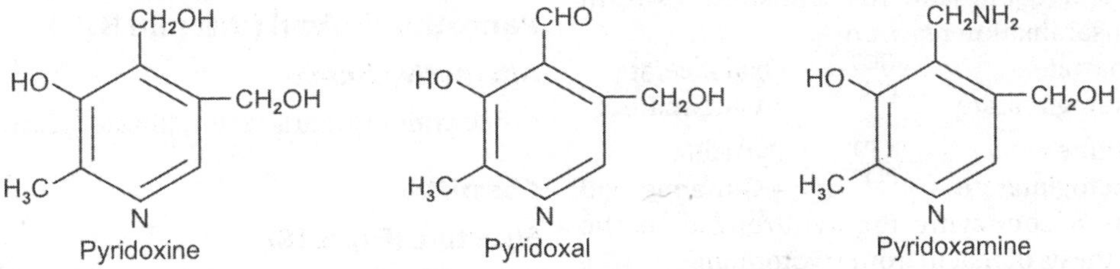

Fig. 8.17: Structure of pyridoxine.

Sources
- *Plant:* Yeast, rice polishings, seeds, cereals
- *Animal:* Liver, eggs, fish, meat.

Metabolism
Biosynthesis, absorption, storage, and excretion
Humans cannot synthesize this vitamin. Intestinal bacteria can synthesize it. It is readily absorbed from the small intestine. It is not stored. Major urinary metabolite is 4-pyridoxic acid. Pyridoxal and pyridoxamine are excreted in small amount in urine.

Coenzyme
Pyridoxal phosphate (PLP) is the major coenzyme of pyridoxine.

Functions
Biochemical
Pyridoxal phosphate acts as a coenzyme for several enzymes in metabolism.

Carbohydrate metabolism
It acts as an integral part of the enzyme phosphorylase in the breakdown of glycogen (glycogenolysis).

Lipid metabolism
It is required as a coenzyme with condensing enzyme for chain elongation of fatty acids.

Amino acid metabolism
- It is a coenzyme for decarboxylase which catalyzes decarboxylation of certain amino acids to form biogenic amines.

  Tryptophan → Serotonin
  Tyrosine → Catecholamines
  Histidine → Histamine
  Glutamic acid → Glutamine

- It is a coenzyme for transaminases in transamination reaction.

  Aspartate + α-ketoglutarate $\xrightarrow{\text{SGOT}}_{\text{PLP}}$ Oxaloacetate + Glutamate

  Alanine + α-ketoglutarate $\xrightarrow{\text{SGPT}}_{\text{PLP}}$ Pyruvate + Glutamic acid

- It is a coenzyme for kynurenase in the synthesis of niacin from tryptophan.

  Tryptophan → Niacin

- It acts as a coenzyme in the transulfuration reaction in the transfer of sulfur from homocysteine to serine to form cysteine.

  Homocysteine → Cysteine

- *Heme synthesis:* It is required for the synthesis of δ aminolevulinic acid (ALA) which is an important intermediate in the synthesis of porphyrin and heme.

  Glycine + Succinyl-CoA → ALA → Heme

Others
- Essential for growth of infants
- Used for treatment of nausea and vomiting in pregnancy, radiation sickness, muscular dystrophy (therapeutic use).

Daily Requirements (RDA)
- *Adults:* 1.6–2 mg/day
- *Children:* 0.6–1.2 mg/day

Deficiency
Causes
- Lactation
- Alcoholism
- Isoniazid therapy for tuberculosis

Symptoms
- Epileptiform convulsion, peripheral neuropathy
- Irritability, depression, mental confusion
- Pyridoxine responsive anemia
- Inborn error of metabolism, e.g., cystathioninuria.
- Xanthurenic acid is excreted more in urine.

Antivitamins/Antagonists
- Deoxypyridoxine
- Isoniazid (antituberculosis drug)

Pantothenic Acid (Vitamin B_5)
Alternative Names
Chick antidermatitis factor, filtrate factor.

Chemistry
Structure (Fig. 8.18)
It consists of β-alanine and pantoic acid linked through a peptide bond.

$HO-CH_2-\underset{\underset{CH_3}{|}}{\overset{\overset{CH_3}{|}}{C}}-\underset{\underset{}{}}{\overset{\overset{OH}{|}}{CH}}-\overset{\overset{O}{\|}}{C}-NH-CH_2-CH_2-COOH$

Fig. 8.18: Structure of pantothenic acid.

Properties
- Pale yellow viscous oil
- Soluble in water
- Heat stable

Sources
- *Plant:* Jelly, yeast, rice polishings, wheat germ, leafy vegetables
- *Animal:* Milk, meat, egg, liver.

Metabolism

Biosynthesis, absorption, storage, and excretion
Human cannot synthesize this vitamin. Intestinal bacteria can contribute fair amount. It is absorbed readily from the small intestine. It is not stored. It is excreted mainly in urine and sweat and to minor extent in milk.

Coenzyme
Coenzyme of pantothenic acid is coenzyme A.

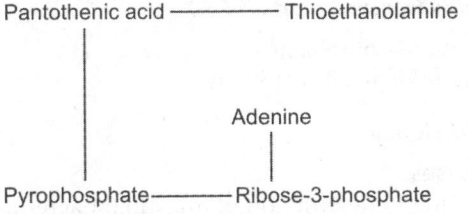

It can occur in two forms:
1. Oxidized (-SS) form: CoA
2. Reduced (-SH) form: CoA - SH

Functions

Biochemical

Action of acetyl-CoA (active acetate)
Coenzyme A readily combines with acetate to form acetyl-CoA, which participates in a number of metabolic reactions.
- *Carbohydrate metabolism:* It condenses with oxaloacetate to form citric acid which initiates TCA cycle.
  Oxaloacetate + Acetyl-CoA → Citric acid
- *Lipid metabolism:* It is the starting compound for the synthesis of cholesterol.
  Acetyl-CoA → Cholesterol
- Acetyl-CoA and malonyl-CoA are used in the synthesis and elongation of fatty acids.

Action of succinyl-CoA (active succinate)
α-ketoglutarate undergoes oxidative decarboxylation in TCA cycle to form active succinate (Succinyl-CoA). It is involved in important metabolic reactions.
- *Lipid metabolism*
  - Succinyl-CoA is involved in:
    - β-oxidation of fatty acids
    - Biosynthesis of fatty acids
    - Degradation of ketone bodies
- *Amino acid metabolism:* Activation of branched chain amino acids may involve coenzyme A.
- *Heme synthesis:* Succinyl-CoA and glycine combine to form ALA—the first step in heme synthesis.
  Succinyl-CoA → α-amino levulinic acid (ALA) + Glycine

Others
It plays an important role in adrenocortical function.

Daily Requirements (RDA)
- *Adults:* 5–10 mg/day
- *Children:* 4–5 mg/day

Deficiency

In Humans
Deficiency of pantothenic acid in human is rare due to its wide distribution in food stuffs and its synthesis to a little extent by intestinal bacteria. However, the burning foot syndrome has been detected. (Dr Gopalan, NIN). Its symptoms are:
- Numbness and pain in the toes
- Fatigue
- Sleep disturbances

In Animals
Dermatitis and toughness of feathers, retardation of growth, depigmentation and spectacled condition of the eye are observed in chicks.

Antivitamins/Antagonists
- Pantoyl taurine
- Methyl pantothenate

Biotin (Vitamin B_7)

Alternative Names
Anti-egg white injury factor, vitamin H.

Chemistry
Structure (Fig. 8.19)
It consists of fused imidazole and thiophene ring with a fatty acid chain and sulfur.

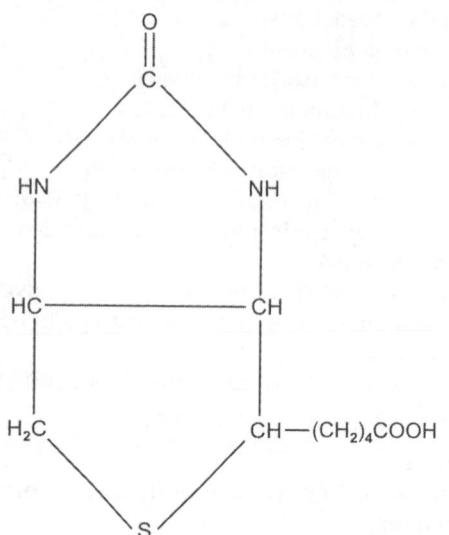

Fig. 8.19: Structure of biotin.

Properties
- It is soluble in water and alcohol.
- It forms colorless crystalline needles.
- It is destroyed by acids and alkalis only on rigorous treatment.

Sources
- *Animal:* Egg yolk, liver and kidney, milk
- *Plant:* Yeast, vegetables, grains

Metabolism
Biosynthesis, absorption, storage, and excretion
Humans cannot synthesize this vitamin. It is synthesized by intestinal bacteria. It is readily absorbed from the small intestine. It may be stored to a limited extent in liver and kidneys. It is excreted in urine, feces, and milk.

Coenzyme
Coenzyme form of biotin is biocytin.

Functions
Biochemical
Multienzyme complexes containing biocytin as coenzyme catalyze CO_2 transfer reactions (CO_2 fixation reactions/carboxylation reactions) in metabolism.
- Biotin acts as a coenzyme for acetyl-CoA carboxylase which converts acetyl-CoA to malonyl-CoA. It is the first step of de novo fatty acid synthesis in the extramitochondrial pathway.
$$\text{Acetyl-CoA} \rightarrow \text{Malonyl-CoA}$$
- It acts as a coenzyme for pyruvate carboxylase which converts pyruvate to oxaloacetate in gluconeogenesis.
$$\text{Pyruvate} \rightarrow \text{Oxaloacetate}$$
- It acts as a coenzyme with propionyl-CoA carboxylase which converts propionyl-CoA to methyl malonyl-CoA.
$$\text{Propionyl-CoA} \rightarrow \text{Methyl malonyl-CoA}$$

> **Note**
> Biotin is not involved in the fixation of CO_2 for the formation of carbon-6 of purine ring.

Others
It prevents a skin condition induced by feeding a diet of egg white to experimental animals.

Daily Requirements (RDA)
- *Adults:* 50–60 µg/day
- *Children:* 20–40 µg/day

Deficiency
Causes
- Due to destruction of intestinal bacteria by sulfonamide drugs.
- Due to large intake of raw egg white which contains the glycoprotein avidin (egg white injury factor) that interferes with absorption of biotin.

Symptoms
Dermatitis, loss of hair (alopecia), depression, hallucination, paralysis, muscle pain, anorexia, nausea, anemia.

Antivitamins/Antagonists
- Avidin
- Desthiobiotin
- Biotin sulfonic acid

Folic Acid

Alternative Names
Folacin; Pteroylglutamic acid (PGA).

Chemistry
Structure (Fig. 8.20)
The term folic acid refers to a group of compounds which contain the following structural unit:
  Pteridine - Para-aminobenzoic acid (PABA) - Glutamic acid.

Properties
- It is a yellow crystalline substance.
- It is slightly soluble in water.
- It is inactivated by light.

Sources
- *Plant:* Whole grains, cereals, green leafy vegetables, yeast
- *Animal:* Liver, kidney, eggs

Metabolism
Biosynthesis, absorption, storage, and excretion
Humans cannot synthesize this vitamin. Bacteria in the intestine can synthesize it. Folate derivatives ingested in the diet are converted to monoglutamate folates for absorption. Most of these are reduced to tetrahydrofolates in the intestinal cells by folate reductase. Methyl tetrahydrofolates enter portal blood and then carried to liver. It is stored in liver. It is excreted in urine and feces as 5-methyl-H_4 folate.

Coenzyme
Coenzyme of folic acid is tetrahydrofolate (FH_4) or H_4 folate. It is 5, 6, 7, 8 tetrahydrofolate.

$$\text{Folic acid} \xrightarrow{\text{Dihydrofolate reductase}} \text{Tetrahydrofolate } (FH_4)$$

Functions
Biochemical
One carbon metabolism
Definition: It refers to a group of biochemical reactions which are involved in the transfer of one carbon units or moieties formed in the metabolic pathways with the help of enzymes and coenzymes.

Folic acid coenzyme FH_4 helps in the transfer of one carbon (C-1) moieties or units (one carbon metabolism) to form new compounds.

Tetrahydrofolate (FH_4) may receive one carbon unit (C-1) namely formyl (CHO), methyl (CH_3), methenyl (–CH), methylene (–CH_2), formino (–CH=NH), hydroxymethyl (–CH_2OH) groups on its N_5 and/or N_{10} position from different substrates during catabolism. It then acts as a carrier or donor of these C-1 groups to other substrate forming new compounds. Thus it acts as a coenzyme for many transferase enzymes (N5-formyl tetrahydrofolate is known as folinic acid or citrovorum factor).

Reactions in which one carbon unit is transferred by FH_4 carrier
- Glycine → Serine
- Ethanolamine → Choline
- Homocysteine → Methionine
- Uracil → Thymine
- Nicotinamide → N-methyl nicotinamide
- Biosynthesis of histidine
- Biosynthesis of purines

> **Note**
> Other one carbon units CH_3 transfer by SAM-P. 181.

Others
- Necessary for hemopoiesis
- Required for normal growth of microorganisms and many animal species.

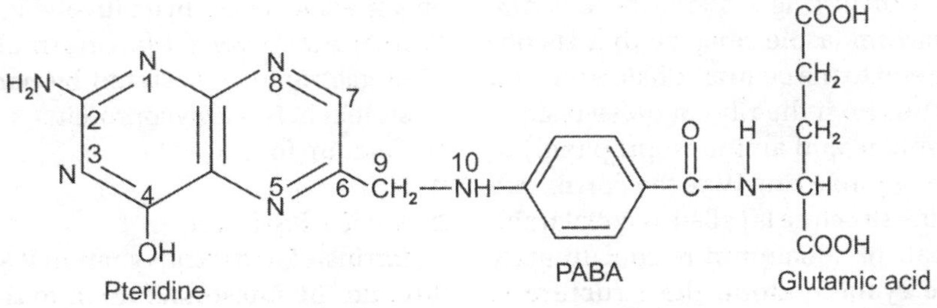

Fig. 8.20: Structure of folic acid.

Section 2: Chemistry of Biomolecules

Daily Requirements (RDA)
- *Adults:* 400–500 µg/day
- *Children:* 100–300 µg/day

Deficiency
Causes
- Decreased dietary intake
- Decreased intestinal absorption
- Effect of drugs
- Alcoholism

Symptoms
- Macrocytic anemia with megablastic changes in bone marrow
- Glossitis
- Gastrointestinal disorders
- Growth retardation
- Lethargy
- Reproduction defects in women

Test to detect deficiency
Formiminoglutamic acid (FIGLU) test (histidine load test) (*refer* Chapter 13)

Antivitamins/Antagonists
- Aminopterin
- Amethopterin (methotrexate)
 (both are anticancer drugs. They inhibit DNA synthesis).

Cobalamin (Vitamin B$_{12}$)

Alternative Names
Antipernicious anemia factor, extrinsic factor of Castle.

Chemistry
Structure (Fig. 8.21)
The central portion of the molecule consists of 4 reduced and substituted pyrrole rings surrounding a single cobalt atom. This central structure is called as *Corrin ring* system.

Below the Corrin ring system, there is a 5, 6-dimethylbenzimidazole riboside that is connected at one end to the central cobalt atom and at the other end (from the ribofuranose residue through phosphate and amino isopropanol) to a side chain on pyrrole ring IV of the corrin ring system. Now the structure is called as cobalamin.

If the cobalt of cobalamin is coordinately linked to the cyanide atom, the structure is

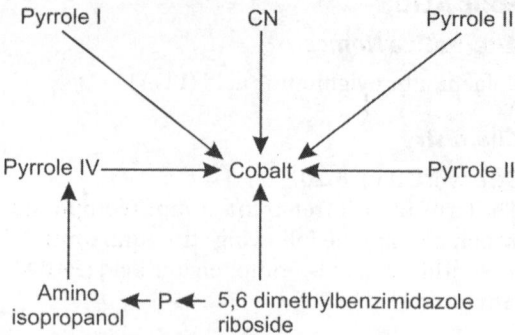

Fig. 8.21: Structure of vitamin B$_{12}$.

called as cyanocobalamin. This is commercial form of vitamin B$_{12}$.

Molecular formula: $C_{63} H_{90} N_{14} O_{14} PCO$.

Properties
- It is soluble in water and alcohol.
- It is a dark red compound.
- It is tasteless and odorless.

Sources
It is present only in foods of animal origin and completely absent in all vegetarian sources.
- *Rich:* Liver, kidney
- *Good:* Meat, fish, eggs
- *Fair:* Milk and dairy products

> **Note**
> Vegetarians get vitamin B$_{12}$ synthesized by intestinal bacteria only.

Metabolism
Biosynthesis
Intestinal bacteria can synthesize B$_{12}$. Human cannot synthesize it.

Absorption
Vitamin B$_{12}$ (extrinsic factor of Castle) is absorbed from the ileum. Its absorption depends on a specific mechanism involving:
- *Intrinsic factor (IF):* A normal constituent of gastric juice secreted by parietal cells of stomach. It is a glycoprotein.
- Calcium ions (Ca^{2+})
- HCl
- A releasing factor

Intrinsic factor binds vitamin B$_{12}$ for transport through the intestinal lumen to the absorptive site in the ileum. In the ileum, a 'receptor' site accomplishes the removal of B_{12} from intrinsic factor in presence of Ca^{2+} ions and a releasing factor (RF) secreted by duodenum. B_{12} now enters ileal mucosal cells for absorption into circulation.

Transport
Vitamin B_{12} is transported in the blood in association with specific proteins namely transcobalamins.

Storage
It is mainly stored in liver bound to transcobalamin I.

Excretion
It is not excreted in urine under ordinary conditions.

Coenzymes
Coenzymes of vitamin B_{12} are known as cobamide coenzymes. Cobamide coenzymes do not contain the cyano group attached to cobalt but a different group is linked to cobalt. There are two forms of cobamide coenzymes in humans.
- Deoxyadenosylcobalamin
- Methylcobalamin

Functions
Biochemical
- *Conversion of methyl malonyl-CoA to succinyl-CoA:* Vitamin B_{12} functions as a coenzyme (Deoxyadenosyl cobalamin) for the enzyme isomerase which converts methyl malonyl-CoA to succinyl-CoA.

$$\text{Methyl-malonyl CoA} \xrightarrow[\text{Deoxyadenosyl cobalamin}]{\text{Isomerase}} \text{Succinyl-CoA}$$

Note
Normal healthy individuals excrete < 2 mg of methyl malonic acid in urine which is not detectable. But in vitamin B_{12} deficiency, methyl malonic acid accumulates and its excretion is increased in urine. This condition is known as methyl malonic aciduria.

- *Conversion of homocysteine to methionine:* It acts as a coenzyme (methyl cobalamin) in the methylation of homocysteine to methionine. In this reaction H_4 folate acts as CH_3 carrier. In vitamin B_{12} deficiency, transfer of CH_3 from

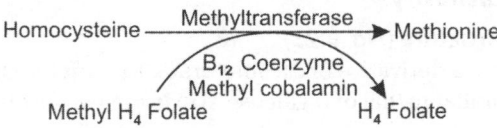

Fig. 8.22: Methyl trap (folate trap).

methyl FH_4 is blocked. Thus FH_4 is trapped as methyl FH_4 (folate trap, methyl trap) **(Fig. 8.22)**. This reaction is common to both folic acid and vitamin B_{12}.

Others
- Vitamin B_{12} along with folic acid is required for the development of red blood cells beyond megaloblastic stage (erythropoiesis).
- It cures the neurological symptoms of pernicious anemia.
- It stimulates the appetite and general health of the subject.

Daily Requirements (RDA)
- *Adults:* 3 µg/day
- *Children:* 1–2 µg/day

Deficiency Symptoms
- *Pernicious anemia:* It involves hematological manifestations (reduction in the number of RBCs) with neurological changes (degenerative changes in spinal cord).
- Mucosal atropy of stomach
- Glossitis, stomatitis, pharyngitis
- Severe metabolic acidosis in children
- Homocystinuria and methylmalonic aciduria

Test to Detect Deficiency
- Estimation of vitamin B_{12} in serum
- Methyl malonic acid in urine

Note
Both folic acid and vitamin B_{12} are hematopoietic vitamins.

■ NON B-COMPLEX VITAMIN

Vitamin C
Ascorbic acid

Alternative Name
Antiscorbutic vitamin

Chemistry

Structure (Fig. 8.23)
It is a derivative of carbohydrate. Its structure is similar to that of L-glucose. It exists in two forms:

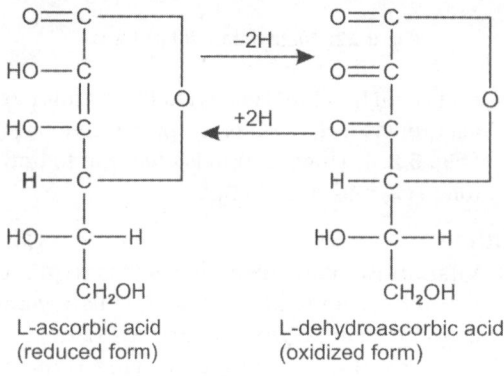

Fig. 8.23: Structure of vitamin C.

Properties
- It is a white crystalline substance.
- It is freely soluble in water.
- Its biological activities are due to its reversible oxidation-reduction.
- It is lost during processing and storage.

Sources
- *Animal:* Adrenal gland, corpus luteum, liver
- *Plant:* Citrus fruits (lemon, orange), amla, bananas, pineapple, strawberries, cabbage, cauliflower, tomatoes, green peas, beans, rose.

> **Note**
> Milk is poor source of vitamin C.

Metabolism

Biosynthesis
Man and other primates cannot synthesize this vitamin due to absence of enzyme L-gulonolactone oxidase. Hence the entire requirement must be supplied by the diet. Nonprimates can synthesize it from glucose by uronic acid pathway.

$$\text{Glucose} \rightarrow \text{Ascorbic acid}$$

Absorption
It is readily absorbed from the small intestine, peritoneum and subcutaneous tissue.

Storage
It is not stored.

Excretion
About 25–50% of the ingested vitamin is excreted in the urine as such. Rest being converted to inactive compounds and excreted in the urine. It is also secreted in the milk.

Functions

Biochemical

Amino acid metabolism
- It is a coenzyme with the enzyme p-hydroxy phenylpyruvate hydroxylase which catalyzes the hydroxylation and conversion of p-hydroxyphenylpyruvate to homogentisic acid (tyrosine metabolism).

$$\text{p-hydroxyphenyl pyruvate} \rightarrow \text{Homogentisic acid}$$

- It is required as a coenzyme for the enzyme dopamine hydroxylase which catalyzes the conversion of dopamine to norepinephrine.

$$\text{Dopamine} \rightarrow \text{Norepinephrine}$$

- Tryptophan $\rightarrow$ Serotonin

Lipid metabolism
It helps in the action of the enzyme hydrolase (a mono-oxygenase) which catalyzes oxidation of long chain fatty acids to form hydroxy fatty acids.

Electron transport system
Enzymes such as ascorbic acid oxidase, cytochrome oxidase, flavin transhydrogenase participate in the electron transport system of microsomes, where ascorbic acid takes part between NADH and cytochrome b.

Formation of active folate (FH_4)
It is required in the conversion of folic acid to folinic acid (citrovorum factor).

Synthesis of bile acids
It is involved in the synthesis of bile acids from cholesterol.

Iron metabolism
Ascorbic acid in food helps in the absorption of iron by converting the ferric iron to the ferrous form. It is necessary for the formation of tissue ferritin. It also helps in mobilization of iron from its storage form ferritin.

Collagen synthesis
Vitamin C helps in the formation of hydroxyproline from proline and hydroxylysine from lysine. Hydroxyproline and hydroxylysine are components of collagen in connective tissue.

Proline → Hydroxyproline
Lysine → Hydroxylysine

Activities of fibroblasts/osteoblasts
It is needed for the activities of fibroblasts, osteoblasts which are responsible for formation of mucopolysaccharides of connective tissues, osteoid formation, dentin and intercellular cement substance of capillaries.

Antioxidant
It can prevent cancer due to its action as antioxidant.

Immunity
It induces synthesis of immunoglobulins (antibodies).

Others
Plays an important role in the body against stress.

Therapeutic uses
Used for treatment of scurvy **(Fig. 8.24)**, infectious diseases (tuberculosis, streptococcal infections), allergic conditions (common cold), wound healing.

Daily Requirements (RDA)
- *Adults:* 75 mg/day
- *Children:* 40 mg/day

Deficiency

Causes
Its deficiency produces a disease called 'Scurvy' due to failure to deposit intercellular substance.

Symptoms
- *Hemorrhage:* Capillaries are fragile and tend to bleed. Internal hemorrhage may occur.

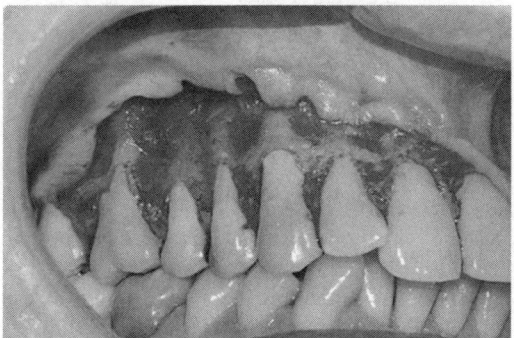

Fig. 8.24: Scurvy.
(For color version, see Plate 2)

- *Oral cavity:* Gums become swollen spongy and painful. Poor dentine formation leads to defective teeth. Wound healing may be delayed.
- *Bone:* Bones become weak and fracture occurs due to failure of osteoblasts to form the intercellular substance osteoid. Hemorrhage into joint cavities and painful swelling of joints may also occur.
- *Anemia:* Microcytic hypochromic anemia is seen.
- *Toxicity:* May occur at very high dose.

VITAMIN-LIKE COMPOUNDS
Some compounds are present in food as accessory food factors. They are not well established vitamins but perform several important functions in the body.

Examples
- *Lipoic acid:* It is a sulfur-containing fatty acid. It exists in oxidized and reduced forms. It is widely distributed in natural foods. It acts as a coenzyme in the oxidative decarboxylation of pyruvic acid and α-ketoglutaric acid. No deficiency symptoms have been identified.
- *Choline:* It is trimethyl hydroxy ethanolamine. It is present in many dietary sources, such as liver, eggs, milk, cereals, etc. It is a constituent of lecithin (phospholipid). It acts as a lipotropic factor to prevent fatty liver formation. It is involved in one carbon metabolism. Acetylcholine is required for transmission of nerve impulse.
- *Inositol:* It is hexahydroxycyclohexane. It is present in meat, milk, nuts, and vegetables. It exists in the form of phospholipids in animal tissues and as phytic acid in plants. It acts as a lipotropic factor and as second messenger for some hormones.
- *PABA:* It is one of the structural constituents of vitamin folic acid. It is synthesized by the bacteria and is essential for growth. It is the competitive inhibitor of sulfanilamide drug. It is a bacteriostatic agent.
- *Vitamin P (bioflavonoids)*
  - Antioxidant
  - Maintains capillary permeability

Differences between fat-soluble and water-soluble vitamins is given in **Table 8.1**.

Section 2: Chemistry of Biomolecules

Table 8.1: Differences between fat-soluble vitamins and water-soluble vitamins.

Features	Fat-soluble vitamins	Water-soluble vitamins
Solubility	Soluble in fat solvents but insoluble in water	Soluble in water
Absorption	Requires bile salts; absorbed along with lipids	Simple absorption (except vitamin B_{12})
Storage	Stored in liver	Not stored (except vitamin B_{12})
Excretion	Not excreted	Excreted
Coenzyme	Vitamin K only acts as coenzyme	All act as coenzymes
Deficiency	Occurs only when stores are depleted	Occurs rapidly as there is no storage (except vitamin B_{12})
Toxicity	Hypervitaminosis may occur	Very rare (excess is excreted)

■ ANTIVITAMINS

Antivitamins are compounds which have structural similarity to vitamins. They act as antagonists to vitamins and cause vitamin deficiency. List of antivitamins is given in the **Table 8.2** and list of vitamins is given in **Table 8.3**.

Table 8.2: Antivitamins.

Vitamins	Antivitamins
Vitamins A, D, and E	Nil
Vitamin K	Warfarin (Dicumarol)
Thiamine	Oxythiamine, pyrithiamine
Riboflavin	Dichlororiboflavin, isoriboflavin
Niacin	3-acetyl pyridine
Pyridoxine	Isoniazid, deoxypyridoxine
Pantothenic acid	Pantoyl taurine
Biotin	Desthiobiotin, avidin
Folic acid	Aminopterin, amethopterin
Vitamin B_{12}	Nil
Vitamin C	Nil

Table 8.3: Vitamins.

Sl. No.	Vitamins	Sources	Functions	RDA (adults)	Deficiency symptoms	Toxicity symptoms
1.	Vitamin A	Fish liver oils, milk, carrots, yellow/red, green leafy vegetables	Vision (rhodopsin cycle), reproduction, growth, immunity, antioxidant, skin structure	5,000 IU	Night blindness (nyctalopia) Xerophthalmia Bitot spots, scaly skin	Hypervitaminosis A
2.	Vitamin D	Cod liver, oil, egg, yolk, Sunlight as activator	Calcification of bone, calcium homeostasis	400 IU	Rickets in children, osteomalacia in adults	Hypervitaminosis D
3.	Vitamin E	Vegetable and seed, oils, eggs	Antioxidant, scavenger of free radicals	20–25 IU	Muscular dystrophy, sterility in rats	Not established

Contd...

Contd...

Sl. No.	Vitamins	Sources	Functions	RDA (adults)	Deficiency symptoms	Toxicity symptoms
4.	Vitamin K	Green leafy vegetables, liver	Blood clotting (coagulation) (vitamin K cycle)	50–100 µg	Hemorrhage	Hemolytic anemia, jaundice
5.	Vitamin (B_1)	Whole grains leafy, vegetables, nuts, meat, eggs	Coenzyme—TPP oxidative decarboxylation (carbohydrate metabolism)	1–1.5 mg	Beriberi, Wernicke, Korsakoff syndrome	Not established
6.	Riboflavin (B_2)	Germinating seeds, green leafy, vegetables, liver, egg, milk	Coenzymes—FMN, FAD—Oxidation—reduction reactions in carbohydrate, lipid, and protein metabolism	1.3–1.8 mg	Cheilosis, glossitis, stomatitis, dermatitis	Not established
7.	Niacin (B_3)	Liver, meat, fish, green vegetables, legumes, nuts, coffee, tea	Coenzymes, NAD, NADP oxidation, and energy reactions	16–20 mg	Pellagra (3Ds syndrome)	Not established
8.	Pantothenic acid (B_5)	Wheat germs cereals liver, meat, eggs, milk, yeast	Coenzymes—coenzyme A (Acyl carrier—Acetyl-CoA and succinyl-CoA in carbohydrate, lipid and protein metabolism)	5–10 mg	Burning feet syndrome	Not established
9.	Pyridoxine (B_6)	Vegetables, cereals, liver, meat, egg	Coenzyme–PLP–transamination in protein metabolism. Heme synthesis, decarboxylation	1.6–2 mg	Peripheral neuropathy, anemia	Not established
10.	Biotin (B_7)	Vegetables, liver, egg yolk, milk, grains	Coenzymes—Biocytin for carboxylation	50–60 µg	Dermatitis anorexia, nausea	Not established
11.	Folic acid (B_9)	Whole grains, green leafy, vegetables, liver, egg yolk	Coenzymes FH_4, one carbon metabolism, synthesis of protein	400–500 µg	Megaloblastic anemia, neural tube defects, gastrointestinal disorders	Not established
12.	Cobalamin (B_{12})	Present in animal sources only. Meat, egg, liver, fish	Coenzymes • Methylcobalamin • Deoxyadenosine cobalamin ▪ Protein metabolism	3 µg	Pernicious anemia, neuropathy, methylmalonic aciduria	Not established
13.	Vitamin C (ascorbic acid)	Citrus fruits, amla, tomatoes, strawberries, bananas, liver	Antioxidant, synthesis of collagen, absorption of iron, dental structures, immunity	60–75 mg	Scurvy	Not established

Section 3 Metabolism

9 Introduction to Metabolism

Chapter Outline
- Definition
- Phases of Metabolism
- Importance
- Methods of Studying (Investigating) Metabolism
- Type of Reactions in Metabolic Pathways
- Additional Information

■ DEFINITION

Metabolism refers to the sequence of chemical changes undergone by the food stuffs after absorption from the gastrointestinal tract.

Digestion → Absorption → Metabolism

■ PHASES OF METABOLISM

Reaction pathways that comprise metabolism are mainly divided into two phases:
1. Anabolism
2. Catabolism
   (Amphibolism refers to both the phases)

Anabolism

It refers to biosynthetic processes whereby larger molecules are synthesized from small molecules. In this phase energy is utilized.

Small molecules $\xrightarrow[\text{+ Energy}]{\text{Anabolism}}$ Large molecules

e.g., Glucose → Glycogen

Catabolism

It consists of degradative processes whereby larger molecules are degraded to simple molecules. Energy is liberated in this phase.

Large molecules $\xrightarrow{\text{Catabolism}}$ Small molecules + Energy

e.g., Glucose → Pyruvate/Lactate

Thus, metabolism can be represented as:

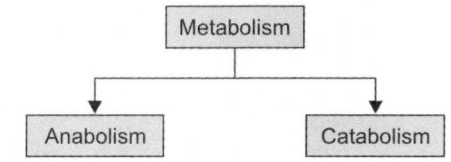

Amphibolism, e.g., Krebs cycle.

■ IMPORTANCE

- Metabolism is the overall process through which living systems acquire and utilize energy to carry out their various functions.
- Derangements of certain reactions of metabolism are frequently associated with pathological states, e.g., diabetes mellitus occurs due to defective carbohydrate metabolism.

■ METHODS OF STUDYING (INVESTIGATING) METABOLISM

Feeding Animals with Chemicals

This method consists in feeding or injecting a normal animal with the chemical under investigation. It is followed by demonstration of an increase in one or more metabolites of that chemical in the blood, excreta or tissues.

Radioactive Isotopic Techniques

The substance under investigation is tagged (labelled) with a radioactive isotope which acts as a tracer substance. The tracer substance in the body can be detected by Geiger-Muller counter or liquid scintillation counter.

Isotope	Used to investigate
^{14}C Glucose	Carbohydrate metabolism
^{14}C Acetate	Lipid metabolism
^{15}C Leucine	Protein metabolism
^{3}H Thymidine	Nucleic acid metabolism
^{59}Fe, ^{131}I, ^{60}Co	Mineral metabolism

Other methods such as Warburg's tissue slice technique and respiratory exchange experiment can also be used.

TYPE OF REACTIONS IN METABOLIC PATHWAYS

Almost all the reactions that occur in metabolic pathways can be classified into four major categories. Among them oxidations and reductions are predominant:
- Oxidation and reduction
- Group-transfer reactions
- Isomerization and rearrangement
- Reactions that make or break carbon-carbon bonds

Oxidation

It can be defined as:
- Addition of oxygen atoms

$$CH_3CHO \xrightarrow{+O} CH_3COOH$$

- Loss of hydrogen

$$CH_3CH_2OH \xrightarrow{-H} CH_3CHO$$

- Loss of electrons

$$Fe^{++} \xrightarrow{-e} Fe^{+++}$$

Reduction

It is the reversal of oxidation.

Mechanism of Oxidation-Reduction

- Oxidation is always accompanied by reduction

$$A_{red} + B_{ox} \rightarrow A_{ox} + B_{red}$$

- Electrons pass from reductant (which has lower affinity for electrons) to oxidant (which has higher affinity for electrons).
  Oxidizing agent (oxidant) = Electron acceptor
  Reducing agent (reductant) = Electron donor
- Affinity for electrons by the oxidant is called as redox potential. It is symbolically represented as E_o.

- In the laboratory (in vitro) various oxidations and reductions are carried out by some specific agents under particular temperature and pressure.

ADDITIONAL INFORMATION

Antimetabolities

Definition

Antimetabolities are the chemical substances or drugs which inhibit normal metabolism. They are usually structural analogues of metabolites. For examples, Functions:
- Function as competitive inhibitors, e.g., MDH (*refer* Chapter 7)
- Act as antivitamins, e.g., Dicumarol (*refer* Chapter 8)
- Act as anticancer agents, e.g., 5-fluorouracil, 6-mercaptopurine, cytarabine, aminopterin (methotrexate), amethopterin

Key Enzymes

Allosteric enzymes are utilized by the body to regulate metabolic pathways. Such a regulatory enzyme in a particular pathway is called the key enzyme or rate limiting enzyme.
For example, Glycolysis:

$$Fructose-6-P + ATP \xrightarrow{Phosphofructokinase} Fructose\ 1,6\ bisphosphate + ADP$$

Multienzyme Complex

It contains several enzymes packed into one assembly. It catalyzes a single or a sequence of consecutive reactions of a metabolic pathway. It increases the efficiency of the overall metabolic pathway. For example:
- Pyruvate dehydrogenase complex (*refer* Chapter 11)
- α-ketoglutarate dehydrogenase complex (*refer* Chapter 11)
- Fatty acid synthase complex (*refer* Chapter 12).

10 Biological Oxidation, Electron Transport Chain, and Bioenergetics

Chapter Outline
- Biological Oxidation
- Electron Transport Chain
- Oxidative Phosphorylation
- Bioenergetics
- Additional Information

BIOLOGICAL OXIDATION

In the body, various oxidations and reductions are effected at physiological temperature with the help of enzymes, coenzymes, hydrogen and electron carrier systems. They occur not in a single step but in several steps for proper utilization and storage of energy.

Alternative Names
Cellular respiration/internal respiration.

Enzymes Involved in Biological Oxidation

All the enzymes involved in biological oxidations are known as oxidoreductases. They are divided into four major groups:

Oxidases
Enzymes that catalyze removal of hydrogen from a substrate but use only oxygen as a hydrogen acceptor are known as oxidases. They are conjugated proteins containing prosthetic group. Water or hydrogen peroxide is formed as a product.

$$AH_2 + 1/2 O_2 \rightarrow A + H_2O$$

E.g.,:
- *Cytochrome oxidase:* It is the terminal component of electron transport chain. It contains heme as prosthetic group. It is also known as cytochrome aa_3.
- *Tyrosinase:* It is a copper containing enzyme involved in metabolism of tyrosine.

Note
Some flavoprotein enzymes containing FMN or FAD also belong to this group of oxidases, e.g., L-amino acid oxidase (FMN), Xanthine oxidase (FAD).

Dehydrogenases
These enzymes catalyze removal of hydrogen from a substrate, but cannot use oxygen as acceptor.
- NAD^+ *linked dehydrogenases:* Present in electron transport chain, glycolysis, TCA cycle.
- $NADP^+$ *linked dehydrogenases:* Involved in reductive synthesis of fatty acids, steroids, etc.
- *FMN-linked dehydrogenases:* Present in electron transport chain.
- *FAD-linked dehydrogenases:* Present in electron transport chain.
- *Cytochromes:* Except cytochrome oxidase, all cytochromes fall under the group, e.g., Cytochrome b, c1, c, occur in the electron transport chain.

Hydroperoxidases
They catalyze oxidation using hydrogen peroxide or organic peroxide as substrate. They protect the body against harmful peroxides which can form free radicals.

They are of two subgroups, e.g.,
1. *Peroxidases:* They reduce peroxides using electron acceptor.
$$H_2O_2 + AH_2 \rightarrow 2H_2O + A$$
e.g., Glutathione peroxidase.

2. *Catalases:* They reduce peroxides using hydrogen peroxide as electron donor and electron acceptor.
$$2H_2O_2 \rightarrow 2H_2O + O_2$$

Oxygenases

These enzymes catalyze direct transfer and incorporation of oxygen into the substrate. They are involved in the synthesis or degradation of different metabolites.

They are divided into two subgroups.
1. *Mono-oxygenases (mixed function oxidases, hydroxylases):* These incorporate only one atom of molecular oxygen into the substrate forming hydroxyl group on it. The other oxygen atom is reduced to water in the presence of additional electron donor or cosubstrate.
$$A - H + O_2 + BH_2 \rightarrow A - OH + H_2O + B$$
e.g.,
 - *Cytochrome P 450:* It is present in microsomes of liver involved in metabolism of drugs such as aniline morphine. It is also present in mitochondria of testis, ovary, adrenal, placenta involved in synthesis of steroid hormones.
 - *Phenylalanine hydroxylase:* It is involved in the conversion of phenylalanine to tyrosine.
2. *Dioxygenases:* These catalyze the incorporation of both atoms of molecular oxygen into the substrate.
$$A + O_2 \rightarrow AO_2$$
e.g.,
 - *Homogentisate dioxygenase (homogentisate oxidase):* It is involved in tyrosine metabolism.
 - *Tryptophan dioxygenase (tryptophan pyrrolase):* It is involved in tryptophan metabolism.

Importance

- Biological oxidation reductions are vital for existence and functioning of cells.
- Living systems derive most of their energy from them.
- They are important reactions in cellular respiration which occur through electron transport chain.
- Many drugs, pollutants and chemical carcinogens are metabolized by the reactions involving those enzymes.

■ ELECTRON TRANSPORT CHAIN

Definition

Electron transport chain (ETC) is a sequence of carriers or acceptors which collect and transport electrons from reducing equivalents formed from different substrates to oxygen to form water with synthesis of ATP **(Fig. 10.1)**.

Alternative Name

Respiratory chain.

Site

It is located in the inner membrane of the mitochondria: Mitochondria is known as the powerhouse of the cell because it contains the machinery for trapping energy in the form of ATP.

Organization (Components)

ETC is a multicomponent system. It consists of the following (electron carriers) organized

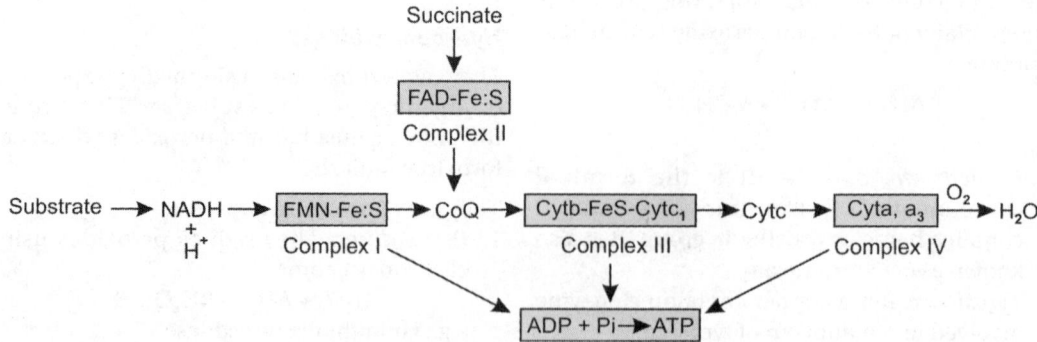

Fig. 10.1: Electron transport chain.

into four major complexes. It is arranged in increasing order of redox determine (CoQ and FeS are present as individual components).
- Complex-I: NADH-CoQ reductase
- Complex-II: Succinate-CoQ reductase
- Complex-III: CoQ-Cytochrome C reductase
- Complex-IV: Cytochrome oxidase (cytochrome aa_3)

Note

NADH produced in the cytosol enters the mitochondria via two shuttle pathways:
1. Glycerol-phosphate shuttle
2. Malate-aspartate shuttle

Steps

1. Electrons from NADH are transferred to CoQ by complex-I (NADH-CoQ reductase) via FMN and FeS.
2. Complex-II (Succinate-CoQ reductase) transfers electrons from succinate to CoQ via FAD and FeS.
3. Complex-III (CoQ - Cytochrome C reductase) transfers electrons from CoQ to cytochrome C via cytochrome b, FeS and cytochrome c_1.
4. Complex-IV (Cytochrome oxidase) transfers electrons from cytochrome c to the final electron acceptor O_2 to form water.

Clinical Importance

Absence or deficiency of certain oxidoreductase enzymes in ETC may result in the following clinical disorders:
- Infantile mitochondrial myopathy
- Renal dysfunction

■ OXIDATIVE PHOSPHORYLATION

Definition

The process by which ADP is phosphorylated by Pi (inorganic phosphate) to ATP in ETC is known as oxidative phosphorylation. ATP is known as energy currency of the cell.

Site

Formation of ATP occurs at three sites at ETC by ATP synthase also called as *complex-V*.
- Complex-I
- Complex-III
- Complex-IV

Steps

The components of ETC are arranged sequentially in the order of increasing redox potential. A redox potential of 0.2 volt between two components of ETC results in the formation of one molecule of ATP through transfer of reducing equivalent.

P:O ratio is defined as the number of ATP synthesized per atom of oxygen consumed.

Note

ATP synthesis—two concepts:
1. **Conventional concept:**
   - When a substrate is oxidized through NAD linked dehydrogenases at ETC, 3 molecules of ATP are formed by per atom of oxygen ($1/2 O_2$) utilized. (P:O ratio = 3).
   - When a substrate is oxidized through FAD linked dehydrogenases at ETC, 2 molecules of ATP are formed per atom of oxygen ($1/2 O_2$) utilized. (P:O ratio = 2).
2. **Current concept:**
   ATP synthesis (current concept)
   - NADH in ETC: 2.5 ATP
   - FADH in ETC: 1.5 ATP
   (No change in substrate level phosphorylation)
   Thus:
   - Complete oxidation of glucose (one molecule).
     – Glycolysis (Aerobic): 7 ATP (Net)
     – Link reaction: 5 ATP (Net)
     – Citric acid cycle: 10 ATP (Per turn)–(Net), 20 ATP (Total)–Net
     – (Glucose → CO_2 + H_2O): 32 ATP–(Net).
   - β–oxidation of fatty acid (palmitic acid) = 106 ATP–Net.

Mechanism

Three hypotheses have been proposed to explain the mechanism of oxidative phosphorylation.
1. *Chemical coupling hypothesis:* It involves direct chemical coupling at all stages of the process.
2. *Conformational coupling hypothesis:* Mitochondrial cristae undergo conformational changes representing high energy states.
3. *Chemiosmotic theory:* It is the widly accepted mechanism of oxidative phosphorylation proposed by Peter Mitchell in 1961. The transport of electron through ETC generates hydrogen ions (protons) which are translocated from the matrix to the inner membrane space through the inner

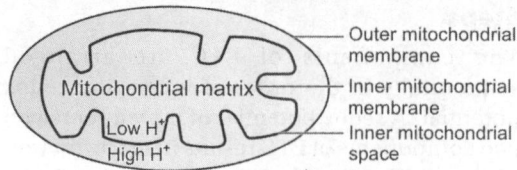

Fig. 10.2: Chemiosmotic theory.

mitochondrial membrane. This process results in an electrochemical (proton) gradient due to accumulation of more hydrogen ions on the outerside of inner mitochondrial membrane than the innerside. The proton gradient developed is used to synthesize ATP from ADP and Pi by ATP synthase (**Fig. 10.2**).

Agents which Inhibit ETC and/or Oxidative Phosphorylation

They can be divided into three types:
1. *Inhibitors of ETC:* They inhibit oxidation as well as phosphorylation. They occur at 3 sites of ATP formation of ETC.
   - *Complex-I:* Rotenone (fish poison), Piericidin (antibiotic), Amobarbital (barbiturates)
   - *Complex-III:* Antimycin A, dimercaprol
   - *Complex-IV:* Cyanide, carbon monoxide, H_2S
2. *Inhibitors of oxidative phosphorylation:* These agents inhibit a step in oxidative phosphorylation, e.g., oligomycin, atractyloside
3. *Uncouplers of oxidative phosphorylation:* These agents uncouple (dissociate) oxidative phosphorylation from ETC, i.e., They prevent the formation of energy but permit oxidation to proceed with generation of heat.
   - Examples: 2, 4 dinitrophenol, 2,4 dinitrocresol, pentachlorophenol.
   - Physiological uncouplers (thyroxine, long chain free fatty acids).

Importance

- ATP is the energy currency of the cell. It is the major storage form of energy in the body.
- ETC is responsible for a large proportion of total ATP production.

■ BIOENERGETICS

Definition

Bioenergetics is the study of energy changes accompanying biochemical reactions in the body.

Alternative Name

Biochemical thermodynamics.

Sources of Energy

Suitable fuel is required to provide the energy that enables the body to carry out its normal functions.
- Glucose is formed by photosynthesis from CO_2 and H_2O utilizing solar radiation.

$$CO_2 + H_2O + E \rightarrow Glucose$$

- Glucose is oxidized to CO_2 and H_2O in the biological systems and the stored energy is released.

$$Glucose \rightarrow CO_2 + H_2O + energy$$

Acetyl-CoA and all other products of metabolism of lipids, proteins are oxidized to CO_2 and H_2O through citric acid cycle. Energy liberated during this phase is stored in the form of high energy compounds.

Free energy: It is that portion of the total energy change in a system that is available for doing work. It is represented as ΔG.

Types of Reactions Involving Energy

- *Exergonic reaction:* It indicates loss (liberation) of energy. It occurs during catabolism

$$A \xrightarrow{-E} B$$

- *Endergonic reaction:* It indicates gain of energy. It occurs during anabolism.

$$C \xrightarrow{+E} D$$

Release of Stored Energy and its Uses

Energy stored is released when necessary to drive different functions of the body.

Exergonic reactions → *Endergonic reactions:* Synthetic reactions, nerve excitation, active transport, muscular contraction, etc.

Chapter 10: Biological Oxidation, Electron Transport Chain, and Bioenergetics

Energy Compounds

All organisms must obtain free energy from the environment. Energy compounds are formed in the body through different processes. They are involved in energy capture and transfer.

Process	Energy compounds formed
Oxidative phosphorylation	ATP
Substrate level phosphorylation	ATP, GTP
Transphosphorylation	Creatine phosphate

Types

All the energy compounds found in the body are of two types based on their standard free energy of hydrolysis of the terminal phosphate of ATP.

High-energy Compounds

These compounds release more calories of energy (at least 7,000 C/mol or 7.0 C/mol) on hydrolysis. (High energy bond is noted as ~ E. Higher energy phosphate is designated as ~ P), for example:

- *ATP (adenosine triphosphate):* It is a nucleotide. It is the energy currency of the cell. It gives up to 7,300 calories during release of one phosphate.

    ATP → ADP + Pi + 7,300 calories (7.3 C)

- *Phosphagens:* Creatine phosphate
- *Acyl phosphates:* 1, 3 diphosphoglycerate
- *Enol phosphate:* Phosphoenol pyruvate
- *S-adenosylmethionine.*

Low-energy Compounds

These compounds release less energy (<7,000 C/mol or 7.0 C/mol) compared to high energy compounds, e.g.:

- *Adenosine diphosphate (ADP):* It is formed during hydrolysis of ATP. It is also a nucleotide. It contains one low-energy phosphate bond. It gives up 6,600 calories during release.

    ADP → AMP + Pi + 6,600 calories (6.6 C)

- *Adenosine monophosphate (AMP):* It is formed during hydrolysis of ADP. It contains only one low energy bond. It gives up 3,000 calories during release.

    AMP → Adenine + Ribose + Pi + 3,000 (3.0 C) calories

- *Others:*
    - Glucose 1-phosphate
    - Glucose 6-phosphate
    - Fructose 6-phosphate
    - Glycerol 3-phosphate

Importance

- Biologic systems utilize chemical energy to carry out the living processes.
- Organism obtains this energy from its body.
- Excess energy results in obesity. Malnutrition is associated with deficiency of energy.

■ ADDITIONAL INFORMATION

Substrate-level Phosphorylation

The process in which ATP is produced directly during substrate level oxidation in a metabolic pathway is known as substrate level phosphorylation. It may occur in cytosol or mitochondria:

- 1, 3 bisphosphoglycerate $\xrightarrow{\text{Glycolysis}}$ 3 phosphoglycerate + ATP
- Phosphoenol pyruvate $\xrightarrow{\text{Glycolysis}}$ pyruvate + ATP
- Succinyl-CoA $\xrightarrow{\text{Citric acid cycle}}$ succinate + GTP → ATP

11. Digestion, Absorption, and Metabolism of Carbohydrates

Chapter Outline

- Digestion
- Absorption
- Metabolism of Glucose
- Alternative Pathways of Glucose Catabolism
- Metabolism of Other Sugars
- Blood Sugar Regulation
- Glucose Tolerance Test (GTT)
- Additional Information

■ INTRODUCTION

Dietary carbohydrates provide a major portion of the daily caloric requirement. They consist of mostly polysaccharides, disaccharides and to minor extent monosaccharides. Monosaccharides need not be hydrolyzed for absorption, but disaccharides and polysaccharides require digestion by enzymes in the gastrointestinal tract before absorption.

■ DIGESTION (FIG. 11.1)

Mouth

α-amylase present in saliva (salivary amylase, optimum pH 6.7) hydrolyzes α - 1,4 glycosidic linkages of starch and glycogen producing smaller molecules namely maltose (disaccharide), maltotriose, and α-limit dextrin (branched oligosaccharides).

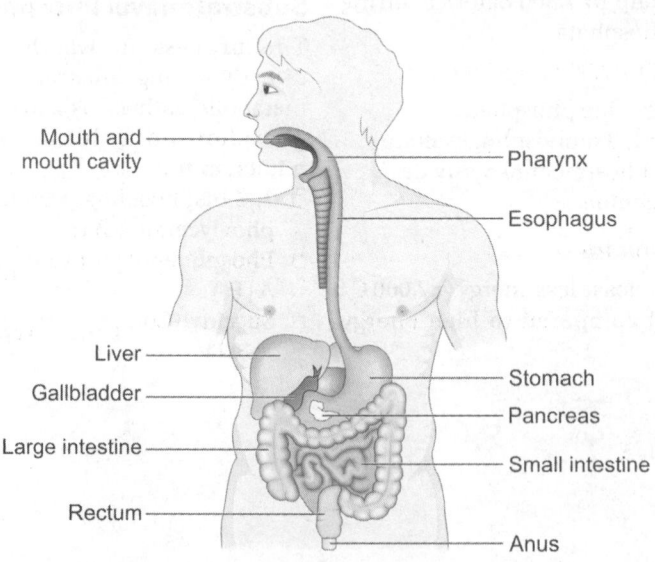

Fig. 11.1: Digestive system.

Starch/glycogen → Maltose + Maltotriose + α- Limit dextrin.

Stomach

No carbohydrate splitting enzymes are present in gastric juice. But some dietary sucrose may be hydrolyzed to glucose and fructose by hydrochloric acid.

Small Intestine

Enzymes present in the small intestine act on the partially digested carbohydrates.

Pancreatic α-amylase (optimum pH 7.1)

It hydrolyzes α-1,4 glycosidic linkages producing maltose maltotriose, isomaltose, α-limit dextrin, nonbranched oligosaccharide.

Starch/Glycogen → Maltose + Maltotriose + α-limit dextrin + Nonbranched oligosaccharide + Isomaltose.

Brush Border Enzymes

Isomaltase

It hydrolyzes α 1,6 glycosidic linkages thus splitting isomaltose at branch points producing glucose.

Isomaltose $\xrightarrow{\text{Isomaltase}}$ Glucose + Glucose

α-limit dextrin $\xrightarrow{\text{Dextrinase}}$ Glucose + Maltose

Disaccharidases

These enzymes will hydrolyze disaccharides to monosaccharides.

- Maltase hydrolyzes maltose to glucose

  Maltose $\xrightarrow{\text{Maltase}}$ Glucose + Glucose

- Lactase hydrolyzes lactose to glucose and galactose

  Lactose $\xrightarrow{\text{Lactase}}$ Glucose + Glucose

- Sucrase hydrolyzes sucrose to glucose and fructose

  Sucrose $\xrightarrow{\text{Sucrase}}$ Glucose + Fructose

Thus, the final products of digestion of carbohydrates are monosaccharides.

Cellulose (polysaccharide) is not digested by human beings because of absence of enzyme hydrolase (cellulase).

> **Clinical Importance: Disorders**
>
> Intestinal disaccharidase deficiencies are encountered frequently in humans, e.g., lactose intolerance.

Lactose Intolerance

It is the major disorder of digestion of carbohydrates. It refers to intolerance to lactose (milk sugar).

Cause

Due to deficiency of lactase, lactose is not converted to glucose and galactose in the small intestine. Accumulated lactose is fermented by intestinal bacteria forming gas (methane, CO_2) and other products (lactate).

Lactose $\xrightarrow{\text{Lactase}}$ Glucose + Galactose

Symptoms

Osmotic diarrhea, flatulence (increased intestinal motility, cramps and irritation).

Diagnosis

- Lactose tolerance test.
- Radiological examination with barium meal.

Treatment

Restrict lactose, milk products containing lactose. Administer lactase (present in yoghurt or commercial preparation) and oral rehydration therapy (ORT).

■ ABSORPTION

Glucose, fructose and galactose are the major monosaccharides resulting from digestion of dietary carbohydrates. They are absorbed almost entirely from the small intestine (duodenum and upper jejunum). They are transported from the lumen into mucosal cells by different transport mechanisms involving specific carrier proteins (Glucose transporters - GLUT). These sugars leave the cell at the basolateral membrane and reach the capillaries by facilitated diffusion via a common transporter **(Fig. 11.2)**.

Inhibitors

- *Ouabain:* Inhibitor of sodium pump
- *Phlorhizin:* Inhibitor of glucose absorption in the kidney

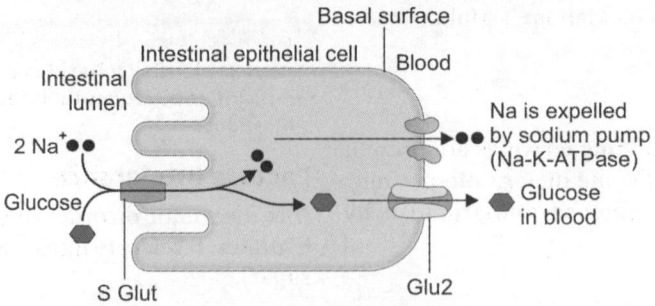

Fig. 11.2: Glucose absorption.

Disorders
They arise due to malabsorption of sugars caused by deficiency of disaccharidases, e.g., lactose malabsorption syndrome.

■ METABOLISM OF GLUCOSE

It can be divided into two parts:
1. Catabolism of glucose
2. Anabolism of glucose

Catabolism of Glucose (Major Pathways)

Catabolism (degradation/breakdown) of glucose can be studied under three heads:
1. Glycolysis
2. Link reaction
3. Citric acid cycle

Glycolysis (Fig. 11.3)

Glycolysis is the first part of major catabolic pathway for the complete oxidation of glucose.

Alternative name
- Embden-Meyerhof pathway/Embden-Meyerhof-Parnas pathway (EMP)
- Meaning:
  Glyco = Sweet; Lysis = Loosening/split (Greek).

Definition
Degradation of glucose to pyruvate (in aerobic conditions) or lactate (in anaerobic conditions) is known as glycolysis.

Glucose → Pyruvate (Aerobic)
         → Lactate (Anaerobic)

Site
- *Organ:* It occurs almost in all tissues
- *Cell:* Cytosol

Conditions
Aerobic and anaerobic conditions.

Pathway*
Glycolysis can be divided into three phases.

Energy investment phase
- Glucose is first phosphorylated by ATP to glucose 6-phosphate by the specific enzyme glucokinase in liver and also by nonspecific enzyme hexokinase in liver, and extra-hepatic tissues.
- Glucose 6-phosphate is converted to fructose 6-phosphate by phosphohexose isomerase.
- Fructose 6-phosphate is phosphorylated with ATP by phosphofructokinase to form fructose 1,6-bisphosphate.

Splitting phase
- Fructose 1,6-bisphosphate is split by the enzyme aldolase into glyceraldehyde 3-phosphate and dihydroxyacetone phosphate.
- Glyceraldehyde 3-phosphate and dihydroxyacetone phosphate are interconverted by phosphotriose isomerase.

Energy generation phase
- Glyceraldehyde 3-phosphate is oxidized to 1,3-bisphosphoglycerate by glyceraldehyde 3-phosphate dehydrogenase with NAD as coenzyme.
- 1,3-bisphosphoglycerate is converted to 3-phosphoglycerate by phosphoglycerate kinase.
- 3-phosphoglycerate is converted to 2-phosphoglycerate by phosphoglycerate mutase.
- Enolase catalyzes elimination of water from 2-phosphoglycerate to form phosphoenol pyruvate.

---
* Refers to steps/reactions throughout the book

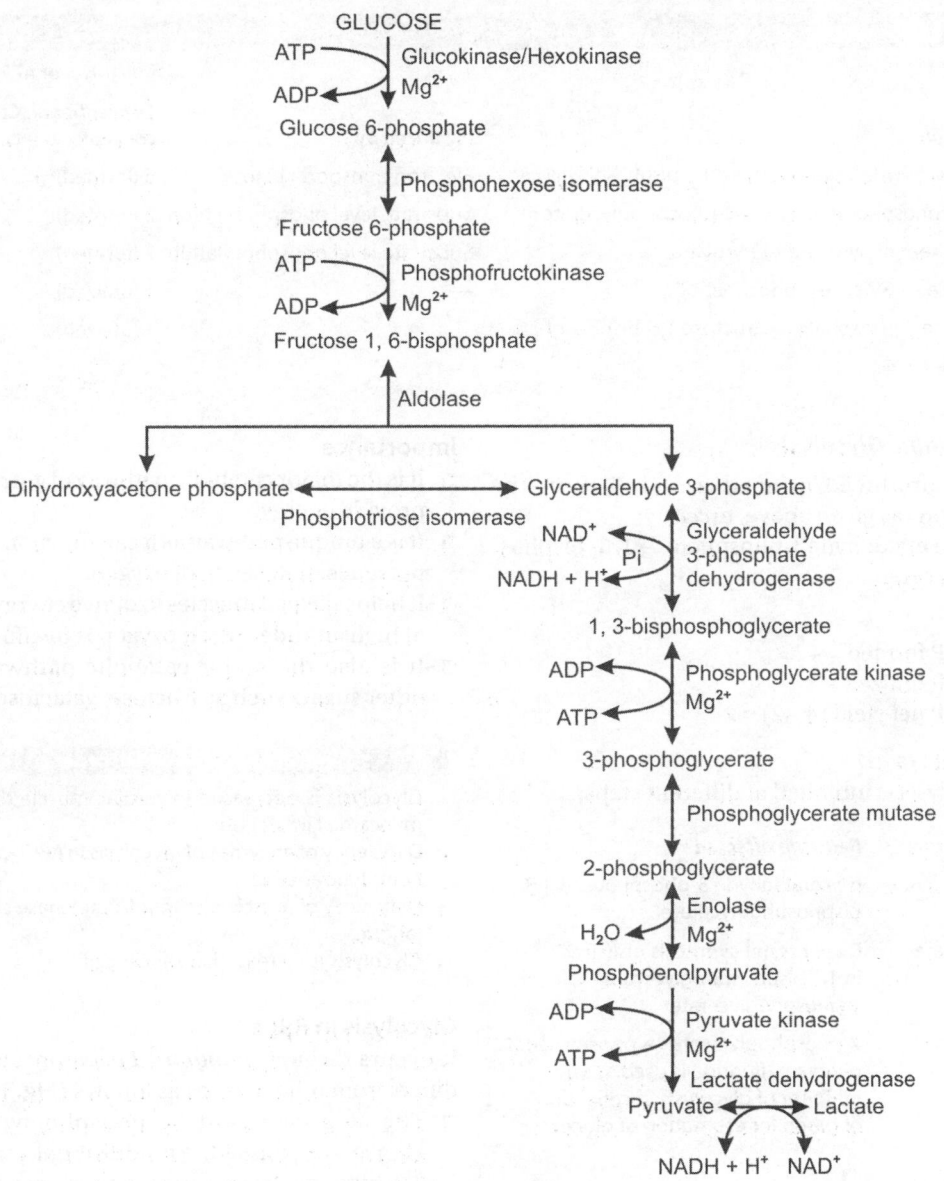

Fig. 11.3: Glycolysis.

- Phosphoenol pyruvate is converted to pyruvate by pyruvate kinase through transfer of high energy phosphate to ADP to form ATP.

Types

Degradation of pyruvate depends on the presence or absence of oxygen in the tissues.

Thus glycolysis is of two types:
1. *Aerobic glycolysis:* In presence of oxygen, pyruvate is oxidatively converted to acetyl-CoA which then enters citric acid cycle producing CO_2 and H_2O.
2. *Anaerobic glycolysis:* In absence of oxygen, pyruvate is reduced to lactate by the enzyme lactate dehydrogenase (LDH).

Energetics

Aerobic Glycolysis

It is shown in **Table 11.1**.

Section 3: Metabolism

Table 11.1: Energetics—aerobic glycolysis.

Reaction	Produced by	No. of ATP Conventional concept	No. of ATP Current concept
Glyceraldehyde 3-phosphate → 1,3-bisphosphoglycerate	Electron transport chain	6 (formed)	5
1,3-bisphosphoglycerate → 3-phosphoglycerate	Substrate level phosphorylation	2 (formed)	2
Phosphoenol pyruvate → Pyruvate	Substrate level phosphorylation	2 (formed)	2
Glucose → Glucose 6-phosphate	—	1 (utilized)	1
Fructose 6-phosphate → Fructose 1,6-bisphosphate		1 (utilized)	1
ATPs net yield		8	7

Anaerobic Glycolysis

ATPs produced/utilized are similar in the reactions as given above, *except*
Glyceraldehyde 3-phosphate → 1, 3- bisphosphoglycerate.

Thus,
- ATP formed = 4
- ATP utilized = 2
- ATP net yield (4 – 2) = 2

Inhibitors

Glycolysis is inhibited at different steps:

Inhibitors	Reaction affected
Iodoacetate	Glyceraldehyde 3-phosphate → 1,3, bisphosphoglycerate
Arsenate	Prevents net synthesis of ATP in 1,3 bisphosphoglycerate → 3-phosphoglycerate
Fluoride	2-phosphoglycerate → phosphoenol pyruvate (fluoride is used as an inhibitor of glycolysis in collection of blood for estimation of glucose)

Regulation

It is regulated at three steps (irreversible reaction) catalyzed by the following enzymes.

Enzyme	Activation	Inhibition
1. a. Hexokinase (present in all tissues)	–	Glucose 6 phosphate
b. Glucokinase (present in liver)	Insulin	Glucagon
2. Phosphofructokinase (regulatory enzyme)	Insulin, AMP	Glucagon, ATP
3. Pyruvate kinase	Insulin	Glucagon, ATP

Importance

- It is the major catabolic pathway of glucose to provide energy.
- It is a unique pathway as it can function in the presence or absence of oxygen.
- It helps skeletal muscles to derive energy even at high altitudes when oxygen is insufficient.
- It is also the major catabolic pathway for other sugars such as fructose, galactose, etc.

Clinical Importance: Disorders

- Glycolysis is decreased in cardiac muscle during myocardial infarction.
- Deficiency of enzymes of glycolysis in RBCs causes hemolytic anemia.
- Deficiency of muscle phosphofructokinase causes fatigue.
- Glycolysis is increased in cancer cells.

Glycolysis in RBCs

It occurs through *Rapoport Luebering cycle*. It differs from other tissues as follows **(Fig. 11.4)**:
- The step catalyzed by phosphoglycerate kinase is bypassed. An additional enzyme 2,3-bisphosphoglycerate mutase catalyzes, conversion of 1,3 bisphosphoglycerate to 2,3 bisphosphoglycerate (2, 3-BPG).
- 2,3-BPG is converted to 3-phosphoglycerate by 2,3-bisphosphoglycerate phosphatase.
- It terminates in formation of lactate because RBCs lack mitochondria.

Importance

- 2,3 bisphosphoglycerate formed in this reaction in RBCs causes a decrease in affinity of oxygen and displacement of the oxyhemoglobin dissociation curve to the right. It thus helps oxyhemoglobin to unload

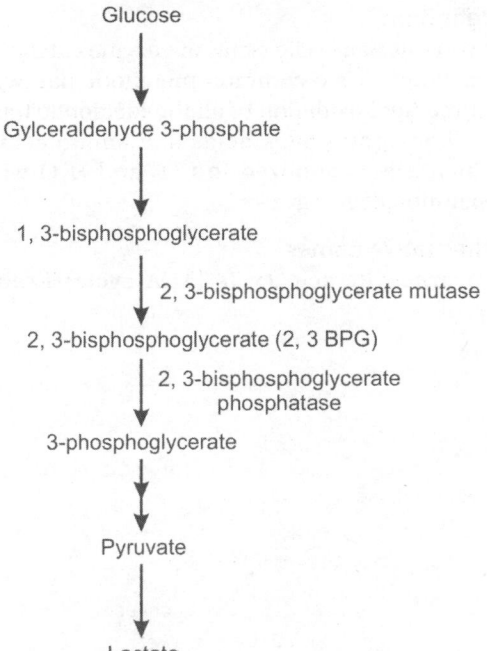

Fig. 11.4: Rapoport Luebering cycle.

oxygen to tissues. It is increased in hypoxia and anemia.
- RBCs depend entirely on glucose for energy through glycolysis.
- Deficiency of enzymes of glycolysis in RBCs causes hemolytic anemia.
- It is a shunt pathway of glycolysis to use minimum ATP in RBCs.

Link Reaction
It refers to conversion of pyruvate to acetyl-CoA. It links glycolysis with citric acid cycle (**Fig. 11.5**).

Site
- *Organ:* Most tissues
- *Cell:* Mitochondria

Conditions
It occurs in aerobic conditions only.
(Pyruvic acid formed in glycolysis under aerobic conditions in the cytosol of the cell is then transported to mitochondria through a special transporter).

Pathway
Pyruvate is converted to acetyl-CoA (active acetate) by oxidative decarboxylation. This reaction is catalyzed by a multienzyme complex known as pyruvate dehydrogenase complex. It is a combination of 3 enzymes with cofactors.

Enzymes
- Pyruvate dehydrogenase
- Dihydrolipoyl transacetylase
- Dihydrolipoyl dehydrogenase

Cofactors
Thiamine pyrophosphate (TPP)
FAD, NAD, lipoic acid, CoA - SH, Mg^{++}

Energetics
Two molecules of pyruvic acid are converted to two molecules of acetyl-CoA.

	Conventional concept	Current concept
ATP produced	6	5
ATP utilized	Nil	Nil
Net ATP yield	6	5

Inhibitors
- Arsenite
- Vitamin B_1 (thiamine) deficiency: Both inhibit pyruvate dehydrogenase.

Regulation
Pyruvate dehydrogenase is regulated by end-product inhibition and covalent modification.

Disorders (Clinical Importance)

Lactic acidosis	It is a metabolic disorder of carbohydrates
Cause	Due to deficiency of pyruvate dehydrogenase or due to increased glycolysis. It occurs in hypoxia, shock, diabetes mellitus, strenuous exercise
Symptoms	Accumulation of lactic acid in blood, pH is low. It is lethal
Diagnosis	Estimation of lactic acid in blood

Importance
- It is a link reaction connecting glycolysis and citric acid cycle. It produces energy.

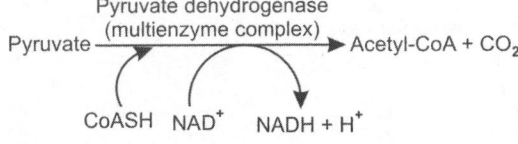

Fig. 11.5: Link reaction.

- It is an example of oxidative decarboxylation.
- It is also an example of reactions catalyzed by a multienzyme complex.
- Pyruvate formed from other sources is also disposed by this process.

Citric Acid Cycle (Fig. 11.6)

It is the final part of complete oxidation of glucose. It produces largest number of ATP in the body.

Definition

It consists of a cyclic series of enzyme catalyzed reactions. It is a common metabolic pathway for the final oxidation of all the metabolic fuels (carbohydrates, fatty acids and amino acids) which are catabolized to CO_2 and H_2O with liberation of energy.

Alternative names

Tricarboxylic acid cycle (TCA cycle)/Kreb's cycle.

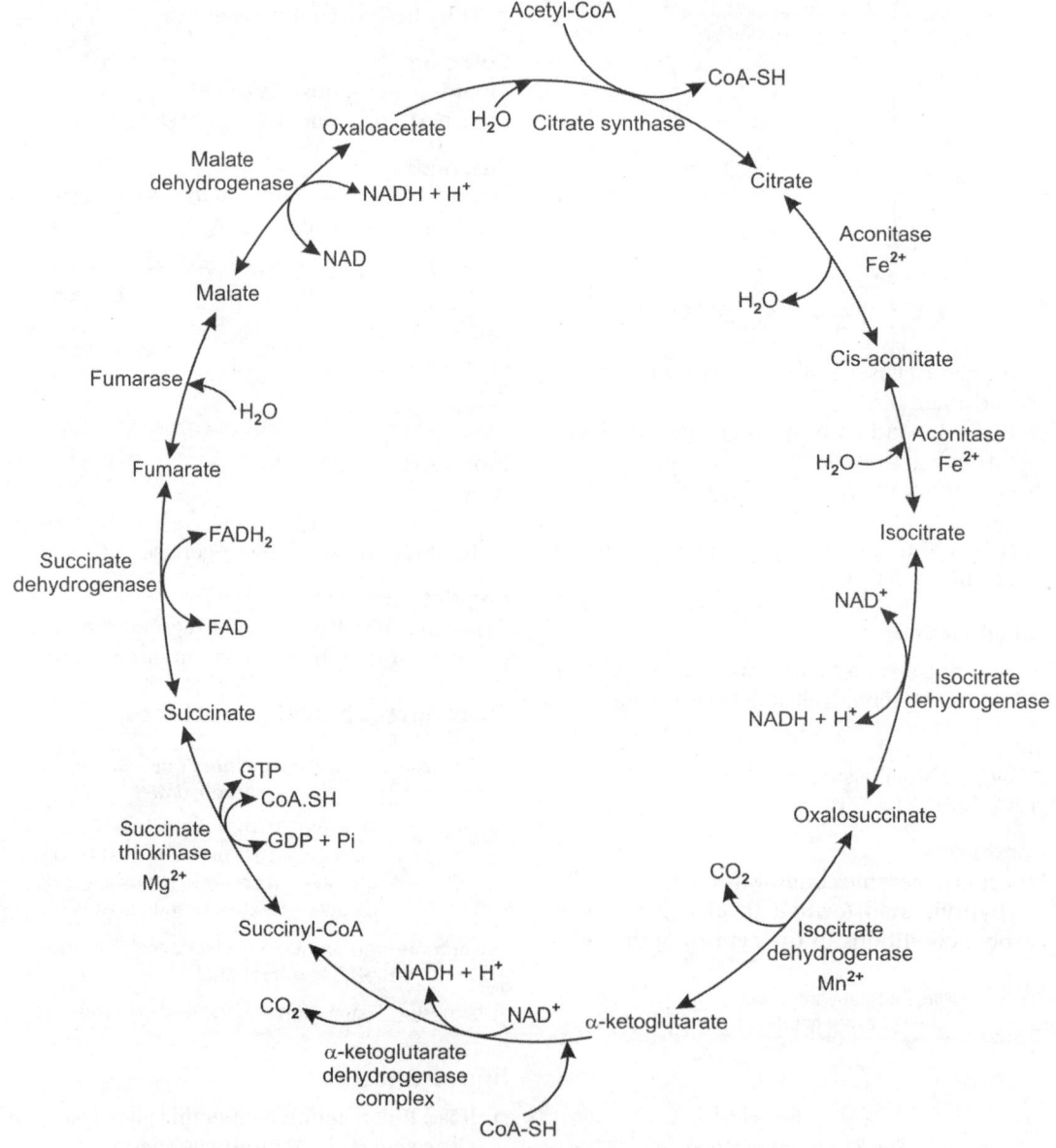

Fig. 11.6: Citric acid cycle.

Chapter 11: Digestion, Absorption, and Metabolism of Carbohydrates

Proposed by: Hans Krebs (1937) (N.P. 1953).

Site
- *Organ:* Occurs in most tissues
- *Cell:* Mitochondria

Condition
Occurs in aerobic conditions only.

Pathway
- *Condensation:* Acetyl-CoA condenses with oxaloacetate to form citrate catalyzed by citrate synthase.
- *Dehydration and rehydration:* Citrate is dehydrated to cis-aconitate which is then rehydrated to isocitrate. Both steps are catalyzed by aconitase requiring Fe^{++}.
- *Dehydrogenation and decarboxylation:* Isocitrate undergoes dehydrogenation to form oxalosuccinate which is decarboxylated to form α-ketoglutarate, both reactions being catalyzed by isocitrate dehydrogenase.
- *Decarboxylation:* α-ketoglutarate undergoes decarboxylation to form succinyl-CoA, being catalyzed by α-ketoglutarate dehydrogenase (multienzyme complex) which requires cofactors, thiamine pyrophosphate (TPP), lipoate, NAD^+, FAD, and CoA.
- *Substrate level phosphorylation:* Succinyl-CoA is converted to succinate by succinate thiokinase. In this reaction GDP is converted to GTP at substrate level phosphorylation.
- *Oxidation:* Succinate is oxidized by succinate dehydrogenase to form fumarate.
- *Hydration:* Fumarate is hydrated to form malate by fumarase.
- *Oxidation:* Malate is oxidized to oxaloacetate catalyzed by malate dehydrogenase in the presence of NAD^+.
- *Condensation and recycling:* Oxaloacetate combines with acetyl-CoA and the cycle continues again.

Inhibitors

Inhibitors	Reaction affected
Fluoroacetate	Citrate → cis-aconitate
Arsenite	α-ketoglutarate → Succinyl-CoA
Malonate	Succinic acid → Fumaric acid

Regulation
- Respiratory control through electron transport chain and oxidative phosphorylation is the overall control of citric acid cycle.
- Reactions catalyzed by citrate synthase, isocitrate dehydrogenase and α-ketoglutarate dehydrogenase are also possible sites for regulation.

Energetics
Each pyruvate molecule produces 2 molecules of acetyl-CoA which enter citric acid cycle producing 20 ATPs. Thus 1 molecule of acetyl-CoA produces 10 ATPs per turn of citric acid cycle (current concept) **(Table 11.2)**.

Biomedical importance
- It is the final common pathway for oxidation of not only carbohydrates, but also lipids and proteins.
- TCA cycle as amphibolic pathway: Amphibolism is a metabolic pathway which involves both catabolic (degradation) and synthetic pathway, e.g., citric acid cycle.
  - *Catabolic nature:* It is the final oxidative (catabolic) pathway for producing energy from carbohydrates, lipids and proteins.

$$Glucose \rightarrow CO_2 + H_2O + ATP$$

  - *Anabolic nature:* It is provides various intermediates for the synthesis of several compounds in the body.
  - Oxaloacetate → Aspartate ⎫ Non-essential
  - α-ketoglutarate → Glutamate ⎭ amino acids
  - Succinyl-CoA → Porphyrins → Heme
  - Citrate → Acetyl-CoA → Fatty acids

Disorders (Clinical Importance)
Deficiency of fumarase in citric acid cycle has been reported very rarely in humans.

Total ATP (net) formed during complete oxidation of one molecule of glucose to $CO_2 + H_2O$.

	Conventional concept	Current concept
Aerobic glycolysis	8	7
Link reaction	6	5
Krebs cycle	24	20
	38	32

Note
Glucose can also be catabolized by alternate pathways.

Table 11.2: Energetics: citric acid cycle.

Reactions	ATP produced by	No. of ATP Conventional concept	No. of ATP Current concept
Isocitrate → Oxalosuccinate	Electron transport chain	6	5
α-ketoglutarate → Succinyl-CoA	Electron transport chain	6	5
Succinyl-CoA → Succinate	Substrate level phosphorylation	2	2
Succinate → Fumarate	Electron transport chain	4	3
Malate → Oxaloacetate	Electron transport chain	6	5
	ATP formed	24	20
	ATP utilized	Nil	Nil
	ATP net yield	24	20

ALTERNATIVE PATHWAYS OF GLUCOSE CATABOLISM

There are two alternative pathways of catabolism (oxidation) of glucose.
1. Hexose monophosphate (HMP) shunt
2. Uronic acid pathway.

Hexose Monophosphate Shunt

It is one of the alternative pathways of glucose catabolism (oxidation) **(Fig. 11.7)**.

Alternative Names

- Pentose phosphate pathway
- Phosphogluconate pathway

Site

- *Organs:* Liver, adipose tissue, lactating mammary gland, erythrocytes, testes, adrenal cortex, thyroid
- *Cell:* Cytosol

Pathway

It can be divided into two phases:

Oxidative phase

In this phase, glucose is converted to ribulose 5-phosphate (ketopentose) through various steps with the formation of NADPH.
- Glucose is phosphorylated to glucose 6-phosphate.
- Glucose-6-phosphate is dehydrogenated to 6-phosphogluconolactone by glucose 6 phosphate dehydrogenase.
- 6-phosphogluconolactone is hydrolyzed to 6-phosphogluconate by gluconolactone hydrolase.
- 6-phosphogluconate is converted to ribulose 5-phosphate (ketopentose) via 3 - keto 6-phosphogluconate in presence of NADP which is reduced to NADPH.

Nonoxidative phase

In this phase, pentoses undergo rearrangements and the products formed finally enter glycolytic pathway.
- Ribulose 5-phosphate serves as substrate for two different enzymes:
  - It is converted to xylulose 5-phosphate (ketopentose) by epimerase.
  - It is also converted to ribose 5-phosphate (aldopentose) by ketoisomerase.
- Transketolase catalyzes interconversion between xylulose 5-phosphate and ribose 5-phosphate forming sedoheptulose 7-phosphate and glyceraldehyde 3-phosphate.
- Transaldolase catalyzes interconversion between sedoheptulose 7-phosphate and glyceraldehyde 3-phosphate forming erythrose 4-phosphate and fructose 6-phosphate.
- Transketolase also catalyzes synthesis of fructose 6-phosphate and glyceraldehyde 3-phosphate by combining erythrose 4-phosphate and xylulose 5-phosphate.
- Finally fructose 6-phosphate and glyceraldehyde 3-phosphate enter glycolytic pathway for further catabolism.

Chapter 11: Digestion, Absorption, and Metabolism of Carbohydrates

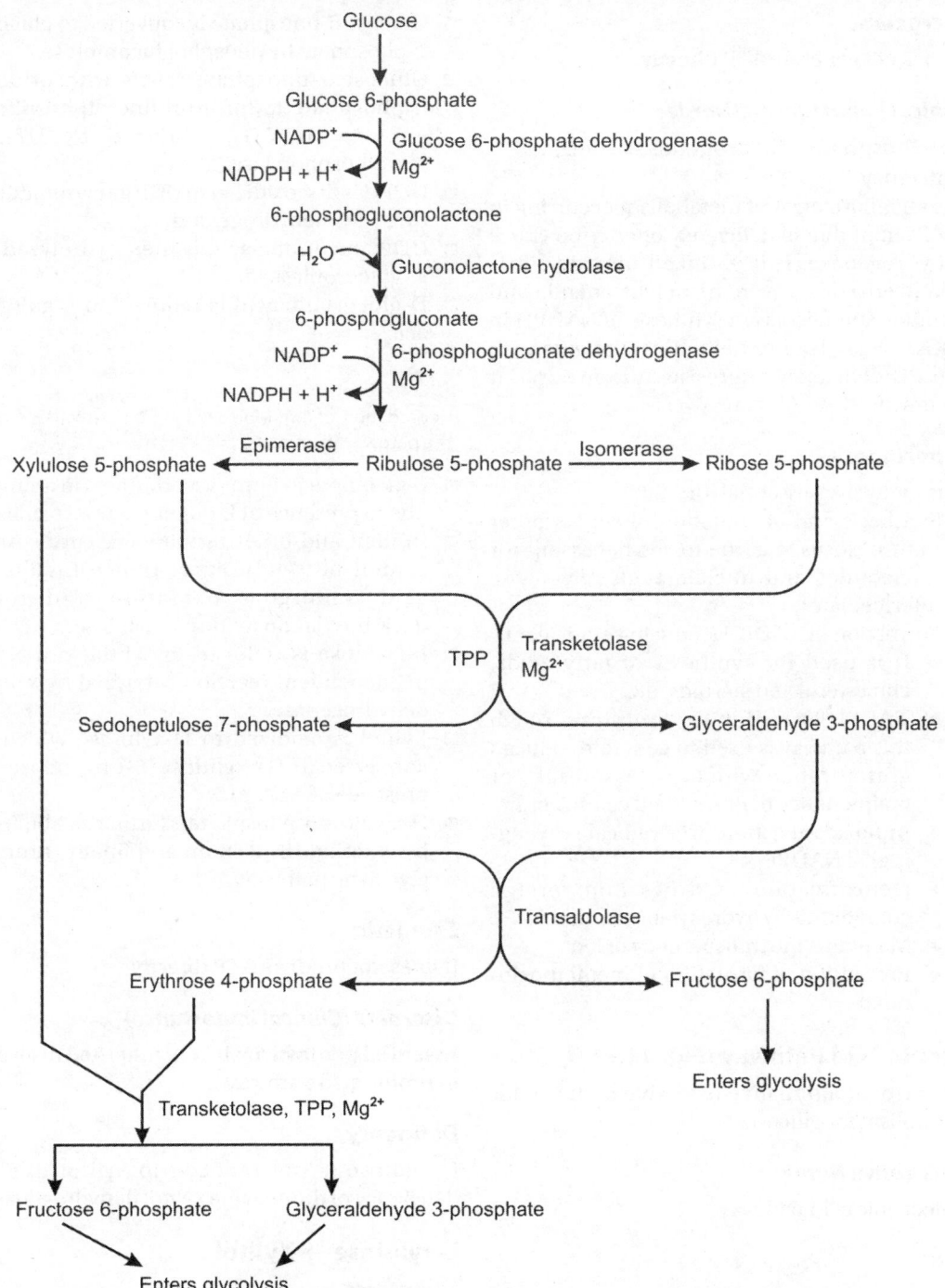

Fig. 11.7: Hexose monophosphate shunt.

Regulation
- Mainly regulated by the level of NADP$^+$
- Step catalyzed by G-6-PD is the rate limiting step.

Energetics
It does not generate ATP directly.

Clinical Importance: Disorder
G-6-Phosphate dehydrogenase (G6PD) deficiency
It is an inborn error of metabolism occurring in HMP shunt due to deficiency of enzyme G-6-P dehydrogenase. It is X linked disorder. It is characterized by severe hemolytic anemia and jaundice and decreased synthesis of NADPH in RBCs. It may lead to hemolysis. Patients with G-6-PD deficiency are resistant to malaria. It occurs mostly in Africans.

Importance
This pathway is essential for:
- Synthesis and degradation of sugars other than hexoses, e.g., pentoses necessary for nucleotides and nucleic acids, glycolytic intermediates.
- Formation of NADPH (reducing equivalent).
  - It is used for synthesis of fatty acids, cholesterol and steroids, etc.
  - NADPH formed in erythrocytes through this pathway is used to generate reduced glutathione, which is essential for maintenance of normal red cell structure.
  - Antioxidant action (free radical scavenging) of $NADP^+$.
  - Detoxification of drugs and foreign compounds by hydroxylation with $NADP^+$.
  - Maintains the transparency of lens
  - Prevention of formation of methemoglobin.

Uronic Acid Pathway (Fig. 11.8)
It is also an alternative oxidative pathway for catabolism for glucose.

Alternative Name
Glucuronic acid pathway.

Site
- *Organs:* Liver
- *Cell:* Cytosol

Pathway
- Glucose is phosphorylated to glucose 6-phosphate.
- Glucose 6-phosphate is converted to glucose 1-phosphate by phosphoglucomutase.
- Glucose 1-phosphate reacts with uridine triphosphate to form uridine diphosphate glucose (UDPG) catalyzed by UDPG pyrophosphorylase.
- UDPG is first oxidized to UDP glucuronic acid by UDPG dehydrogenase.
- UDP glucuronic acid is then hydrolyzed to D-glucuronic acid.
- D-glucuronic acid is reduced to L-gulonic acid.

Note
Degradation of L-gulonic acid in humans varies from the pathway in animals.

- L-gulonic acid forms ascorbic acid in animals due to presence of L-gulonolactone oxidase.
- In men and other primates, ascorbic acid cannot be synthesized. Hence L-gulonic acid undergoes oxidation and then decarboxylation to form L-xylulose.
- L-xylulose is reduced to xylitol in a NADpH dependent reaction catalyzed by xylitol dehydrogenase.
- Xylitol is oxidized to D-xylulose which is converted to D-xylulose 5-phosphate in presence of ATP.
- D-xylulose 5-phosphate is further catabolized by entering HMP shunt and finally through glycolytic pathway.

Energetics
It does not produce ATP directly.

Disorders (Clinical Importance)
Essential pentosuria: It is an inherited disorder in uronic acid pathway.

Deficiency
L-xylulose is not reduced to xylitol due to deficiency of the enzyme xylitol dehydrogenase.

L-xylulose → Xylitol
Symptoms
It is asymptomatic. L-xylulose is highly excreted in urine.

Diagnosis
L-xylulose in urine can be detected by Bial's test.

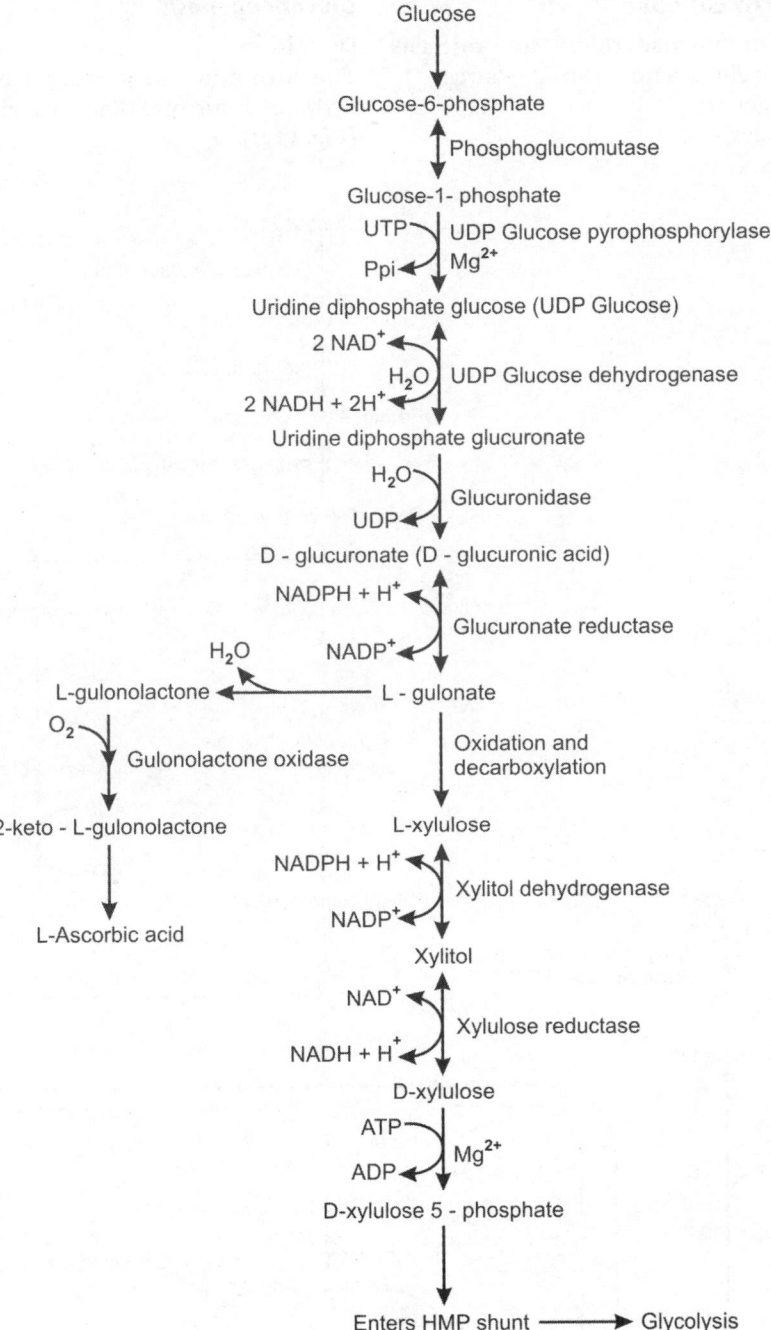

Fig. 11.8: Uronic acid pathway.

Treatment

It is a benign (harmless) condition.

Importance

❏ Glucuronic acid is used:
- In the detoxification of bilirubin and some drugs.
- As constituents of mucopolysaccharides.

❏ This pathway leads to synthesis of ascorbic acid in animals.

Anabolism of Glucose

Anabolism of glucose refers to synthesis (formation) of glucose from various sources:
- Gluconeogenesis
- Glycogenolysis
- Other sugars

Gluconeogenesis

Definition

The formation of glucose from noncarbohydrate precursors is known as gluconeogenesis **(Fig. 11.9)**.

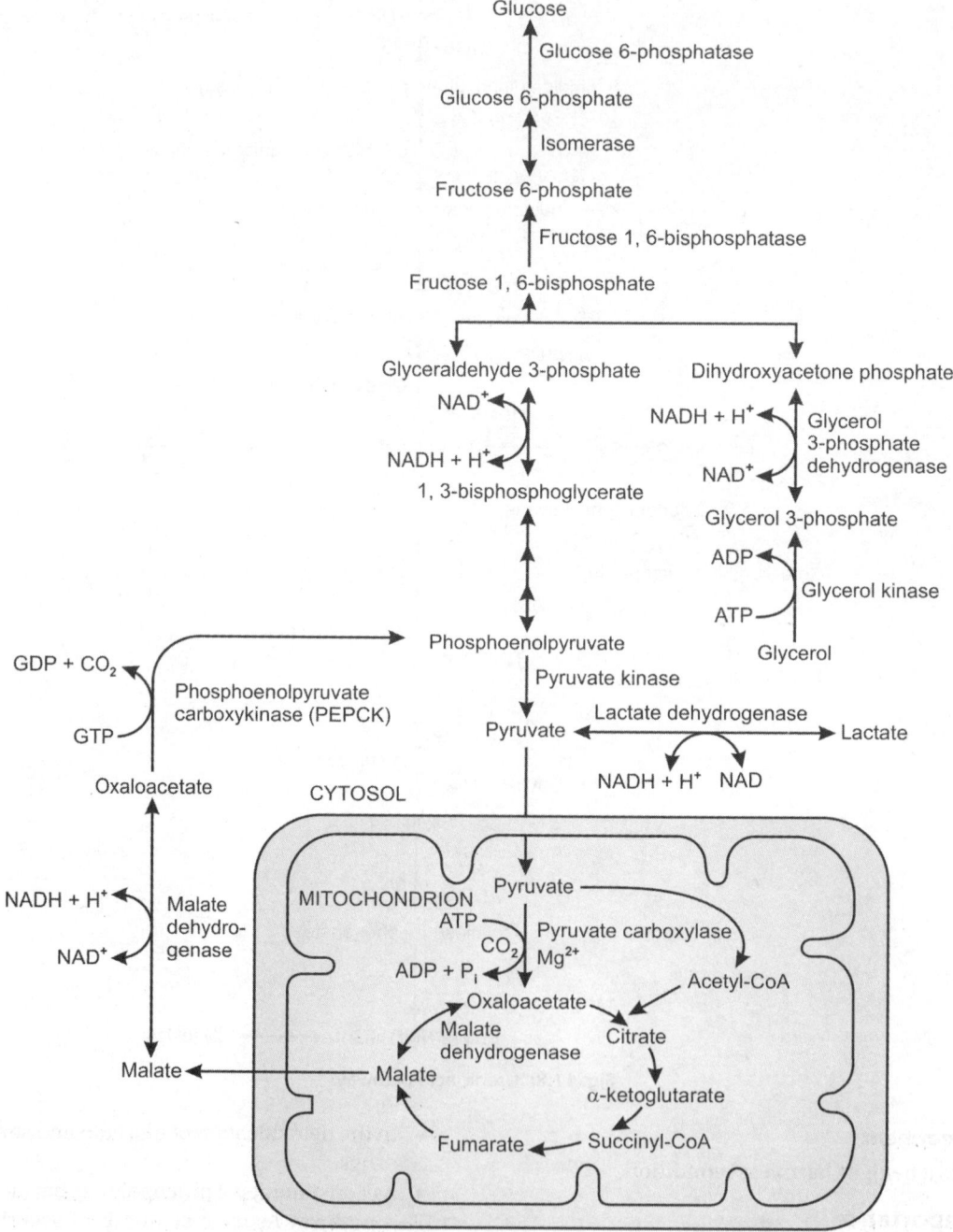

Fig. 11.9: Gluconeogenesis.

Noncarbohydrate precursors are: Pyruvate, lactate, glycerol, glucogenic amino acids, propionate, intermediates of citric acid cycle.

Site
- *Organs:* Approximately 90% of gluconeogenesis occurs in the liver and 10% of it in kidneys.
- *Cell:* Mitochondria and cytosol.

Pathway
Conversion of pyruvate to glucose

In cytosol

Pyruvate cannot be converted to phosphoenolpyruvate (PEP) by pyruvate kinase because this reaction is irreversible. But it can be converted to phosphoenol pyruvate by different route. Pyruvate enters mitochondria from cytosol.

In mitochondria
- Pyruvate is converted to oxaloacetate by pyruvate carboxylase in the presence of ATP, biotin and CO_2.
- Oxaloacetate is impermeable to mitochondrial membrane. It is converted to malate via citric acid cycle.
- Malate then enters cytosol.

In cytosol
- Malate is again oxidized to oxaloacetate by malate dehydrogenase.
- Oxaloacetate is converted to phosphoenolpyruvate by phosphoenolpyruvate carboxykinase (PEPCK).
- Phosphoenolpyruvate is converted to fructose 1,6 - bisphosphate as in glycolytic pathway.
- Fructose 1, 6 bisphosphate is converted to fructose 6 - phosphate by a specific enzyme fructose 1, 6 bisphosphatase.
- Fructose 6-phosphate is converted to glucose 6-phosphate as in glycolic pathway.
- Glucose 6-phosphate is converted to glucose by a specific enzyme glucose 6-phosphatase.

Conversion of lactate to glucose (Cori cycle)

Cori cycle (Fig. 11.10)

Alternative name: Lactic acid cycle.

Lactate is produced in skeletal muscle via anaerobic glycolysis. It is carried to the liver through blood and is converted to glucose by gluconeogenesis which then returns to the skeletal muscles for energy.

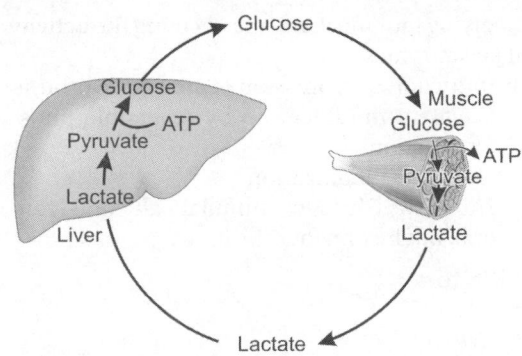

Fig. 11.10: The Cori cycle.

Definition: The cycle involving the synthesis of glucose from lactate formed in the skeletal muscles and to reuse of glucose thus synthesized by the muscles for energy is known as Cori cycle.

Importance:
- Cori cycle links gluconeogenesis with anaerobic glycolysis
- It is important in red blood cells.
- It produces energy.

Conversion of glucogenic amino acids to glucose (glucose alanine cycle)

Glucogenic amino acids after transamination or deamination liberate either pyruvic acid or intermediate compounds of the citric acid cycle. These compounds are converted to malate and finally converted to glucose as explained earlier.

Conversion of glycerol to glucose

Glycerol is phosphorylated to glycerol 3-phosphate by glycerol kinase. Glycerol 3-phosphate is converted to dihydroxyacetone phosphate by glycerol 3 phosphate dehydrogenase. Dihydroxyacetone phosphate is converted to glucose as given in the **Figure 11.9**.

Conversion of propionate to glucose

It is also a substrate for gluconeogenesis.

Energetics

Two molecules of pyruvate are converted to one molecule of glucose by utilizing 6 molecules of ATP.

Regulation

Glycolysis and gluconeogenesis share the same pathway but operates in the opposite directions. Thus their pathway is regulated reciprocally

involving four mechanisms affecting the activity of key enzymes.
- Induction or repression of enzyme synthesis
- Covalent modification by reversible phosphorylation
- Allosteric modification
- *Hormone:* Glucagon stimulate gluconeogenesis, but insulin inhibits it.

Inhibitors
- Ethanol
- ADP

Importance
- It meets the requirements of glucose in the body when glucose is not available in sufficient amount from diet or glucose formed from glycogen stores is not enough.
- It enables the maintenance of blood glucose level during fasting.
- It clears certain metabolites (lactate, glycerol, etc.) from the blood.
- It has reciprocal relationship to glycolysis.

Clinical Importance: Disorder
Defective enzymes of gluconeogenesis lead to hypoglycemia and lactic acidosis.

Glycogenolysis (refer Below)
Glycogen Metabolism

It consists of two phases:
1. Glycogenesis
2. Glycogenolysis

Glycogenesis
Glycogen is a branched homopolysaccharide.

Definition
Synthesis of glycogen from glucose in the liver and muscle is known as glycogenesis (**Fig. 11.11**).
$$\text{Glucose} \rightarrow \text{Glycogen}$$

Site
- *Organ(s):* It occurs practically in all the tissues of the body, but the major sites are liver and muscles.
- *Cell:* Cytosol

Pathway
- Glucose is first phosphorylated to glucose 6-phosphate by glucokinase in liver and hexokinase in peripheral tissues, such as muscles.
- Glucose 6-phosphate is then converted to glucose 1-phosphate by phosphoglucomutase.

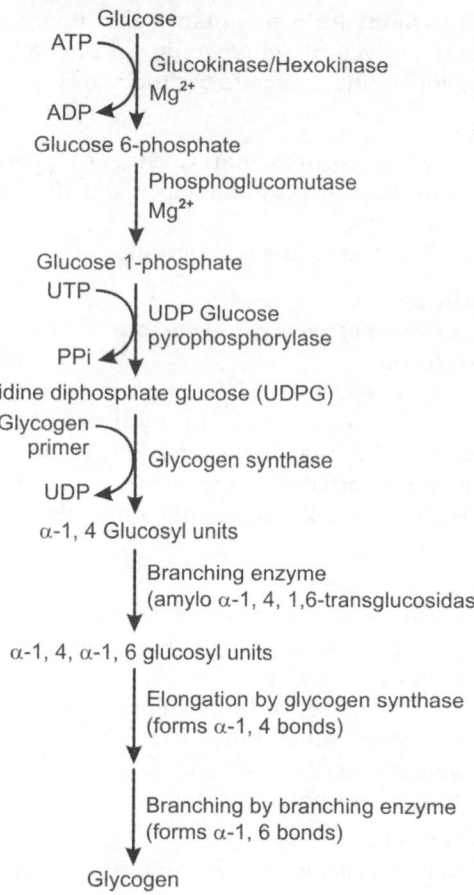

Fig. 11.11: Glycogenesis.

- Glucose 1-phosphate reacts with uridine triphosphate (UTP) to form uridine diphosphate glucose (UDPG) catalyzed by the enzyme UDPG pyrophosphorylase.
- Glycogen synthase catalyzes transfer of the activated glucose molecule (glucosyl - moiety) of UDPG to a pre-existing glycogen molecule (glycogen primer) at its non-reducing (outer) end to form α-1, 4-glucosyl unit.
- The glycogen chain thus gradually lengthens with the successive additions of glucose moieties having α-1, 4 linkages (straight chain).
- Once the growing glycogen chain reaches a minimum of 11 glucose moieties, a branching enzyme (amylo α 1, 4 → 1,6 transglucosidase) transfers a part of the chain with a minimum of 6 glucose residues to another chain to form α 1, 6 linkage thus establishing a branched point.
- The branches of glycogen molecule grow by further addition of α 1, 4 glucosyl residues and further branching.

Energetics: 2 ATP are utilized.

Glycogenolysis

Definition
Breakdown of glycogen to glucose in liver, and to lactate in extrahepatic tissues, such as muscles is known as glycogenolysis **(Fig. 11.12)**.

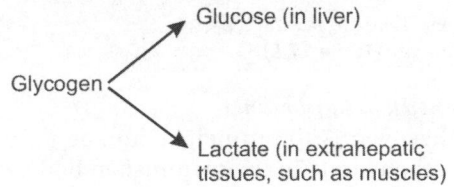

Site
- *Organ(s):* Liver and extrahepatic tissues like muscles.
- *Cell:* Cytosol

Pathway
1. a. Glycogen phosphorylase breaks α 1, 4 linkage in glycogen molecule and removes glucose 1-phosphate.
   b. The removal of glucose residues continues until 4 glucosyl residues remain on either side of α 1, 6 linkage.
   c. 3 of these glucosyl residues may be shifted to a different chain by debranching

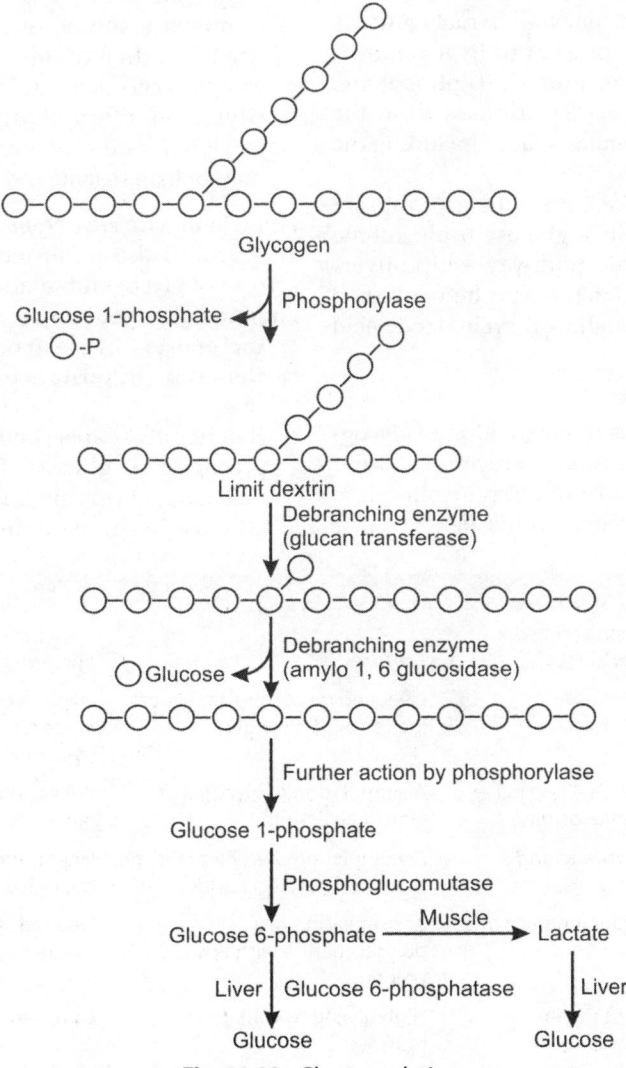

Fig. 11.12: Glycogenolysis.

enzyme (glucan transferase) thus exposing α-1, 6 linkage.
d. α-1, 6, linkage is then hydrolytically split by the debranching enzyme (amylo 1, 6 glucosidase) and releases a free glucose. Thus branches are removed.
e. Further, action of phosphorylase continues to provide glucose-1-phosphate.
2. Glucose-1-phosphate is then converted to glucose 6-phosphate by phosphoglucomutase.

Note

All the above steps are similar in the liver and muscles. The pathway hereafter differs.

3. a. *Liver:* A specific enzyme namely glucose 6-phosphatase present in liver removes phosphate from glucose 6-phosphate. Free glucose formed diffuses from the cells to extracellular spaces including the blood.
b. *Muscles:* Glucose 6-phosphatase is absent in muscles. Hence glucose 6-phosphate enters glycolytic pathway and converted to lactate. Lactate can be converted to glucose through Cori cycle (lactic acid cycle).

Regulation
Cyclic AMP integrates the regulation of glycogenolysis and glycogenesis in a reciprocal order by promoting the activation of phosphorylase and inhibition of glycogen synthase.

Clinical Importance: Disorders of Glycogen Metabolism

Glycogen storage diseases
Definition: It refers to a group of inborn errors of glycogen metabolism. They are characterized by deposition of abnormal quantity or altered type of glycogen in tissues.
Types: There are several types
Examples: **(Table 11.3)**

Biomedical importance
❏ Glycogen is the principal storage form of carbohydrate in the mammalian body. It is stored mainly in the liver and muscles.
❏ Glycogen present in the liver serves as immediate source of blood glucose to be used in other tissues for energy. Muscle glycogen serves the needs of that organ only.
❏ Glycogen storage diseases occur due to deficiencies of enzymes of glycogen metabolism in liver and muscles.

von Gierke's disease (type 1)
It is one of the inherited disorders (inborn errors) of glycogen metabolism. It is the most common glycogen storage disease.
❏ **Incidence:** 1 in 2 lakh persons.
❏ **Genetics (inheritance):** Autosomal recessive.
❏ **Biochemical cause:** Body cannot breakdown glycogen to glucose for energy. Due to deficiency of enzyme glucose-6-phosphatase. Glucose 6 phosphate is not converted

Table 11.3: Glycogen storage diseases.

Sl. No.	Name	Cause (enzyme deficiency)	Features	Symptoms
1.	von Gierke's disease	Glucose-6-phosphatase	Liver and renal tubular cells are loaded with glycogen	Hypoglycemia, lactic acidemia, ketosis, hyperlipidemia, hyperuricemia (*see* above)
2.	Pompe's disease	α 1→ 4 and α 1→ 6-glucosidase	Accumulation of glycogen in almost all tissues	Enlargement of heart, heart failure. No hypoglycemia
3.	Cori's disease	Debranching enzyme	Accumulation of a characteristic branched polysaccharide	Hepatomegaly, moderate hypoglycemia
4.	Andersen's disease	Branching enzyme	Accumulation of a polysaccharide with few branch points	Death due to cardiac or liver failure
5.	Mc Ardle's syndrome	Muscle phosphorylase	High glycogen content in muscles	Diminished exercise tolerance
6.	Her's disease	Liver phosphorylase	High glycogen content in liver	Hypoglycemia

to glucose in the liver and released into blood.

Glucose 6–phosphate → Glucose.

- **Symptoms:**
  - Hypoglycemia
    Clinical
    - Enlarged liver, swollen belly
    - Fatigue
    - Constant hunger
    - Weak muscles
    - Muscle pain
  - Lactic acidosis
  - Hyperlipidemia
  - Hyperuricemia

Diagnosis: Estimation of G-6-phosphatase in blood.

Treatment: To give small quantity of food at frequent intervals.

Metabolism of Other Sugars

Fructose metabolism

It is a monosaccharide (ketohexose). Fructose is absorbed by facilitated diffusion from small intestine and reaches liver through portal blood. It is metabolized as follows **(Fig. 11.13)**:

Site
- *Organ:* Liver, kidney, intestine
- *Cell:* Cytosol

Major pathway
Fructose is converted to fructose 1-phosphate by fructokinase. Fructose 1-P is split into D- glyceraldehyde and dihydroxyacetone phosphate by aldolase B. D-glyceraldehyde can be converted to D-glyceraldehyde 3-P by triokinase. Glyceraldehyde 3-P and dihydroxyacetone-P can enter glycolysis and be degraded or they may combine by aldolase A and be converted to glucose by gluconeogenesis.

Minor pathway
It occurs in all cells. Fructose is phosphorylated to fructose 6-P by hexokinase. Fructose 6-phosphate can be converted to glucose **(Fig. 11.13)**.

Importance
- It forms glucose in liver.
- It is source of energy for sperms.
- It stimulates fatty acid synthesis.
- Glucose can be converted to fructose via sorbitol. Fructose and sorbitol accumulate in the lens of diabetics causing diabetic cataract.

Clinical importance: Disorders (inborn errors of metabolism)

Essential fructosuria

Cause: It occurs due to deficiency of fructokinase. Hence fructose is not converted to fructose 1-P.

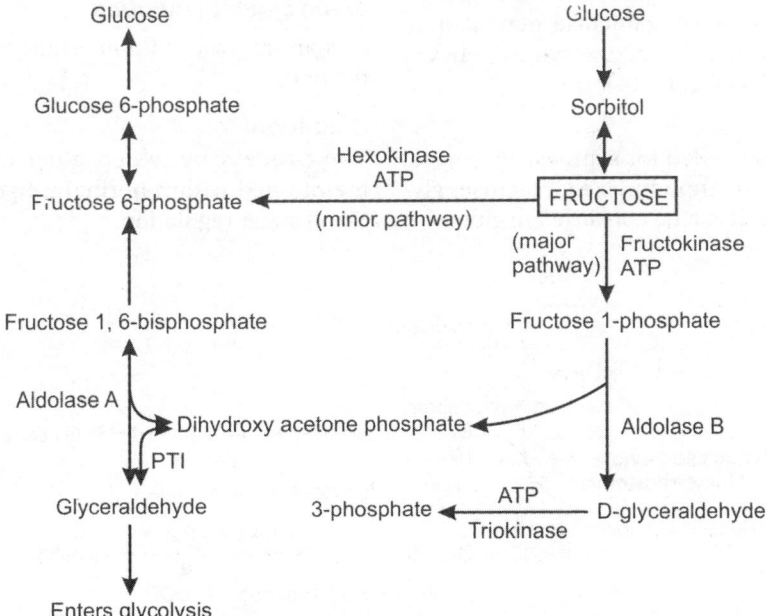

Fig. 11.13: Fructose metabolism.

Symptoms: Fructose is highly excreted in the urine.

Diagnosis: Detection of fructose in urine by qualitative test and chromatography.

Treatment: Restriction of dietary fructose and sucrose.

Hereditary fructose intolerance

Cause: It occurs due to deficiency of aldolase B and thus fructose 1-P is not converted to glyceraldehyde and dihydroxy acetone-P.

Symptoms: Hypoglycemia, hepatic failure.

Diagnosis: Detection of fructose in urine by qualitative test and chromatography.

Treatment: Diet free from fructose and sucrose.

Galactose metabolism

It is a monosaccharide (aldohexose).

Site
- *Organ:* Liver
- *Cell:* Cytosol

Pathway

Galactose is phosphorylated by galactokinase to form galactose 1-p. Galactose 1-p reacts with UDP glucose to form UDP galactose and glucose 1-p by galactose 1-p uridyl transferase. UDP galactose can be converted to UDP glucose by uridine diphosphate galactose epimerase. UDP glucose can form glycogen which is degraded to form glucose. UDP galactose may also be converted to lactose by lactose synthase in the mammary gland **(Fig. 11.14)**.

Importance
- Galactose is needed for synthesis of several biochemical compounds, e.g., lactose, glycolipids, etc. It can be converted to glucose.
- Galactose tolerance test (liver function test) is based on the conversion of galactose to glucose in the liver.

Clinical importance: Disorders (inborn errors of metabolism)

Deficiency of any of the enzymes involved galactose metabolism results in galactosemia. There are three types of galactosemia.

Galactosemia I (classic)

It is the major type of galactosemia.

Cause: It occurs due to deficiency of galactose 1-P uridyl transferase involved in the reaction.

$$\text{Galactose 1-P} \rightarrow \text{UDP galactose}$$

Symptoms: Galactose level is increased in blood and in urine. Galactose is converted to galactitol in eye lens which causes cataract. Hepatosplenomegaly, jaundice, mental retardation, hypoglycemia are other symptoms.

Diagnosis: Identification of galactose in urine by qualitative test and chromatography.

Treatment: Diet free of galactose and lactose.

Galactosemia II

Due to galactokinase deficiency.

Galactosemia III

Due to UDP-Galactose 4-epimerase deficiency.

Blood Sugar Regulation

It is an important homeostatic mechanism in the body.

Definition

The process by which glucose in blood is maintained within normal range is known as blood sugar regulation.

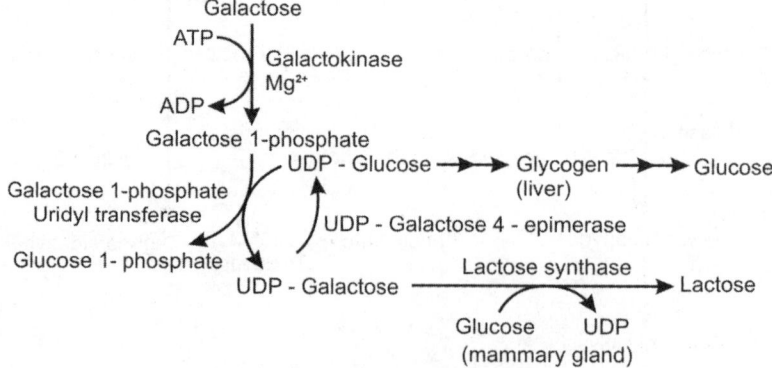

Fig. 11.14: Galactose metabolism.

Blood glucose level is the net result of two processes **(Fig. 11.15)**.
1. Addition of glucose to blood
2. Withdrawal of glucose from blood.

Regulatory mechanisms
Blood glucose level is most efficiently regulated by mechanisms in which liver, extrahepatic tissues and hormones play important roles.

Role of liver
Liver is the principal organ in regulating the blood glucose concentration. It is freely permeable to glucose via GLUT 2 transporter.

During hyperglycemia
- Glucose is drawn from blood for glycolysis, HMP shunt, etc.
- Glucose is converted to glycogen (glycogenesis) for its storage.

During hypoglycemia
- Glucose is released from glycogen (glycogenolysis) due to presence of glucose 6-phosphatase.
- Synthesis of glucose from noncarbohydrate precursors (gluconeogenesis) occurs.

Role of extrahepatic tissues
Extrahepatic tissues (except brain) are relatively impermeable to glucose and therefore insulin is required for the uptake of glucose into these cells.

Muscle
- *During hyperglycemia:* Increase in blood glucose promotes glycogenesis and oxidation of glucose in muscle as in exercise.
- *During hypoglycemia:* Muscle glycogen cannot serve directly as a source of glucose due to absence of glucose 6-phosphatase. But it can provide glucose (muscle glycogenolysis) to blood via Cori cycle.

Kidney
- *During hyperglycemia:* As renal tubules could not reabsorb all the filtered sugar, the excess is excreted in the urine.
- *During hypoglycemia:* Kidney possesses some capacity for forming of glucose from non-carbohydrate precursors (gluconeogenesis).

Role of hormones

Hormone which decreases blood sugar (hypoglycemic hormone)

Insulin
It is secreted by β cells of islets of Langerhans of pancreas as direct response to hyperglycemia. Some amino acids, free fatty acids, ketone bodies and drugs such as tolbutamide also cause secretion of insulin.
Effects of insulin are:
- *Glucose update by tissues:* Glucose entry into hepatic cells does not require insulin, but insulin is required for the uptake of glucose by muscles and adipose tissue through GLUT 4.
- *Glucose utilization:* Insulin increases glycolysis in muscles and liver, enhances glycogenesis and stimulates HMP shunt.
- *Glucose production:* Insulin decreases gluconeogenesis and inhibits glycogenolysis.

Hormones which increase blood sugar (hyperglycemic hormones)
- *Glucagon:* It is secreted by α-cells of islets of Langerhans of pancreas being stimulated by hypoglycemia. It causes glycogenolysis in liver and also enhances gluconeogenesis.
- *Anterior pituitary hormones (growth hormone, ACTH):* These hormones elevate the blood sugar level by antagonizing the action of insulin.
- *Glucocorticoids:* These hormones secreted by adrenal cortex, cause increased gluconeogenesis from amino acids due to increased

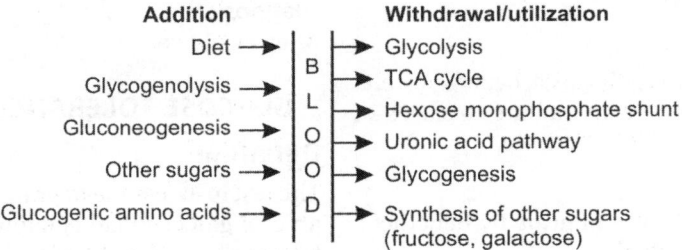

Fig. 11.15: Sources and utilization of glucose from blood.

protein catabolism in the tissues. They also inhibit utilization of glucose in extrahepatic tissues.
- *Epinephrine:* It is secreted by adrenal medulla due to stressful stimuli. It increases glycogenolysis in liver and muscle.
- *Thyroxine:* It increases absorption of glucose from small intestine. It also accelerates hepatic glycogenolysis and gluconeogenesis with consequent rise in blood sugar.

Clinical Importance: Disorders of Blood Sugar Regulation

It occurs due to defective carbohydrate metabolism. It may be of two types: (1) Hyperglycemia; (2) Hypoglycemia.
Normal level: Plasma glucose (F) 70–110 mg/dL.

Hyperglycemia

It refers to increased level of glucose in blood above normal level. It may be caused by deficiency of insulin, hyperactivity of pituitary, thyroid, adrenal, glucose infusion, and drugs, such as salicylates, oral contraceptives. Its major syndrome is diabetes mellitus.

Diabetes mellitus

It is a chornic metabolic disease in which blood sugar level is elevated (hyperglycemia). It occurs due to deficiency of insulin or factors which oppose insulin action.

Types

It is mainly divided into two types:
1. **Insulin dependent diabetes mellitus (IDDM):** It occurs in youngsters (<30 years). It is due to deficiency or absence of insulin (Type I: DM).
2. **Noninsulin dependent diabetes mellitus (NIDDM):** It occurs in old people (above 30 years). It is due to aging, stress, and sedentary life (Type II: DM).

Clinical symptoms

Glucosuria, polyuria, polydipsia, hyperglycemia, coma. Long-term effects include diseases of kidney, eye muscles, infection, etc.

Diagnosis

- Detection of glucose in urine by Benedict's test/drystrip method
- Estimation of glucose in blood (colorimetric method)
- Glucose tolerance test (*refer* below)
- Glycosylated hemoglobin (HbA_{1C})
  - *Definition:* Glycosylated hemoglobin (HbA_{1C}) is glucose combined product of normal adult hemoglobin (HbA_1).
    When glucose level is increased in the blood (as in diabetes mellitus), hemoglobin may undergo glycosylation with glucose. It is a nonenzymatic, post-translational process. It remain in the RBCs throughout their life span (120 days) and is not removed from hemoglobin. Thus HbA_{1C} level in the blood reveals the mean glucose level over the previous 8–10 weeks (half life period of RBC).
  - *Diagnostic use:*
    - Normal level of HbA_{1C} in blood = 4–6%
    - Abnormal level:
      - 6–6.5%—impaired glucose tolerance.
      - Above 7%—poor control of diabetes.

  HbA_{1C} is thus used as a valuable diagnostic aid in monitoring the treatment of diabetes mellitus.

Treatment

- Insulin
- Drugs
- Diet
- Exercise

Hypoglycemia

It refers to the decrease in blood glucose level below normal (<40 mg/100 mL). It may occur due to over-dosage of insulin, insulinoma, hyposecretions of pituitary, thyroid, adrenal, and severe exercise, etc. It induces symptoms, such as sweating, hunger, convulsion, unconsciousness, and coma.

Diagnosis

As given above.

GLUCOSE TOLERANCE TEST (GTT)

Definition

The test to assess the tolerance of the body after an oral glucose load is known as oral glucose tolerance test **(Fig. 11.16)**.

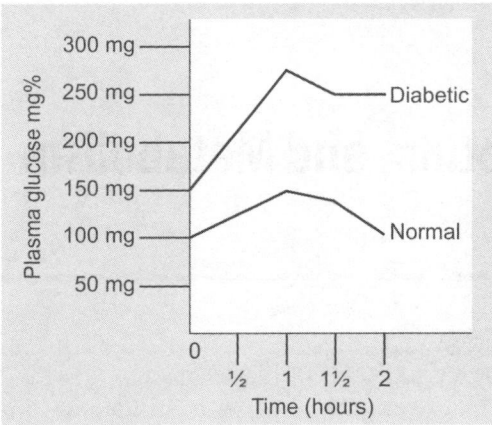

Fig. 11.16: Glucose tolerance test (GTT).

Importance

- It is used to assess the response to oral glucose load.
- It is a valuable aid to detect diabetes mellitus.
- It is used to rule out renal glycosuria.
- It can also be used to know the hyper or hypoactivity of pancreas, pituitary, thyroid, etc.

Test

Prerequisites

The test is performed after an overnight fast (12 hours). The patient should be on carbohydrate rich diet for at least three days and avoid drugs which may influence carbohydrate metabolism for at least two days prior to test.

Procedure

- At fasting state (8 AM) samples of venous blood and urine collected in two separate test tubes.
- About 75 g of glucose dissolved in 250 mL of water is given to the patient to drink.
- Samples of venous blood and urine are collected at 1/2 hr, 1 hr, 1^1/$_2$ hr and 2 hr after administration of glucose.
- Amount of glucose in all 5 samples of blood are estimated separately by true sugar method (GOD - POD method). All samples of urine are tested separately for glucose by Benedict's qualitative test.
- A curve is plotted with glucose values against timing.

Interpretation

Various types of curves are obtained.

Normal Curve

Fasting glucose value is within normal limit. Peak value is reached within one hour. Fasting level returns by 2 hour. No glucose is detected in any specimen of urine.

Diabetic Curve

Fasting glucose level is increased. High value (more than normal) is reached after 1–1 1/2 hour. Urine may give positive Benedict's test. Glucose level may or may not reach normal depending on the severity of diabetes mellitus.

Note
Abnormal curves are also observed in other diseases or conditions, e.g., renal glycosuria, gastrectomy, hyper activities of pituitary, thyroid and adrenal glands.

ADDITIONAL INFORMATION

Glycosuria

Definition

Excretion of detectable amount of sugar in the urine is known as glycosuria. It occurs when blood sugar level rises beyond the renal threshold (180 mg/100 mL).

Types

- **Diabetic glycosuria:** It occurs in the patients suffering from diabetes mellitus when their blood sugar level goes beyond renal threshold. It is a pathological condition.
- **Renal glycosuria:** It occurs due to diminished tubular reabsorption of glucose and lower renal threshold. It is a benign condition.
- **Alimentary glycosuria:** It occurs due to increased rate of absorption of glucose from the intestine which rises above the renal threshold. It is also a benign condition.

Diagnosis: Test for glycosuria.

Urine → Benedict's test
Urine → Dipstick test

12 Digestion, Absorption, and Metabolism of Lipids

Chapter Outline
- Digestion
- Absorption
- Transport and Storage
- Metabolism
- Lipid disorders

■ INTRODUCTION

An adult human ingests 60–150 g of lipids daily. This consists of mostly triglycerides (90%) and the remainder is cholesterol, cholesterol esters, phospholipids and free fatty acids.

■ DIGESTION

Digestion of fat (triglycerides/triacylglycerol) (**Fig. 12.1**).

Mouth

A lingual lipase is secreted by the dorsal surface of the tongue (Ebner's glands) but this enzyme is not much significant in the human. It initiates hydrolysis of fats.

Stomach

The stomach secretes gastric lipase. Low pH is not favorable for its action. It is able to digest only a limited amount (30%) of triacylglycerols by hydrolysis. The released short and medium chain fatty acids are absorbed via the stomach wall and enter the portal vein, whereas longer chain fatty acids are passed onto the duodenum along with partially digested triacylglycerols. The latter are made soluble in the duodenum through emulsification with bile salts to form minute particles known as micelles.

Intestine

Most part of hydrolysis of fats takes place in the small intestine where higher pH is optimum for pancreatic lipase. The latter is controlled by hormones, such as cholecystokinin. Pancreatic lipase acts on the emulsified fat droplets. It can hydrolyze ester linkage at 1 and 3 positions of triacylglycerols to form fatty acids and 2-monoacylglycerols. But by action of an enzyme isomerase, 2-monoacylglycerols are slowly converted to 1-monoacylglycerols. Thus finally less than one fourth of the triacylglycerols only is completely broken down to fatty acids and glycerol.

■ ABSORPTION

Bergstrom theory is the recent and accepted theory on the absorption of lipids (**Fig. 12.1**). It is described below:

- Fatty acids, 2-monoacylglycerols and 1-monoacylglycerols are transported to intestinal mucosal cells, where they are absorbed into the intestinal epithelium. The bile salts are passed onto the ileum, where most are absorbed into enterohepatic circulation.
- Within the intestinal wall, 1-monoacylglycerols are hydrolyzed to produce free glycerol and fatty acid by an intestinal lipase (different from pancreatic lipase). 2-monoacylglycerols are reconverted to triacylglycerol via the monoacylglycerol pathway.
- Triacylglycerol synthesized in the intestinal mucosa is not transported to any extent in the portal venous blood. But it generates chylomicrons that form a milky fluid (chyle), which is collected by the lymphatic vessels (lacteals) of the abdominal region via the thoracic duct.
- The free glycerol released in the intestinal lumen is not reutilized but passes directly

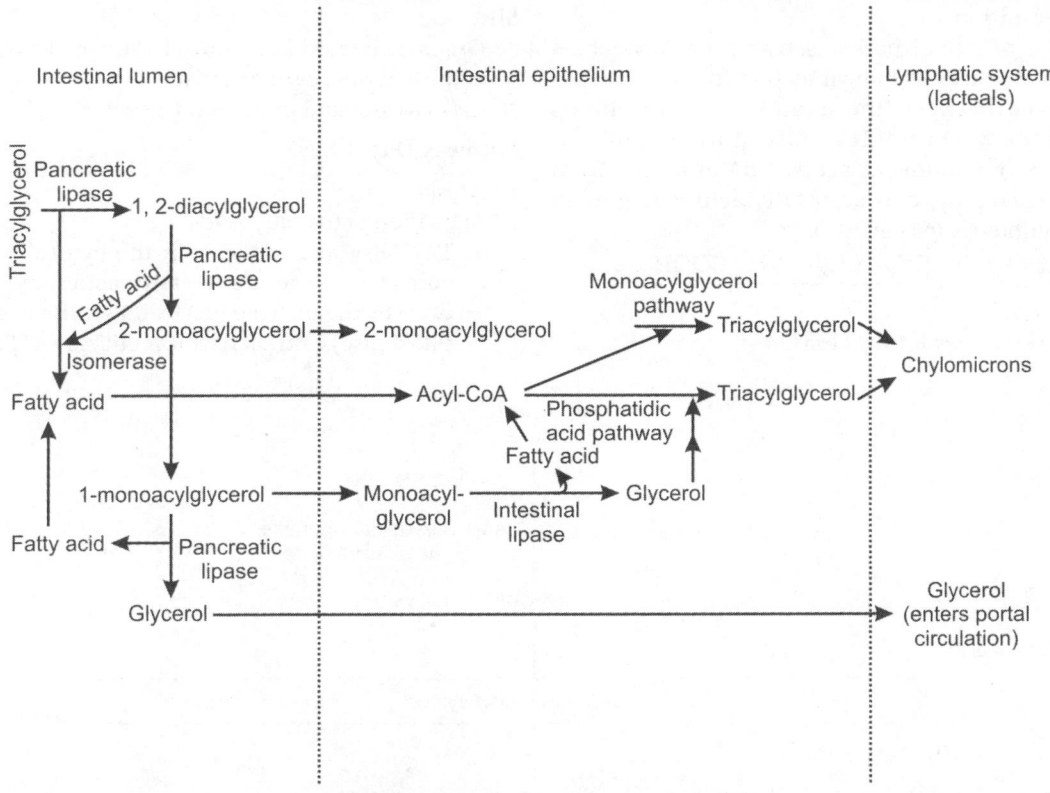

Fig. 12.1: Digestion and absorption of lipids.

to the portal vein. However, the glycerol released within the intestinal cells can be reutilized for triacylglycerol synthesis after activation to glycerol 3-phosphate by ATP.

Clinical Importance: Disorders
Steatorrhea It refers to increased fat content in feces. It occurs due to biliary obstruction, diseases of pancreas, tropical sprue (normally <5% of ingested fat is excreted in feces). **Chyluria and Chylothorax** These abnormalities occur due to obstruction to transportation phase in lacteals. Milky urine appears in chyluria and milky pleural effusion occurs in chylothorax.

■ TRANSPORT AND STORAGE

Lipids are insoluble in water, hence they must be combined with amphipathic lipids and proteins to make water-soluble for transport between the tissues and blood plasma.

Triacylglycerol is the main storage from lipids in adipose tissue (Brown adipose tissue is the site of nonshivering thermogenesis. It is found in hibernating animals. It is also present in humans and is responsible for diet-induced thermogenesis. It is due to presence of a protein, thermogenin).

■ METABOLISM

Metabolism of lipids can be mainly divided into:
- Metabolism of fatty acids
- Metabolism of triacylglycerol
- Metabolism of phospholipids and glycolipids
- Metabolism of cholesterol
- Metabolism of lipoproteins

Metabolism of Fatty Acids

It comprises:
- Catabolism of fatty acids
- Formation and utilization of ketone bodies
- Biosynthesis of fatty acids

Catabolism of Fatty Acids

Major pathways

β-oxidation of saturated fatty acids with even number of carbon atoms, e.g., palmitic acid (16C).

Definition

The principal pathway by which fatty acids are oxidized is known as β-oxidation. It takes place between the α and β carbon atoms of the fatty acid. It results in the removal of 2 carbon atoms as acetyl-CoA at a time from the carboxyl end until fatty acid is degraded completely to acetyl-CoA.

$$\underset{\hphantom{R - CH_2 -\ }\beta\hphantom{\ - CH_2 -\ }\alpha\hphantom{\ - COOH}}{R - CH_2 - CH_2 - CH_2 - COOH}$$

Proposed by: Knoop (1951).

Site

- *Organs:* Liver, kidney, muscle, lungs, testis, adipose tissue, cardiac muscle
- *Cell:* Cytosol and mitochondria.

Pathway (Fig. 12.2)

In cytosol
1. Activation of the fatty acids
   a. The fatty acid present in the cytosol is converted to an active fatty acid (acyl-CoA) by the enzyme (acyl-CoA synthetase thiokinase) with coenzyme A utilizing ATP.

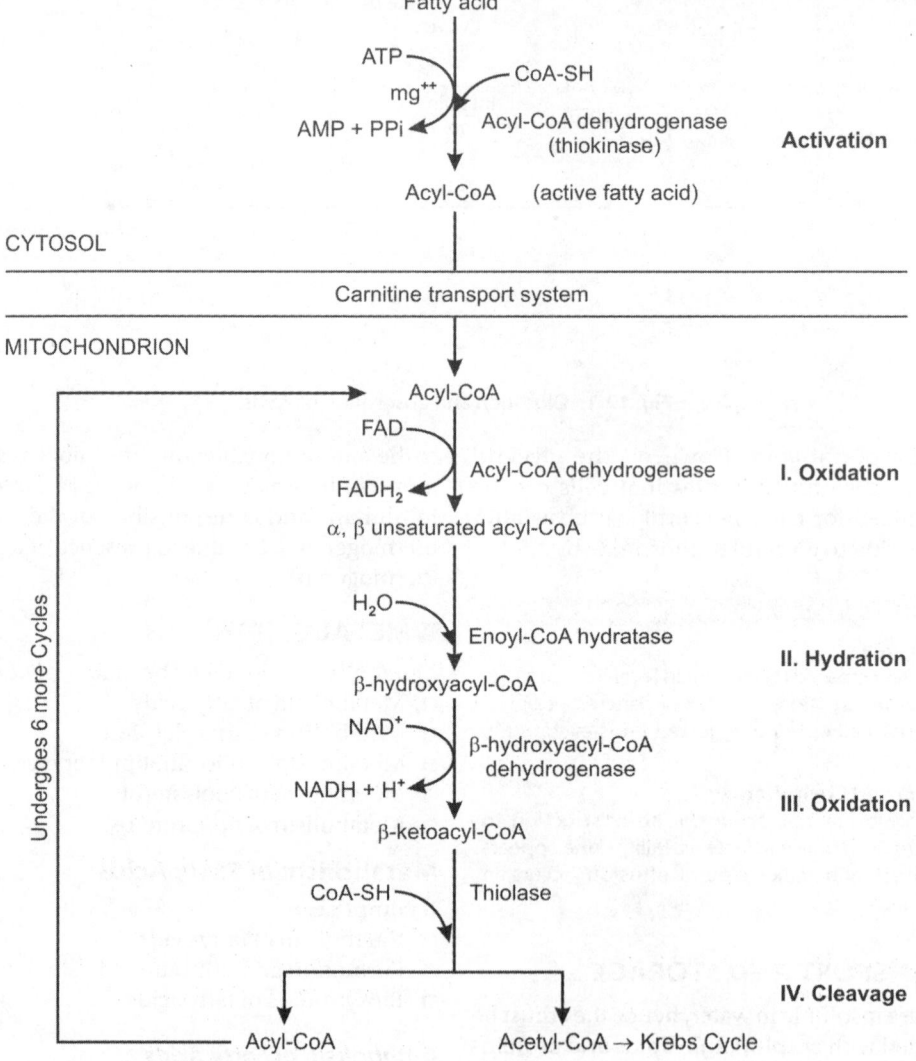

Fig. 12.2: β-oxidation of fatty acids (saturated FA with even number carbon atoms).

Fatty acid + ATP + CoA → Acyl-CoA + PPi + AMP (Active fatty acid)

b. From cytosol, acyl-CoA enters the mitochondria via carnitine transport system.

In mitochondria
- β-oxidation of acyl-CoA involves the following four steps:
  - *Oxidation:* Acyl-CoA is converted to Δ^2, trans-enoyl-CoA catalyzed by acyl-CoA dehydrogenase containing FAD as coenzyme.
  - *Hydration:* Δ^2 trans-enoyl-CoA is then hydrated to form β-hydroxy acyl-CoA by enoyl-CoA hydratase.
  - *Oxidation:* β-hydroxy acyl-CoA is converted to β-keto acyl-CoA by dehydrogenation being catalyzed by β-hydroxy acyl-CoA dehydrogenase in the presence of NAD^+.
  - *Cleavage:* Finally β-keto acyl-CoA is split between α and β position by thiolase with the addition of one molecule of CoA. The products of this reaction are acetyl-CoA and acyl-CoA.

Acyl-CoA (which contains 2 carbon atoms less than the original acyl-CoA molecule) undergoes further degradation (6 more cycles) by β-oxidation.

Thus original fatty acid is degraded completely to acetyl-CoA which enters citric acid cycle and gets oxidized to CO_2 and H_2O.

Energetics (Table 12.1)

Complete oxidation of palmitic acid produces ATP as follows:

Palmitic acid → Acetyl-CoA + H_2O

Summary: Complete oxidation of palmitic acid produces ATP as follows:

	Conventional concept	Current concept
Total ATP produced	131	108
Total ATP utilized	2	2
Net ATP yield	129	106

Regulation
- The whole pathway is regulated by the process of transport of fatty acyl-CoA into the mitochondria.
- ATP level regulates the entry of acetyl-CoA into citric acid cycle.

Table 12.1: Energetics.

	No. of ATPs produced/utilized	
	Conventional concept	Current concept
7 NADH × 3 or 2.5	21	17.5
7 $FADH_2$ × 2 or 1.5	14	10.5
Each acetyl-CoA provides 12 ATPs when converted to CO_2 + H_2O by citric acid cycle.		
8 Acetyl-CoA × 12 (10)	96	80
Total energy yield from one molecule of palmitic acid (Palmitic acid → Palmitoyl-CoA)	131	108
No. ATPs utilized (activation of FA)	2	2
Net energy yield of ATPs	(131 – 2) = 129	(108 – 2) = 106

Importance
- β-oxidation of FA produces large quantities of ATP.
- Increased FA oxidation occurs in starvation and diabetes mellitus leading to ketone body production.

Clinical Importance: Disorders
- *Carnitine deficiency:* It is caused due to inadequate synthesis, renal leakage and hemodialysis. It leads to hypoglycemia.
- *Inherited defects* in the enzymes of β-oxidation also lead to hypoglycemia, coma, fatty liver.
- *Jamaican vomiting sickness:* It occurs due to eating of the unripe fruit (which contains toxin hypoglycin) of ackee tree. It inactivates acyl-CoA dehydrogenase thus inhibiting β-oxidation. It leads to hypoglycemia vomiting, convulsions, coma and death.
- *Zellweger's syndrome:* A modified form of β-oxidation is present in peroxisomes. It involves oxidation of long chain fatty acids leading to the formation of acetyl-CoA and H_2O_2. Zellweger's syndrome is an inherited disorder which occurs due to absence of peroxisomes in all the tissues. Long chain fatty acids accumulate in brain, liver, kidney and hence known as cerebrohepatorenal syndrome.

β-oxidation of saturated fatty acids with odd number of carbon atoms, e.g., Valeric acid (5C):
Fatty acids having odd number of

carbon atoms are oxidized to acetyl-CoA by β-oxidation until propionyl-CoA (3 carbon residue) is formed. Propionyl-CoA is then converted to succinyl-CoA which enters citric acid cycle and gets oxidized to CO_2 and water **(Fig. 12.3)**.

Energetics

Less energy is produced.

Disorders

Two types of inheritable disorders (methylmalonic acidemia) may occur due to deficiency of Vitamin B_{12} or enzyme mutase. Methylmalonic acid accumulates in both the cases and is highly excreted in urine. It causes metabolic acidosis, damages central nervous system (CNS) and retards growth.

Oxidation of Unsaturated Fatty Acids (e.g., Linoleic Acid)

It occurs by a modified β-oxidation pathway, utilizing additional enzymes, isomerase and reductase, etc. It produces less energy.

Minor Pathways
α-oxidation

It occurs in microsomes of brain and liver. It involves removal of one carbon (α-carbon) at a time from the carboxyl end of fatty acid. This pathway is important in the catabolism of branched chain and odd chain fatty acids. It does not produce high energy phosphates. Refsum's disease occurs due to deficiency of enzyme phytanate α-oxidase which converts phytanic acid in food stuffs by oxidation. It produces mainly neurological symptoms.

ω-oxidation

It occurs in liver microsomes. It involves oxidation of terminal (ω) methyl group of fatty acid to CH_2OH which is oxidized to carboxyl group to form dicarboxylic acids. Further catabolism takes place by β-oxidation.

Metabolism of Ketone Bodies

It comprises two phases.
1. Formation of ketone bodies (ketogenesis)
2. Utilization of ketone bodies (ketolysis)

The ketone bodies are:
- Acetone: $CH_3 - CO - CH_3$
- Acetoacetate: $CH_3 - CO - CH_2 - COOH$
- β-hydroxybutyrate: $CH_3 - \underset{OH}{CH} - CH_2 - COOH$

Formation of Ketone Bodies (Ketogenesis)
Definition

Formation of ketone bodies from fatty acids is known as ketogenesis **(Fig. 12.4)**.

Site
- *Organ:* Liver
- *Cell:* Mitochondria

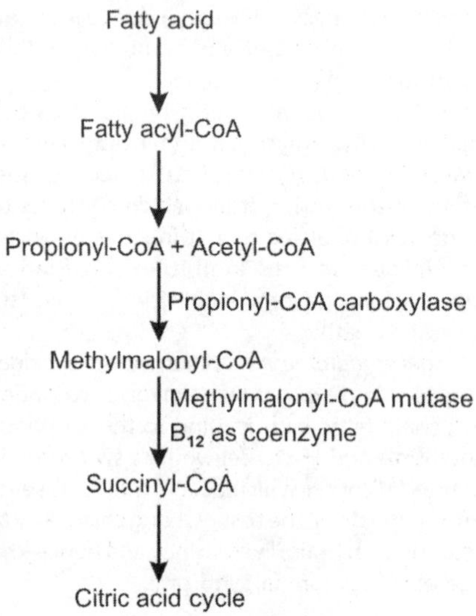

Fatty acid
↓
Fatty acyl-CoA
↓
Propionyl-CoA + Acetyl-CoA
↓ Propionyl-CoA carboxylase
Methylmalonyl-CoA
↓ Methylmalonyl-CoA mutase
  B_{12} as coenzyme
Succinyl-CoA
↓
Citric acid cycle

Fig. 12.3: β-oxidation (saturated FA with odd number carbon atoms).

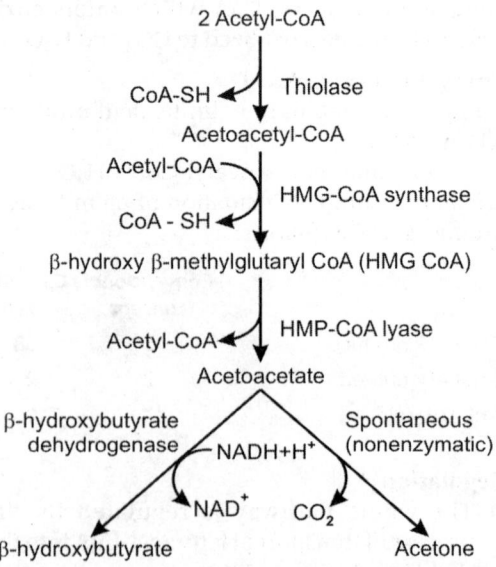

Fig. 12.4: Formation of ketone bodies (ketogenesis).

Pathway
- Two molecules of acetyl-CoA condense to form acetoacetyl-CoA by reversal of thiolase reaction.
- Acetoacetyl-CoA condenses with another molecule of acetyl-CoA to form β-hydroxy-β-methylglutaryl-CoA (HMG-CoA) catalyzed by HMG-CoA synthase.
- HMG-CoA is cleaved to produce acetoacetate and acetyl-CoA by HMG-CoA lyase.
- Acetoacetate undergoes the following pathways:
  - It is reduced to β-hydroxybutyrate by β-hydroxybutyrate dehydrogenase.
  - It undergoes spontaneous decarboxylation to form acetone.

Regulation
Ketogenesis is regulated at the three steps:
1. Mobilization of free fatty acids from adipose tissue
2. Activity of carnitine palmitoyl transferase - I in liver
3. Partition of acetyl-CoA between the pathway of ketogenesis and citric acid cycle.

Utilization of ketone bodies (ketolysis)
Definition
Utilization or catabolism of ketone bodies is known as ketolysis **(Fig. 12.5)**.

Site
- *Organ:* Extrahepatic tissues (e.g., muscle)
- *Cell:* Mitochondria

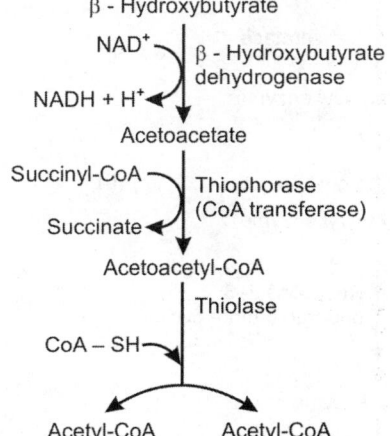

Fig. 12.5: Utilization of ketone bodies (ketolysis).

Pathway
- β-hydroxybutyrate is oxidized to acetoacetate by dehydrogenase.
- Acetoacetate reacts with succinyl-CoA to form acetoacetyl-CoA, catalyzed by CoA transferase (Thiophorase).
- Acetoacetyl-CoA is split to acetyl-CoA by thiolase.
- Acetyl-CoA is oxidized in the citric acid cycle to form CO_2, H_2O and ATP.
- Acetone is difficult to be oxidized and is mostly volatilized in the lungs.

Clinical Importance
During normal metabolism of fatty acids, production of ketone bodies in the liver and its catabolism in the extrahepatic tissues is normal. Ketone bodies are not utilized in the liver due to deficiency of enzyme thiophorase. They are the important sources of energy for the extrahepatic tissues.

Normal level
Blood: <1 mg/100 mL
Urine: <1 mg/24 hours

During starvation and diabetes mellitus, more than normal quantity of ketone bodies are formed in the liver. Thus large quantities of ketone bodies are present in the blood (ketonemia) and also highly excreted in the urine (ketonuria). The overall condition (ketonemia + ketonuria) is known as ketosis. As the ketone bodies are moderately strong acids, ketosis may lead to diabetic ketoacidosis which is fatal as in uncontrolled diabetes mellitus.

Diabetic ketoacidosis (DKA): It is a serious complication of diabetes mellitus.

Cause: It occurs due to deficiency of insulin. Hence body breaks down fat which leads to the increased formation of (keto) acids in the blood leading to DKA (metabolic acidosis).

Symptoms: Thirst, frequent urination abdominal pain, nausea, Kussmaul's respiration (fruity odor breath), weakness, confusion, coma.

Diagnosis: Rothera's test (to detect ketone bodies in the urine).

Treatment: Insulin therapy, fluid and electrolyte therapy.

Ketogenic substances: (a) FFA, (b) Proteins.

Antiketogenic substances: (a) All carbohydrates, (b) Insulin.

Treatment: Regulate ketogenic/antiketogenic ratio in the diet.

Test for detection of ketone bodies in urine: Rothera's test.

Biosynthesis of Fatty Acids

It can be studied as follows:
- Biosynthesis of short chain saturated fatty acids (de novo synthesis)—Lipogenesis.
- Biosynthesis of long chain saturated fatty acids (elongation of short chain fatty acids).
- Biosynthesis of unsaturated fatty acids and its derivatives (eicosanoids).

Biosynthesis of short chain saturated fatty acids (lipogenesis)

Extramitochondrial pathway (Fig. 12.6) (de novo synthesis)

Site
- Organ: Present in many tissues including adipose tissue, liver, kidney, brain, lung and mammary gland.
- Cell: Cytosol

Pathway: It can be divided into two stage.

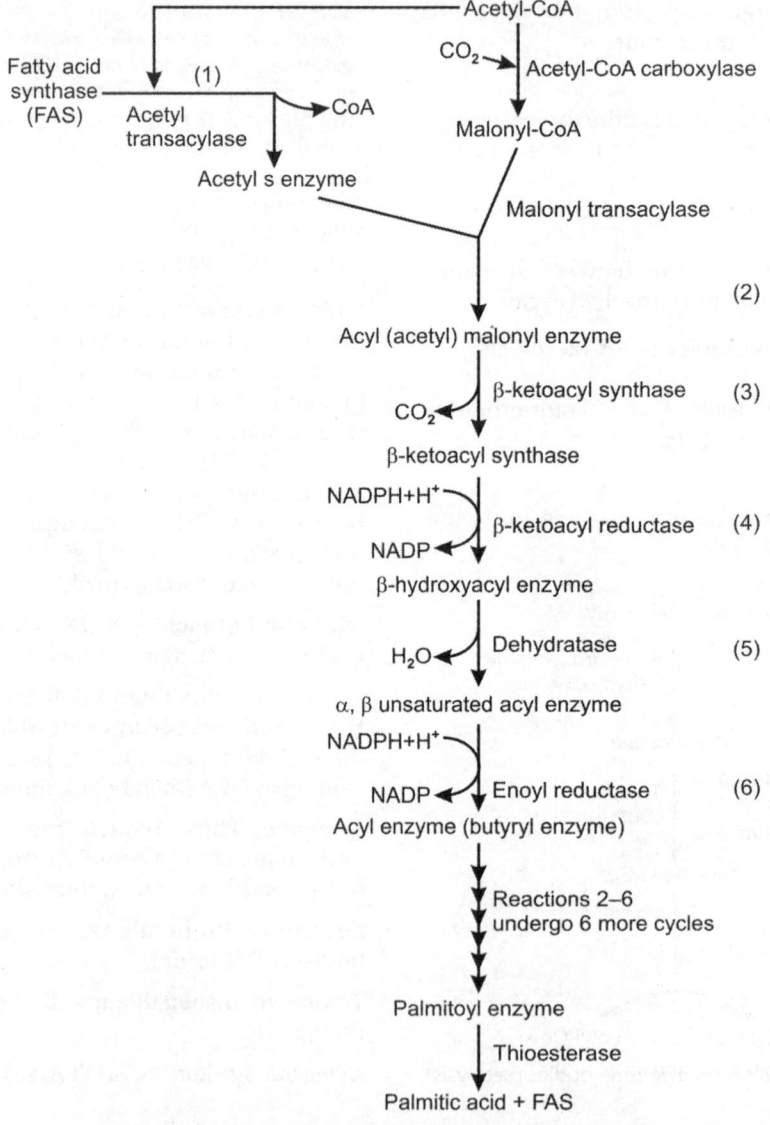

Fig. 12.6: Biosynthesis of fatty acid (de novo synthesis).

- Formation of malonyl-CoA:
  - Acetyl-CoA formed in mitochondria is converted to citrate which is transferred to cytosol, where citrate is converted to acetyl-CoA.
  - In the cytosol, acetyl-CoA is carboxylated to form malonyl-CoA by acetyl-CoA carboxylase in the presence of biotin ATP and CO_2.
- Reactions of fatty acid synthase (FAS) complex: The rest of the steps are catalyzed by the enzyme fatty acid synthase. It is a multienzyme complex. It is present as dimer. Each monomer contains seven enzymes and an acyl carrier protein (ACP) attached to 4-phosphopantetheine containing SH group. Both monomers are connected as 'head-to-tail' configuration.
- Binding of acetyl-CoA and malonyl-CoA.
  - Acetyl-CoA (a priming molecule) combines with cysteine - SH group of one monomer catalyzed by acetyl transacylase.
  - Malonyl-CoA combines with the adjacent - SH group on the pantetheine of ACP of other monomer, catalyzed by malonyl transacylase.
    The product formed due to the above two reactions is acetyl (acyl) malonyl enzyme.
- *Condensation:* Acetyl group is transferred from the cysteine - SH group to malonyl group with liberation of CO_2. This reaction is catalyzed by β-ketoacyl synthase. The product formed is-β-ketoacyl enzyme (Acetoacetyl enzyme).
- *Reduction:* β-ketoacyl enzyme is reduced by β-ketoacyl reductase utilizing NADPH to form β-hydroxyacyl enzyme.
- *Dehydration:* β-hydroxyacyl enzyme is dehydrated to form 2, 3-unsaturated acyl-enzyme by dehydratase.
- *Reduction:* Unsaturated acyl enzyme is reduced to form (saturated) acyl enzyme by enoyl reductase.
    Butyryl group of the saturated acyl enzyme is transferred to cys-SH.
    The sequence of reactions (2-6) is repeated 6 cycles more until palmitoyl group (saturated 16 carbon acyl radical) is formed.
- *Termination:* Palmitoyl group is released from the enzyme by a thioesterase to form palmitic acid (16C).

Energetics
7 ATP utilized.

Regulation
- *Nutritional control:* Rate is higher in the well-fed state, but is depressed during starvation, on a high fat diet or in diabetes mellitus.
- *Enzymatic control:* The rate limiting enzyme is acetyl-CoA carboxylase which catalyzes
Acetyl-CoA → Malonyl -CoA
Acetyl-CoA carboxylase is an allosteric enzyme. It is activated by citrate and inhibited by long chain acyl-CoA molecules.
- *Hormonal control:*
  - Insulin activates acetyl-CoA carboxylase in the short-term by dephosphorylation and in the long-term by induction of synthesis
  - Glucagon and epinephrine have opposite actions to insulin.

Clinical Importance

- It may be of little importance in human and critical diseases of this pathway have not been reported.
- Its variations in activity in humans may decide the extent and nature of obesity.
- One of the effects of type I insulin dependent diabetes mellitus (IDDM) is inhibition of lipogenesis.

Biosynthesis of long chain saturated fatty acids (elongation of short chain saturated fatty acids)
There are two systems for elongation of short chain saturated fatty acids:
1. *Microsomal system:* This is the major pathway for elongation of existing fatty acids. Acyl-CoA compounds are converted to higher fatty acids by means of malonyl-CoA along with NADPH (**Fig. 12.6**).
Palmitic acid (16C) → Stearic acid (18C)
2. *Mitochondrial system:* In this pathway, the incorporation of acetyl-CoA into long chain fatty acids occurs.

Biosynthesis of unsaturated fatty acids
This can be studied under the three heads.
- *Biosynthesis of monounsaturated fatty acids:* An enzyme system catalyzes the conversion of saturated to unsaturated fatty acids.
Stearic acid → Oleic acid
- *Biosynthesis of polyunsaturated fatty acids:*

- Linoleic acid, α-linolenic acid and arachidonic acid are polyunsaturated fatty acids. They are essential fatty acids.
- Linoleic acid and α-linolenic acid must be supplied in the diet for the synthesis of other polyunsaturated fatty acids in the body.
- Linoleic acid can be converted to arachidonic acid as follows:

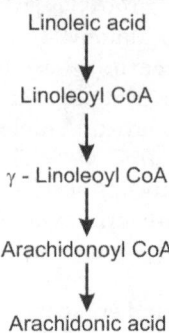

☐ Metabolism of eicosanoids (Prostaglandins).

Synthesis
Arachidonic acid is formed from the phospholipids in the cell membrane due to action of phospholipase A_2. Eicosanoids are formed from arachidonic acid by two pathways.

The Cyclooxygenase Pathway (Fig. 12.7)
Site: Seminal vesicles, lung, liver, brain, renal medulla, heart, adipose tissue, GI tract.

Pathway: Arachidonic acid is catalyzed by enzyme cyclooxygenase and peroxidase (multienzyme complex prostaglandin endoperoxide synthase) in the presence of O_2, reduced glutathione, FH_4 to form prostaglandins and thromboxanes.

Aspirin inhibits cyclooxygenase. Cyclooxygenase is known as suicide enzyme as it switches of PG synthesis due to self-catalyzed destruction.

The Lipooxygenase Pathway (Fig. 12.8)
Site: Leukocytes, mast cells, platelets and macrophages.

Phospholipids (in cell membrane)
↓ Phospholipase A_2
Arachidonic acid
↓ Cyclooxygenase and peroxidase
Prostaglandins and thromboxanes

Fig. 12.7: Cyclooxygenase pathway.

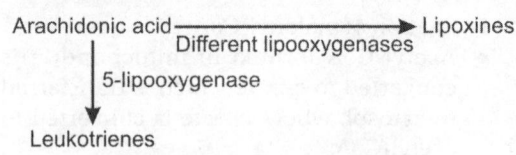

Fig. 12.8: Lipooxygenase pathway.

Pathway: Arachidonic acid is converted to leukotrienes and lipoxines by lipoxygenases.

Metabolism of Triacylglycerols
Triacylglycerols are the major lipids in the diet as well as in fat depots. They are also the major energy storing lipids. Triacylglycerols play an important role in lipid transport, storage and in various diseases, such as obesity, diabetes mellitus and hyperlipoproteinemia.

Digestion and Absorption
Refer page 148

Synthesis (Fig. 12.9)
Site
☐ *Organs:* Mostly in liver and adipose tissue
☐ *Cell:* Cytosol, endoplasmic reticulum, mitochondria.

Pathway
☐ Fatty acids are activated to acyl-CoA by acyl-CoA synthetase.
☐ Two molecules of acyl-CoA combine with glycerol 3-phosphate to form phosphatidate (1,2 diacylglycerol 3-phosphate) catalyzed by acyl transferase.
☐ Phosphatidate is then converted to 1, 2 diacylglycerol by phosphohydrolase.
☐ Finally another molecule of acyl-CoA is esterified with 1,2 diacylglycerol to form triacylglycerol, catalyzed by acyl transferase.

Catabolism
Site
Adipose tissue

Pathway
Triacylglycerols undergo hydrolysis in the adipose tissue by lipase to give free fatty acids and glycerol. Free fatty acids reach plasma and combine with albumin and is transported to tissues such as liver, kidney, heart, muscle, lung, testis, brain and adipose tissue for oxidation or re-esterification.

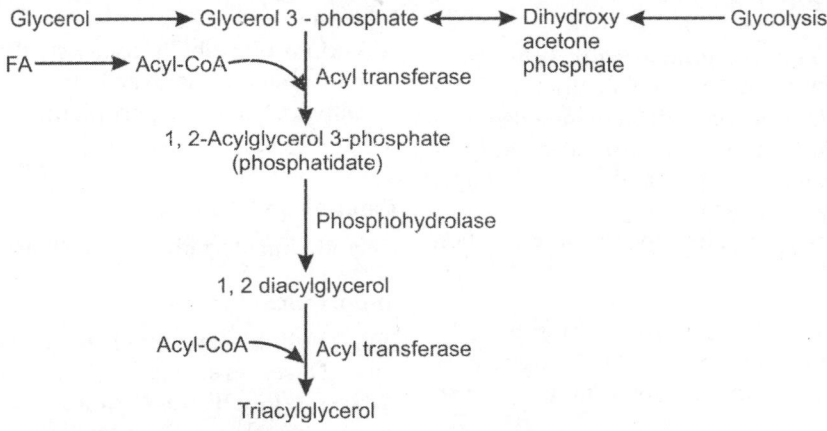

Fig. 12.9: Synthesis of triacylglycerol.

Glycerol is utilized in liver, kidney, intestine, brown adipose tissue lactating mammary gland where the activating enzyme glycerol kinase is present.

Importance
- Phosphatidate and 1,2 diacyl glycerol formed in this pathway are utilized for phospholipids synthesis.
- Triacylglycerol serve as major energy store in adipose tissue.

Fatty Liver and Lipotropic Factor

Fatty Liver (Figs. 12.10A and B)

Alternative name: hepatic steatosis
Liver is not a storage organ for fat. It can store up to 5% of fat only. If it exceeds this amount, fat will build up in the liver leading to fatty liver.

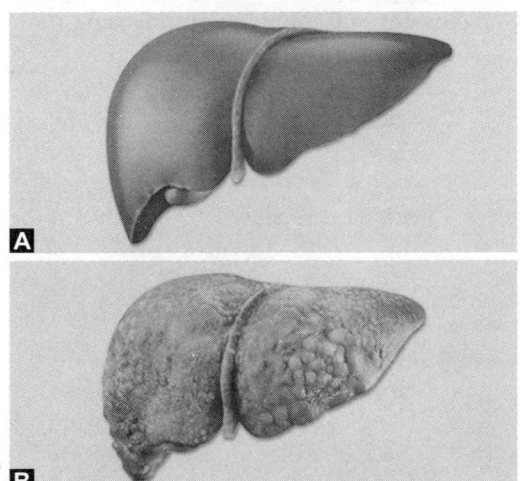

Figs. 12.10A and B: (A) Healthy liver and (B) Fatty liver.
(For color version, see Plate 3)

Definition: Accumulation of fat (triacylglyerol) in the liver beyond normal level is known as fatty liver.

Causative agents:
1. Hormones: Insulin, thyroid hormones
2. Deficiency of vitamin E and selenium
3. Chemicals (puromycin, CCl_4)
4. Alcoholism
5. Deficiency of lipotropic factors

Symptoms:
1. Enlarged liver
2. Elevation of liver enzymes (SGPT, rGT)
3. Liver cirrhosis

Types: Two types—
1. Fatty liver diseases (FLD)
   a. *Due to increased synthesis of triacylglycerols:* It results from mobilization of fat from adipose tissue or from the hydrolysis of lipoprotein triacylglycerol by lipoprotein lipase in extrahepatic tissues. It occurs in starvation and feeding of high fat diet, uncontrolled diabetes mellitus.
   b. *Due to metabolic block in the production of lipoproteins:* It occurs due to defective apoprotein synthesis or provision of phospholipids or secretary mechanism itself.
2. Nonalcoholic fatty liver disease (NAFLD): It is the most common liver disease. High fat diet and uncontrolled diabetes are the causes.

Treatment/prevention of fatty liver
- Avoid saturated fats
- Avoid alcohol
- Lipotropic factors
- Drugs

Lipotropic Factors

Definition: Lipotropic factors are substances which remove or decrease deposition of fat in the liver by interaction with fat metabolism.

Lipotropic factors: They are produced naturally in the body, e.g., choline, methionine, betaine, inositol, folic acid, vitamin B_{12}.

They are mostly required for transmethylation reaction.

Uses: Used for treatment of fatty liver.

Mechanism of action: Lipotropic factors have the ability to remove and prevent fat deposits. They are required for normal mobilization of fat from liver.

- *Choline:* Required for phospholipid synthesis.
- *Betaine:* It is required for choline synthesis (methyl group donor for choline synthesis).
- *Methionine:* Required for transmethylation reaction.
- *Inositol:* Necessary for phospholipid synthesis.

Metabolism of Phospholipids

Digestion and Absorption

Phospholipids may be absorbed from the intestine without digestion. It may also be absorbed after hydrolysis by phospholipases. Some phospholipids may be incorporated in synthesis of chylomicrons and VLDL in intestinal mucosal cell and carried in lymphatic vessels.

Synthesis (Fig. 12.11)

Site
- *Organ:* Liver
- *Cell:* Endoplasmic reticulum

Pathway
- Various phospholipids are synthesized from phosphatidate as given below.

Dihydroxyacetone phosphate $\xrightarrow{\text{Several Steps}}$ Plasmalogen

Catabolism

Degradation of lecithin (*refer* Chapter 3).

Importance

Phospholipids are involved in causation of several diseases such as:
- Respiratory distress syndrome (lack of lung surfactant) (*refer* Chapter 3)
- Multiple sclerosis (demyelination)

Metabolism of Glycolipids

Cerebrosides

Synthesis

Sphingosine $\xrightarrow{\text{Acyl CoA}}$ Ceramide $\xrightarrow{\text{UDP Galactose}}$ Cerebroside

Catabolism

Galactosyl ceramide $\xrightarrow{\beta\text{-Galactosidase}}$

Ceramide $\xrightarrow{\text{Ceramidase}}$ Sphingosine + FA

Gangliosides

Synthesis

Ceramide $\xrightarrow[\text{Sialic acid}]{\text{UDP Glucose/UDP Galactose}}$ Gangliosides

Catabolism

Gangliosides → Ceramide + Sphingosine + FFA

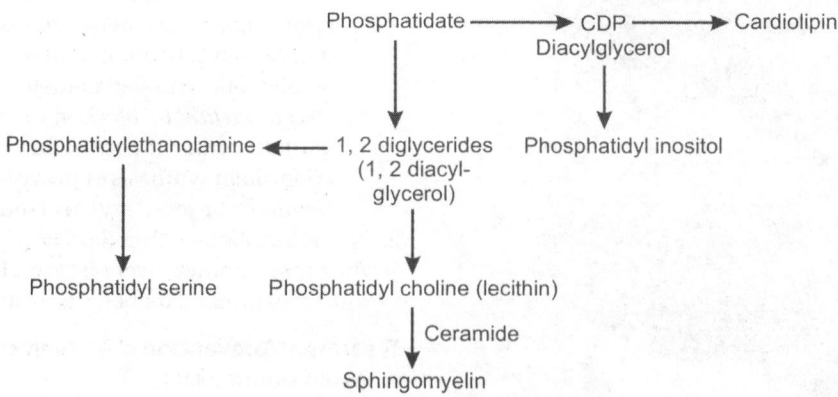

Fig. 12.11: Synthesis of phospholipids.

Clinical Importance

Sphingolipidoses: These are lipid storage disorders which occur due to inability to break down sphingolipids in lysosomes due to inherited defects in hydrolase enzymes. These are often manifested in childhood. These diseases belong to a group of lysosomal storage disorders, e.g.,
- Gaucher's disease ⎫
- Tay–Sach's disease ⎬ (*refer* Chapter 3)
- Niemann–Pick's disease ⎭

Cholesterol Metabolism

Digestion and Absorption

Cholesterol is mostly present in the diet as cholesterol ester.

They are hydrolyzed by cholesterol esterase (secreted by pancreas) in the lumen of the intestine and are absorbed in nonesterified free form.

Metabolism

It consists of two phases:
1. Biosynthesis
2. Catabolism (degradation and utilization)

Biosynthesis

Slightly more than half of the cholesterol of the body is due to synthesis (about 700 mg/day) and the remaining part is provided by the normal diet.

Site

- *Organ:* Liver, intestine, and other tissues containing nucleated cells
- *Cell:* Microsomes (endoplasmic reticulum) and cytosol

Pathway (Fig. 12.12)

Cholesterol biosynthesis occurs in the five major stages:

Formation of mevalonate

- *Condensation:* Two molecules of acetyl-CoA in the cytosol condense to form acetoacetyl-CoA catalyzed by thiolase.
- *Condensation:* Acetoacetyl-CoA condenses with another molecule of acetyl-CoA to form β-hydroxy β-methylglutaryl-CoA (HMG-CoA) catalyzed by HMG-CoA synthase.
- *Reduction:* HMG-CoA is converted to mevalonate by reduction with NADPH

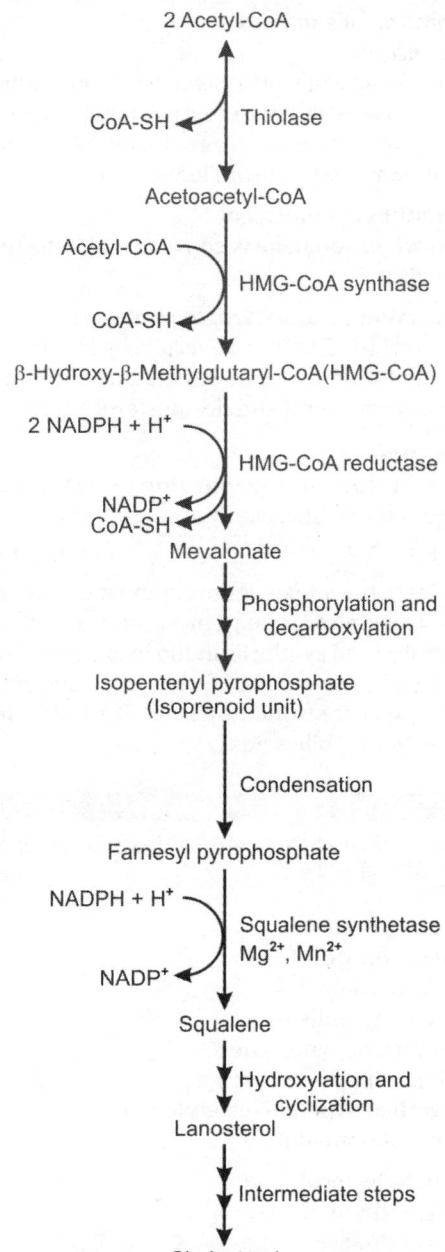

Fig. 12.12: Biosynthesis of cholesterol.

catalyzed by HMG-CoA reductase in the microsomes.

Formation of isoprenoid unit

Phosphorylation and decarboxylation: Mevalonate after three successive phosphorylation with ATP followed by decarboxylation gives isopentenyl pyrophosphate.

Formation of squalene

Condensation:
- Three molecules of isopentenyl pyrophosphate condense to form farnesyl pyrophosphate.
- Two molecules of farnesyl pyrophosphate condense to form squalene.

Formation of lanosterol

Cyclization: Squalene is converted to lanosterol by cyclization.

Conversion of lanosterol to cholesterol

Lanosterol is finally converted to cholesterol through formation of intermediate compounds such as zymosterol and desmosterol, etc.

Regulation

- The rate limiting enzyme is HMG-CoA reductase which catalyzes the reaction.

  HMG-CoA $\xrightarrow{\text{HMG-CoA reductase}}$ Mevalonate

  - It is the site of action of most cholesterol lowering drugs, e.g., mevastatin, rovastatin.
- Cholesterol synthesis in the liver is regulated partly by the influx of dietary cholesterol.
- It is also controlled by feedback inhibition, hormones, bile acids.

Clinical Importance

Normal level of cholesterol (total) in serum/ plasma = 150–200 mg/100 mL.

Abnormalities

Hypercholesterolemia
1. Atherosclerosis
2. Hypothyroidism
3. Nephrotic syndrome
4. Hyperlipoproteinemia
5. Familial hypercholesterolemia
6. Diabetes mellitus

Hypocholesterolemia
1. Hyperthyroidism
2. Liver disease
3. Malabsorption syndrome
4. Malnutrition

Factors controlling cholesterol level in blood

- *Heredity:* It has an important role in cholesterol level in individuals.
- *Diet:* Increased fat in diet increases cholesterol level. Saturated fatty acids increase cholesterol level whereas polyunsaturated fatty acids decrease it. Excess calorie increases cholesterol level. Dietary fibers induce reduction in cholesterol level.
- *Physical activity:* Regular physical exercise decreases cholesterol level.
- *Lifestyle:* Smoking, alcohol, etc., increase cholesterol level.
- Certain drugs (statin drugs) decrease cholesterol level, e.g., lovastatin.

Catabolism

Degradation (Fig. 12.13)

About 1 g cholesterol is eliminated from the body every day. It is excreted after conversion to bile acids and neutral steroids.

Conversion to bile acids

Site: Liver and small intestine

This is the major pathway of cholesterol catabolism. 50% of cholesterol is converted to bile acids and excreted in feces (**Fig. 12.14**).

Pathway

In the liver
- Cholesterol is converted to 7α-hydroxycholesterol, catalyzed by 7α-hydroxylase in the presence of NADPH—oxygen and cytochrome p450.
- Through two separate pathways, 7α-hydroxy cholesterol leads to the formation of two primary bile acids, namely:
  - Cholic acid
  - Chenodeoxycholic acid

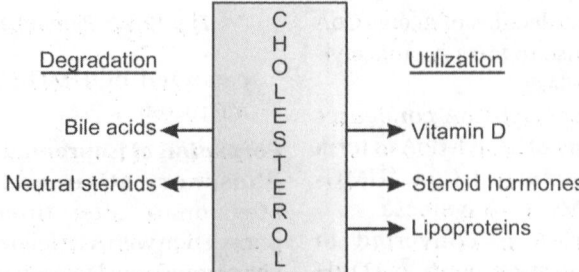

Fig. 12.13: Degradation of cholesterol.

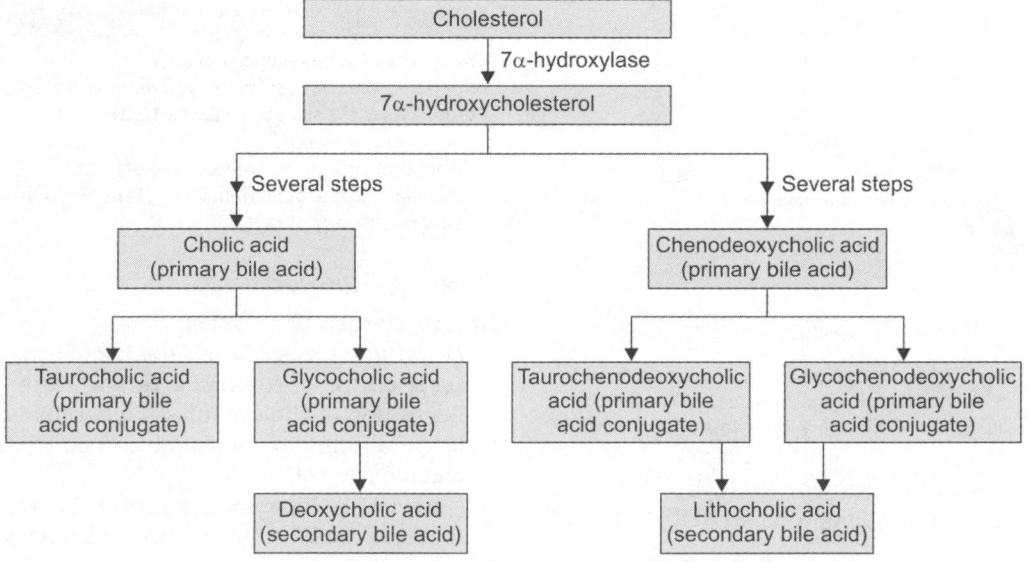

Fig. 12.14: Biosynthesis of bile acids.

- These primary bile acids form conjugates with taurine or glycine as follows:
  - Cholic acid is converted to taurocholic acid and glycocholic acid (primary bile acids conjugates).
  - Similarly chenodeoxycholic acid is converted to taurochenodeoxycholic acid and glycochenodeoxycholic acid (primary bile acids conjugates).
- The primary bile acids and their conjugates enter the bile. Since bile contains sodium and potassium and pH is alkaline, these bile acids and their conjugates exist as bile salts.

In the small intestine

Primary bile acids enter the small intestine and a portion of it gets converted to secondary bile acids by the intestinal bacteria, due to deconjugation and 7 α-hydroxylation. 98.99% primary and secondary bile acids are absorbed exclusively in the ileum and enter portal blood reaching liver. This continuous circuit of bile salts is known as enterohepatic circulation. A small fraction of the bile salts escapes absorption and is eliminated in the feces.

Regulation
- The principal rate limiting step is the reaction catalyzed by 7α-hydroxylase.
- Bile acids exert a feedback inhibition on 7α-hydroxylase.

Conversion to neutral sterols
About 10% of cholesterol is converted to neutral sterols (e.g., coprosterol) in the lower part of the intestine by the bacterial flora and excreted in feces.

Utilization (Fig. 12.13)
Conversion to steroid hormones:
- Adrenocortical hormones are formed from cholesterol
- *Sex hormones:* Androgens, estrogens and progesterone are also synthesized from cholesterol.

Conversion to vitamin D
Cholesterol is converted to 7-dehydro-cholesterol. The latter is converted to vitamin D in the skin due to UV light of sun's rays.

Lipoproteins

Cholesterol is a constituent of lipoproteins.

Metabolism of Lipoproteins (Fig. 12.15)

Lipids are dynamic molecules. They are in a constant state of synthesis, degradation and removal from the plasma. Lipids are transported in the blood as plasma lipoproteins. There are four major groups of lipoproteins.
1. Chylomicrons
2. Very low-density lipoproteins (VLDL)

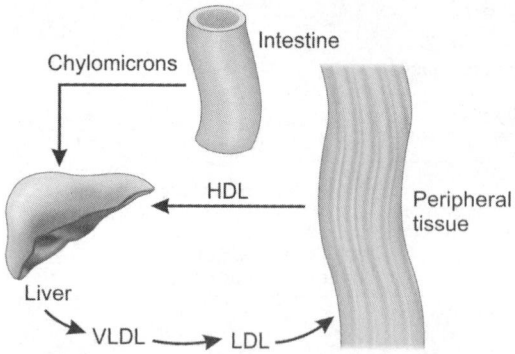

Fig. 12.15: Lipoproteins metabolism (cutline). (HDL: high-density lipoprotein; LDL: low-density lipoprotein; VLDL: very low-density lipoprotein)

3. Low-density lipoproteins (LDL)
4. High-density lipoproteins (HDL)

Each lipoprotein has two components:
1. Lipid (cholesterol, triglycerides and phospholipids)
2. Protein (apoprotein/apolipoprotein)

(Composition of each component present in various lipoproteins is given in Chapter 3)

- *Chylomicrons:* They contain highest amount of lipids (99%) and lowest quantity (1%) of proteins. They are synthesized in the intestine and exogenous (dietary) triacylglycerol is transported by them to various tissues.
- *Very low-density lipoproteins (VLDL):* It is a triacylglycerol rich lipoprotein synthesized mainly in the liver. They are involved in the transport of endogenously synthesized triacylglycerol from the liver to the extrahepatic tissues.
- *Low-density lipoprotein (LDL):* It is a cholesterol-rich lipoprotein. It is formed from VLDL via IDL (intermediate density lipoproteins). It transports cholesterol from the liver to the extrahepatic tissues. LDL cholesterol is known as bad cholesterol.
- *High-density lipoproteins (HDL):* They contain highest amount of protein and lowest amount of lipids. They are synthesized and secreted by the liver and intestine. They transport cholesterol from peripheral tissues to the liver for excretion through a process known as reverse cholesterol transport. HDL cholesterol is known as good cholesterol as it is inversely related to cardiovascular disease (CVD).

Clinical Importance

Disorders of plasma lipoproteins
Hyperlipoproteinemias: There are five types based on Frederikson's classification **(Table 12.2)**.
Hypolipoproteinemias:
- Abetalipoproteinemias: Absence of LDL
- Familial α-lipoprotein deficiency (Tangier disease): Low or absence of HDL.

Other Lipid Disorders

Atherosclerosis (Fig. 12.16)
- *Definition:* It refers to hardening of arteries (especially coronary arteries) due to deposition of cholesterol and other lipids. It leads to formation of plaque and narrowing and blocking of arteries.
- *Causes:* Hyperlipoproteinemias **(Table 12.2)**, diabetes mellitus, nephrotic syndrome and

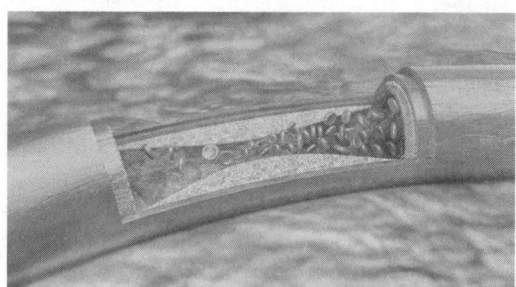

Fig. 12.16: Atherosclerosis.
(For color version, see Plate 3)

Table 12.2: Type of hyperlipoproteinemias.

Type	Features
I	Deficiency of lipoprotein lipase, chylomicrons increased, no increased risk of coronary heart disease (CHD)
IIA	Familial hypercholesterolemia occurs due to deficiency of LDL receptors, LDL increased, risk due to atherosclerosis and CHD
IIB	Overproduction of Apo-B, LDL and VLDL increased, risk due to atherosclerosis
III	Deficiency in clearance of remnants by the liver, IDL increased. Causes hypercholesterolemia, xanthomas, atherosclerosis
IV	Overproduction/decreased catabolism of VLDL, VLDL increased, associated with CHD
V	Secondary to other causes, chylomicrons and VLDL increased, may/may not increase atherosclerosis

hypothyroidism. Other factors include excessive smoking, hypertension, lack of physical activity, obesity, consumption of saturated fat, age and genetic factors.
- *Effect:* It is the main causative factor of coronary heart disease (CHD) and cerebrovascular disease (stroke).
- *Diagnosis:* Cholesterol and LDL cholesterol (bad cholesterol) are elevated, HDL cholesterol (good cholesterol) is inversely related to CHD.
- *Treatment:* Lovastatin, clofibrate.

Obesity

Definition: Obesity is a complex disorder involving an excessive amount of fat in the body. It occurs when a person's body mass index (BMI) is above 25 (normal 20–25).

Causes:
- Excess food intake
- Junk foods
- Lack of exercise
- Certain medications
- Leptin resistance
- Hormone imbalance
- Genetics

Symptoms:
- Pain in the back and joints
- Snoring
- Overeating
- Pot belly

Effects: It increases of risk of diseases and health problems, e.g., diabetes mellitus, heart diseases, hypertension, etc.

Prevention:
- Regular exercise
- Healthy eating plan
- Monitoring weight regularly

Treatment:
- Diet
- Exercise
- Medications, e.g., leptin (body weight regulating hormone)
- Surgery (liposuction)

Diagnosis of Lipid Disorders

Lipid profile

Lipid profile forms an important group of investigations for mostly cardiovascular diseases. It includes the following investigations which should be measured in blood at fasting state (10–12 hours after a meal).
- Total cholesterol
- LDL cholesterol
- HDL cholesterol
- Triglycerides (triacylglycerol)
- $\dfrac{\text{Total cholesterol}}{\text{HDL cholesterol}}$ Ratio
- Lipoprotein (a)

Patients values are interpreted with reference to established normal values (reference value) to arrive at a diagnosis by the clinicians (*refer* Appendix G: Normal value chart).

13. Digestion, Absorption, and Metabolism of Proteins

Chapter Outline
- Digestion
- Absorption
- Metabolism of Amino Acids (General Pathways)
- Urea Cycle (Urea Biosynthesis)
- Metabolism of Nonessential Amino Acids
- Metabolism of Essential Amino Acids
- Additional Information

■ INTRODUCTION

Proteins taken in the diet may be of animal or plant sources. The total daily protein load to be digested consists of about 70–100 g of dietary proteins and 35–200 g of endogenous proteins.

■ DIGESTION

There is no digestion of proteins in the mouth. The process of protein digestion can be divided into three phases:
1. Gastric phase
2. Pancreatic phase
3. Intestinal phase

Gastric Phase

Proteins get denatured by HCl present in the gastric juice (pH2). Denaturation makes proteins more susceptible to hydrolysis by proteases (proteolytic enzymes). Pepsin (an endopeptidase formed from proenzyme pepsinogen) hydrolyzes the denatured proteins into larger polypeptides.

$$\text{Proteins} \rightarrow \text{Larger polypeptides}$$

(The enzyme rennin present in the stomach of infants and children converts milk protein casein to calcium paracaseinate which can be effectively digested by pepsin. It is absent in adults).

Pancreatic Phase

Pancreatic juice is rich in proenzymes of:
- *Endopeptidases:* Trypsin, chymotrypsin and elastase
- *Exopeptidase:* Carboxypeptidase

They are activated after they reach the lumen of the small intestine by hormones namely cholecystokinin and secretin.

Action of Endopeptidases

Trypsin, chymotrypsin and elastase split peptide bonds at the interior of larger polypeptides.

Action of Exopeptidases

Carboxypeptidase splits of successive amino acids from the carboxy terminal of the larger peptides.

The combined action of pancreatic peptidases results in the formation of small peptides and free amino acids.

$$\text{Larger polypeptides} \rightarrow \text{Small peptides} + \text{Free amino acids}$$

Intestinal Phase

Final digestion of small peptides is carried out by enzymes of small intestine namely aminopeptidases and dipeptidases.

Aminopeptidase: It is an exopeptidase. It splits peptide bonds next to amino terminal of amino acids of small peptides.

$$\text{Small peptides} \rightarrow \text{Dipeptides} + \text{Amino acids}$$

Dipeptidases: Complete digestion of dipeptides to amino acids occurs due to action of dipeptidases.

$$\text{Dipeptides} \rightarrow \text{Amino acids}$$

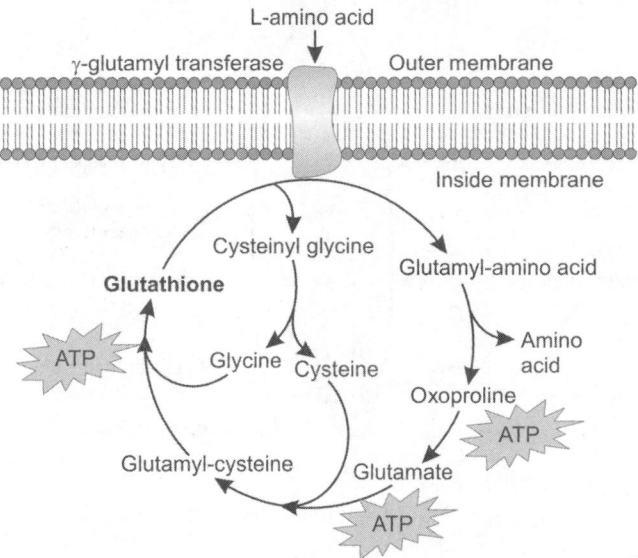

Fig. 13.1: γ glutamyl cycle (Meister cycle).

■ ABSORPTION

Normally the dietary proteins are almost completely digested to their constituent amino acids. They are absorbed from the small intestine to reach liver via portal blood. D-amino acids are absorbed slowly through simple diffusion. L-amino acids are absorbed more rapidly by active transport with the aid of transporters. Meister proposed a mechanism known as Meister cycle or γ-glutamyl cycle to explain the absorption of L-amino acids **(Fig. 13.1)**.

Changes in the Large Intestine

Undigested protein passes into the large intestine where bacteria act through fermentation and putrefaction. Thus amino acids undergo following changes, producing toxic amines or other toxic compounds. For example:
- Lysine → Cadaverine
- Tyrosine → Tyramine
- Histidine → Histamine
- Tryptophan → Indole + Skatole (responsible for odor of feces)
- Cysteine → Mercaptans + H_2S

Also large intestine produces ammonia due to bacterial action on nitrogenous substances. High protein diet also may lead to ammonia intoxication.

> **Clinical Importance: Disorders**
>
> Absorption of unhydrolyzed polypeptides may cause immunologic reactions as in non-tropical sprue. *Hartnup disease* may occur due to defect in absorption of neutral amino acids (*refer* page 184).

Storage

Amino acids ingested in excess of requirement or liberated by catabolism of proteins are degraded and not stored.

Amino Acid Pool

A mixture of endogenous and exogenous amino acids constitutes a reservoir of amino acids called as amino acid pool of the body. It is not a single compartment but represents several compartments. It has also 100 g of free amino acids. It is maintained by two ways **(Fig. 13.2)**.

■ METABOLISM OF AMINO ACIDS (GENERAL PATHWAYS)

Amino groups from amino acids are removed by some metabolic reactions and carbon skeleton is converted into intermediates.

Anabolism: It refers to synthesis of amino acids and proteins (*refer* to respective pages of amino acid metabolism and protein biosynthesis).

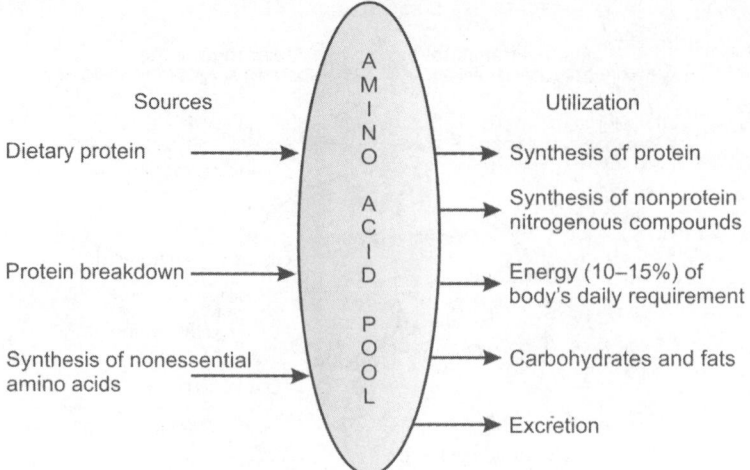

Fig. 13.2: Amino acid pool.

Catabolism: It involves:
- Removal/transfer of amino groups and disposal of amino groups
- Disposal of carbon skeleton

Removal of Amino Groups from Amino Acids

It takes place by one of the following reactions.

Transamination

Definition
Process of transfer of an amino group from an amino acid to a keto acid resulting in the formation of a new amino acid and new keto acid is called as transamination. Transamination is catalyzed by the enzyme transaminase (aminotransferase) with pyridoxal phosphate as coenzyme.

Examples
There are two important transaminases in the body.
- SGOT (serum glutamate oxaloacetate transaminase)/AST (aspartate aminotransferase)

    Aspartate + α-ketoglutarate $\xrightleftharpoons{\text{SGOT}}$
    Oxaloacetate + Glutamate

- SGPT (serum gultamate pyruvate transaminase)/ALT (alanine aminotransferase)

    Alanine + α-ketoglutarate $\xrightleftharpoons{\text{SGPT}}$
    Pyruvate + Glutamate

Importance
- Both enzymes are increased in serum in myocardial infarction and liver diseases.
- All amino acids except lysine, threonine and proline participate in transamination.
- It is a reversible reaction
- It requires pyridoxal phosphate as coenzyme
- Free ammonia is not liberated but transfer of amino group only occurs
- It is the initiating point of amino acid metabolism
- It provides nonessential amino acids.

Deamination

Removal of amino group from amino acids is called as deamination. It is of two types:
- *Oxidative deamination:* This process involves oxidation (dehydrogenation) first and then hydrolysis liberating ammonia and keto acid.

    Amino acid → Imino acid → Keto acid + NH_3

    This reaction is catalyzed by enzymes called amino acid oxidases with FAD as coenzyme, which occur in mammalian liver and kidneys.

    Specific examples: *Refer*
    - Alanine metabolism
    - Glutamic acid metabolism

- *Nonoxidative deamination:* It involves deamination without oxidation catalyzed by enzyme amino acid dehydratase, with pyridoxal phosphate as coenzyme, e.g., *refer* metabolism of serine and threonine.

Transdeamination

This process is a combination of transamination and deamination (*refer* to glutamic acid metabolism).

Disposal of Amino Group (Ammonia Metabolism)

Ammonia released from amino acids may be utilized for anabolic purpose or catabolic purpose.

Synthetic (Anabolic) Pathway
- Formation of purines and pyrimidines
- Formation of new amino acids

Catabolic Pathway
- *Glutamine pathway:* If ammonia is formed in excess, it has to be removed as it is toxic in the cells. This is carried out by detoxification, e.g., formation of glutamine from ammonia by glutamine synthetase.

  Glutamic acid + NH_3 → Glutamine

  This reaction takes place in extrarenal tissues. Glutamine formed thus passed from tissues via blood to kidneys where it is hydrolyzed to glutamic acid by glutaminase.

  Glutamine + H_2O → Glutamic acid + NH_3

  Ammonia is excreted in urine.
- *Direct excretion of ammonia:* When ammonia is not required for metabolic synthetic purpose, it is excreted directly in urine (40% of total ammonia).
- *Formation of urea* (**Fig. 13.3**).

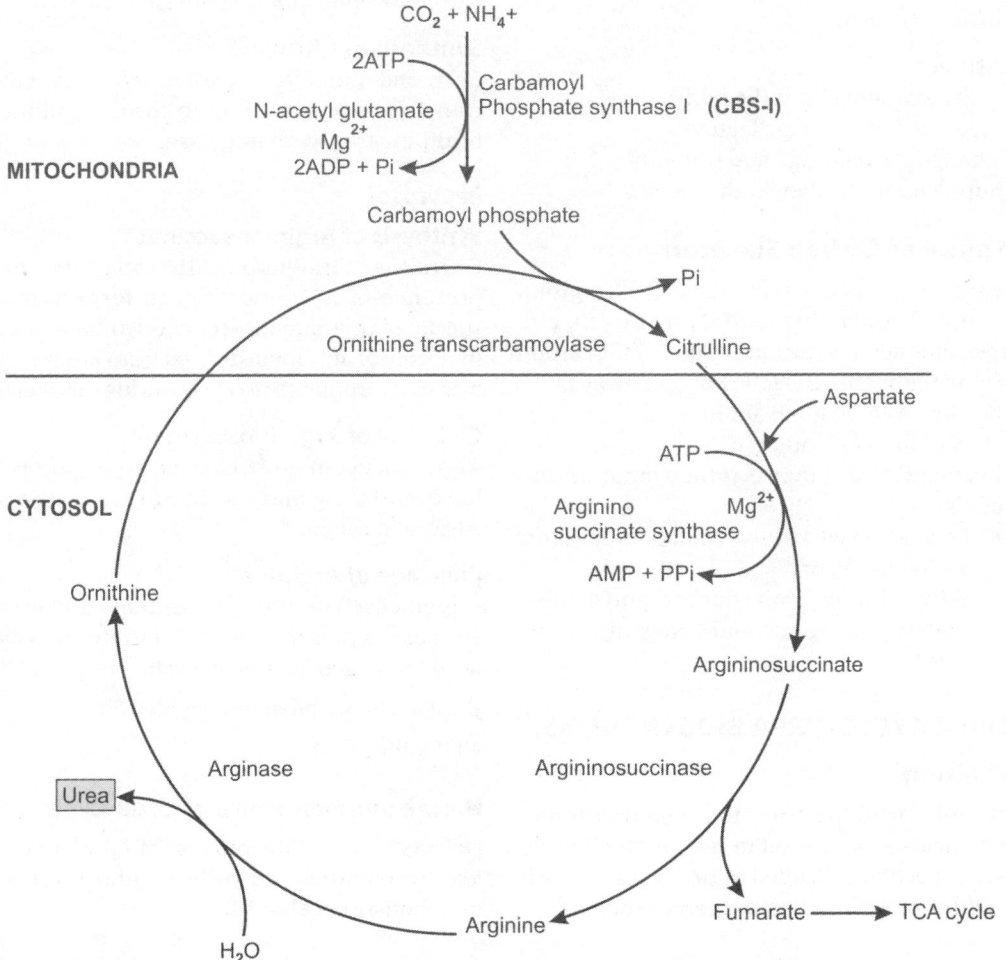

Fig. 13.3: Urea cycle.

Ammonia Intoxication/Ammonia toxicity

Ammonia intoxication is a life-threatening problem. Ammonia is formed in the body by (a) enteric bacteria (b) degradation from amino acids in the tissues. It is a highly toxic product. Its normal level in blood is 10–20 μg/dL. Hence excess ammonia should be removed from circulation promptly (via) urea cycle, etc.

Effects
- Severely impaired hepatic function
- Liver cirrhosis

Clinical symptoms
- Tremor
- Slurred speech
- Blurred vision
- Coma
- Ultimately death

Treatment
Detoxify ammonia from the body:
- Take medication, e.g., lactulose
- Change the diet, e.g., add probiotics
- Supplement the diet/limit proteins

Disposal of Carbon Skeleton

The amino acid after removal of amino group (ammonia) containing carbon, hydrogen, and oxygen are called as carbon skeleton. This carbon skeleton undergoes the following pathways:
- Formation of original amino acid
- Oxidation to CO_2 and H_2O
- Formation of glucose (glucogenic amino acids) or
  - Formation of ketone bodies (ketogenic amino acids) or
  - Formation of both glucose and ketone bodies (glucogenic and ketogenic amino acid).

■ UREA CYCLE (UREA BIOSYNTHESIS)

Definition

Ammonia resulting from the deamination of amino acids is converted to urea in the liver by a cyclic mechanism called as urea cycle. Urea is the end-product of protein catabolism.

Alternative Names
- Krebs–Hensleit cycle (named after the discoverers Krebs and Hensleit, 1932).
- Ornithine cycle

Site
- *Organ:* Liver
- *Cell:* Cytosol and mitochondria

Pathway (Fig. 13.3)

In Mitochondria

Synthesis of Carbamoyl Phosphate

CO_2 condenses with one molecule of ammonia in the presence of ATP and cofactor Mg^{++} and N-acetyl glutamate to form carbamoyl phosphate. This reaction is catalyzed by carbamoyl phosphate synthase I (CPS-I).

Synthesis of Citrulline

Carbamoyl moiety of carbamoyl phosphate is transferred to ornithine to form citrulline by ornithine transcarbamoylase.

In Cytosol

Synthesis of Argininosuccinate

Citrulline condenses with aspartate in the presence of ATP and Mg^{2+} to form argininosuccinate by argininosuccinate synthase. Second molecule of ammonia derived from amino group of aspartate enters urea cycle during this reaction.

Cleavage of Argininosuccinate

Argininosuccinate is cleaved to arginine and fumarate by argininosuccinase (fumarate enters citric acid cycle).

Cleavage of Arginine

Arginine is hydrolyzed to ornithine and urea by arginase in presence of Mn^{2+}. Ornithine is again used for urea formation in cyclic way (**Fig. 13.3**).

Regulation: Regulatory enzyme CPS-I

ATP utilized = 4

Metabolic Disorders of Urea Cycle

Defects in any of the enzymes in the urea cycle lead to metabolic disorders (inborn errors of metabolism) (**Table 13.1**).

Table 13.1: Urea cycle disorders.

Disorders	Defect (Enzyme Deficiency)	Symptoms	Treatment
Hyperammonemia Type - I	Carbamoyl phosphate synthase I	All disorders of urea cycle result in hyperammonemia leading to ammonia intoxi cation (tremor, slurred speech, blurred vision, coma)	Low protein diet to ingest as frequent small meals to avoid sudden increase in blood ammonia levels
Hyperammonemia Type - II	Ornithine transcarbamoylase		
Citrullinemia	Argininosuccinate synthase	Clinical symptoms common to all urea cycle	
Argininosuccinic aciduria	Argininosuccinase	Disorders include vomiting, intermittent ataxia	
Hyperargininemia	Arginase	Irritability, lethargy and mental retardation	

Clinical Importance

Urea

Normal level in blood = 15–40 mg/100 mL
* *Increased in:* Renal diseases and high protein diet
* *Decreased in:* Pregnancy and some liver diseases and low protein diet
* *Normal level in urine:* 15–30 g/day
* *Increased in:* Renal diseases
* *Decreased in:* Low protein diet and liver disease

Note: Urea clearance test is a renal function test

METABOLISM OF NONESSENTIAL AMINO ACIDS

Glycine

Glycine is a neutral, nonessential and glucogenic amino acid. It is the simplest amino acid.

Synthesis

It can be synthesized in the mammalian body by the following routes:

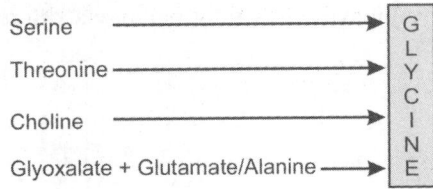

Catabolism

Major pathway

Glycine is reversibly split into CO_2 and NH_4^+ by glycine synthase complex present in liver mitochondria and forms $N^{5,10} CH_2FH_4$.

Glycine + NAD^+ ↔ CO_2 + NH_4^+ + NADH + H^+

Other pathways

□ Glycine is first reversibly converted to serine which is degraded to form pyruvate.
  Glycine ↔ Serine ↔ Pyruvate
  (precursor for glucose)
□ Glycine is converted to glyoxylate which is oxidized to oxalate or formate.

Utilization

Glycine participates in the biosynthesis of several physiologically important compounds (for details, refer below).

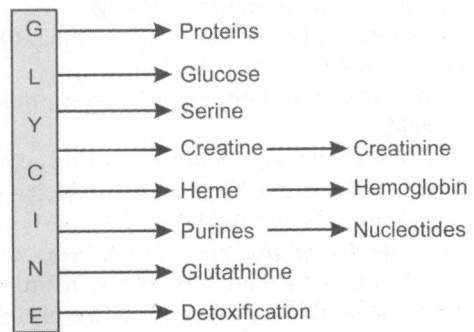

Compounds Formed from Glycine

1. *Synthesis of glutathione:* Glutathione is a tripeptide formed from three amino acids namely glutamic acid, cysteine, and glycine (γ-glutamyl cysteinyl glycine).
2. *Synthesis of purine:* Glycine molecule is utilized to form C_4, C_5, and N_7 of purine ring.

3. *Synthesis of heme:* Glycine condenses with succinyl-CoA to form δ aminolevulinate which is the precursur for the synthesis of heme.

   Glycine + Succinyl-CoA → δ aminolevulinate → heme

4. *Synthesis of creatinine* (*refer* page 177).
   a. There amino acids namely glycine, arginine, and methionine are required for the synthesis of creatinine. The quanidine groups of arginine is transferred to glycine to form guanidoacetate, being catalyzed by transamidinase.
   b. In the liver, S-adenosyl methionine (active methionine) donates methyl group to guanidoacetate to produce creatine (anhydride of creatinine).
   c. Creatine is reversibly phosphorylated to creatine phosphate (phosphocreatine) by creatine kinase. It is stored in muscle as high energy compound.
   d. Creatinine is formed from creatine or creatine phosphate by spontaneous cyclization.
   Importance: Creatinine is excreted in the urine as a waste product and is proportional to total body mass. Blood creatinine level (normal range: 0.6–1.2 mg/100 mL) is a good indicator of kidney function. Creatinine clearance test is used as a renal function test to assess glomerular filtration rate (GFR).

5. *Detoxication:* Glycine acts as a conjugating agent in detoxication:
   a. It detoxicates benzoic acid to hippuric acid.
      Glycine + Benzoic acid → Hippuric acid
   b. Bile acids are conjugated with glycine or taurine to be excreted (*refer* page 161).

6. *Constituent of proteins, hormones, and enzymes:* Glycine is an important constituent amino acid of body tissue proteins, protein hormones, and enzymes.

> **Clinical Importance: Disorders**
>
> ❖ **Glycinuria:** It occurs probably from a defect in renal tubular reabsorption. Plasma glycine level is normal. But high urinary excretion of glycine occurs and leads to formation of oxalate renal stones.
>
> *Contd...*

Contd...

> ❖ **Primary hyperoxaluria:** It is an inherited disorder. It may occur due to impairment of oxidation of glyoxylate to formate. Gyoxalate formed from glycine is converted to oxalate. It leads to calcium oxalate urolithiasis and urinary infection.

Alanine (α-Alanine)

Alanine is a neutral, nonessential and glucogenic amino acid.

Synthesis

Glutamate + Pyruvate $\xrightarrow[\text{Transamination}]{\text{SGPT}}$ α-ketoglutarate + Alanine

Catabolism

Transamination of alanine forms pyruvate which is then decarboxylated to acetyl-CoA.

Alanine $\xrightarrow{\text{Transamination}}$ Pyruvate $\xrightarrow{-CO_2-}$ Acetyl-CoA

Utilization

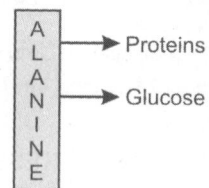

Disorder

Nil.

Serine

Serine is a neutral, nonessential and glucogenic amino acid.

Synthesis

Serine biosynthesis may occur via different routes.

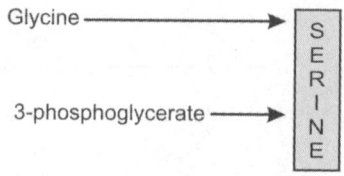

Catabolism

Serine is degraded via glycine.

Serine ↔ Glycine → Follows catabolic pathway of glycine

Utilization

It is involved in the synthesis of several compounds of physiological importance.

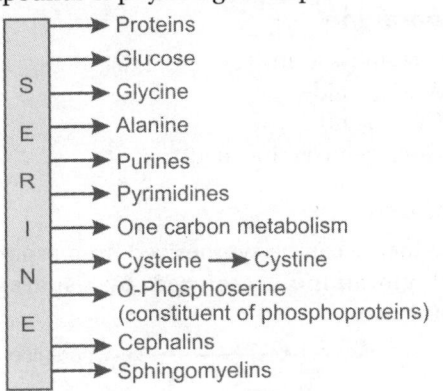

Disorder

Nil.

Glutamic Acid

Glutamic acid is a/an:
- Acidic
- Nonessential
- Glucogenic amino acid

Synthesis

It is formed in the body through different routes:

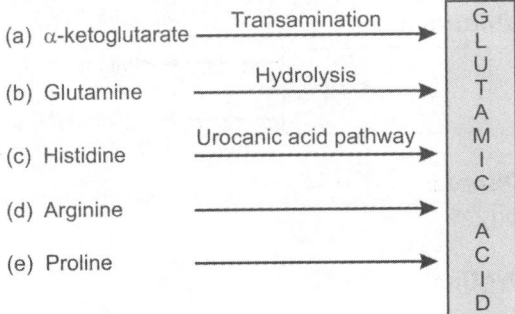

Catabolism

- On transmination with pyruvic acid, it forms α-ketoglutarate and alanine. This reaction is catalyzed by SGPT requiring pyridoxal phosphate as coenzyme.

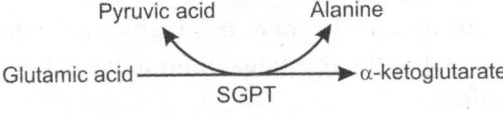

- By oxidative deamination, it forms alanine and ammonia. Alanine follows its usual catabolic pathway.

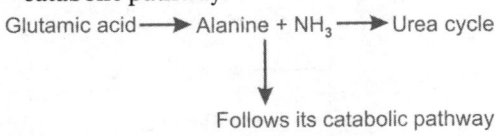

Utilization

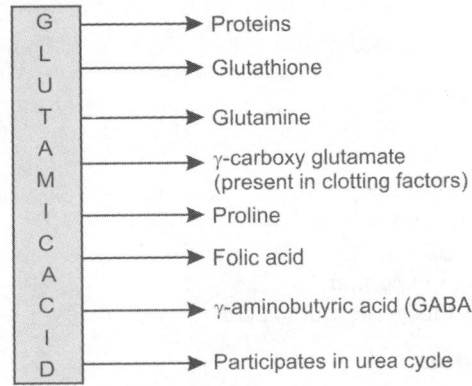

γ-Aminobutyric Acid (GABA)

Glutamate is decarboxylated to form GABA by PLP dependent glutamate decarboxylase. It is the major inhibitory neurotransmitter. Deficiency of GABA may lead to convulsions.

Disorder

Nil.

Aspartic Acid

Aspartic acid is a/an:
- Acidic
- Nonessential
- Glucogenic amino acid

Synthesis

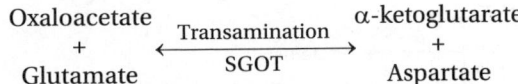

Catabolism

- Aspartic acid is converted to oxaloacetate by transamination.

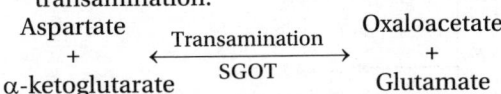

Utilization

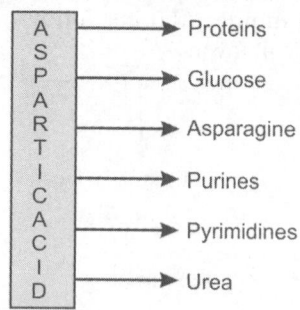

Disorder
Nil.

Glutamine

Glutamine is a/an:
☐ Acidic amide
☐ Nonessential
☐ Glucogenic amino acid

Synthesis

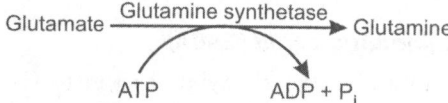

Catabolism

Glutamine is deamidated by glutaminase in the kidneys liberating free ammonia and glutamic acid. Glutamic acid then follows its catabolic pathway.

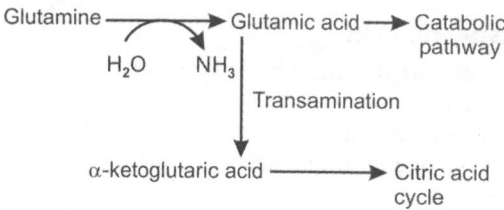

Utilization

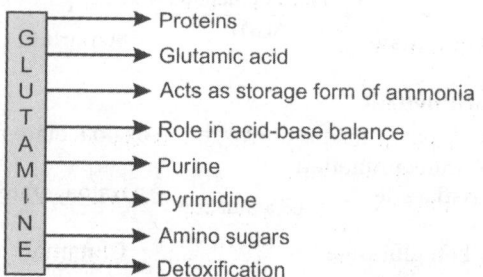

Disorder
Nil.

Asparagine

Asparagine is a/an:
☐ Acidic amide
☐ Nonessential
☐ Glucogenic amino acid

Synthesis

Asparagine can be synthesized from aspartate and glutamine, catalyzed by asparagine synthetase.

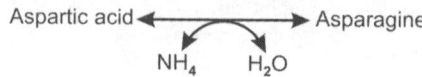

Catabolism

Asparagine is degraded to oxaloacetate via aspartate.

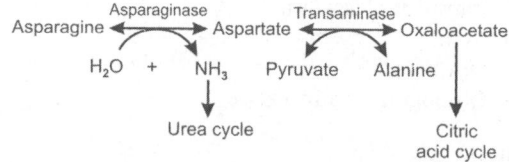

Utilization

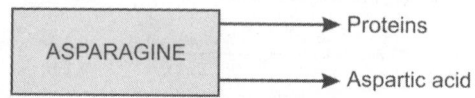

Disorder
Nil.

Proline

Proline is a:
☐ Neutral
☐ Nonessential
☐ Glucogenic amino acid

Synthesis

Glutamate → Proline

Proline is formed from glutamate by reversal of the reactions of proline catabolic pathway.

Catabolism

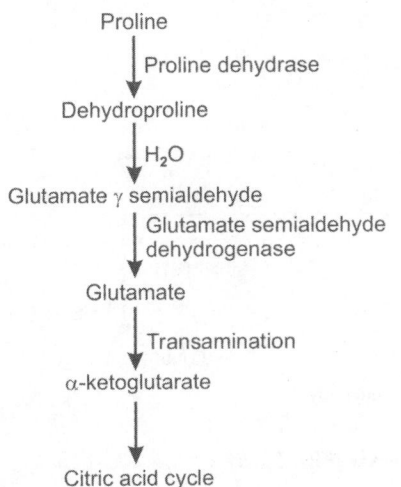

(Proline does not undergo direct transamination).

Utilization

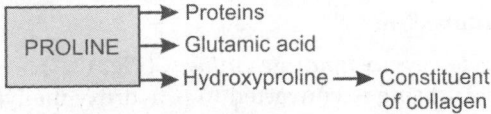

Clinical Importance: Disorders

- *Hyperprolinemia Type I:* It occurs due to deficiency of proline dehydrase.
- *Hyperprolinemia Type II:* Defective enzyme is glutamate semialdehyde dehydrogenase in this disorder.

Cysteine

Cysteine is a:
- Neutral
- Nonessential
- Glucogenic amino acid

It is one of the sulfur containing amino acids present in protein.

Synthesis

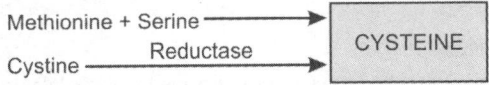

Catabolism

Cysteine is degraded by two different routes:

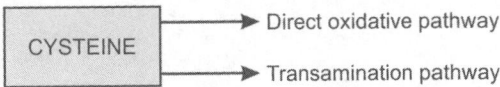

Direct oxidative pathway (cysteine sulfinate pathway) (Fig. 13.4)

- Cysteine is converted to cysteine sulfinate catalyzed by cysteine dioxygenase.
- Cysteine sulfinate undergoes transamination to sulfinyl pyruvate.
- Sulfinyl pyruvate is converted to pyruvate and sulfite, catalyzed by desulfinase.

Transamination pathway (3-mercaptopyruvate pathway) (Fig. 13.5)

- Cysteine is transaminated to form 3-mercaptopyruvate.
- 3-mercaptopyruvate may be reduced to 3 mercaptolactate by lactate dehydrogenase.
- It may undergo desulfuration to form pyruvate and H_2S.

Utilization

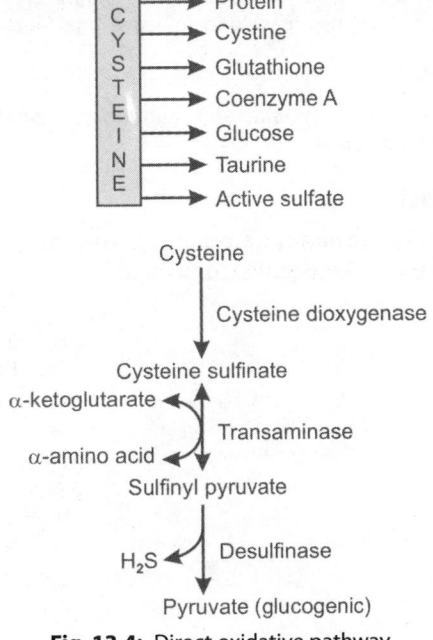

Fig. 13.4: Direct oxidative pathway.

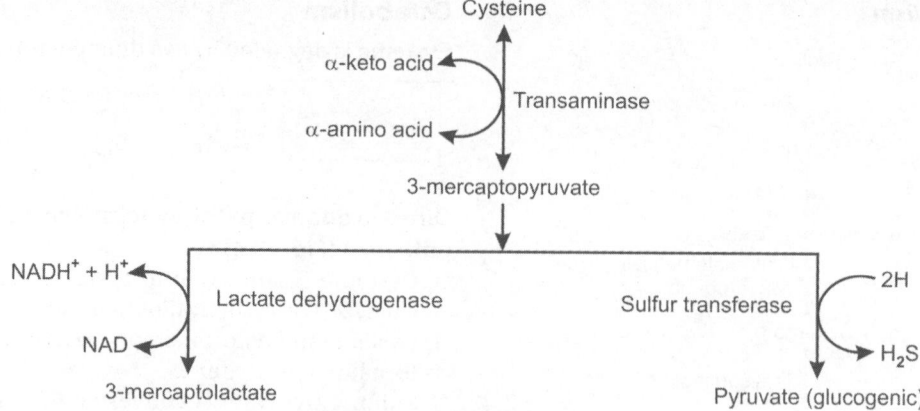

Fig. 13.5: Transamination pathway.

Clinical Importance: Disorders

- *Cystinuria:* It occurs due to defect in the renal reabsorption mechanism of cystine along with lysine, arginine, and ornithine. It is accompanied by high excretion of cystine along with other three amino acids. Cystine calculi are formed in the renal tubules.
- *Cystinosis:* It is a rare lysosomal disorder (cystine storage disease). It occurs due to defect in the carrier-mediated transport of cystine. Symptoms are aminoaciduria, deposition of cystine crystals in tissues and organs, and defective renal function.

> **Note**
> Metabolism of cysteine and methionine should be studied together.

Tyrosine

Tyrosine is a neutral, aromatic, nonessential and glucogenic-ketogenic amino acid.

Synthesis (Fig. 13.6)

Tyrosine is synthesized from phenylalanine by the reaction catalyzed by phenylalanine hydroxylase.

Phenylalanine $\xrightarrow{\text{Phenylalanine hydroxylase}}$ Tyrosine

Catabolism

Acetoacetate-fumarate pathway (**Fig. 13.7**).
- Tyrosine is converted to p-hydroxyphenyl-pyruvate by transamination catalyzed by tyrosine transaminase.
- Hydroxylation of p-hydroxyphenyl pyruvate and side chain migration forms homogentisate.
- Oxidative breaking of the benzene ring of homogentisate catalyzed by homogentisate oxidase results in the formation of maleylacetoacetate.

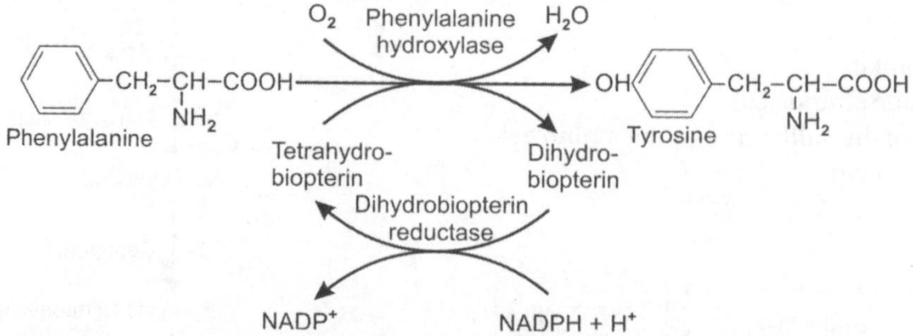

Fig. 13.6: Synthesis of tyrosine from phenylalanine: Phenylalanine is hydroxylated to tyrosine by phenylalanine hydroxylase utilizing the coenzyme biopterin (its active form is tetrahydrobioptein). During this reaction tetrahydrobiopterin is oxidized to dihydrobiopterin. Dihydrobiopterin is converted to tetrahydrobioptein by an NADPH dependent dihydrobiopterin reductase.

- Isomerization of maleylacetoacetate forms fumarylacetoacetate, being catalyzed by maleylacetoacetate cis-trans isomerase.
- Fumarylacetoacetate is hydrolyzed to form fumarate and acetoacetate.
- Formation and uses/functions of some of the above compounds are given below.

Melanin

Melanin is the pigment of skin, hair, and eye. It is formed from tyrosine in melanocytes.

Dopamine, Epinephrine (Adrenaline) and Norepinephrine (Noradrenaline)

These are catecholamines formed from tyrosine.

Parkinson's disease occurs due to decreased production of dopamine. Epinephrine and norepinephrine are hormones which regulate carbohydrate and lipid metabolism (*refer* to respective pages for more details). Pheochromocytoma is a tumor in adrenal gland which secrete more epinephrine (E) and norepinephrine (NE).

Thyroid Hormones (T_3, T_4)

Formation and functions of thyroid hormones (*refer* Chapter 25).

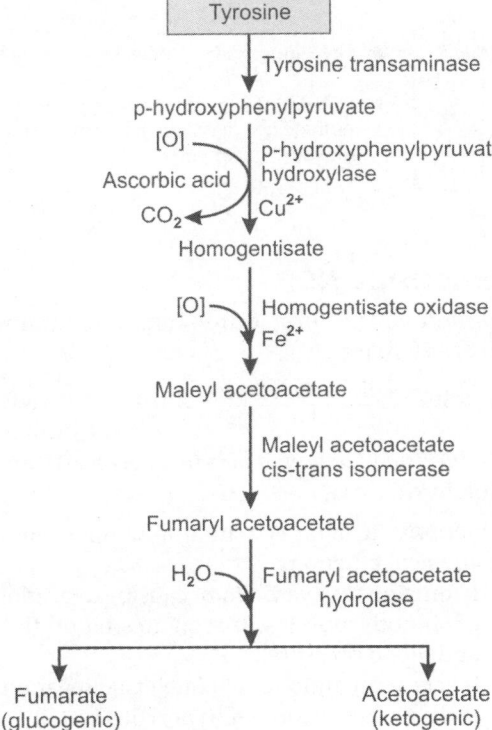

Fig. 13.7: Catabolism of tyrosine.

Utilization (Fig. 13.8)

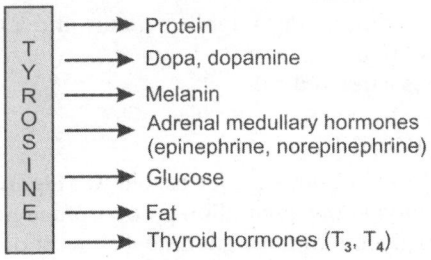

Clinical Importance: Disorders

Inborn Errors of Metabolism
Phenylketonuria
Refer page 188.

Alkaptonuria
It is the first IEM discovered by Garrod.

Incidence: 2–5/million birth.
Alternative name. Black urine disease.

Defect: Homogentisate is not converted to maleyl-acetoacetate due to deficiency of homogentisate oxidase.

Homogentisate → Maleylacetoacetate

Symptoms: Darkening of urine in air due to oxidation of homogentisate to brownish-black pigment; pigmentation of connective tissue (ochronosis) and arthritis.

Diagnosis: Urine changes to black color in air.

Treatment: Low phenylalanine in the diet. Benedict's test gives positive reaction.

Contd...

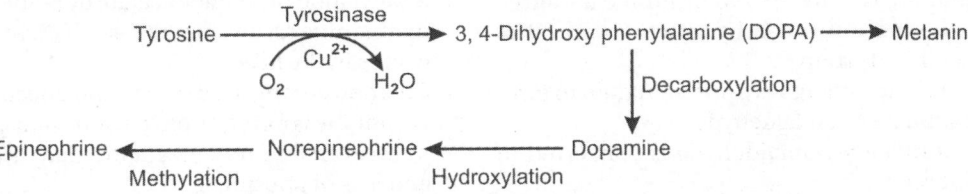

Fig. 13.8: Compounds formed from tyrosine.

Contd...

Albinism
It is an inborn error of tyrosine metabolism. There are different forms of albinism.

Incidence: 1 in 2,000. It is a autosomal disease.

Defect: Due to deficiency of the enzyme tyrosinase, tyrosine is not converted to melanin.

Symptoms: Less pigmentation in skin and eyes, sensitivity to sunlight, increased susceptibility to skin cancer, photophobia. Protect the body from sunlight.

Treatment: Gene transfer.

Tyrosinemia
Several types have been reported.

> **Note**
> Metabolism of tyrosine and phenylalanine should be studies together.

METABOLISM OF ESSENTIAL AMINO ACIDS

Arginine
Arginine is a:
- Basic
- Semiessential
- Glucogenic amino acid

Synthesis
It is a semiessential amino acid. It is not essential for adults but becomes essential during growing period in humans.
- It is formed in the urea cycle as follows:
  Argininosuccinate $\xrightarrow{\text{Argininosuccinase}}$ Arginine + Fumarate
- It is also synthesized in the kidney.

Catabolism

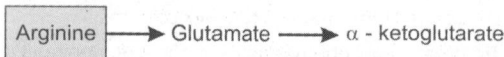

Pathway
- Arginine is converted to ornithine and urea by arginase through hydrolytic removal of guanidino group.
- Ornithine undergoes transamination to form glutamate γ-semialdehyde.
- Glutamate-γ-semialdehyde is converted to glutamate.
- Glutamate is transaminated to form α-ketoglutarate which then enters citric acid cycle or gluconeogenesis.

Utilization

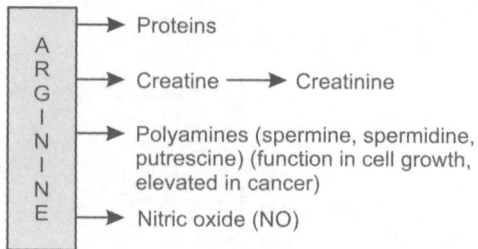

Nitric Oxide (NO)
Formation: It is formed from arginine (amino acid) as follows:

Arginine $\xrightarrow[O_2]{\text{Nitric oxide synthase}}$ Nitric Oxide (NO) + Citrulline

Mechanism of action: It acts through cGMP and protein kinase G.

Functions: It acts as a mediator for several biomedical functions.
- It functions as a vasodilator causing relaxation of smooth muscles. It regulates blood flow and blood pressure.
- It acts as an inhibitor of platelet aggregation.
- It is a neurotransmitter in nervous system.
- It mediates the bactericidal action of macrophages.

Harmful effects:
- It is also an automobile exhaust and a toxic pollutant.
- It is a free radical.

Creatinine
It is formed from arginine as follows **(Fig. 13.9)**:
- Transfer of a guanidino group from arginine to glycine to form guanidoacetate. It occurs in the kidney.
- Methylation of guanidoacetate by S-adenosyl methionine results in synthesis of creatine. It occurs in the liver.
- Creatine is converted to creatine phosphate.
- Creatinine is formed from creatine phosphate by irreversible nonenzymatic dehydration and loss of phosphate.

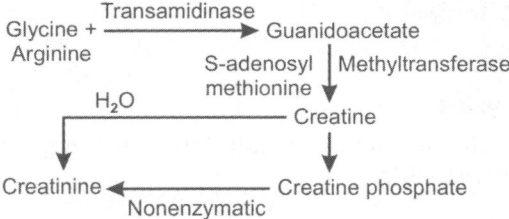

Fig. 13.9: Formation of creatinine.

Creatine and creatine phosphate (energy reserve) are present in muscle, brain, and blood. Creatinine is the anhydride of creatine. The 24 hour excretion of creatinine in the urine of a given subject is constant from day-to-day and proportionate to muscle mass. Creatinine clearance test is an important renal function test.

Clinical Importance: Disorders
❖ *Hyperornithinemia:* It results due to impaired transport of ornithine into mitochondria. It is accompanied by defective urea formation with consequent ammonemia and ornithinemia. ❖ *Hyperargininemia:* Refer page 169.

Histidine

Histidine is a neutral, semiessential, and glucogenic amino acid.

Synthesis

It is a semiessential amino acid as it may be synthesized at low amount insufficient for normal growth. For growing humans, it becomes essential and should be supplied in the diet.

Catabolism

Urocanate pathway (Fig. 13.10)

❑ Histidine is deaminated by histidase to form urocanate.
❑ Urocanate is converted to 4-imidazolone-5-propionate by urocanase.
❑ Hydrolysis of 4-imidazolone 5-propionate forms N-formiminoglutamate (Figlu).
❑ Transfer of formimino group of Figlu to tetrahydrofolate forms N_5 formimino H_4 folate. Glutamate is liberated. In deficiency of folic acid, figlu accumulates and excreted in urine. Thus *figlu test* (estimation of folic acid in urine) is used as a test for folic acid deficiency.
❑ Glutamate is converted to α-ketoglutarate by transamination.

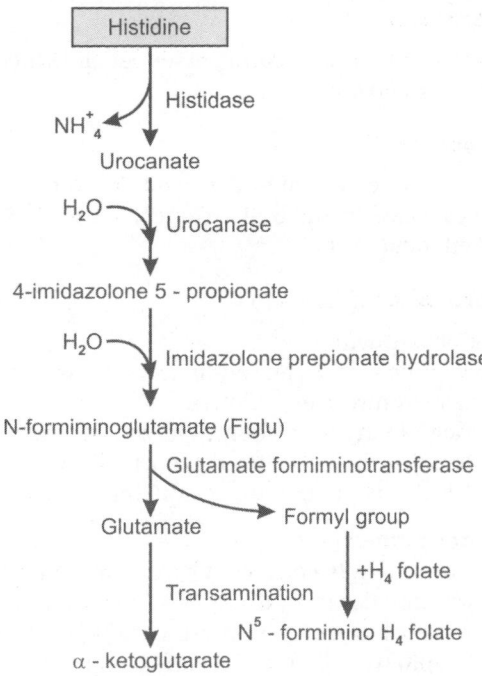

Fig. 13.10: Catabolism of histidine (urocanate pathway).

Utilization

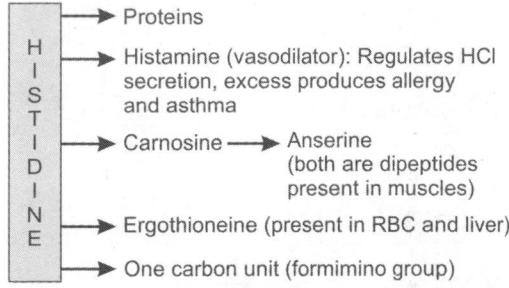

Clinical Importance: Disorders
❖ *Histidinemia:* It results due to deficiency of histidase—it is characterized by elevated level of histidine in blood and urine. ❖ *Urocanic aciduria:* It occurs due to defective urocanase. It is accompanied by elevated excretion of urocanate.

Threonine

Threonine is a/an neutral, essential and glucogenic amino acid.

Synthesis

As it is an essential amino acid, it cannot be synthesized in the body. Hence, it should be taken in the diet.

Catabolism (Fig. 13.11)

Major pathway

Threonine is first cleaved to acetaldehyde and glycine by threonine aldolase.
- Acetaldehyde is then oxidized to acetate which is then converted to acetyl-CoA.
- Glycine is catabolized as explained earlier.

Minor pathway
- Threonine is converted by deamination to α-ketobutyrate by threonine dehydratase.
- α-ketobutyrate is then catabolized to propionyl-CoA by an enzyme complex.

Threonine → α-ketobutyrate → Propionyl-CoA

Note
Threonine does not undergo transamination.

Utilization

It is a constituent of proteins. It can be converted to glycine.

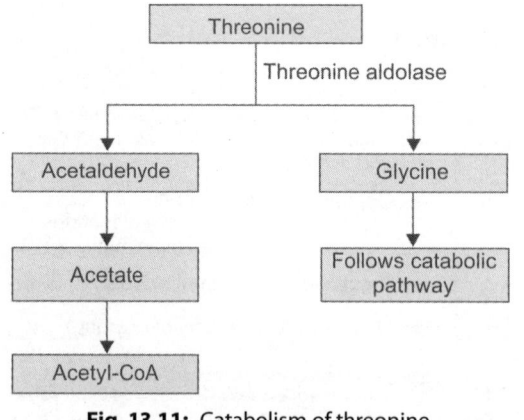

Fig. 13.11: Catabolism of threonine.

Disorder

Nil.

Lysine

Lysine is a/an basic, essential, and ketogenic amino acid.

Synthesis

It cannot be synthesized in the body as it is an essential amino acid. Thus it has to be included in the diet. Vegetable proteins are deficient in lysine.

Catabolism

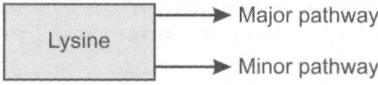

Major pathway (Fig. 13.12)
- Lysine is converted to α-aminoadipate via intermediate compounds.
- α-aminoadipate forms α-ketoadipate by transamination.
- α-ketoadipate undergoes further reactions leading to formation of acetoacetyl-CoA. (lysine does not undergo transamination)

Minor pathway
- It is converted to a cyclic compound namely pipecolate by removal of α-amino group.
- Pipecolate joins the major pathway at the level of semialdehyde intermediate compound.

Utilization

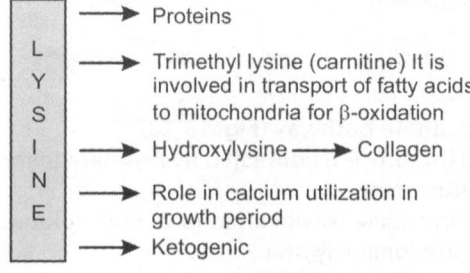

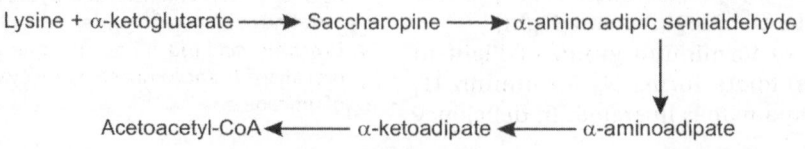

Fig. 13.12: Metabolism of lysine.

Clinical Importance: Disorders

- Periodic hyperlysinemia with associated hyperammonemia
- Persistent hyperlysinemia without hyperammonemia.
  Both disorders may result from impaired conversion of lysine to saccharopine.

Valine, Leucine, Isoleucine (Branched Chain Amino Acids)

- *Valine:* Neutral, essential, and glucogenic amino acid.
- *Leucine:* Neutral, essential, and ketogenic amino acid.
- *Isoleucine:* Neutral, essential, glucogenic, and ketogenic amino acid.

All these three amino acids have common features regarding structures. Hence their metabolism will be discussed as a group.

Synthesis

All are essential amino acids. They cannot be synthesized in the body and hence they are taken in the diet.

Catabolism

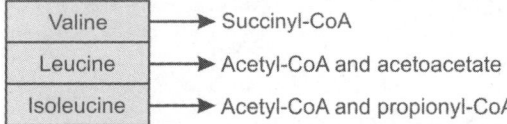

Catabolism of all of them initially involves the same reactions; subsequently each amino acid skeleton follows a unique pathway (Fig. 13.13).

Pathway

- All the three branched chain amino acids are converted to their corresponding α-keto acids by transamination catalyzed by transaminase.
- The resulting α-ketoacids enter mitochondria. Here they are oxidatively decarboxylated to branched chain α-ketoacyl-CoA thioesters. This reaction is catalyzed by α-keto acid dehydrogenase (a multienzyme complex).
- α-ketoacyl-CoA thioesters are converted to the corresponding α, β unsaturated acyl-CoA thioesters.

Note

- All the above three reactions are similar for three branched amino acids.
- Thereafter the resulting, α, β unsaturated acyl-CoA thioesters are degraded by distinct pathways.
- α, β-unsaturated acyl-CoA thioester
  - Formed from valine is known as methylacrylyl-CoA. It is finally catabolized to succinyl-CoA.
  - Formed from leucine is known as β-methylcrotonyl-CoA. It is finally catabolized to acetyl-CoA and acetoacetate.
  - Formed from isoleucine is known as tiglyl-CoA. It is finally catabolized to acetyl-CoA and propionyl-CoA.

Utilization

They are constituents of proteins.

Clinical Importance: Disorders

- Maple syrup urine disease (branched chain ketonuria)
  - *Incidence:* 1 in 1,85,000 births.
  - *Defect:* Conversion of all three branched chain keto acids to CO_2 and acyl-CoA thioesters does not occur due to deficiency of α-keto acid dehydrogenase.
  - Branched chain keto acids → Acyl-CoA thioesters + CO_2
  - *Symptoms:* Urine has odor of maple sugar or burnt sugar. Patients may not take food, may vomit, and exhibit lethargy convulsion and mental retardation.
  - *Diagnosis:* Detection of branched chain amino acids in urine by chromatography.
  - *Treatment:* Diet without branched chain amino acids.
- *Isovaleric acidemia:* Isovaleryl-CoA dehydrogenase is deficient in this disorder.
- *Methylmalonic acidemia:* Methylmalonyl-CoA is not converted to succinyl-CoA due to deficiency of vitamin B_{12} coenzyme.

Methionine

Methionine is a/an neutral, essential, and glucogenic ketogenic amino acid. It is also one of the sulfur containing amino acids.

Synthesis

It cannot be synthesized in the body as it is an essential amino acid. It has to be supplied in the diet.

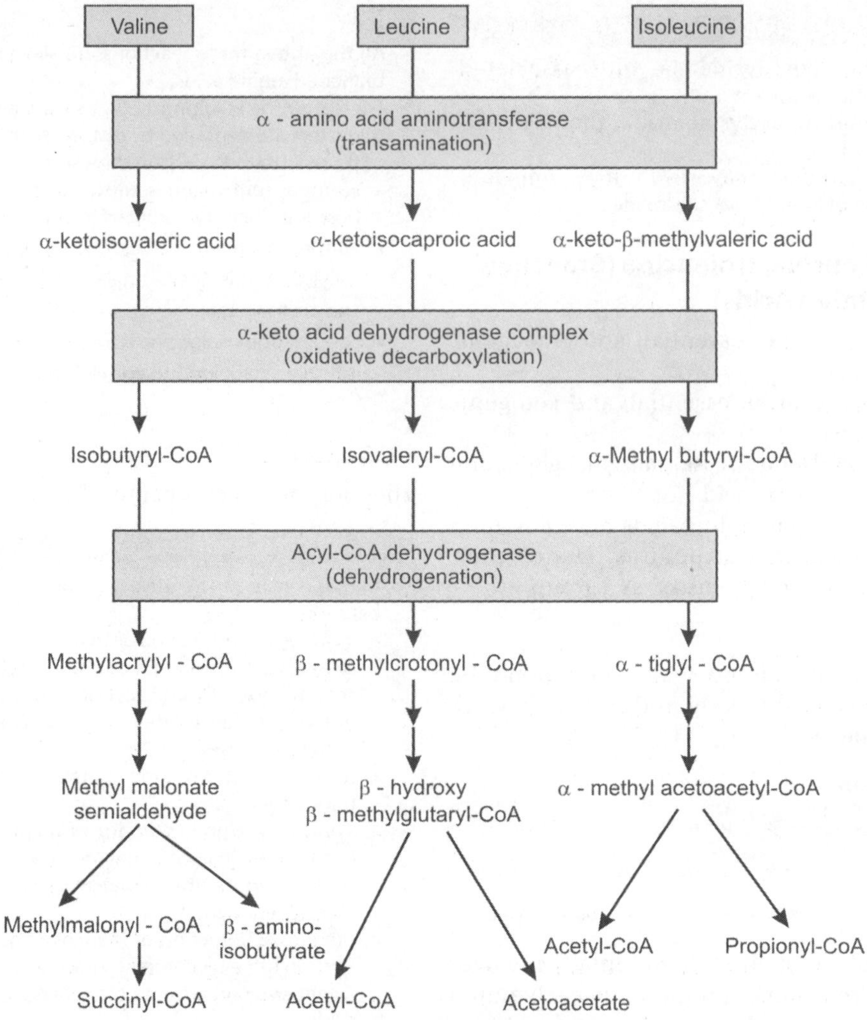

Section 3: Metabolism

Fig. 13.13: Catabolism of branched chain amino acids.

Catabolism

- Methionine condenses with ATP to form S-adenosyl methionine (active methionine/SAM).
- The activated methyl group is transferred to an acceptor by methyl transferase. The resulting compound is S-adenosyl homocysteine.
- Hydrolysis of S-adenosyl homocysteine forms homocysteine and adenosine.
- Homocysteine condenses with serine to form cystathionine (Transsulfuration).
- Cystathionine is hydrolyzed to cysteine and homoserine by cystathioninase (Transsulfuration).
- Homoserine is converted to α-ketobutyrate by homoserine deaminase.
- α-ketobutyrate undergoes oxidative decarboxylation to form propionyl-CoA **(Fig. 13.14)**.

Utilization

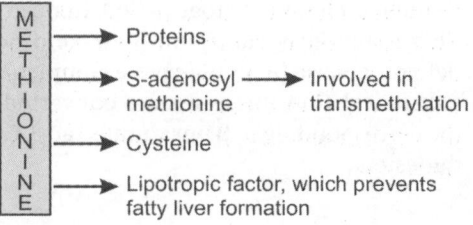

Chapter 13: Digestion, Absorption, and Metabolism of Proteins

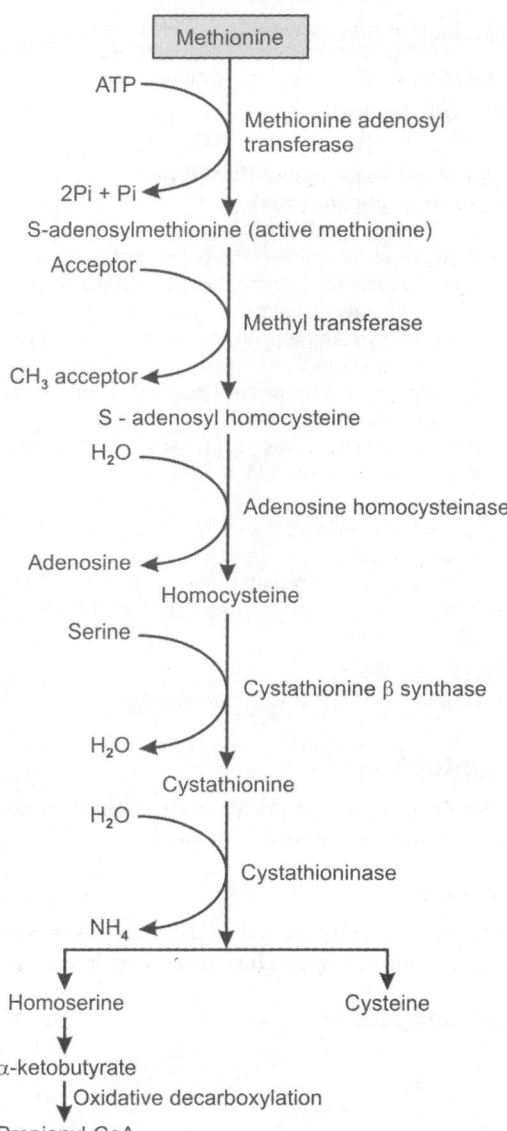

Fig. 13.14: Catabolism of methionine.

Clinical Importance: Disorders

Homocystinuria: It is an inborn error of methionine of metabolism.
- *Incidence:* 1 in 1,60,000 births
- *Types:* Four types of homocystinuria have been reported.

Type I Homocystinuria: It is an important inborn errors of matthiasiam metabolism.
- *Enzyme deficiency:* Cystathionine β-synthase is deficient which catalyzes
  Homocysteine → Cystathionine

Contd...

Contd...
- *Biochemical changes:* Plasma methionine level is elevated. High excretion of homocysteine and also S-adenosyl methionine in urine occur.
- *Clinical symptoms:* Thrombosis, osteoporosis, dislocated lenses, mental retardation. Relationship between heart attack and elevated level of homocysteine in blood is established recently.
- *Diagnosis:* Estimation of homocysteine in blood.
- *Treatment:* A diet low in methionine and high in cysteine is recommended.

(Types II, III, IV homocystinuria occur due to defects in remethylation cycle).

Transmethylation

Definition

It is an example of one carbon metabolism.

Methionine (amino acid) is converted to active methionine (S-adenosyl methionine) by transferase and ATP. The latter transfers a methyl group (CH_3– one carbon moiety) to an acceptor compound to form a new compound.

Methionine → S-adenosyl methionine

For example,
- Serine $\xrightarrow{CH_3}$ Choline
- Norepinephrine $\xrightarrow{CH_3}$ Epinephrine
- Guanidoacetate $\xrightarrow{CH_3}$ Creatine
- Acetyl serotonin $\xrightarrow{CH_3}$ Serotonin
- Nicotinamide $\xrightarrow{CH_3}$ N-methylnicotinamide

Importance

- Several physiologically important compounds are formed by this process, e.g., choline, epinephrine, etc.
- Many compounds become functionally active only after methylation.
- Protein methylation protects the proteins from degradation.
- It is involved in one carbon metabolism.

Phenylalanine

Phenylalanine is a/an neutral, aromatic, essential, and glucogenic-ketogenic amino acid.

Synthesis

It cannot be synthesized in the body as it is an essential amino acid. It has to be supplied in the diet.

Catabolism

Major pathway
(Conversion of phenylalanine to tyrosine)
Phenylalanine hydroxylase.
Phenylalanine → Tyrosine → follows its catabolic pathway
(*refer* to tyrosine metabolism)

Note
Metabolism of phenylalanine and tyrosine should be studied together.

Minor pathway (Fig. 13.15)

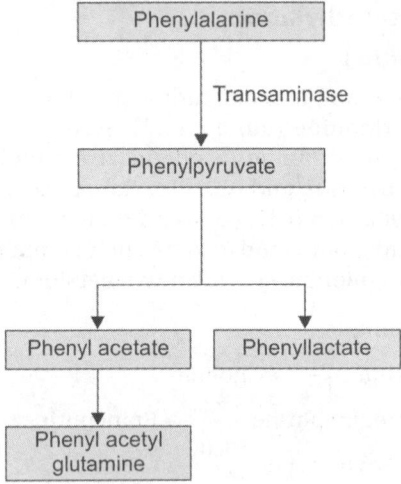

Fig. 13.15: Minor pathway.

Note
The above reactions occur in the liver of normal individuals but are of minor significance. But in phenylketonuria, this alternative pathway is very active.

Utilization

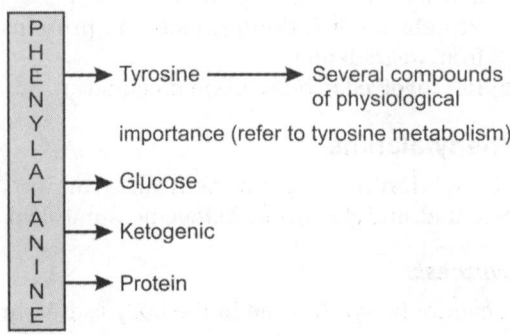

Clinical Importance: Disorders

Inborn errors of phenylalanine metabolism.

Phenylketonuria
There are five types of phenylketonuria.

Classic phenylketonuria (PKU Type I hyperphenylalaninemia)
- *Incidence:* 1 in 10,000 births.
- *Defect:* Phenylalanine is not converted to tyrosine due to deficiency of phenylalanine hydroxylase.
  Phenylalanine → Tyrosine
  As phenylalanine is not converted to tyrosine, alternative catabolite compounds are produced, e.g., phenylpyruvate, phenyllactate, etc. **(Fig. 13.15)** and exhered more in urine.
- *Symptoms:* Mental retardation, seizures, psychoses, eczema, and mousy odor in urine.
- *Diagnosis*
  - Ferric chloride test
  - Guthrie test
  - Chromatography with urine
- *Treatment:* A diet containing low levels of phenylalanine.

Other disorders
Refer page 175 (Tyrosine metabolism).

Tryptophan

Tryptophan is a neutral, aromatic, essential, and glucogenic ketogenic amino acid.

Synthesis
It cannot be synthesized in the body as it is an essential amino acid. It has to be taken in the diet.

Catabolism

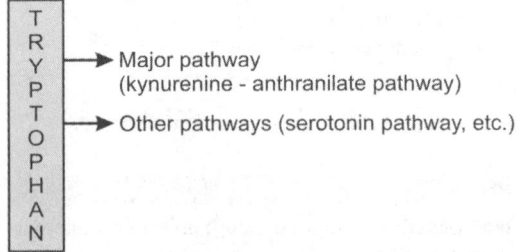

Major pathway (kynurenine-anthranilate pathway) (Fig. 13.16)
It occurs mostly in the liver.
- Tryptophan is converted to N-formylkynurenine by tryptophan oxygenase (tryptophan pyrrolase).

Chapter 13: Digestion, Absorption, and Metabolism of Proteins

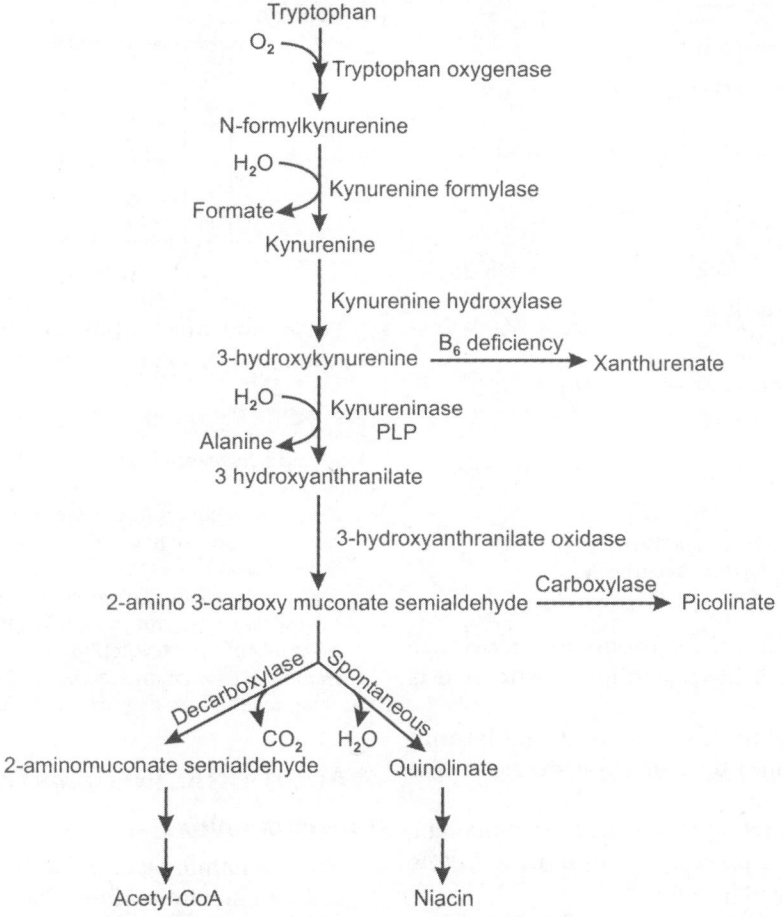

Fig. 13.16: Catabolism of tryptophan (major pathway).

- Hydrolytic removal of formal group of formylkynurenine by kynurenine formylase produces kynurenine and formate.
- Kynurenine may be hydrolyzed to 3 hydroxy kynurenine by kynurenine hydroxylase.
- 3-hydroxykynurenine is oxidized to 3-hydroxyanthranilate by kynureninase.
  (Kynureninase is a pyridoxal phosphate dependent enzyme. In vitamin B_6 deficiency, 3-hydroxykynurenine is diverted to form xanthurenate).
- 3-hydroxyanthranilate is converted to 2-amino 3-carboxy muconate semialdehyde
  - It may be converted to niacin.
  - It may be degraded in several steps to form acetyl-CoA.
  - It may be converted to picolinate which is excreted in urine.

Importance
- Vitamin niacin (nicotinic acid) is formed in this pathway. Hence deficiency of tryptophan produces pellagra like symptoms.
- *Hartnup disease:* It occurs due to defect in intestinal and renal transport of neutral amino acids including tryptophan (*refer* page 184).

Other pathways
Serotonin pathway (Fig. 13.17)
- Tryptophan is hydroxylated to 5-hydroxytryptophan by tryptophan hydroxylase.
- 5-hydroxytryptophan is decarboxylated to serotonin (5-hydroxytryptamine) by pyridoxal dependent decarboxylase.
- **Serotonin:**
  - It may be catabolized to 5-hydroxyindole-acetic acid (5-HIAA) through oxidative

Section 3: Metabolism

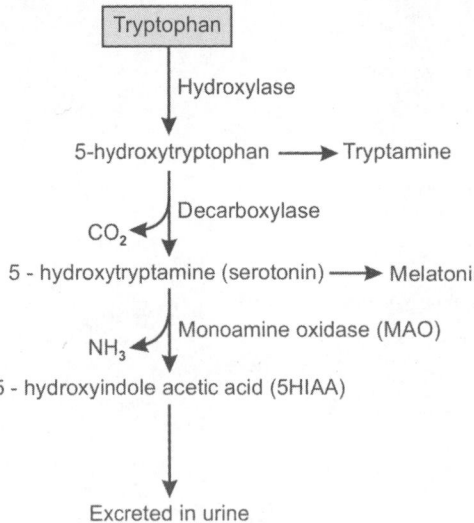

Fig. 13.17: Catabolism of tryptophan (serotonin pathway).

Utilization

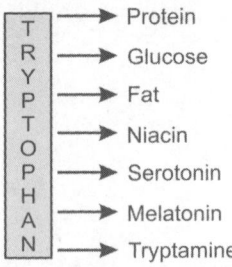

Formation and importance of the above compounds (*refer* to respective pages).

Clinical Importance: Disorders

Hartnup's disease: It is an inborn error of tryptophan metabolism.
- *Defect*: It occurs due to defect in intestinal and renal transport of neutral amino acids specifically tryptophan.
- *Symptoms*: Pellagra like symptoms appear because synthesis of vitamin niacin is affected due to nonavailability of tryptophan.
- *Diagnosis*: Estimation of tryptophan/niacin.
- *Treatment*: To take diet rich in tryptophan/niacin.

deamination by monoamino oxidase (MAO). 5-hydroxyindole acetic acid is excreted in urine.
- It may be converted to melatonin (hormone) by acetyl transferase in the pineal gland.
- It may be converted to methoxytryptamine which is excreted as 5-methoxyindole acetate conjugate.
- It is produced by argentaffin cells of gastrointestinal tract. It is a neurotransmitter. It is also powerful vasoconstrictor. It controls behavior, sleep, body temperature, and blood pressure. It is increased in tumor malignant carcinoid syndrome (Argentaffinomas). It can be diagnosed by estimating 5HIAA in urine. It produces symptoms, such as respiratory distress, sweating, and hypertension.

Minor pathways

These pathways usually occur in the liver, kidney, and fecal flora.

Tryptamine is oxidized to indole pyruvic acid, and then to indole 3 acetic acid. These two catabolites are the principal products excreted in the urine.

Indole or indoxyl derivatives of tryptophan are also excreted in urine.

■ ADDITIONAL INFORMATION

Catecholamines

Amines containing a catechol ring (group) are called as catecholamines. They are organic compounds, e.g., dopamine, epinephrine (adrenaline), norepinephrine (noradrenaline).

They are released into blood in response to physical or emotional stress. They function as:
❏ Neurotransmitters
❏ Transfer of signals
❏ Hormones

(*Refer* phenylalanine and tyrosine metabolism)

Indoleamines

They are amine derivatives of indole. They are a group of monoamine neurotransmitters. They are involved in mood and sleep, e.g., tryptophan, serotonin, melatonin (*refer* tryptophan metabolism).

Biogenic Amines (Table 13.2)

Biogenic amines are organic compounds formed by decarboxylation of amino acids.

Table 13.2: Biogenic amines.

Sl. No.	Amine	Amino acids	Function of amines
1.	Histamine	Histidine	Vasodilator
2.	GABA	Glutamic acid	Neurotransmitter
3.	Tyramine	Tyrosine	Vasoconstrictor
4.	Dopamine	Phenylalanine	For synthesis of E and NE
5.	Tryptamine	Tryptophan	Elevates BP
6.	Serotonin	Tryptophan	Increases cerebral activity
7.	Melatonin	Tryptophan	Circadian rhythm

$$R-\underset{NH_2}{CH}-COOH \xrightarrow[-CO_2]{\text{Decarboxylase}} R-CH_2-NH_2$$

Amino acid   Amine

- **Polyamines:** *Refer* to arginine metabolism page 176.

Biogenic amines having multiple amino groups are known as polyamines. They are formed from arginine as follows:

Arginine → ornithine → polyamines, e.g., putrescine, spermidine, and spermine.

They are present in high concentration in semen. They are involved in the synthesis of DNA, RNA and proteins. They act as growth factors in cell proliferation and growth. Clinically, they are used in the diagnosis and treatment of cancer.

- Specialized products formed from amino acids (*refer* Chapter 4)
- List of inborn errors of metabolism (*refer* Appendix C: Inborn errors of metabolism)

14. Integration of Metabolism

Chapter Outline
- Definition
- Metabolic Pathways
- Integration of Metabolism

INTRODUCTION

Metabolism of major energy nutrients, such as carbohydrates, lipids, and proteins are mostly interconvertible to give energy or to be stored in the body depending on the physiological needs. The metabolic pathways are closely integrated and actually occur simultaneously in the body. Similarly each organ has metabolic relationship with the rest of the body.

DEFINITION

The coordination between metabolic pathways of carbohydrate, lipid, and protein is known as integration of metabolism. This process is well regulated to meet the energy requirements of the body under various conditions.

METABOLIC PATHWAYS

Catabolic pathways:
- Glycolysis
- Citric acid cycle
- Fatty acid oxidation
- Degradation of amino acids
- Hexose monophosphate shunt
- Uronic acid pathway

Anabolic pathways:
- Gluconeogenesis
- Biosynthesis of fatty acids
- Biosynthesis of amino acids/proteins

Regulation of Metabolic Pathways

Three principal nutrients namely carbohydrates, lipids, and proteins are interconvertible in the body.

1. **Carbohydrates:**
   - They can form lipids
     Glucose → Acetyl-CoA → Fatty acid
   - They can form amino acids (nonessential)
     Glucose → Intermediates → Transmination → Amino acid
2. **Lipids:** Glycerol can be converted to glucose via gluconeogeneses (other lipids cannot form carbohydrates).
3. **Proteins:**
   - They can form glucose through glucogenic amino acids.
   - They can form lipids through ketogenic amino acids.

INTEGRATION OF METABOLISM (FIG. 14.1)

It can be studied at two levels:
1. Metabolism in starvation
2. Metabolism at well fed state (absorptive state)

Metabolism in Starvation

The metabolic changes in starvation are mostly opposite to changes occurring in well fed state.

Liver

- *Carbohydrate metabolism:* The liver acts as the most vital organ in maintaining the blood sugar level during starvation. Increased gluconeogenesis and enhanced glycogenolysis supply glucose to the tissues.
- *Lipid metabolism:* Oxidation of fatty acids is enhanced with increased formation of ketone bodies, as citric acid cycle cannot utilize excess production of acetyl-CoA. The energy demands of the brain are met by ketone bodies.

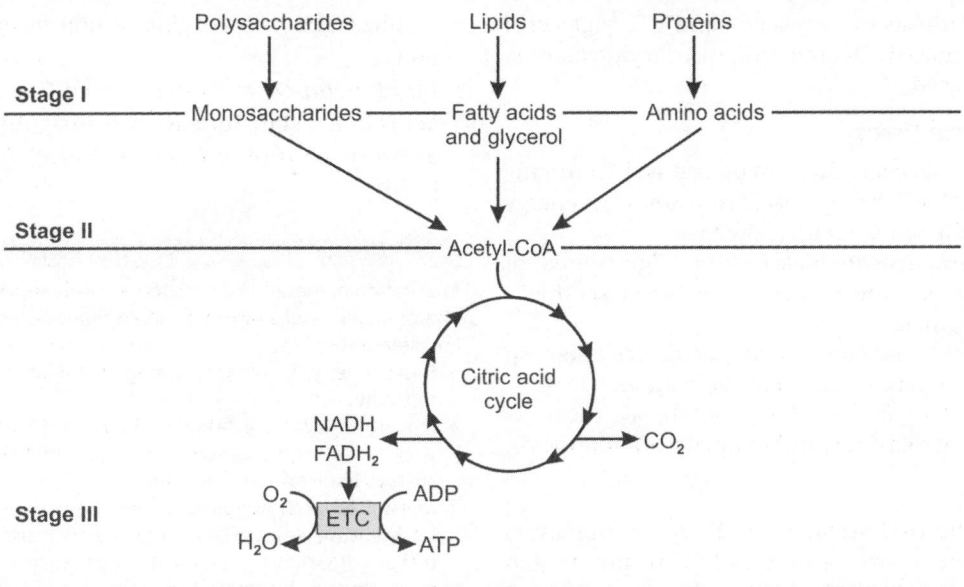

Fig. 14.1: Integration of metabolism.

Adipose Tissue

- *Carbohydrate metabolism:* Uptake of glucose and its metabolism is reduced.
- *Lipid metabolism*
  Degradation of triacylglycerol is increased leading to elevated fatty acids and glycerol. Fatty acids are utilized in various tissues except brain. Glycerol is utilized for synthesis of glucose by gluconeogenesis in the liver. Also, synthesis of fatty acids and triglycerides is reduced.

Skeletal Muscle

- *Carbohydrate metabolism:* Glucose uptake and its metabolism are very much reduced.
- *Lipid metabolism:* Muscle can utilize both fatty acids and ketone bodies as sources of energy. But on prolonged starvation, it can utilize fatty acids only.
- *Protein metabolism:* In the beginning of starvation, muscle proteins are degraded to liberate amino acids which are utilized for the synthesis of glucose via gluconeogenesis. But during prolonged starvation, protein degradation is depressed.

Brain

Normally, the brain is adapted to utilize glucose as the preferable source of energy. In initial stage of starvation, it depends mostly on glucose formed via gluconeogenesis from the amino acids liberated from degradation of muscle proteins. But during prolonged starvation, the brain adapts itself to derive energy from ketone bodies.

Metabolism in Well Fed (Absorptive) State

The various tissues and organs of the body function in well coordinated manner to meet their metabolic needs.

Liver

The liver serves as the major metabolic organ. The food constituents reaching the liver after absorption are processed and distributed to various tissues/organs for utilization.

- *Carbohydrate metabolism:*
  - Glycolysis, glycogenesis and HMP, hunt are increased
  - Gluconeogenesis is decreased
- *Lipid metabolism:* Synthesis of fatty acids and triacyl glycerol is increased.
- *Protein metabolism:* Degradation of amino and synthesis of protein is increased.

Adipose Tissue

It is the energy storage tissue for fat:

- *Carbohydrate metabolism:* Glucose uptake is increased leading to increased glycolysis and HMP shunt.
- *Lipid metabolism*

Synthesis of fatty acids and triacylglycerol is increased. Degradation of triacylglycerol is decreased.

Skeletal Tissue

Role of skeletal muscle in utilization of nutrients is variable. Resting muscle consumes less energy than the muscle during exercise.
- *Carbohydrate metabolism:* High uptake of glucose and increased glycogen synthesis take place.
- *Lipid metabolism:* Fatty acids are taken up from the circulation for utilization.
- *Protein metabolism:* Protein synthesis is increased due to higher uptake of amino acids.

Brain

It is the vital organ in the body. Through it is smaller in size, it utilizes 20% of the oxygen consumed by the body.
- *Carbohydrate metabolism:* Glucose is the only source of energy to the brain in fed state. It utilizes about 60% of glucose utilized by the body.
- *Lipid metabolism:* Utilization of free fatty acids in fed state for energy is insignificant as they cannot cross the blood-brain barrier.

Clinical Importance

Integration of metabolism ensures a steady supply of energy in all tissues or organs at all times (fed state and starvation).
- Excess energy is stored as glycogen and fat in well fed state.
- During starvation, fatty acids are utilized in preference to glucose to spare glucose for tissues, such as brain and erythrocytes.
- *Clinical aspects:* Regulatory mechanisms of the body ensure a supply of suitable fuel to all tissues/organs. Breakdown of these mechanisms due to hormonal imbalance or metabolic defects may lead to various pathological symptoms of starvation syndrome.

15 Digestion, Absorption, and Metabolism of Nucleic Acids

Chapter Outline
- Digestion
- Absorption
- Metabolism

■ DIGESTION

Nucleic acids are present in the diet as nucleoproteins.

Stomach

Nucleoproteins are hydrolyzed to nucleic acids and proteins by the proteolytic enzymes present in the stomach.

Nucleoproteins → Nucleic acid + Proteins

(The proteins thus liberated follow their digestion, absorption, and metabolic pathway).

Small Intestine

- The liberated nucleic acids are degraded to polynucleotides by the enzymes secreted by the pancreas and present in the small intestine.

  RNA $\xrightarrow{\text{Ribonucleases}}$ Polyribonucleotides

  DNA $\xrightarrow{\text{Deoxyribonucleases}}$ Polydeoxyribonucleotides

- Polynucleotides are converted to mononucleotides by polynucleotidases secreted by intestinal mucosa.

  Polynucleotides $\xrightarrow{\text{Polynucleotidases}}$ Mononucleotides

- Mononucleotides are hydrolyzed by nucleotidases (phosphatases) present in intestinal juice to nucleosides and phosphate.
  Mononucleotide → Nucleoside + Phosphate

■ ABSORPTION

There are two routes of absorption of nucleosides:

- They may be absorbed as such in the small intestine and then degraded to its constituents (bases + sugars) by nucleosidases present in liver, kidney, spleen, bone marrow, etc.
- They may be further broken to its constituents by phosphorylases present in the small intestine itself and then absorbed.

(Phosphate and sugars formed follow their absorption and utilization).

■ METABOLISM

DNA and RNA contain two types of nucleotides.
1. Purine nucleotides
2. Pyrimidine nucleotides

Metabolism of Purine Nucleotides

- Purine ribonucleotide = Purine + Ribose + Phosphate
- Purine deoxyribonucleotide = Purine + Deoxyribose + Phosphate

Biosynthesis of Purine Ribonucleotides

There are two pathways by which purine ribonucleotides can be synthesized in the body.
1. De novo pathway
2. Salvage pathway

De novo pathway (Fig. 15.1)

It is the main pathway by which purine nucleotides are formed in the body.

Site
- *Organ:* Mainly liver
- *Cell:* Cytosol

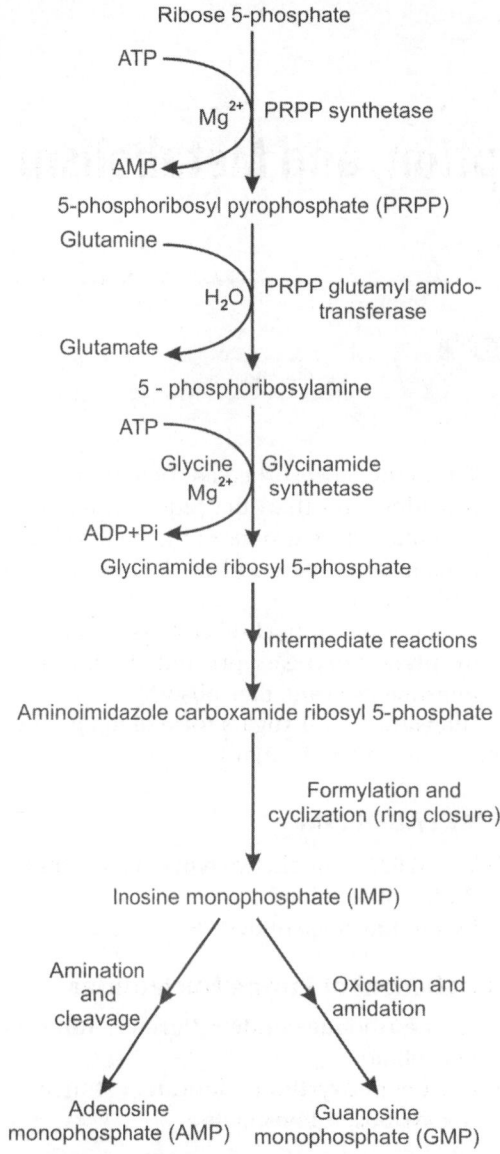

Pathway

- Ribose 5-phosphate is converted to 5-phosphoribosyl pyrophosphate (PRPP) by PRPP synthetase in presence of ATP and Mg^{2+}.
- PRPP reacts with glutamine to form 5-phosphoribosylamine catalyzed by PRPP glutamyl amino transferase.
- 5-phosphoribosylamine combines with glycine to produce glycinamide ribosyl 5-phosphate by glycinamide synthetase.
- By a series of reactions, glycinamide ribosyl 5-phosphate is converted to aminoimidazole carboxamide ribosyl 5-phosphate.
- Aminoimidazole carboxamide ribosyl 5-phosphate is formylated and undergoes further cyclization (ring closure) to form inosine monophosphate (IMP).
- IMP is the precursor for the synthesis of purine ribonucleotides:
  - IMP, on amination and cleavage forms adenosine monophosphate (AMP)
  - IMP, on oxidation and then amidation forms guanosine monophosphate (GMP).

Energetics

Total ATPs consumed = 6

Regulation

Purine biosynthesis is regulated by:
- The pool size of PRPP
- Feedback inhibition of PRPP glutamyl amino transferase by the end products (AMP and GMP).

Inhibitors

Antifolate drugs (e.g., methotrexate) and glutamine analogues inhibit synthesis of purine nucleotides and function as anticancer drugs (antimetabolites).

Fig. 15.1: Biosynthesis of purine ribonucleotides.

Sources of atoms of purine ring (Fig. 15.2)

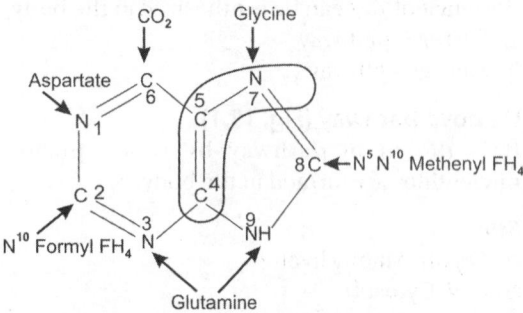

Fig. 15.2: Sources of atoms of purine ring.

Salvage pathway

Salvage pathways are alternate pathways by which purine nucleotides are formed from purines.

- Adenine + PRPP $\xrightarrow{\text{Adenine phosphoribosyl transferase}}$ AMP + PPi
  - Guanine + PRPP → GMP + PPi
  - Hypoxanthine + PRPP → IMP + PPi
  - Both reactions are catalyzed by hypoxanthine-guanine and phosphoribosyl transferase (HGPRT)

Importance
- It requires less energy than de novo pathway.
- Purine is utilized economically.
- It is important in erythrocytes and brain where de novo pathway is not operative.

Clinical Importance: Disorders
Lesch–Nyhan syndrome: It is a genetic disorder of purine salvage pathway, discovered by Lesch and Nyhan in 1964. It affects mostly males only.
- *Cause:* It occurs due to deficiency of the enzyme hypoxanthine-guanine phosphoribosyl transferase (HGPRT) an enzyme of purine salvage pathway. Thus, PRPP is not used in salvage pathway and hence results in overproduction of purine and uric acid leading to gouty arthritis.
- *Symptoms:* Hyperuricemia, uric acid lithiasis mental retardation, self-mutilation (urge to bite their fingers or lips).
- *Treatment:* Allopurinol

Synthesis of Purine Deoxyribonucleotides
Purine ribonucleotides can be converted to purine deoxyribonucleotides.

Catabolism of Purine Ribonucleotides (Fig. 15.3)

Site
- *Organ:* Mainly in the liver
- *Cell:* Cytosol

Pathway
1. Purine nucleotide is converted to purine nucleoside by the enzyme nucleotidase. Thus:
   Adenosine monophosphate → Adenosine (AMP) + Pi
   Guanosine monophosphate → Guanosine (GMP) + Pi
2. a. Adenosine is deaminated to inosine by adenosine deaminase.
   b. Inosine is hydrolyzed to hypoxanthine and ribose 1-phosphate by phosphorylase.
   c. Hypoxanthine is oxidized to xanthine by xanthine oxidase.
3. a. Guanosine is hydrolyzed to guanine and ribose 1-phosphate by phosphorylase.
   b. Guanine is converted to xanthine by guanase.
   Xanthine is the common intermediate compound formed during catabolism of purine ribonucleotides (AMP and GMP).
4. Xanthine is oxidized to uric acid by xanthine oxidase.

Note
- Uric acid is the end product of purine catabolism in humans, birds, some animals and is excreted in urine.
- However in other organisms, uric acid is further degraded to other substances, such as allantoin, allantoic acid and is excreted in urine.
- Uricotelic organisms: Organisms which excrete nitrogenous waste products in the form of uric acid, e.g., birds.

Catabolism of Purine Deoxyribonucleotides
These are also degraded by the same catabolic pathway and enzymes as given above.

Normal level of uric acid
- Blood = 3–7 mg/100 mL (male). It is slightly lower in women.
- Urine = 400–700 mg/day.

Clinical Importance: Disorders
Hyperuricemia: Gout (**Fig.15.4**).

Definition: It is a chronic metabolic disorder of purine-catabolism, due to excessive production of uric acid and its subsequent deposition as sodium urate crystals (tophi) in the joints, kidneys, etc.

Prevalence: 1 in 3,000 (mostly males).

Types: There are two types of gout.
1. Primary gout: It is an inborn error of purine catabolism. Defect in PRPP synthetase (superactive) and deficiency of HGPRT may lead to overproduction of purine and hence increased catabolism of purine resulting in more formation of uric acid. It may be associated with increased excretion of uric acid.
2. Secondary gout: It occurs secondary to an increase in purine catabolism leading to over-production of uric acid as in leukemias and renal failure or decreased excretion of uric acid.

Symptoms: Inflammation in the joints resulting in painful gouty arthritis. Uric acid level in blood is increased (hyperuricemia) urinary calculi, typhi (sodium urate crystals) in soft tissues.

Treatment:
- Low purine diet
- Uricosuric drug, e.g., allopurinol

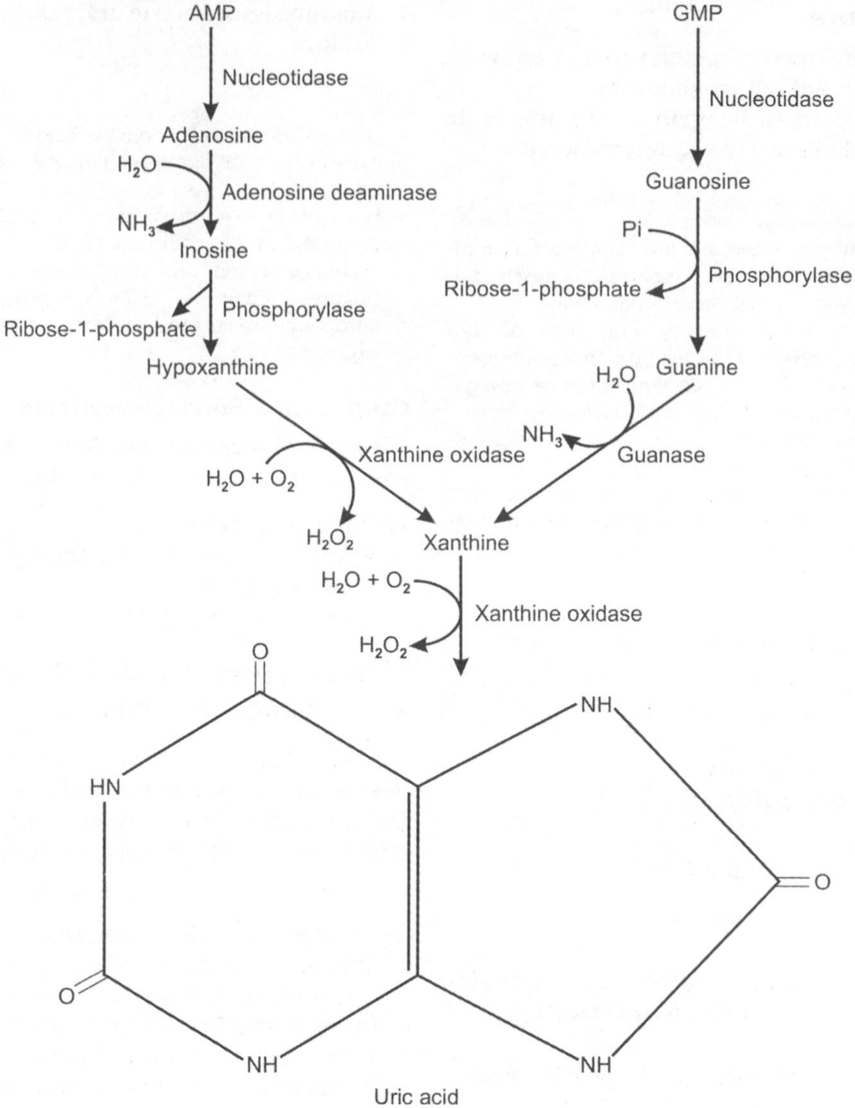

Section 3: Metabolism

Fig. 15.3: Catabolism of purine ribonucleotides.

Other examples:
- Lesch–Nyhan syndrome
- Von Gierke's disease

Hypouricemia: Xanthinuria

Causes: Production of uric acid is stopped or decreased.
- Due to deficiency of xanthine oxidase or liver damage
- Excretion of uric acid is increased.

Changes:
- Hypouricemia
- More excretion of xanthine, hypoxanthine in urine.

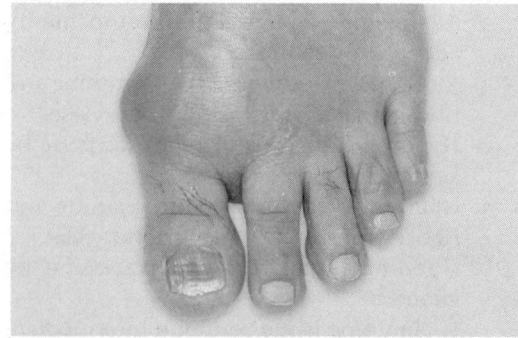

Fig. 15.4: Gout.
(For color version, see Plate 3)

Symptoms: Xanthine calculi (urinary stones) may be formed in the urinary tract.

Severe combined immunodeficiency disease (SCID): It occurs due to adenosine deaminase deficiency. In this condition, both T cells and B cells are not functional.

Metabolism of Pyrimidine Nucleotides

- Pyrimidine ribonucleotide = Pyrimidine + Ribose + Phosphate
- Pyrimidine deoxyribonucleotide = Pyrimidine + Deoxyribose + Phosphate

Synthesis of Pyrimidine Ribonucleotides (Fig. 15.5)

De novo synthesis
Site
Organ: Liver
Cell: Cytosol

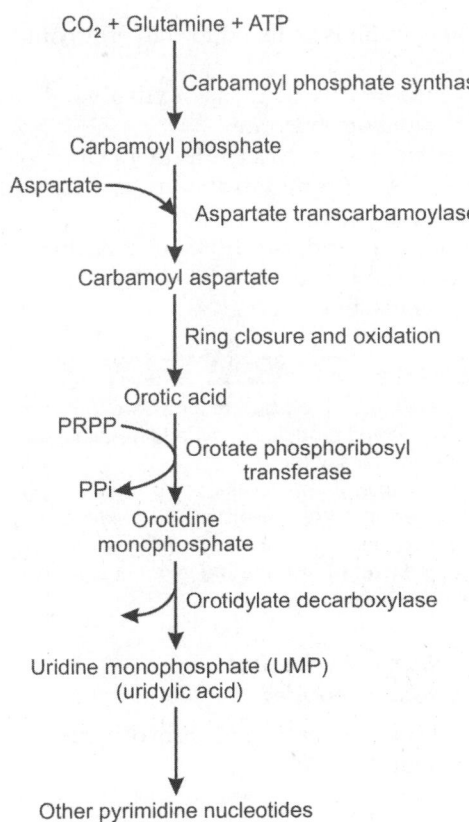

Fig. 15.5: Biosynthesis of pyrimidine ribonucleotides.

Sources of atoms of pyrimidine ring (Fig.15.6):

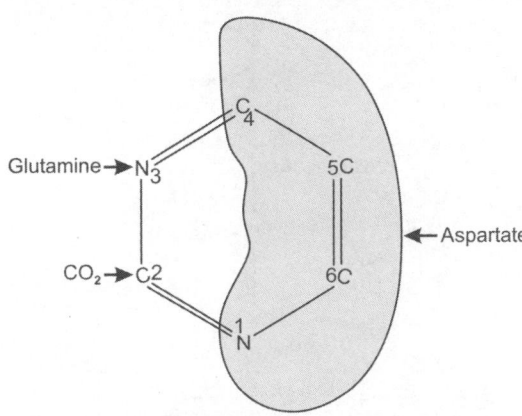

Fig. 15.6: Sources of atoms of pyrimidine.

Pathway
- Carbamoyl phosphate is first formed from glutamine, ATP, and CO_2 by the action of carbamoyl phosphate synthase II (CPS-II).
- Carbamoyl phosphate condenses with aspartate to form carbamoyl aspartate catalyzed by aspartate transcarbamoylase.
- Ring closure of carbamoyl aspartate and its oxidation produces orotic acid.
- Orotic acid is converted to uridylic acid (UMP) by phosphorylation and then decarboxylation.
- UMP is the precursor for the synthesis of other pyrimidine nucleotides.

Regulation
CPS-II and aspartate transcarbamoylase are regulatory enzymes.

Inhibitors
- 5-fluorouracil
- Methotrexate

These agents may be used as anticancer agents.

Clinical Importance: Disorders
Orotic Aciduria ❖ *Type I orotic aciduria:* It occurs due to deficiency of both orotate phosphoribosyl transferase and orotidylate decarboxylase. ❖ *Type II orotic aciduria:* It occurs due to deficiency of only orotidylate decarboxylase. Both types of disorders show orotic aciduria, severe anemia, and retarded growth. They can be treated by oral uridine.

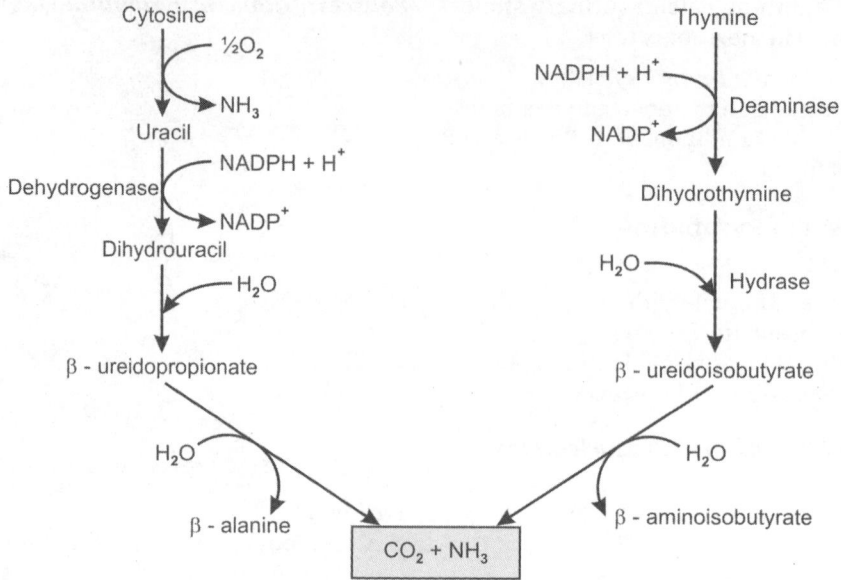

Fig. 15.7: Catabolism of pyrimidine ribonucleotides.

Salvage pathway

Pyrimidine nucleotides are also synthesized by salvage pathways.

Uracil + Ribose 1-P → Uridine → UMP

Synthesis of Pyrimidine Deoxyribonucleotides

Pyrimidine ribonucleotides can be converted to pyrimidine deoxyribonucleotides.

Catabolism of Pyrimidine Ribonucleotides (Fig. 15.7)

Steps

1. a. Pyrimidine nucleotides are dephosphorylated to form pyrimidine nucleosides.
   b. Pyrimide nucleosides are degraded to ribose 1-phosphate and free bases.
2. a. Cytosine is deaminated to form uracil
   b. Uracil is then reduced to dihydrouracil by NADPH.
   c. Dihydrouracil is hydrolyzed to β-ureidopropionate. β-ureidopropionate is further hydrolyzed to form β-alanine, CO_2 and NH_3.
3. a. Thymine is reduced to dihydrothymine by NADPH.
   b. Dihydrothymine is hydrolyzed to β-ureidoisobutyrate.
   c. β-ureidoisobutyrate is further hydrolyzed to form β-aminoisobutyrate, CO_2 and NH_3.
4. Thus, the end products of pyrimidine catabolism are CO_2, NH_3, β-alanine, β-aminoisobutyrate.

> **Clinical Importance: Disorders**
>
> Clinically detectable abnormalities are very rare because the end products of pyrimidine catabolism are highly water soluble.
> For example, *β-aminoisobutyric aciduria:* It may occur as an inherited disorder due to deficiency of the enzyme transaminase. β-aminoisobutyrate is highly excreted in urine in leukemia and X-ray radiation exposure.

Catabolism of Pyrimidine Deoxyribonucleotides

It also occurs similar to catabolism of pyrimidine ribonucleotides.

16 Metabolism of Hemoglobin

Chapter Outline
- Biosynthesis of Hemoglobin
- Catabolism of Hemoglobin
- Jaundice

Metabolism of hemoglobin can be studied under two phases:
1. Biosynthesis of hemoglobin
2. Catabolism of hemoglobin

BIOSYNTHESIS OF HEMOGLOBIN (FIG. 16.1)

Approximately 6 g hemoglobin is produced each day. It is a hemoprotein.

Site

- *Organ:* Mainly in immature erythrocytes and liver and, to some extent, in other tissues except mature erythrocytes.
- *Cell:* Mitochondria and cytosol.

Pathway

It consists of three stages:
1. Synthesis of protoporphyrin III (IX)
2. Synthesis of heme
3. Synthesis of hemoglobin

Synthesis of Protoporphyrin III (IX)

In mitochondria
- Succinyl-CoA and glycine condense to form α-amino-β-ketoadipate.
- α-amino β-ketoadipate is rapidly decarboxylated to form δ-aminolevulinate. (ALA).
  Both reactions occur in mitochondria and are catalyzed by ALA synthase. Reaction in 1 requires pyridoxal phosphate as coenzyme.
- δ-aminolevulinate comes out of mitochondria and enters into the cytosol.

In cytosol
- Two molecules of ALA condense to form a molecule of porphobilinogen (PBG). This reaction is catalyzed by ALA dehydratase.
- PBG is converted to uroporphyrinogen III by uroporphyrinogen I synthase and uroporphyrinogen III synthase.
- Uroporphyrinogen III is decarboxylated to coproporphyrinogen III by uroporphyrinogen decarboxylase.

In mitochondria
- Coproporphyrinogen III enters mitochondria and is converted to protoporphyrinogen III by coproporphyrinogen oxidase.
- Protoporphyrinogen III is oxidized to protoporphyrin III (protoporphyrin IX) by protoporphyrinogen oxidase.

Synthesis of Heme

Ferrous iron (Fe^{2+}) is incorporated into protoporphyrin III (IX) to form heme, catalyzed by heme synthase (ferrochelatase).

Synthesis of Hemoglobin

The heme gets attached to globin to form hemoglobin.

Regulation: ALA synthase is the regulatory enzyme in heme biosynthesis.

Inhibitors: (a) Lead: Inhibits ALA dehydratase as in lead poisoning, (b) Oxygen, (c) Glucose, (d) Steroids, (e) Iron, (f) Hematin.

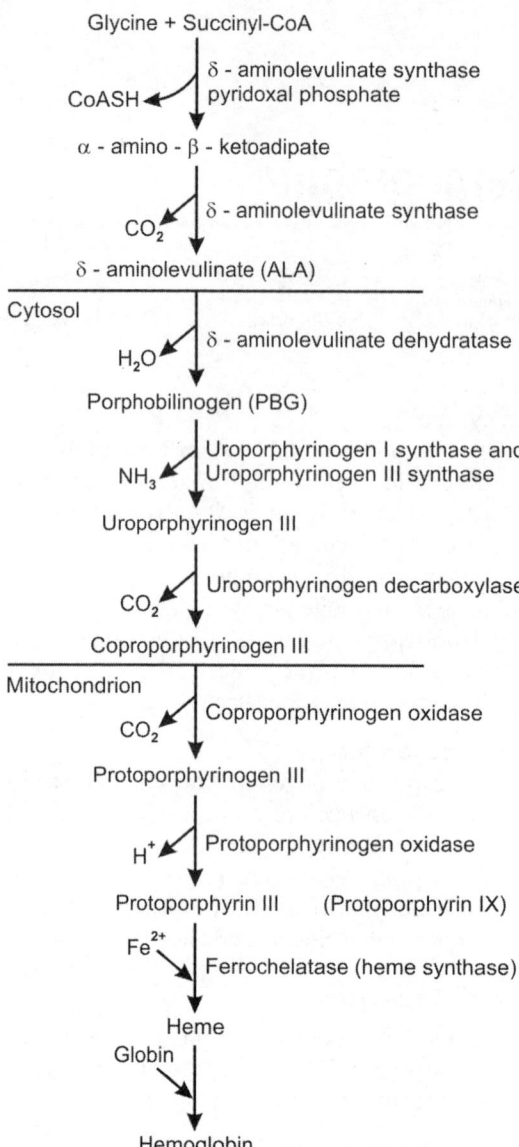

Fig. 16.1: Biosynthesis of hemoglobin.

> **Clinical Importance: Disorders**
>
> Defects in heme biosynthesis may result in clinical disorders known as porphyrias.

Porphyrias

Definition

These are a group of inborn errors of metabolism occurring due to deficiency of enzymes in the biosynthesis of heme. These are mainly divided into three groups based on the type of organ affected.

Examples (Table 16.1)
Treatment

These patients must avoid any anesthetics, drugs, alcohol. They are advised to take more carbohydrate or hematin to reduce the production of heme precursors. They may use sunscreen to avoid visible light.

Acute Intermittent Porphyria

It is an inborn error metabolism of hemoglobin.

Cause: It occurs in biosynthetic pathway of hemoglobin due to deficiency of enzyme uroporphyrinogen I synthase (porphobilinogen deaminase).

Incidence: 1 in 2,000.

Symptoms: Abdominal pain, constipation, neuropsychiatric symptoms. Urine turns red/brown on exposure to air.

Diagnosis: Measurement of porphobilinogen in urine.

Treatment: Administration of hematin.

> **Note**
>
> Acquired porphyria occurs due to some toxic chemicals or secondary to some diseases or metal poisoning (lead) or drugs.

CATABOLISM OF HEMOGLOBIN (FIG. 16.2)

Formation and Excretion of Bile Pigments

In the human body, the average life of a red blood cell is about 120 days. An adult human degrades approximately 6 g of hemoglobin every day which produces 250–350 mg bilirubin (1 g Hb gives 35 mg bilirubin approximately).

Site

- *Organ:* Reticuloendothelial system (bone marrow, spleen, and liver)
- *Cell:* Microsomes (ER)

Catabolism of hemoglobin can be considered under two stages.

Chapter 16: Metabolism of Hemoglobin

Table 16.1: Porphyrias.

Types and examples	Defective enzymes	Clinical symptoms
1. Hepatic porphyria		
• Acute intermittent porphyria	Uroporphyrinogen I synthase	Abdominal pain Neuropsychiatric symptoms
• Porphyria cutanea tarda	Uroporphyrinogen decarboxylase	Photosensitivity
• Variegate porphyria	Protoporphyrinogen oxidase	Abdominal pain, photosensitivity, neuropsychiatric symptoms
2. Erythropoietic porphyria		
• Congenital erythropoietic porphyria	Uroporphyrinogen II synthase	Photosensitivity
3. Erythrohepatic porphyria		
• Protoporphyria	Ferrochelatase	Photosensitivity

1. Conversion of hemoglobin to bile pigments
2. Excretion of bile pigments

Conversion of Hemoglobin to Bile Pigments

❐ Hemoglobin is hydrolyzed to form heme and globin (globin may be reutilized to form Hb or degraded to individual amino acids). Heme is converted to hemin by heme oxygenase system. Hemin is then oxidized to biliverdin with liberation of iron.
❐ Biliverdin is reduced to bilirubin by bilirubin reductase. It is unconjugated bilirubin and is insoluble in water. It is transported in the blood in combination with albumin (bilirubin-albumin complex) to the liver.

Excretion of Bile Pigments

In the liver, bilirubin is conjugated with glucuronic acid to form bilirubin diglucuronide (conjugated bilirubin) by the enzyme bilirubin glucuronyl transferase.

Bilirubin diglucuronide is excreted in bile and reaches the large intestine, where it is reduced by bacterial action to a group of colorless compounds called urobilinogens. Most of the urobilinogens are excreted in feces where it is oxidized by air to stercobilin which gives brown color to the feces. A small fraction of urobilinogens not reduced in the large intestine is returned to liver through portal circulation (enterohepatic circulation) while the remainder is transferred to kidney where it converted to urobilin and excreted. This pigment gives straw color to the urine.

Clinical Importance

Normal Levels in Blood

❐ Total bilirubin = 0.2–1 mg/100 mL
❐ Direct (conjugated) bilirubin = 0.0–0.2 mg/100 mL
❐ Indirect (unconjugated) bilirubin = 0.2–0.8 mg/100 mL.

Abnormal Levels (Disorders)

When total bilirubin level in blood exceeds 1 mg/100 mL, a clinical condition known as hyperbilirubinemia occurs.

Causes

Hyperbilirubinemia may occur due to:
❐ Overproduction of bilirubin than the liver can excrete normally.
❐ Failure of damaged liver to excrete bilirubin produced in normal amounts.
❐ Obstruction to the excretory ducts of the liver by prevention of excretion of bilirubin.

Types

Unconjugated (indirect) hyperbilirubinemias:
❐ *Cause:* Overproduction of bilirubin or due to damaged liver
  • Due to acquired defect
    ▪ Neonatal (physiological) jaundice: It is a clinical condition due to increased bilirubin level in newborn babies. It is not a genetic disease.
    Alternative name: Physiologic jaundice.
    Cause: Neonatal jaundice is caused by increased hemolysis due to immature hepatic system for uptake, conjugation

Section 3: Metabolism

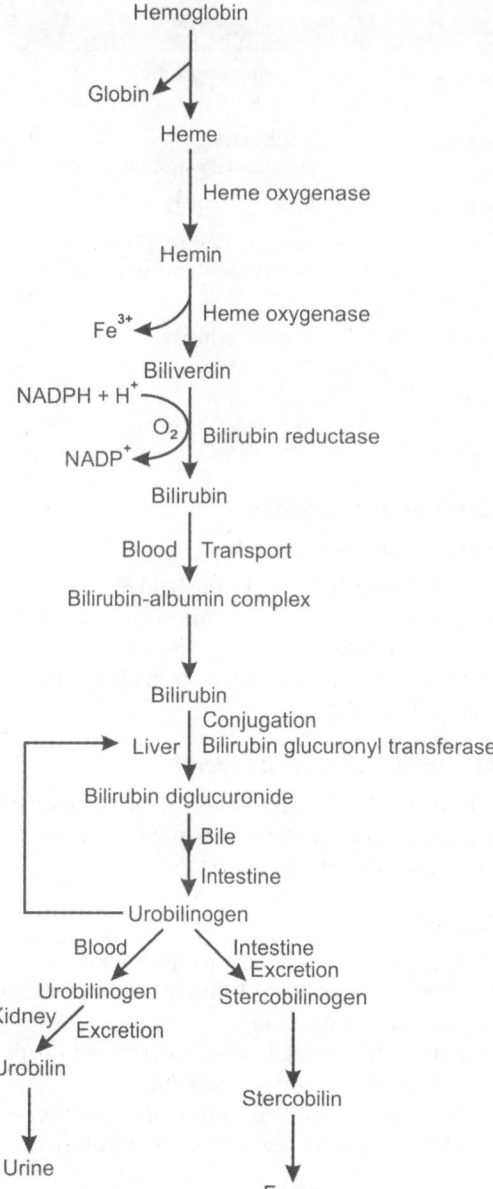

Fig. 16.2: Catabolism of hemoglobin.

and secretion of bilirubin. Also the activity of enzyme UDP-glucuronyl transferase is low in the newborn babies.

Effects:
a. Serum unconjugated bilirubin is highly elevated which can cross the blood-brain barrier which results in kernicterus (hyperbilirubinimic toxic encephalopathy).

b. Mental retardation.

Treatment:
a. Phenobarbital (drug)
b. Blood transfusion
c. *Phototherapy:* Patient is exposed to blue light (420–470 mm) and toxic conjugated bilirubin gets converted to nontoxic isomer lumirubin by photoisomerization which can be easily excreted by kidneys.
- Due to toxic effects by hepatitis, virus infections, chemicals, etc.
- Due to inherited abnormalities
  - Crigler–Najjar syndrome - type I
  - Crigler–Najjar syndrome - type II
  - Gilbert syndrome

Conjugated (direct) hyperbilirubinemia:
❏ *Cause:* Obstruction to hepatic or common bile duct.
- Dubin–Johnson syndrome
- Rotor syndrome
❏ *Symptom:* Jaundice (for both types)

■ JAUNDICE (FIG. 16.3 AND TABLE 16.2)

Definition

It is an abnormality of bilirubin metabolism. It is characterized by yellowish discoloration of eyes (sclera, conjunctiva), skin and mucous membrane. It occurs when the level of total bilirubin reaches 2 mg/100 mL of blood. It is a symptom and not a disease.

Alternative name: Icterus.

Type: It is divided into three major types (Table 16.2).

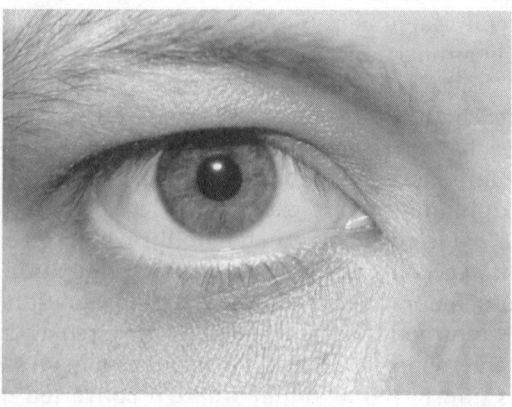

Fig. 16.3: Jaundice.
(For color version, see Plate 3)

Table 16.2: Types, causes, and laboratory diagnosis of jaundice.

Sl. No.	Types	Causes	Laboratory diagnosis
1.	Prehepatic jaundice (hemolytic jaundice)	It occurs due to increased breakdown of hemoglobin as in incompatible blood transfusion, hemolytic anemias, malaria, etc. Liver is unable to conjugate all the increased bilirubin formed	*Blood* Unconjugated bilirubin increased; VDB reaction—indirect +; ALP—normal, SGOT, SGPT—normal *Urine* Urobilinogen increased; bilirubin absent *Feces* Stercobilinogen increased; dark colored
2.	Hepatic jaundice (toxic/infective jaundice)	It occurs due to disease of the parenchymal cells of the liver as in chronic hepatitis, viral hepatitis, toxic hepatitis, drugs. There is a defect in the conjugation process	*Blood* Both conjugated and unconjugated bilirubin increased; VDB—delayed Direct + (Biphasic), ALP—normal/moderately increased. SGOT, SGPT—increased *Urine* Urobilinogen decreased; bilirubin present; dark colored *Feces* Stercobilinogen decreased; stool-pale color
3.	Posthepatic jaundice (obstructive jaundice)	It occurs due to obstruction to the flow of bile in the extrahepatic ducts as in carcinoma of head of pancreas, gallstone formation. Excretion of conjugated bilirubin is prevented	*Blood* Conjugated bilirubin increased; VDB—direct + ALP—highly increased. SGOT, SGPT—normal *Urine* Urobilinogen absent, bilirubin present; dark colored *Feces* Stercobilinogen—Trace/absent; stool—clay color

SGOT: serum glutamic oxaloacetic transaminase; SGPT: serum glutamic pyruvic transaminase; ALP: alkaline phosphatase; VDB: van den Bergh

17. Mineral Metabolism

Chapter Outline
- Definition
- Alternative Name
- Biomedical Importance/Functions
- Classification
- Abnormal States
- Macrominerals
- Sodium (Na⁺)
- Potassium (K⁺)
- Chloride (Cl⁻)
- Calcium (Ca)
- Phosphorus (P)
- Magnesium (Mg)
- Sulfur (S)
- Microminerals (Trace Elements)
- Iron (Fe)
- Iodine (I)
- Copper (Cu)
- Zinc (Zn)
- Manganese (Mn)
- Molybdenum (Mo)
- Fluoride (F)
- Cobalt (Co)
- Chromium (Cr)
- Selenium (Se)
- Nonessential Trace Elements

DEFINITION

Minerals are inorganic elements required in very small quantities for growth and maintenance of normal functions of the body.

ALTERNATIVE NAME

Accessary food factors.

BIOMEDICAL IMPORTANCE/FUNCTIONS

- They provide a suitable medium for protoplasmic activity.
- They play a primary role in osmotic phenomenon.
- They maintain acid-base balance.
- They are essential for formation and growth of certain tissues, such as bone and teeth.
- They are part of specialized physiological compounds, such as hemoglobin, thyroxine, etc.
- They are cofactors or activators of several enzymes.
- They do not provide energy.

CLASSIFICATION (FIG. 17.1)

The minerals present in the human body are divided into two major groups depending on their requirements for the body.
1. *Macrominerals*
2. *Microminerals:* This group is further sub-classified in **Figure 17.1**.

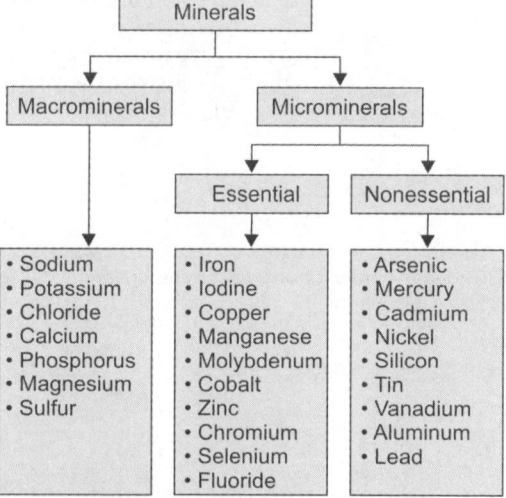

Fig. 17.1: Classification of minerals.

ABNORMAL STATES

Deficiency may produce deficiency symptoms and excess may produce toxicity.

MACROMINERALS (TABLE 17.1)

Definition

The inorganic elements taken in the diet in more than 100 mg daily are macrominerals. They form 60–80% of all inorganic matter in the body.

Chapter 17: Mineral Metabolism

Table 17.1: Macrominerals.

Sl. No.	Macrominerals	Sources	Functions	RDA (adults)	Deficiency symptoms	Toxicity symptoms
1.	Sodium	Common salt, (table salt) salted foods, meat, milk, vegetables	Chief cation of ECF, osmotic pressure, water and acid base balance muscle function, cell membrane permeability	1–5 g	Overhydration, diarrhea, vomiting, Addison's disease	Dehydration, edema, hypertension, Cushing syndrome
2.	Potassium	Vegetables, fruits, nuts, meat, coconut, water	Chief cation of ICF, water and acid base balance, neuromuscular irritability controls activity of heart muscle	3–4 g	Muscular weakness, cardiac arrhythmias	Mental confusion
3.	Chloride	Common salt (table salt) salted foods	Chief anion of ECF, HCl formation, acid base balance	1–5 g	As for sodium	As for sodium
4.	Calcium	Milk, dairy products, legumes, leafy, vegetables, dry fruits	Calcification of bones and teeth, muscle contraction, nerve transmission, blood clotting cofactor of enzymes, e.g., glycogen synthase, hormone, function	800–1,200 mg	Osteoporosis, tetany, rickets, osteomalacia	Renal stones, bone pain muscular and neurological disorders
5.	Phosphorus	Milk, dairy products, cereals, vegetables, meat, eggs	Calcification of bones and teeth, constituent of nucleic coenzymes. Constituent of high energy compounds	1–1.2 g	Muscle weakness, skeletal deformations, cardiac, arrhythmias	Metastatic calcification
6.	Magnesium	Vegetables, cereals, fruits, milk	Component of bones and teeth, cofactor of enzymes, e.g., kinases, nerve impulse transmission	300 mg	Neuromuscular weakness	Lethargy, drowsiness
7.	Sulfur	Sulfur containing amino acids	Constituent of sulfur containing amino acids and vitamins (thiamin, biotin, heparin, chondroitin sulfates)	Adequate amount of sulfur containing amino acids	Not established	Not established

(ECF: extracellular fluid; ICF: intracellular fluid)

Alternative Names

Principal minerals/Principal elements.

Examples

- Sodium
- Potassium
- Chloride
- Calcium
- Phosphorus
- Magnesium
- Sulfur

General Functions

- They are structural elements of tissues.
- They maintain osmotic pressure.
- They regulate acid-base balance.
- They are involved in the development and growth of bones and teeth.
- They are involved in neuromuscular function and blood coagulation.

■ SODIUM (Na⁺)

Sources

It is widely distributed in food stuffs:
- *Rich:* Common salt (sodium chloride)
- *Good:* Meat, milk, salty foods
- *Poor:* Vegetables, fruits, cereals

Distribution in the Body

Total sodium content of the body is 100 g. It is the major cation (Na^+) of extracellular fluid. It exists in the body in association with the anions—chloride (Cl^-), bicarbonate (HCO_3^-).

Functions

- It maintains normal water balance by regulating osmotic pressure of the body fluids and thus protects the body against excessive fluid loss.
- It regulates acid-base balance in association with chloride and bicarbonate.
- As sodium pump ($Na^+ - K^+$ ATPase), it is involved in the absorption of glucose, galactose and amino acids from the small intestine.
- It maintains normal neuromuscular irritability.
- It initiates and maintains heartbeat.
- It plays an important role in the permeability of cells.

Metabolism

It is normally completely absorbed from ileum. Less than 2% of unabsorbed sodium is eliminated in feces. It is excreted mainly in urine (95%) and to a minor extent via skin (through perspiration). Excess sodium is lost through skin during exercise, environmental heat and fever leading to heat cramps.

Normal blood level: 135–145 mEq/L

Abnormal States

Hypernatremia

Causes	Toxicity symptoms
a. Dehydration	Edema
b. Cushing's syndrome	Hypertension
c. Excess ACTH	Cardiac failure

Hyponatremia

Causes	Deficiency symptoms
a. Excess water intake	Decrease in blood pressure, drowsiness
b. Diarrhea, vomiting	Thirst
c. Addison's disease	Lethargy
d. Renal disease	Tremors
e. Severe burns, accidents	Coma

Daily Requirement (RDA)

Adults 1–5 g as sodium chloride (NaCl).

■ POTASSIUM (K⁺)

Sources

Potassium is found in almost all foods—both plant and animal sources.

Plant: Green leafy vegetables, bananas, orange, coffee, tea, tender coconut water.

Animal: Chicken, beef, liver.

Distribution in the Body

Total body potassium is 200 g. It is the major cation (K^+) in the intracellular fluid.

Functions

- It regulates osmotic pressure and water balance.
- It maintains acid-base balance.
- It is essential for all membrane functions (cell permeability).
- It has an important role in muscular contraction especially cardiac muscle.
- It has a role in the conduction of nerve impulse.
- It is an activator of glycolytic enzyme pyruvate kinase.
- Protein synthesis in ribosomes depends on potassium.

Metabolism

Normally potassium in food is almost completely absorbed from the small intestine. Excretion of potassium is mainly through urine and is related with the maintenance of acid-base balance.

Normal blood level: 3.5–5.0 mEq/L

Abnormal States
Hyperkalemia

Causes	Toxicity symptoms
a. Dehydration	Depression of CNS
b. Respiratory acidosis	Weakness
c. Addison's disease	Numbness
d. Chronic renal failure	Cardiac arrest

Hypokalemia

Causes	Deficiency symptoms
a. Diarrhea and vomiting	Muscular weakness
b. Metabolic alkalosis	Tachycardia and heart enlargement, irritabilities, paralysis
c. Cushing's syndrome	
d. Diuretics	

Adults daily requirement (RDA): 2–4 g

■ CHLORIDE (Cl⁻)

Sources

Rich: Common salt/table salt (sodium chloride), milk, meat, eggs, leafy vegetables, whole grains.

Distribution in the Body

It is the major anion of extracellular fluid (Cl⁻).

Functions

- It regulates osmotic pressure and water balance.
- It maintains acid-base balance.
- It is essential for production of HCl in gastric juice.
- It is an activator of enzyme salivary amylase.
- It is involved in chloride shift.

Metabolism

It is normally absorbed by the GI tract. It is mainly eliminated in the urine and minor part through perspiration.

Normal blood level: 95–105 mEq/L

Hyperchloremia

Causes	Toxicity symptoms
a. Dehydration	Mostly similar to hypernatremia
b. Excess saline therapy	
c. Cushing's syndrome	
d. Respiratory acidosis	

Hypochloremia

Causes	Deficiency symptoms
a. Vomiting	Mostly similar to hyponatremia
b. Diarrhea	
c. Addison's disease	
d. Renal disease	
e. Excess sweating	

Adults daily requirement (RDA): 1–5 g as sodium chloride (NaCl).

■ CALCIUM (Ca)

Sources

- *Rich:* Milk and dairy products
- *Good:* Egg yolk, beans, nuts, cabbages, green leafy vegetables
- *Poor:* Meat, cereals

Distribution in the Body

It is the most abundant mineral in the body. An adult contains 1,200 g of calcium. It forms 2% of total body weight and is mainly in bones and teeth.

Functions

Calcium performs a number of important physiological and biochemical functions in the body.

- *Mineralization of bones and teeth:* Calcium along with phosphorus is essential for formation of bones and teeth.
- *Blood coagulation:* Ionized calcium is necessary for blood coagulation, producing substances for thromboplastic activity of blood.
- *Activation of enzymes in metabolism:*

- Some enzymes are activated directly by calcium, e.g., pancreatic lipase, rennin, enzymes of coagulation.
- Some enzymes are activated indirectly by calmodulin (calcium regulatory protein), e.g:
  - Adenylyl cyclase
  - Ca^{++} dependent protein kinase
  - Ca^{++}, Mg^{++} ATPase
  - Glycogen synthase
  - Phospholipase A_2
  - Pyruvate carboxylase
  - Pyruvate dehydrogenase
  - Myosin kinase
  - Pyruvate kinase
- *Second messenger of hormone action:* It functions as a second messenger for action of many hormones, e.g., gastrin, vasopressin.
- *Muscle-nerve function:* It has an important role in:
  - Muscular contraction
  - Excitability of nerves
  - Neuromuscular transmission
- *Cell permeability:* It is essential for maintaining cell permeability.
- Required for hydrolysis of casein of milk in infants.
- *Pharmacological action (therapeutic uses):*
  - Calcium lactate or calcium gluconate is used for the treatment of rickets and osteomalacia.
  - Calcium gluconate is used for the immediate relief of tetany.

Metabolism

Absorption

Calcium is taken in the diet as calcium salts (calcium phosphate, calcium carbonate, calcium oxalate). Only 30% of dietary calcium is absorbed actively from duodenum and proximal jejunum. It is governed by many factors.

Factors Assisting

- *Intestinal pH:* Acidic pH favors absorption because calcium salts are soluble in acidic pH.
- *Vitamin D:* It promotes absorption of calcium.
- *Relationship with phosphorus:* Ca:P ratio 1:1.2 to 1.5 in the diet is most favorable for absorption of both.
- High protein diet increases absorption of calcium.

Factors Inhibiting

- *Intestinal pH:* Alkaline pH decreases absorption of calcium because calcium salts are insoluble in it.
- *Substances present in food:* Any substance present in food which can form insoluble salt with calcium will interfere with the absorption of calcium, e.g.:
  - Phytic acid present in cereals
  - Oxalic acid present in vegetables
  - Fatty acids (by forming calcium salts of fatty acids-calcium soaps).

Excretion

It is excreted as follows:
- In feces = As mostly unabsorbed calcium
- In urine = 50–200 mg/day
- In sweat = 15 mg/day

Normal level: 9–11 mg/100 mL plasma
It is present in three forms in plasma:
1. Ionized (diffusible) = 4 mg% (40%)
2. Protein bound (nondiffusible) = 3–5 mg% (60%)
3. In combination = 0–0.2 mg% (negligible) with citrate (diffusible).

Regulation of Blood Calcium Level

Regulation of Serum Calcium (Calcium Homeostasis)

Calcium is mostly present in plasma (or serum) in the range 9–11 mg/100 mL. It is maintained by the coordinate activity of the hormones, PTH, calcitriol and calcitonin.

PTH plays a major role in the regulation of calcium. If calcium concentration falls, secretion of PTH is increased. It acts on osteoclasts and increases bone resorption. In also increases reabsorption of calcium from the kidney. It also activates vitamin D and converts it to calcitriol. Calcitriol promotes intestinal absorption of calcium. The net effect of all these processes is to increase serum calcium level **(Fig. 17.2)**.

Calcitonin is secreted when serum calcium level is increased. Its action is to lower serum calcium level by promoting deposition of calcium by the osteoblasts of the bone.

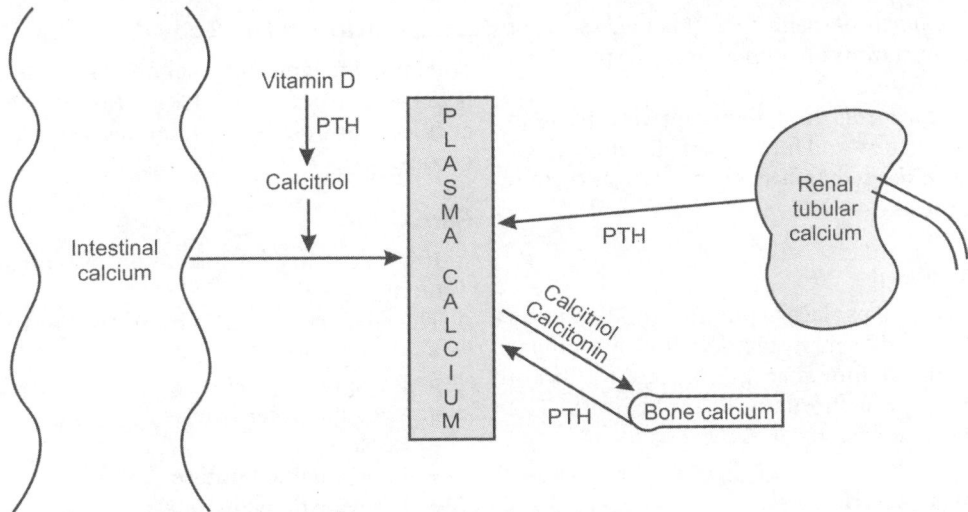

Fig. 17.2: Regulation of blood calcium.

> **Note**
> Teeth calcium is not used in this process.

Abnormal States

Failure to maintain blood calcium level may result in clinical disorders.

Hypercalcemia

Causes	Toxicity symptoms
a. Hyperparathyroidism	Lethargy
b. Vitamin D intoxication	Depression
c. Malignancy	Bone pain
d. Paget's disease	Urinary calculi

Hypocalcemia

Causes	Deficiency symptoms
a. Hypoparathyroidism	Hypocalcemia <7 mg%
b. Vitamin D deficiency	Results in tetany
c. Renal disease	Muscular and neurological disorders

Daily Requirement (RDA)

- Adult (male and female) = 800 mg
- Women during pregnancy and lactation = 1,200 mg
- Children = 1,200 mg
- Infants = 300–500 mg

PHOSPHORUS (P)

Sources

A diet supplying sufficient calcium also supplies an appropriate amount of phosphorus.
- *Rich:* Milk and dairy products
- *Good:* Eggs, beans, nuts, meats, protein-rich foods

Distribution in the Body

It is the fifth abundant element of the body. Total body contains 700 g of phosphorus. It makes up 1% of body weight. It is present in various tissues of the body as inorganic and organic forms.

Functions

- *Mineralization of bones and teeth:* Phosphorus along with calcium is necessary for the formation of bones and teeth.
- *Energy storage and transfer:* It is required for the formation of energy rich compounds, e.g., ATP, GTP, etc.
- *Formation of biologically important compounds:* It is necessary for the formation of phospholipids, phophoproteins, nucleic acids, hexose phosphate, etc.
- *Acid-base balance:* Phosphate buffers maintain acid-base balance.

- *Component of coenzymes:* It is necessary for the formation of coenzyme, e.g., pyridoxal phosphate.
- *Structural role:* It plays an important role in the structure and function of all living cells.
- *Synthesis*: It has a role in DNA and RNA synthesis.

Metabolism

Absorption takes place mainly from midjejunum. It is governed by many factors which are similar to that of calcium absorption. About 2/3rd of absorbed phosphorus appears in urine. The remainder is excreted in feces.

Normal Blood Level

Phosphorus is present in plasma and RBCs in two forms:
1. *Inorganic phosphorus:* 3–5 mg/100 mL
2. *Organic phosphorus:* 14–30 mg/100 mL

Abnormal States

Hyperphosphatemia

Causes	Toxicity symptoms
a. Vitamin D hypervitaminosis	Metastatic Calcification
b. Hypoparathyroidism	

Hypophosphatemia

Causes	Deficiency symptoms
a. Vitamin D deficiency	Rickets
b. Hyperparathyroidism	Osteomalacia

Daily Requirement (RDA)

- Adult (men and women) = 800 mg
- Women during pregnancy and lactation = 1,200 mg
- Infants and children = 300–800 mg.

■ MAGNESIUM (Mg)

Sources

- *Plant:* Leafy vegetables, such as cabbage, cauliflower, fruits
- *Animal:* Egg, dairy products

Distribution in the Body

Total body magnesium is about 25g; 2/3rd of it is present in bones and 1% is present in extracellular fluids and remainder is present in soft tissues.

Functions

- It is necessary for formation of bones and teeth.
- The enzymes activated by magnesium are:
  - Hexokinase
  - Phosphofructokinase
  - Phosphoglycerokinase
  - Enolase
  - Phosphoglucomutase
  - Pyruvate dehydrogenase
  - Transketolase
  - Glucose 6-phosphate dehydrogenase
- It activates all enzyme systems which catalyze transfer of phosphate from ATP, GTP to a substrate (or) from a phosphorylated compound to ADP. Thus the synthesis of carbohydrates, lipids, protein, and nucleic acids and also activation of muscle contraction require magnesium.
- It is necessary for neuromuscular function.

Metabolism

Magnesium in the form of its soluble salts is readily absorbed from the small intestine.

Absorption is affected by (a) large intake of calcium, phosphorus, and protein in the diet (b) consumption of more alcohol (c) acid. It is mostly excreted in feces. It is also excreted in the urine and bile.

Normal Level in Blood

2–3 mg/100 mL.

Abnormal States

Hypermagnesemia

Causes	Toxicity symptoms
a. Renal failure	Muscle weakness depression
b. Increased use of laxatives and antacids	Decreased neuromuscular transmission

Hypomagnesemia

Causes	Deficiency symptoms
a. Rickets	Neuromuscular disturbances and hyperirritability with tremors and convulsions
b. Pregnancy, kwashiorkor	Cardiac arrhythmia
c. Chronic alcoholics	

Daily requirement (RDA): Adult 300 mg.

SULFUR (S)

Sources

The main sources of sulfur for the body are dietary proteins containing amino acids, cystine, cysteine, and methionine. Sulfolipids and glycoprotein also provide sulfur. Free sulfur is present in meat, fish, legumes, egg, liver, and cereals.

Distribution in the Body

About 150–200 g of total body weight is sulfur. It is mainly present as organic compounds.

Functions

- It is a constituent of sulfur containing amino acids which are present in several proteins, e.g., keratin—the protein of hair, hoofs.
- It plays an important role in the structure of proteins and also immunoglobulins.
- It is a constituent of:
  - Enzymes, e.g., thiamine pyrophosphate, CoA-SH, lipoic acid, and NADH-linked dehydrogenase.
  - Vitamins, e.g., thiamine, biotin, pantothenic acid.
  - Hormones, e.g., insulin
  - Bile acids, e.g., taurocholic acid
  - Biological compounds, e.g., glutathione, heparin.
- Sulfur as sulfate is used for the detoxification of certain compounds in the liver, e.g., phenol, indoxyl, skatole and steroids.

Metabolism

The metabolism of sulfur is essentially a matter of cystine and methionine metabolism.

It is excreted almost entirely in urine in three forms (*see* below).

Excretion of sulfur in urine

Form	Compound	Output
Inorganic sulfate	Sulfates of sodium, potassium, calcium, magnesium	70–80%
Organic (ethereal) sulfate	Conjugated sulfates with phenol P-cresol, indole, and skatole	15–25%
Neutral sulfate (unoxidized)	Methionine, cystine, taurocholic acid, thiosulfate, thiocyanate	5%

Normal blood level: Present in three forms
1. Inorganic = 0.5–1.1 mg%
2. Organic (ethereal sulfate) = 0.1–1.0 mg%
3. Neutral sulfate = 1.7–3.5 mg%

Abnormal States

- Renal function impairment
- Intestinal obstruction, leukemia

RDA: Adequate amount of sulfur containing amino acids.

MICROMINERALS (TRACE ELEMENTS)

Definition

Minerals which are required in amount <100 mg/day are called microminerals. They also include some minerals which are slightly toxic and functions of some of them are not well-established **(Table 17.1)**.

Alternative Name

Microelements

Classification

It is classified into two subgroups **(Fig. 17.3)**.

Essential Trace Elements

These trace elements are essential for the body. Their requirement is less than 100 mg/day. Deficiency may lead to severe deficiency symptoms and excess may result in toxic symptoms **(Table 17.2)**.

General Functions

- They are cofactors for a number of enzymes involved in metabolism of carbohydrates, lipids, and proteins.

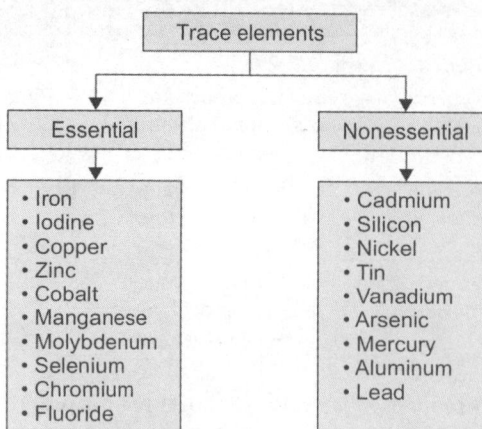

Fig. 17.3: Classification of microminerals.

- They are involved in the formation of many physiologically important compounds: Hemoglobin, vitamin B_{12}, thyroid hormones, etc.

■ IRON (Fe)

Sources

- *Rich:* Liver, kidney, heart, spleen
- *Good:* Egg yolk, nuts, beans, bananas, apples, green leafy vegetables, molasses
- *Poor:* Milk, dairy products, wheat

Distribution in the Body (Fig. 17.4)

An adult man contains only 3–5 g iron in the body. It is distributed in the body as follows:

Table 17.2: Essential trace elements.

Micro-minerals	Sources	Functions	RDA (adults)	Deficiency symptoms	Toxicity symptoms
Iron	Red meat, liver, eggs, fruits such as apples and bananas	• Essential constituent of hemoglobin which is involved in the transport of O_2 and CO_2 in the tissues • Essential component of myoglobin which supplies oxygen to muscles • *Involved in cellular respiration:* Constituent of heme enzymes, e.g., cytochromes, which catalyze biological oxidation and provide energy • Constituent of oxidative enzymes, such as catalases and peroxidases • Necessary for the normal development of RBCs	10 mg	Anemia	Hemosiderosis, hemochromatosis
Iodine	Seafoods, iodized salt	• Constituent of thyroid hormones [thyroxine (T_4) and triiodothyronine (T_3)] • T_3 and T_4 are involved in cellular oxidation, growth and reproduction and the activity of central and autonomous nervous systems	100–150 µg	*Children:* Cretinism *Adults:* Simple goiter, myxedema	Thyrotoxicosis goiter
Copper	Liver, kidney, meat, nuts, dried legumes	• Constituent of enzymes (cytochrome oxidase) tyrosinase cytosolic superoxide dismutase monoamine oxidase, ALA synthase, etc. • Role in iron absorption • Role in synthesis of hemoglobin phospholipids, collagen • Role in bone formation • Maintenance of integrity of myelin sheath	2–3 mg	Menke's syndrome (steely hair syndrome)	Wilson's disease (hepatolenticular degeneration) *see* page 213

Contd...

Contd...

Micro-minerals	Sources	Functions	RDA (adults)	Deficiency symptoms	Toxicity symptoms
		• Constituent of cerebrocuprein, erythrocuprein and hepatocuprein which are present in brain, RBC and liver respectively • Ceruloplasmin is a copper dependent ferroxidase			
Manganese	Cereals, vegetables fruits, nuts, tea	• Cofactor of enzymes, such as hydrolases, decarboxylases, transferase, mitochondrial superoxide dismutase • Role in glycoprotein and proteoglycan synthesis	5–6 mg	Impaired growth and skeletal deformities	Psychotic symptoms and parkinsonism, such as symptoms produced by inhalation
Molybdenum	Cereals legumes	Cofactor of oxidase enzymes (e.g., xanthine oxidase, aldehyde oxidase)	100 µg	Mental retardation	Growth retardation anemia, diarrhea
Cobalt	Foods of animal sources	• A constituent of vitamin B_{12} and its coenzymes • Promotes erythropoiesis	1–2 mg of vitamin B_{12}	Vitamin B_{12} deficiency	Polycythemia
Zinc	Liver, eggs, milk, dairy products, and vegetables	• Cofactor of many enzymes, e.g., lactate dehydrogenase, alkaline phosphatase, carbonic anhydrase, etc. • Maintaining normal levels of vitamin A in blood • Provides immunity	10–15 mg	Hypogonadism, growth failure, impaired wound healing, acrodermatitis enteropathica	Gastrointestinal irritation and vomiting
Chromium	Brewer's yeast, meat, liver, whole grains, nuts, cheese	• An activator of insulin • Known as glucose tolerance factor	50–100 µg	Impaired glucose intolerance	Lung cancer (occupational hazard)
Selenium	Plants in foods, present as selenoamino acids	• Constituent of enzyme such as glutathione peroxidase • Acts as antioxidant with vitamin E • Protects from free radicals and carcinogens	50–200 mg	Keshan disease, alkali disease, congestive heart failure	Hair loss, dermatitis irritability. Garlic like breath, weight loss, occupational hazard
Fluoride	Drinking water tea	• Tooth development, normal maintenance and hardening of dental enamel and prevention of dental caries • Bone development	<2 ppm (2–3 mg)	Dental caries	Above 3 ppm causes toxicity leading to dental fluorosis, skeletal fluorosis

Nonessential trace elements (*refer* page 217)

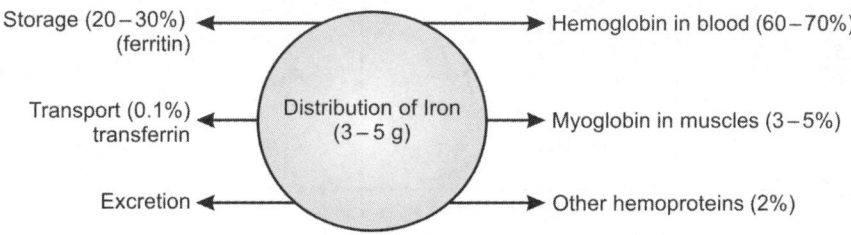

Fig. 17.4: Distribution of iron in the body.

- Hemoglobin (heme protein) = 60–70%
- Myoglobin (heme protein) = 3–5%
- Heme enzymes = 2%
- Storage forms (ferritin) = 20–30%
- Transport form (transferrin) = 0.1%

Biomedical Importance/Functions

Iron performs many vital functions in the body.
- *Oxygen carriage in blood:* It is an essential constituent of hemoglobin which is involved in the transport of oxygen to the tissues.
- *Oxygen supply to muscles:* The muscles store oxygen in combination with myoglobin which also contains iron.
- *Tissue oxidation (cellular respiration):* Iron forms an integral part of all the cytochromes which catalyze biological oxidation and provide energy. Iron also forms a part of prosthetic group of some flavoproteins and thus involved in electron transfer.
- Iron is also present in oxidative enzymes such as catalases and peroxidases.
- Iron is required in sufficient amounts for the normal development of RBCs.

Absorption

Absorption of iron is generally poor. Only 10–15% of dietary iron is absorbed mainly from stomach and duodenum and to a lesser extent throughout the small intestine. Absorption of iron is best explained on the basis of *mucosal block theory*. Iron in food is mostly present in Fe^{3+} as $Fe(OH)_3$. Fe^{3+} is released by gastric HCl and organic acid. Fe^{3+} is converted to Fe^{2+} by ascorbic acid. Ferrous iron on entering the mucosal epithelial cells is oxidized to ferric form by the enzyme ferroxidase which combines with a protein called apoferritin to form ferritin. Apoferritin is unstable and breaks away quickly from ferritin. Ferric iron (Fe^{3+}) released from ferritin is reduced again by ferric reductase to ferrous iron (Fe^{2+}) which leaves the mucosal cells of intestine and enters the plasma (**Fig. 17.5**).

Factors Affecting Iron Absorption

- Absorption of iron occurs mainly in the stomach and duodenum. Impaired absorption takes place in the patients who have total removal of stomach or a part of the intestine.
- A diet high in phosphate causes decreased absorption due to the formation of insoluble ferric phosphate. Very low phosphate in diet favors increased absorption of iron.
- Vitamin C (which has reducing property) increases absorption (reduces ferric to ferrous). That is why citrus fruit which contains vitamin C is given in iron deficiency anemia, because of malabsorption syndrome.
- Phytic acid (present in cereals) decreases absorption.
- Copper deficiency decreases absorption by forming insoluble compounds with iron.
- Proteins of low molecular weight favor absorption.
- Alcohol intake favors iron absorption.
- Acid pH of GI tract increases absorption by converting $Fe(OH)_3$ to Fe^{++}.
- Achlorhydria decreases absorption.
- Administration of alkali decreases absorption.

Transport of Iron in the Plasma

In the plasma, ferrous iron is rapidly oxidized to ferric iron by the action of ferroxidase. Now ferric iron is incorporated into a specific protein called as transferrin or siderophilin to form

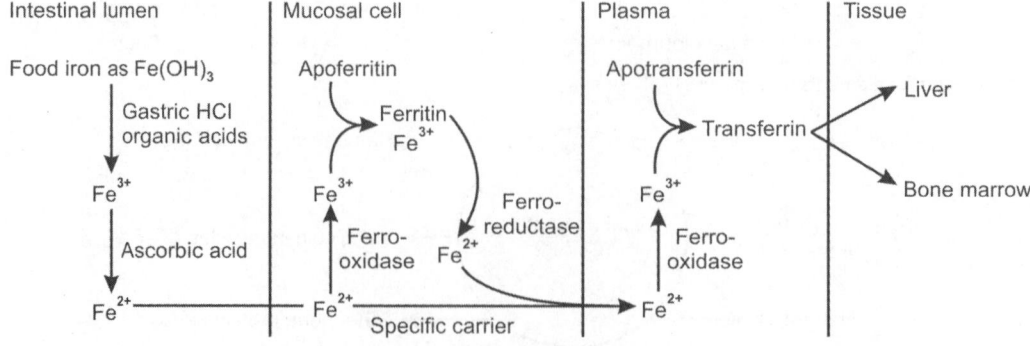

Fig. 17.5: Iron absorption and transport.

iron bound transferrin. It is a ferric protein complex. Transferrin is the main form in which iron is transferred in the blood. Iron is present in plasma only in combination with transferrin. Under normal circumstances almost all of the iron bound to transferrin is taken up readily by bone marrow to synthesize hemoglobin. Also iron bound to transferrin is also released when the tissues need it. It passes out of the capillaries into the cells where it is stored or utilized.

Iron Binding Capacity of Serum

- Quantity of transferrin present = 0.4 g in 100 mL blood
- Quantity of iron actually carried = 100 mg by transferrin

But maximum 330 mg iron can be carried by transferrin. This maximum ability of transferrin to bind iron, i.e., 330 mg/100 mL blood is called as iron binding capacity (IBC). Estimation of IBC in blood is useful for detecting iron deficiency.

Storage

Iron is mainly stored in the liver, spleen, and intestinal mucosa in the form of ferritin. To a small extent, it is also stored in all other reticuloendothelial cells and also other organs, such as adrenals and pancreas.

Excretion

The body stores of iron are conserved efficiently. Only minute quantities are excreted in urine, feces and sweat. Iron is also lost through skin (by means of sweat) hair loss, nail. The bulk of iron in the feces is unabsorbed food iron. Large amounts are lost during menstrual flow. During pregnancy, iron is lost (given) to the fetus.

Daily Excretion in Urine

- Adult (male and female in = 0.5–1.5 mg premenstrual period)
- Female during menstruation = Double the above quantity

Daily Requirement (RDA)

- Male adult = 10 mg
- Female .... (during pregnancy and lactation = 40 mg)
- .... other years = 18 mg
- Children .... = 10–15 mg
- Normal blood level = 50–175 µg%

Abnormalities

Toxicity

- *Hemosiderosis:* When iron is taken in large quantities (in repeated blood transfusion, excessive parenteral iron therapy, excessive hemolysis, less synthesis of hemoglobin) which exceeds the capacity of the body to store it as iron, the excess iron is deposited in the liver in the form of minute particles called as hemosiderin. Hemosiderin is actually a protein combined with colloidal iron oxide. When iron is deposited all over the body, the condition is called as hemosiderosis.
- *Hemochromatosis:* When iron accumulates in the tissues for many years, skin acquires a wheat colored bronze state pigmentation associated with hepatic cirrhosis, pancreatic fibrosis and diabetes. This condition is collectively called as bronze diabetes.
- *Nutritional siderosis:* Bantus (a sect) in South Africa cook their food in iron pots and so consume iron-rich food which results in the deposition of iron in the body especially liver. This disorder is called as nutritional siderosis.

Deficiency

Causes

- In women during pregnancy and lactation
- In children and adolescent girls
- During poor nutrition or malabsorption
- Due to excessive loss of blood as in menstruation intestinal malignancy, and parasite infection.

Symptoms

- Anemia
- Exertion, giddiness, dullness
- Pallor of the skin
- Poor appetite
- Retardation in growth and development

Treatment

- Iron tonics (ferrous sulfates)
- Ferric ammonium citrate sweetened with glycerine

■ IODINE (I)

Sources

Seafoods, drinking water, iodized salt vegetables grown near sea. Soil and water at high attitude are deficient in iodine.

Distribution in the Body

An adult man contains 20-50 mg of iodine. 80% of iodine is in thyroid gland. The rest is distributed in muscles, salivary glands, hair, skin, liver, etc.

Iodine Level in Blood

Normal level in plasma is 4-10 µg/100 mL. Most of this is present in organic form called as protein bound iodine (PBI). It represents the iodine present as circulating thyroid hormones (T_3, T_4). PBI is increased in hyperthyroidism and decreased in hypothyroidism. RBCs not contain iodine.

Absorption

Iodine and iodides are absorbed mostly from small intestine. Organic iodine compounds (T_3, T_4) are absorbed as such or partly broken in the stomach and intestine and absorbed. Absorption also takes place from mucous membranes, skin and lungs.

Storage

Stored in thyroid gland, iodine in thyroid gland is mostly in combined with a protein called thyroglobulin (glycoprotein) and is known as iodothyroglobulin.

Excretion

Excreted mainly as inorganic iodide in urine and less amount through skin, lung, and milk.

Daily Requirement (RDA)

Adults = 100-150 µg

Function

- Required for the synthesis of thyroid hormones T3, T4 (*refer* Chapter 25).
- Thyroid hormones are involved in several biochemicals functions.

Deficiency

In adults: Leads to simple goiter or endemic goiter (enlargement of thyroid gland and thyroid hypertrophy).

In children: Leads to cretinism (retardation of growth).

Treatment for both: (a) Use iodized salt in the diet; (b) Add iodide in drinking water.

Toxicity

Occurs due to over consumption of iodine—thyrotoxicosis (toxicgoiter).

Goitrogenic Substances

Foods, such as cauliflower, radish, and cabbage contain substances called (oxazolidone). It reacts with iodine present in the food and make them unavailable to the body leading to goiter.

■ COPPER (Cu)

Sources

Rich: Liver, kidney, meats, shellfish, nuts, and legumes.

Poor: Milk and its products

Distribution in the Body

Adult human body contains about 100 mg copper. Widely distributed in all the tissues. More in liver.

Storage

Liver

Absorption

Absorption is aided by a copper-containing protein namely metallothionein. A small amount is only absorbed from upper part of the small intestine.

Excretion

Excreted in feces via bile (major route). Traces only in urine.

Plasma Level

- 100-200 µg/100 mL
- Present in RBC and plasma
- Increased during pregnancy and oral contraceptives intake

Copper-containing Proteins

- *Ceruloplasmin:* It is present in plasma in minute quantities. It is a glycoprotein. It is ferroxidase which functions in iron absorption.
- *Erythrocuprein:* Present in erythrocytes (96%)
- *Cerebrocuprein:* Present in brain
- *Hepatocuprein:* Present in liver

◻ *Metallothionein:* Involved in absorption of copper

Functions

◻ An important constituent of several enzymes. For example:

Cytochrome oxidase	Ascorbic acid oxidase
Catalase	Uricase
Peroxidase	Superoxide dismutase
Ferrooxidase I (ceruloplasmin)	Monoamine oxidase
Ferrooxidase II	ALA synthase
Dopamine hydroxylase	

◻ Plays an important role in hemoglobin synthesis and maturation of RBCs.
◻ Necessary for bone formation.
◻ Necessary for formation of myelin sheaths in nervous system
◻ Necessary for melanin formation, phospholipid synthesis, collagen formation
◻ For absorption of iron from gastrointestinal tract.

Daily Requirement (RDA)

Adult 2–3 mg

Deficiency

◻ Deficiency of copper produces a microcytic anemia (similar to iron deficiency, but it cannot be corrected by iron).
◻ Acute hemolysis
◻ Diarrhea with blue green stools
◻ Abnormal kidney function
◻ Hypopigmentation of skin
◻ Neurological abnormality

Inborn Errors of Copper Metabolism

◻ *Menkes disease:* It is due to defective absorption of copper from intestine.
Symptoms are: Steely hair, mental retardation, depigmentation of skin, and hair.
◻ *Wilsons disease (hepatolenticular degeneration):* It is an inborn error of copper metabolism. It is characterized by abnormally large accumulation of copper in the liver and lenticular nucleus of the brain (**Fig. 17.6**).
Incidence: 1 in 50,000
Inheritance: Autosomal recessive
Cause: Mutation of the gene—ATP7B

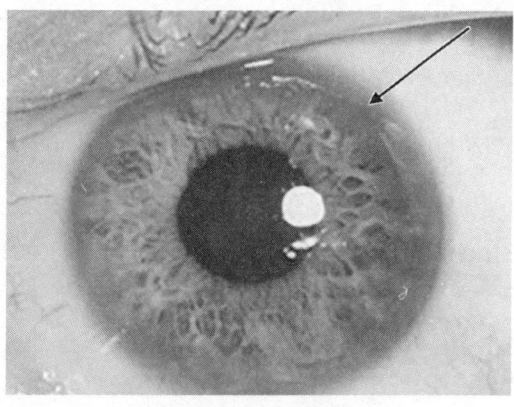

Fig. 17.6: Wilson's disease.
(For color version, see Plate 3)

Effects

◻ Absorption of copper from the intestine may be high.
◻ Ceruloplasmin formation is very low. Hence most of copper cannot bind with sufficient ceruloplasmin. Copper is deposited in other tissues, such as liver, kidneys, and brain.
◻ Serum copper is low
◻ Urine copper is high
◻ Aminoaciduria

Symptoms

◻ Liver failure
◻ Dementia
◻ A brown ring around cornea (Kayser–Fleischer ring)
◻ Abdominal pain, lack of appetite, fatigue
◻ Defective physical coordination

Diagnosis

◻ Measurement of copper in blood and urine
◻ Liver biopsy

Treatment

To administer copper chelating agents, such as penicillamine (to remove copper from tissues).

■ ZINC (Zn)

Sources

Rich: Sea foods

Good: Meat, eggs, liver, and milk

Fair: Cereals, pulses, nuts, oilseeds, vegetables, and fruits.

Distribution

- About 25% body contains zinc.
- Widely distributed in all tissues of the body especially:
  - Skin
  - Prostate
  - Choroid of eyes
  - Bones

Blood Level

- 75–125 µg/100 mL
- Present mostly in red blood cells

Absorption

Poorly absorbed from the intestine.

Excretion

Mostly excreted in faces.

Functions

- A constituent of many enzymes, e.g., carbonic anhydrase, alkaline phosphatase, carboxypeptidase, retinene reductase.
- It maintains normal concentration of vitamin A in plasma.
- Necessary for tissue repair and wound healing.
- Required for the preparation of insulin (zinc is a constituent of crystalline insulin. It increases the duration of insulin action).
- Essential for normal growth and reproduction of animals.
- Provides immunity

Daily Requirement (RDA)

Adult: 15 mg.

Deficiency

- Dwarfism
- Hypogonadism (retarded genital development)
- Loss of taste
- Hepatosplenomegaly
- In leukemia, zinc content of leukocytes is reduced
- Poor wound healing
- Acrodermatitis enteropathica (skin rash)
- Sickle cell disease

Toxicity

- Gastrointestinal irritation
- Vomiting

■ MANGANESE (Mn)

Sources

Rich: Nuts, whole grains, meat
Good: Vegetables, fruits, beguines

Distribution in the Body

- Distributed throughout the body
- Adult man contain 15–20 mg manganese in the body.

Absorption

Through small intestine

Excretion

Mostly excreted in feces

Daily Requirement (RDA)

Adult: 2.5–5 mg

Functions

- Essential for normal bone structure, reproduction and normal functions of CNS.
- Activates a number of enzymes, e.g., arginase (liver) isocitrate dehydrogenaste, phosphoglucomutase
- As a constituent of some enzymes
  - Superoxide dismutase
  - Pyruvate carboxylase
  - Glucose 6 phosphate dehydrogenase

Blood Level

4–20 mg/100 mL

Deficiency

In humans: Not established
In animals: Sterility, bone deformities

Toxicity

Miners inhale more manganese. They develop manganese toxicity leading to neuromuscular symptoms resembling Parkinson's disease.

■ MOLYBDENUM (Mo)

Sources

Liver, kidney, whole grains, leafy vegetables

Absorption

Absorbed by the small intestine

Excretion

Excreted in urine and bile

Functions

- As a constituent of metallo flavoproteins enzymes, e.g., xanthine oxidase, aldehyde oxidase
- It interferes with copper metabolism (diminished copper utilization)

Daily requirement (RDA): Adults 0.15–0.5 mg

Deficiency: It causes xanthinuria (*refer* Chapter 15)

Toxicity: It produces a disease in animals called 'teart'

■ FLUORIDE (F)

Sources

Drinking water, tea, sea fish

Distribution

Mainly in bone, teeth, and kidneys

Daily Requirement (RDA)

Adult: 1–2 ppm (or) 1.5–4 mg

Absorption

Rapidly absorbed from the small intestine

Excretion

Excreted in urine, sweat, intestinal mucosa.

Function

- Normal development of teeth and bones
- In combination with vitamin D, it is required for the treatment of osteoporosis.
- As enzyme inhibitors:
  - *Sodium fluoride:* An inhibitor of glycolytic enzyme enolase.
  - *Fluoroacetate:* Inhibits aconitase an enzyme of citric acid cycle.
  - Fluoride inhibits metabolism of oral bacterial enzymes and diminishes the production of acids which are responsible for dental caries.
- Fluoride forms a protective layer of acid resistant fluorapatite with hydroxyl apatite crystals of the enamel.
- It prevents dental caries.

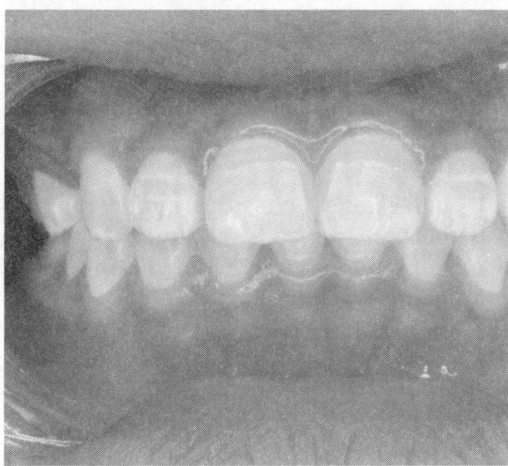

Fig. 17.7: Dental fluorosis.
(For color version, see Plate 3)

Deficiency

Dental caries/dental cavity: Due to bacterial action.

Toxicity

- *Dental fluorosis:* Intake of excess fluoride leads to dental fluorosis (mottled enamel) and discoloration of teeth (**Fig. 17.7**).
- *Skeletal fluorosis:* Workers in the industries of aluminum, steel and fertilizers are exposed to fumes of fluorine and they get fluorosis—the important factor in osteoporosis.
- *Symptoms:* Increased density and hyper calcification of bone of spine, pelvis, and limbs.
- *Treatment:* To use drinking water after removal of excess fluoride.

■ COBALT (Co)

Sources

Liver, pancreas, vitamin B_{12} containing foods.

Absorption

About 70–80% readily absorbed from small intestine.

Excretion

About 65% of ingested cobalt is excreted in urine. Rest in feces.

Distribution

Total body contains 1.1 mg. It is present in all tissues, but mostly in liver, kidney, and bone.

Functions

- It is an essential constituent of vitamin B_{12} (cobalamin) which is required to maintain normal bone marrow formation (RBC formation).
- Certain enzymes require vitamin B_{12} for their activities, e.g., methyl malonyl COA mutase.
- Homocysteine methyl transferase: Stimulates the production of erythropoietin.
- Used for cobalt therapy.

Daily Requirement (RDA)

1–2 mg of vitamin B_{12} containing 0.045–0.09 mg cobalt (adult).

Deficiency

- Deficiency of cobalt (and so vitamin B_{12}) leads to nutritional type of anemia.
- In ruminants (not in other species), deficiency of cobalt results in anorexia.

Toxicity

Excess cobalt leads to polycythemia (increased number of erythrocytes in blood).

■ CHROMIUM (Cr)

Sources

Meat, yeast, whole grains, molasses.

Distribution

Total body contains 6 mg, present in all tissues.

Absorption

Absorbed from small intestine.

Excretion

Mostly in urine. Least in feces and bile.

Functions

- Potentiates the action of insulin (utilization of glucose)
- Improves glucose tolerance in diabetes (glucose tolerance factor)
- Maintains normal cholesterol level in rats.
- Regulations in the incorporation of certain amino acids in heart muscle of rats.

Daily Requirement (RDA)

Adults 0.05–0.2 mg

Deficiency

- Not established well
- May lead to glucose intolerance (deficiency of chromium may be one of the reasons diabetes mellitus)
- May lead to cardiovascular diseases in rats

Toxicity

Inflammation of skin and dermatitis.

■ SELENIUM (Se)

Sources

Meat, liver, kidney, seafood

Distributions

Widely distributed in animal body

Daily Requirement (RDA)

50–200 µg for adults

Functions

- It functions as an antioxidant along with vitamin E (*refer* Chapter 8).
- It is a constituent of glutathione. It catalyzes peroxidation of glutathione. This enzyme is a protective agent against accumulation of H_2O_2 and organic peroxides within the cell.
- Selenocysteine is 21st amino acid.
- Maintains integrity of cell membranes.

Deficiency

- *Human:* Dilation of heart, congestive heart failure, Keshan disease.
- *Rats:* Necrosis of liver
- *Calves lambs:* Muscular dystrophy

Toxicity (selenosis): Occurs in people working in industries of paint, glass and electronics.

- Neuromuscular disorders
- Loss of hair and nails
- Skin lesions
- Garlic odor in breath

NONESSENTIAL TRACE ELEMENTS

Several nonessential trace elements are present in the body entering through various routes. Their functions are not well established yet. But it is supposed that they may have an unbalancing effect on the body's cells. They may affect the absorption and efficient use of other minerals in the body. Most of these elements have toxic effects in the body, though some authors have indicated a positive role for some of these elements. Recent research indicates that dietary intake of essential minerals and trace minerals can protect the body from the effects of toxic elements.

Sources and effects of nonessential trace elements are listed in **Table 17.3**.

Table 17.3: Nonessential trace elements.

Sl. No.	Examples	Sources	Toxic symptoms
1.	Lead	Petrol, paints, cigarettes, lead pipes, newspapers, xerox copies	Mental confusion, convulsions, paralysis, nausea, vomiting, anemia severe—abdominal pain
2.	Mercury	Plastics, paints electrical instruments, fungicides, broken thermometers, dental amalgam	Nervousness, muscle tremors, learning disabilities. Inflammation of mouth and gums, kidney damage, gastritis, vomiting, minamato disease
3.	Cadmium	Air pollutants, cigarette, smoke from industries	Restlessness, headache chest pain increased salivation, vomiting, diarrhea, kidney damage
4.	Aluminum	Cooking vessels, food additives, cosmetics, building materials	Mental status changes, learning and speech disturbances, tremors bone diseases, stroke, heart attack, Alzheimer's disease
5.	Arsenic	Insecticides, fungicides, water pollution	Affects cellular metabolism, muscular paralysis, sensory and visual disturbances

18. Metabolism of Xenobiotics (Detoxication)

> **Chapter Outline**
> - Sources
> - Importance
> - Alternative Names
> - Definition
> - Site
> - Mechanism
> - Types of Detoxication Mechanism

SOURCES

Toxic substances may be formed in the body from two sources:
1. *Endogenous sources:* These are formed during metabolism of some compounds in the body.
2. *Exogenous sources:* Human body is frequently subjected to exposure to various foreign chemicals known as xenobiotics (drugs, food additives or pollutants). These include substances which are not ordinarily ingested or utilized by the organism.

IMPORTANCE

Toxic compounds may cause certain harmful or undesirable effects in the body. They may even prove to be fatal. They can be detoxified by a process known as detoxication. Study of xenobiotic metabolism provides an understanding of pharmacology, toxicology, cancer, etc.

ALTERNATIVE NAMES

Detoxification, biotransformation, metabolism of foreign compounds.

DEFINITION

Detoxication refers to biochemical changes occurring in the body which convert toxic substances to nontoxic or less toxic substances which are easily excretable compounds.

SITE

It occurs mainly in the liver and to a minor extent in kidneys and other organs.

MECHANISM

Various theories have been proposed to explain the mechanism of detoxication.
- *Theory of Sherwin:* Xenobiotics converted to soluble products.
- *Theory of Berczeller:* Xenobiotics converted to compounds having less surface tension.
- *Theory of Quick:* Xenobiotics converted to strong acidic compounds.

TYPES OF DETOXICATION MECHANISM

There are four types of detoxication mechanism which can be grouped under two phases **(Fig. 18.1)**:

Phase I

Some compounds are detoxicated by each of the following processes and excreted.
- Oxidation
- Reduction
- Hydroxylation

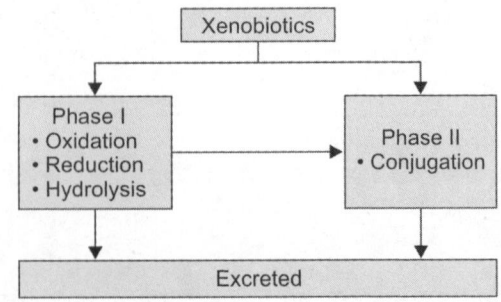

Fig. 18.1: Detoxication.

Oxidation
A large number of foreign substances are destroyed in the body by oxidation.

Alcohols
These are oxidized to corresponding acids
- Methanol → Formic acid
  (Aliphatic)
- Ethyl alcohol → Acetic acid
  (Aliphatic)
- Benzyl alcohol → Benzoic acid
  (Aromatic)
  $\xrightarrow{\text{Conjugation}}$ Excreted

Aldehydes
These are oxidized to corresponding acids:
Benzaldehyde → Benzoic acid

Aromatic hydrocarbons
These are oxidized to corresponding phenols

Benzene → Phenols $\xrightarrow{\text{Conjugation}}$ Excreted

Amines
- Aliphatic amines are oxidized to corresponding acids.
- Aromatic amines are oxidized to corresponding phenols.
  Aniline → p-Amino phenol

Sulfur
Sulfur present in organic sulfur compounds is oxidized to sulfates which may be excreted as inorganic or organic or neutral sulfur.
Sulfur → Sulfates → Inorganic/organic/ neutral sulfur

Reduction
Nitro and aldehyde compounds are detoxicated by reduction.
- Chloral → Trichloroethanol
  ↓
  Conjugated with D glucuronic acid and excreted as corresponding glucuronide
- Picric acid → Picramic acid

Hydrolysis
Certain therapeutic compounds used as drugs and also carcinogens undergo hydrolysis usually in the liver. This type of reaction is catalyzed by monooxygenases (cytochrome P_{450}).

- Digoxin → Sugar + Aglycone
  (Cardiac glycoside)
- Acetyl salicylic acid → Salicyclic acid + Acetic acid
  (Aspirin)
- Atropine → Tropic acid + Tropine

Phase II
Some compounds formed in Phase I may undergo conjugation to be excreted.
- Conjugation

Conjugation
It is a process by which the foreign substances or other metabolites are coupled with conjugating agents and converted to soluble nontoxic derivatives which are easily excreted in urine. This process can occur independently or may follow oxidation, reduction or hydroxylation (Phase I).

Examples
There are mainly eight types of conjugating agents.
1. *Methylation:* Nicotinic acid, nicotinamide, histamine are conjugated by S-adenosyl methionine to form as N-methyl derivatives.

   Nicotinamide → N' Methyl nicotinamide

2. *Acetylation:* Acetylation is done by active acetate (acetyl CoA) catalyzed by the enzyme acetyl transferase.
   Certain drugs are conjugated by acetylation.
   Sulfanilamide → Acetylated sulfanilamide
   Isoniazid (Anti-TB drug) → Acetylated product

3. *Conjugation by sulfuric acid:* Sulfuric acid is used for detoxication of various compounds having phenolic or hydroxyl groups, e.g., substances such as phenol, cresol, indole, and skatole are formed in the gut by the action of intestinal bacteria and are absorbed and transported to liver where they are conjugated with sulfate to form etheral sulfates, which are excreted in urine.
   Phenol/cresol/indole/skatole → Ethereal sulfates

4. *Conjugation with glucuronic acid:* Some compounds are conjugated with glucuronic acid (as UDP glucuronic acid) catalyzed

by the enzyme glucuronyl transferase and excreted as glucuronides, e.g.,
- Bilirubin is converted to bilirubin diglucuronide

  Bilirubin → Bilirubin diglucuronide
- The following compounds are also conjugated with glucuronic acid: phenol.

5. *Conjugation with glycine:* Some acids absorbed from the alimentary tract or arising during metabolism are conjugated with glycine mainly in the liver.
   - Benzoic acid + Glycine → Benzoyl glycine (hippuric acid)
   - Bile acids (cholic acid and deoxycholic acid) → Glycocholic acid

6. *Conjugation with glutamine:* Phenyl acetic acid is conjugated with glutamine to form phenyl acetyl glutamine. It is excreted in urine giving mousy odor as in phenylketonuria.

   Phenyl acetic acid + Glutamine → Phenylacetyl glutamine

7. *Conjugation with thiosulfate:* The highly toxic cyanides produced in the body from tobacco smoke, etc., are detoxified to relatively nontoxic thiocyanates by thiosulfates catalyzed by the enzyme rhodanese.

8. *Conjugation with glutathione:* Carcinogens are conjugated with glutathione catalyzed by the enzyme glutathione transferase.

19 Excretion

Chapter Outline
- Urine
- Feces
- Sweat
- Additional Information

Waste products, such as water, CO_2, and nitrogenous compounds are produced in the body as a result of metabolic activities. These products should be removed promptly to maintain normal health. Retention of these products, unless removed, produces harmful effects in the body.

URINE

The kidneys are the major important organs involved in the excretory system of the body. Formation of urine by the kidneys involves three main stages:
1. Glomerular filtration
2. Tubular reabsorption
3. Tubular secretion

Composition

Urine is a complex fluid-containing several nitrogenous substances.
- *Volume:* A normal adult excretes daily about 1,000–1,800 mL of urine (average 1,500 mL) containing 60 g of solids. Its quantity depends on several factors such as intake of water, diet, and external temperature.
- *Specific gravity:* Normal specific gravity of urine is 1010–1025. It varies depending on the concentration of solutes present in it and food and water intake.
- *Color:* Normal urine is pale yellow or straw or amber color. Normal color is due to the major pigment urobilin. Color change may occur during ingestion of colored foods and in diseases.
- *Odor:* Smell of normal urine is aromatic. It may smell differently after ingestion of certain foods or drugs or compounds.
- *pH:* Normal pH of urine is 4.7–8 (average pH 6.0). It is acidic in high protein intake and becomes alkaline after long standing.

Normal Constituents (*Refer* Appendix H)
- *Urea:* End-product of protein catabolism
- *Creatinine:* Formed from creatine
- *Uric acid:* End-product of purine catabolism
- *Amino acids:* Several amino acids are excreted in urine
- *Sulfates:* Chlorides, oxalates, phosphates and minerals, such as sodium, potassium, calcium, etc.

Abnormal Constituents (Table 19.1)

These constituents appear in the urine in diseases.

Renal function tests: Functions of kidney can be assessed by several tests (*refer* Chapter 24).

FECES

An adult passes 60–250 g daily of moist feces containing solids. Its quantity varies from day-to-day and with diet.

Composition

Water content is 65–80%.

Dry matter contains fat, intestinal secretions, excretion of large intestinal food residues such as cellulose, fruit skin, and seeds, etc. Fat content is increased in steatorrhea.

Section 3: Metabolism

Table 19.1: Abnormal constituents.

Constituent	Conditions/diseases	Test
Glucose	Diabetes mellitus	Benedict's test
Proteins (albumin)	Renal disorders, pregnancy, high protein intake	Heat coagulation test
Hemoglobin (blood)	Hemolysis	Benzidine test
Ketone bodies	Diabetic ketoacidosis, starvation	Rothera's test
Bile salts	Jaundice	Hay's test
Bile pigments	Jaundice	Fouchet's test

Color: Color is brown due to the presence of stercobilin. It depends on food constituents and pathologic state.

Odor: Odor is due to presence of hydrogen sulfide (H_2S), mercaptans, indole, and skatole.

■ PROTEINURIA

It refer to appearance of protein in the urine due to glomerular damage and vascular permeability. Normal level of protein in the urine = 0–150 mg/day. It may appear beyond this level in the urine as in: nephrotic syndrome, inflammation of lower urinary tract, etc.

Tests in urine: Sulfosalicyclic acid test, heat coagulation test.

■ MICROALBUMINURIA

Normal level of albumin in the urine is 0–30 mg/day. If it appears in the range 30–300 mg/day, it is called as microalbuminuria. It is an early indication of nephropathy. It can be tested by heat coagulation test with the urine.

■ GLYCOSURIA

Refer page 147.

■ SWEAT

It is a dilute fluid-containing moist of the diffusible constituents of the plasma. Its pH is 4.5. Its most abundant constituent is sodium chloride. Lactic acid is another constituent. Excessive sodium chloride excretion occurs in sweating and cystic fibrosis (a chronic inherited disease which affects lungs and digestive system).

Section 4: Miscellaneous Topics of Biochemical Importance

20. Energy Metabolism

Chapter Outline
- Energy
- Calorific Value of Foods
- Respiratory Quotient
- Energy Expenditure
- Energy Requirement

ENERGY

Definition
Energy means the capacity to work. It refers to the strength and vitality required for sustained physical and mental activity.

Sources
Human beings get energy from their food in a chemical form which is derived by consuming plants or animal products. The energy is bound in molecules of carbohydrates, fats, and proteins.

Functions
Energy derived from food is used for:
- Involuntary activities, such as absorption, transport of food materials, excretion, respiration, maintenance of body temperature, and osmotic pressure, etc.
- Voluntary activities, such as physical work and exercises.

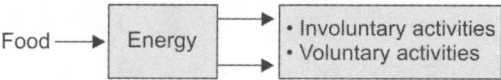

Storage
Energy in excess of immediate requirements of the body is stored as reserves of glycogen in muscles and liver and as fat in adipose tissue. When energy is inadequate to meet expenditure, these reserves along with liable tissue protein reserves are used as metabolic fuels.

Release
The energy is derived from oxidation of food stuffs. Different food stuff release different amounts of energy (in the form of heat) on burning. The amount of heat released provides a measure of the energy content of the food.

CALORIFIC VALUE OF FOODS
The energy released from food stuffs can be expressed in terms of calorific value of foods.

Definition
It is the amount of heat produced on complete burning (combustion) of 1 g of food stuff in the presence of oxygen.

Units of Measurement
The calorific value of foods is measured in calories (or Joules).

Small Calorie (C)
It is the amount of heat required to raise the temperature of 1 g water by 1°C.

Kilocalorie (C)
It is 1,000 times the small calorie, i.e., 1 Kc = 1,000c = C.

> **Note**
> In nutrition, only kilocalorie is used (C).

Energy Value of Foodstuff in the Body

Food materials undergo combustion in the body and liberate energy in the same way as in bomb calorimeter.

The energy values of carbohydrates, fats, and proteins are given below (c/g).

Foodstuffs	Outside the body (bomb calorimeter)	In the body
Carbohydrate	4.1	4.0
Fats	9.4	9.0
Protein	5.4	4.0

■ RESPIRATORY QUOTIENT

Definition

Respiratory quotient (RQ) is the ratio of the volume of carbon dioxide produced to the volume of oxygen utilized by a person as measured by calorimetry.

$$RQ = \frac{\text{Volume of } CO_2 \text{ produced}}{\text{Volume of } O_2 \text{ utilized}}$$

RQ of Different Foodstuff

It depends on the type of foodstuff being metabolized.

RQ of Carbohydrates (e.g., Glucose)

$$C_6H_{12}O_6 + 6O_2 \rightarrow 6CO_2 + 6H_2O$$

Therefore, $RQ = \dfrac{6CO_2}{6O_2} = 1$

RQ of Fats (e.g., Tristearin)

$$2C_{57}H_{110}O_6 + 163\ O_2 \rightarrow 114\ CO_2 + 110\ H_2O$$

Therefore, $RQ = \dfrac{144\ CO_2}{163\ O_2} = 0.7$

RQ of Proteins

RQ of proteins is not easy to determine as proteins are not completely oxidized in the human body such as carbohydrates and fats. But by indirect methods, it has been found:
- RQ of proteins = 0.8
- RQ of mixed diet = 0.85

Importance

- RQ gives some indication of the type of food being metabolized.
- It is low in diabetes mellitus.

■ ENERGY EXPENDITURE

There are three components of energy expenditure:
1. Physical activity (voluntary) **(Table 20.1)**
2. Basal metabolic rate (BMR)
3. Specific dynamic action of food (SDA)

Physical Activity

It is a highly variable factor. Several measurements of energy expenditure of man and women doing a variety of activities have been made by calorimetry and are presented in a series of tables. They provide estimates of the energy output of the individual during his/her various activities in day-to-day life.

Basal Metabolic Rate

When a subject is at complete rest and no physical activity is performed, energy is required only for the activity of the internal organs and to maintain body temperature. The part of energy under basal conditions is called as basal metabolism. It accounts for 60–70% of total expenditure.

Definition

The amount of heat produced in kilocalories under basal conditions per square meter of the body surface per hour is known as basal metabolic rate.

Table 20.1: Energy expenditure for each type of physical activity.

Physical activity	Energy requirement (Cal/hr)
Sitting	25
Standing	30
Reading/writing/eating	40
Car driving	70
Typing	80
Household work	100
Walking (slow)	170
Cycling (slow)	200
Running (moderate)	500
Swimming	700
Walking upstairs	800

Importance

A knowledge of BMR is essential for calculating the calorie requirements and planning of the diet for an individual and population group. It is also helpful in assessment of activity of endocrine glands such as thyroid and adrenals.

Measurement of BMR Using Benedict–Roth Apparatus

It is the commonly used method in the laboratory.

Conditions

- The patient should be in the fasting state.
- He should be awake but completely at physical and mental rest.
- His body temperature should be normal.
- Environmental temperature should be between 25–30°C.

Procedure

It consists of a reservoir (spirometer) filled with pure oxygen. This floats on water present in outer chamber. The patient is allowed to breath in oxygen present in the reservoir for 6 minutes. Carbon dioxide (expired air) is absorbed by the sodalime kept in the cylinder. The volume of oxygen used is recorded on a kymograph.

The height and weight of the subject are measured. Age and sex are noted.

Calculation

$$BMR = \frac{\text{Total heat produced in one hour under basal conditions}}{\text{Total body surface area in square meter}}$$

Note: Total heat produced in one hour under basal conditions may be derived from oxygen consumption.

Total body surface area in square meter may be calculated from nomograph or by using Du Bois surface area formula:

Where A = H 0.725 × W 0.425 × 71.84
  A = Surface area in sq cm
  H = Height in cm
  W = Weight in kg

Normal Values

Values of BMR may be expressed in many ways:
- C/sq m/hour

The normal standard values of BMR for men and women of different ages are available.
- BMR of normal adult male = 40 C/sqm/hr
- BMR of normal adult female = 36 C/sqm/hr
- Percentages above or below the calculated normal values are expressed. This expression is usually followed in the clinical laboratory.

   A percentage of –15% to + 20% is considered to be normal BMR.

Factors which Influence BMR

Table 20.2 shows factors which influence BMR.

Specific Dynamic Action of Foods

When food is eaten, the metabolic activities of the body (digestion, absorption, etc.) are stimulated, resulting in increased heat production, i.e., specific dynamic action of foods (SDA) is due to stimulant action of food stuffs.

Alternative Names

Calorigenic/thermogenic action of foods.

Definition

SDA is the extra amount of heat produced over and above the caloric value of foodstuff when used by the body. This extra heat is drawn from the food store of the body.

Examples

- SDA of carbohydrates = 5 C
  (i.e., carbohydrates containing 100 C when metabolized in the body produces 105 C. This extra 5 C is SDA of carbohydrates).
- SDA of fat = 13 C
- SDA of proteins = 30 C

Importance

- Knowledge of SDA of each food is necessary. It varies with type of food.
- SDA of each food must be provided in the diet in terms of food, in addition to calculated amount of food.
- It is common to add 5–10% to the total calories to provide energy for SDA.
- Protein has highest SDA and carbohydrate has lowest SDA.

Table 20.2: Factors which influence BMR.

Physiological factors	BMR high	BMR low
Age	Children	Adults
Sex	Men	Women
Body surface area	More body surface area	Less body surface area
Climate	Cold climate	Warm climate
Habits	Hard workers, exercise	Sedentary worker
Diet	Nonvegetarian, overnutrition	Vegetarian, undernutrition and starvation
Pregnancy	Later pregnancy	-
Drugs	Caffeine, benzidine	Most anesthetics
Pathological factors (clinical importance)		
Endocrine disorders	Hyperthyroidism, hyperadrenalism	Hypothyroidism, hypoadrenalism
Other diseases	Infections and febrile disease (due to rise in temperature), leukemia and polycythemia (due to increased cellular activity)	Nephrotic syndrome, Addison's disease

ENERGY REQUIREMENT

Food supplies us energy. Sufficient food must be taken to maintain energy balance of a person according to his work **(Table 20.3)**.

Major Factors Affecting Energy Requirement

The following factors should be considered for accurate calculation of the calorie requirement of an individual.
- Supply of calories to maintain BMR
- Supply of calories to meet SDA
- Supply of calories to do physical activity

Other Factors Affecting Energy Requirement

- Age
- Sex
- Climate (environmental temperature)

Table 20.3: Recommended energy intake for various groups of human (Cal/Day).

Light work	2,000–2,500
Moderate work	2,500–3,000
Heavy work	3,000–3,500
Very heavy work	3,500–4,000

- Pregnancy and lactation
- Weight and height

Calculation of Total Calorie Requirement

Based on the following particulars.

Particulars

- Age = 22 years
- Weight = 55 kg
- Sex = Male
- Body surface area = 1.50 sq m
- Height = 162 cm
- BMR = C/sq m/hr

Calculation

- BMR/day = 35 × 1.50 × 24 = 1,260 C
- SDA [(10%) basal requirement] = 126 C
- 8 hours of nonoccupational activity (100 C/hr) = 800 C (walking, light games, washing, dressing, eating)
- 8 hours of sedentary activity (40 C/hr) (sitting, reading and writing) = 320 C

  Total = 2,506 C

Answer: A student requires 2,500 C/day. Similarly, the calorie requirement of any individual can be calculated.

21. Food and Nutrition

> **Chapter Outline**
> - Food
> - Energy-yielding Foods (Primary Foods)
> - Body-building Foods
> - Protective Foods
> - Balanced Diet
> - Milk
> - Diet and Public Health
> - Nutrition
> - Related Terms in Food and Nutrition

■ FOOD

Importance

- Supplies necessary energy for the body to perform its functions.
- Provides materials for growth and repair.
- Maintains health for normal activities.
- Provides sufficient resistance against infection and other diseases.
- Provides some essential compounds which cannot be synthesized by the body, e.g., essential fatty acids, essential amino acids.

Components (Fig. 21.1)

Normal diet can be classified into three major *groups* depending on their role in the body.

■ ENERGY-YIELDING FOODS (PRIMARY FOODS)

They provide energy for the body (**Fig. 21.2**), e.g., carbohydrate, fats, and proteins.

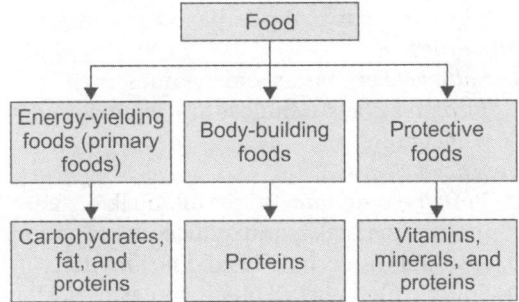

Fig. 21.1: Components of food.

Carbohydrates

They are the most abundant dietary components.

Nutritional Significance

- Carbohydrates are the main energy source in human nutrition. They provide 50–60% of total energy requirement of the body.
- They perform protein sparing action.
- Brain and other parts and central respiratory system are dependent on glucose for energy.

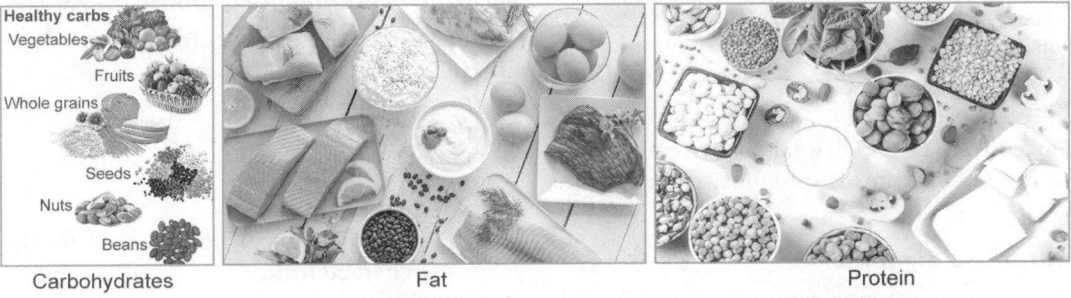

Fig. 21.2: Energy-yielding foods.
(For color version, see Plate 4)

Based on nutritional significance, there are two groups of carbohydrate.
1. *Available carbohydrates:* These can be assimilated and metabolized by the body to give energy. Their caloric value is 4 C/g, e.g., glucose, fructose, galactose, lactose, ... starch, ... glycogen, etc.
2. *Unavailable carbohydrates:* These cannot be assimilated and thus do not provide energy, e.g., dietary fiber.

Dietary fiber
Definition: It refers to all plant cell components (carbohydrates) that cannot be digested by human digestive system due to deficiency of enzyme cellulose. It is unavailable carbohydrate and not a nutrient.

Type: It is of two types based on physical properties.
1. *Soluble fibers:* Fruits and legumes
2. *Insoluble fibers:* Cellulose and lignin found in wheat bran.

Beneficial effects:
- *Roughage action:* Increases bulk of feces, induces peristalsis and reduces constipation.
- Insoluble fibers help in colonic function.
- Soluble fibers lower blood cholesterol, slow emptying of stomach and postprandial rise in blood sugar.
- Eliminates toxic compounds produced by intestinal bacteria.
- Gives satiety value to the foods used as a weight-reducing diet.

Adverse effects:
- Absorption of certain minerals (Mg) is decreased.
- Excess intake produces flatulence.

> **Clinical Importance**
> It reduces incidence of cancer of colon, diverticulosis, diabetes mellitus, atherosclerosis, and cardiovascular diseases (reduces cholesterol level).

Fats

Fats provide 20–25% of total calorie requirement of the body. It has the highest caloric value (9 C/g).

Nutritional Significance

- It provides essential fatty acids (linoleic acid, linolenic acid and arachidonic acid) to the body. ω fatty acids are good for health (*refer* Chapter 3)
- It acts as a solvent for fat-soluble vitamins (vitamin A, D, E and K).
- It increases the palatability of foods by absorbing and retaining flavors.
- It provides a feeling of satiety as it is digested slowly.
- It is the favored cooking medium. The dietary fat may be divided into two types based on whether they are present free or in combination with other substances.
  1. Visible fat (fat consumed as such), e.g., butter, ghee, oils.
  2. Invisible fat (fat present as part of other items), e.g., egg, fish, meat, oil seeds.

Proteins

Proteins are not very important as sources of energy for the body. They provide only 10–15% of the total energy required. Their caloric value is 4 C/g. When sufficient quantities of carbohydrates are present in the diet, amino acids are not oxidized to yield energy (protein sparing effect of carbohydrates). Under conditions of starvation, amino acids may act as energy sources.

Functions

Refer Chapter 4.

■ BODY-BUILDING FOODS

Proteins

The primary function of the proteins is that they form the building blocks for the body tissues. Proteins are the only source of essential amino acids. They are also the major source of nitrogen and sulfur for the body.

Factors which Influence Quantity of Proteins

The quantity of proteins required by the body is affected by three major factors:
1. Protein quality
2. Energy intake
3. Physical activity

Protein quality

Quality of proteins can be assessed by the following characteristics:
- Biological value of proteins
- Amino acid composition of dietary proteins

- Availability of amino acids from foods
- Supplementary amino acids

Biological value of proteins (Table 21.1)
It is a measure of quality of dietary proteins. Dietary proteins differ considerably in the efficiency of their utilization for the synthesis of body proteins.

Definition
It is an expression of a number of the nutritional characteristics of the proteins.

Nutritional characteristics which influence biological value of protein
- Digestibility
- Availability of digested products, i.e., amino acids
- Presence of amount of various essential amino acids.

Evaluation
There are many methods to evaluate the biological value of proteins.
- *Nonprotein utilization:* It is defined as % of food nitrogen that is retained in the body.
- *Protein efficiency ratio (PER):* It involves measurement of weight increase by protein in weaning animals.

Classification of quality of proteins
Based on the above criteria, quality of proteins can be classified into two groups:
1. *Complete proteins (first class proteins/good proteins):* This group of proteins contains all the essential amino acids needed by the human body. It includes all animal proteins. For example:
   - Egg and milk proteins rank highest
   - Meat, fish, poultry proteins occupy next position
2. *Incomplete proteins (second class proteins/poor proteins):* This group of proteins lack some essential amino acids and are of poor quality. It includes plant proteins. For example: Cereals, legumes (peas, beans, soya beans, etc.) and nuts.

Energy intake
The energy derived from carbohydrate and fat affects protein requirements because it spares the use of protein as an energy source.

Physical activity
It increases retention of nitrogen from dietary protein.

Nitrogen Balance
Nitrogen is an extremely important element. It is ingested in the diet mainly in the form of proteins.

Definition
Nitrogen balance refers to the difference between total nitrogen intake and total nitrogen loss in feces, urine and sweat.

Normal adults are in nitrogen equilibrium, i.e., they maintain nitrogen balance (Nitrogen intake = Nitrogen output).

Positive nitrogen balance
It occurs when nitrogen intake exceeds nitrogen excretion. It is observed in:
- Children
- Pregnancy
- Convalescence (recovery after illness)

Negative Nitrogen Balance
It occurs when nitrogen excretion is more than nitrogen intake. It is seen in:
- Inadequate dietary protein intake
- Physiological stresses, such as trauma, burns, illness, surgery
- Kwashiorkor

■ PROTECTIVE FOODS
Vitamins and minerals are known as protective foods. They are present in green vegetables and fruits and also in milk, meat and cereals. They do not provide energy, but are needed for maintenance of health and protection from diseases. Proteins also serve as protective foods.

Table 21.1: Biological value of proteins.

Animal proteins	Plant proteins
Egg = 94	Rice = 68
Fish = 80	Soya beans = 61
Milk = 85	Wheat = 58
Meat = 69	Nut = 54

Vitamins

Vitamins are organic compounds, which are required in minute quantities for the body (for more details, *refer* Chapter 8). There are two groups of vitamins:
1. Fat-soluble vitamins: Vitamin A, D, E, and K
2. Water-soluble vitamins: B-complex vitamins and vitamin C.

Functions

- Essential for health and protection from diseases.
- Act as coenzymes for enzymes in reactions of metabolism.
- Do not provide energy but essential for many chemical processes pertaining to the production and utilization of energy.
- *Clinical:* Deficiency leads to deficiency syndrome and excess leads to toxicity symptoms.

Minerals

Minerals are inorganic compounds which are also required in minute quantities for the body (for more details, *refer* Chapter 17). They have two groups:
1. *Macrominerals:* Sodium, potassium, chloride, calcium, phosphorus, magnesium, sulfur.
2. *Microminerals:* Iron, iodine, copper, zinc, cobalt, manganese, molybdenum, selenium, fluoride, etc.

Functions

They do not supply energy but are necessary for maintenance of certain physiochemical functions which are essential for life.
- Maintain
  - Electrolyte balance
  - Ionic equilibrium
- Act as cofactors for several enzymes involved in metabolic reactions
- *Clinical:* Deficiency leads to deficiency syndrome. Excess may result in toxicity.
- Involved in the formation of body structure and skeleton.

Proteins

Immunoglobulins (γ-globulin fraction of protein) serve as protective agents against infection. They provide immunity to the body (for more details, *refer* Chapter 4).

■ BALANCED DIET

The total solid and liquid foods consumed by an individual or a population group is called as their diet. Foods which could provide adequate nutrients should always be taken in the daily diet. This is known as balanced diet.

Definition

Balanced diet is a mixture of foods in proportionate quantities selected from the different basic food groups so as to supply the essential nutrients required by the body to perform its functions.

Variations

The composition of a balanced diet varies considerably at different ages, different physiological conditions, different occupations and economic status.

Construction of a Balanced Diet

A balanced diet can be constructed based on the following criteria.
- Should be prepared with locally available foods
- Should fit with the local food habits
- Should be within the economic means of the people
- Should be easily digestible
- Should contain enough roughage materials

Such a diet containing the required quantities would perform all the normal functions of the body.

Based on these factors, balanced diet can be constructed for children, adolescents, adults, elders, convalescent people, pregnant women, and lactating women.

The balanced diet should represent the following three food groups in correct amounts.
1. Foods for physical activity and work (sources of energy), e.g.,
   - Simple sugars and complex carbohydrates
   - Fats and oils
2. Foods for body building and growth (protein rich foods), e.g., vegetable proteins, animal proteins.

3. Foods for health and protection from disease, e.g., vitamins and minerals rich foods. All vegetables and fruits.

Composition of Nutrients of a Balanced Diet

The balanced diet for an adult male of 60 kg. requiring 2,500 calories per day should contain the following:

Carbohydrates	400 g
Fats	50 g
Proteins	70 g
Vitamins and minerals as per RDA	

Recommended Dietary Allowance

Recommended dietary allowance (RDA) is an estimate of the daily requirement of nutrient for an individual. It depends on factors such as age, sex, pregnancy, lactation.
(*Refer*: Respective Chapters).

Dietary Goals

Dietary goals are simple nutritional guidelines proposed to decrease diet-related diseases.
- Achieve and maintain an appropriate body weight
- Reduce the calories due to fat
- Reduce the saturated fats
- Increase monounsaturated and polyunsaturated fats
- Reduce consumption of simple carbohydrates
- Increase complex carbohydrates
- Increase dietary fiber
- Reduce cholesterol
- Reduce salt intake
- Better to avoid alcohol

Composition of Important Food Items

Table 21.2 shows the composition of important food items.

■ MILK

Milk, a specialized fluid of the body, is secreted by the mammary gland. It is almost a complete natural food, though it lacks iron and copper. It is an ideal food for the infants though it contains low amount of vitamin C and D.

Table 21.2: Important food items: Composition.

Food groups	Examples
Cereals: They constitute the bulk of the daily diet in developing countries and are main sources of energy	Wheat, rice, maize, etc.
Roots and tubers: They contain large amount of starch	Potatoes
Pulses: They are rich sources of vegetable proteins and B complex vitamins (except B_{12})	Beans, peas
Vegetables, fruits: They are rich in vitamins and minerals	Cabbage, spinach, carrots, etc; mango, guava, papaya
Fats, oil, sugars	Triglycerides, fatty acids, carbohydrates
Meat, fish, egg, meat,	Foods of animal origin (proteins)

Composition

Composition of milk from various species differs in many ways. Water is the major constituent (83–87%). 13–17% is made up of several substances, such as carbohydrate, lipids, proteins, minerals, and vitamins. Differences between the composition of human milk and cow's milk are given in **Table 21.3**.

■ DIET AND PUBLIC HEALTH

A nutritionist (dietician) may be consulted about the diet of an institution or a particular occupational group or a problem in community nutrition. Under such circumstances, the nutritionist has to study all the aspects of their nutrition. Due to intake of a particular diet in a community, the people may be exposed to infection or develop cancer. The nutritionist has to study the etiology, assessment and prevalence based on the previous surveys and advise proper diet.

Food Toxins

Some of the common food stuffs may contain certain toxic compounds. They enter the body through different routes **(Table 21.4)**.

Effect of Processing on Foods

The changes which occur during processing and milling of wheat, rice, vegetables, and fruits are of immense public health importance.

Table 21.3: The composition of human and cow's milk.

Constituents	Human milk	Cow's milk
• Water (%)	87.5	87.0
• Total solids (g%)	12.5	13.5
▪ Carbohydrate (g%)	7.5	5.0
▪ Lipids (g%)	4.0	5.0
▪ Proteins (g%) (caseinogen, lactalbumin, lactoglobulin)	1.5	4.0
▪ Calcium (mg%)	40	130
▪ Phosphorus (mg%)	30	90
▪ Sodium (mg%)	15	60
▪ Potassium (mg%)	55	140
▪ Magnesium (mg%)	5	20
▪ All vitamins present (*except* vitamins C and D in low amounts)	–	–
▪ Calories/100 g	67	69

Effect of Cooking on Foods

Cooking may have different effects on foods.
- It kills most of the pathogenic organisms in food.
- It causes a considerable loss of vitamins and minerals.
- It makes the diet more palatable.

■ NUTRITION

Definition

Nutrition can be defined as the utilization of foods by living organisms.

Normal Nutrition

The basic aim in the practice of nutrition is to provide the essential nutrients in a palatable and assimilable form in quantities sufficient to meet the requirement and prevent deficiency.

Table 21.4: Sources of toxins and its examples.

Sources of toxins	Examples
Toxins normally present in plants	• Goitrogens • Neurotoxins
Contaminants through cultivation	• Pesticides • Insecticides
Contaminants through storage	Aflatoxins
Contaminants through food processing	Mineral oils
Toxins through cooking	Monosodium glutamate
Food adulterants	Keshari dal, mustard oil

Special care is taken to provide for additional requirement during physiological states of growth, pregnancy, lactation, and convalescence.

Nutritional Disorders

The principal or the most obvious cause is the consumption of a diet with insufficient or excess sources of energy or lacking a proper balance of nutrients.

Causes

- Interferences with food intake such as poverty, famine, floods, and alcoholism, drug addiction.
- Psychological factors, such as anorexia nervosa.

They are classified into two groups:

Due to undernutrition

Undernutrition or reduced intake of diet is a problem of developing countries. Many diseases arise due to undernutrition.
- Protein calorie malnutrition (kwashiorkar, marasmus).
- Deficiency diseases of vitamins (xerophthalmia, rickets, etc.)
- Deficiency diseases of minerals (anemia, endemic goiter).

Protein-calorie malnutrition (PCM) or Protein-energy malnutrition (PEM)

Definition

It is a nutritional disorder, which occurs due to insufficient calorie intake and also less protein intake. It is seen in mostly underdeveloped countries.

Chapter 21: Food and Nutrition

Table 21.5: Difference between marasmus and kwashiorkor.

	Marasmus	Kwashiorkor (Fig. 21.3)
Occurrence	In children under one year of age	In children between 1–5 years of age
Cause	Deficiency of calories	Deficient intake of proteins
Symptoms	Growth retardation, muscle wasting, anemia and weakness. No edema Albumin: Normal/slight decrease	Stunted growth, edema (especially on hands and legs) diarrhea, anemia, discoloration of skin and hair. Low serum albumin, fatty liver
Treatment	Protein and calories	Protein rich foods

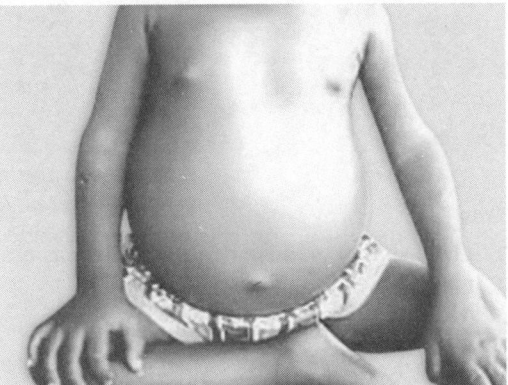

Fig. 21.3: Kwashiorkor.
(For color version, see Plate 4)

Types
There are two forms of protein calorie malnutrition:
1. Kwashiorkor **(Fig. 21.3)**
2. Marasmus

The major differences between these two disorders are given in the **Table 21.5**.

Due to overnutrition
Overnutrition is a physiological status which results from ingestion of more food (surplus calories) than required. It is also undesirable and dangerous for health. For example:
- Obesity, atherosclerosis (*refer* Chapter 13)
- *Toxicity of vitamins:* Hypervitaminosis A and D (*refer* Chapter 8).
- *Toxicity of minerals:* Hemochromatosis (*refer* Chapter 12).

RELATED TERMS IN FOOD AND NUTRITION

Protein Sparing Action of Carbohydrates
As energy content of the diet from carbohydrates is increased, the need for protein decreases. This is known as protein sparing action of carbohydrates.

Mutual Supplementation of Amino Acids
Relative insufficiency of a particular amino acid in vegetable food can be compensated by combination with other vegetable foods which have adequate level of that limiting amino acid, e.g., protein of cereals deficient in lysine and pulses with adequate level of lysine have a mutually supplementary effect.

Glycemic Index
Definition

It is an indicator that ranks carbohydrate containing foods based on their effect on blood sugar level. It is given as GI: 0-100 which represents relative rise in the blood glucose level two hours after consuming particular food item.

Uses
- It indicates the relative rapidity with which the body breaks carbohydrate.
- Glycemic index:
  - 1–55: Low, e.g., starch
  - 56–69: Middle, e.g., mixed carbohydrates
  - 70–100: High, e.g., refined sugar
- It is advised to take low GI index carbohydrate containing foods.

Body Mass Index
The degree of obesity is calculated by means of body mass index (BMI).

$$\text{BMI} = \frac{\text{Body weight (kg)}}{\text{Height (m}^2\text{)}}$$

Normal BMI = 20–25

Importance: refer Chapter 12.

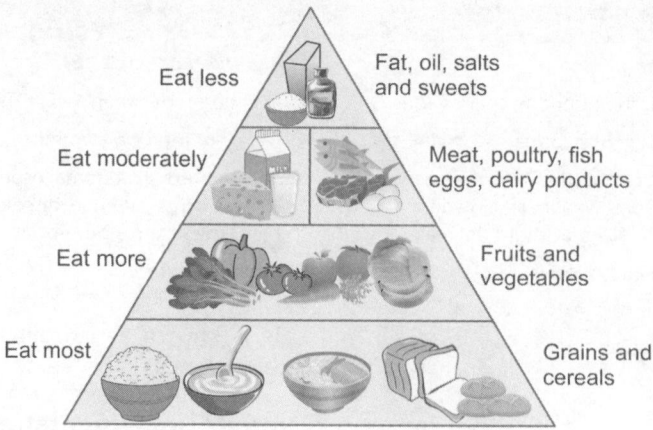

Fig. 21.4: Food pyramid.

Food Pyramid

Definition

A food pyramid is a triangular/pyramid shape diagram which represents the optimal number of servings to be eaten every day from each of the basic food groups. It was first published in Sweden in 1974. Now it is followed with slight modification as a guide for preparation of balanced diet **(Fig. 21.4)**.

Uses

- It is designed to make healthy eating easier.
- It is a guide for balanced diet.

Parenteral Nutrition (Parenteral Therapy)

It refers to medicine in solution administered via a route other than ingestion. It is usually adopted for patients who are unable to take food through mouth.

22. Water (Fluid) and Electrolyte Balance

Chapter Outline
- Water
- Electrolytes
- Regulation of Water and Electrolyte Balance
- Disorders
- Related terms

WATER

Water is the most important inorganic component of the organism. It is the largest constituent of the body. The total body water constitutes 60–70% of adult body weight. This value is higher in men than in women. It decreases with advanced age due to increased fat content. Soft tissue contains more water (80%) than bone (20%).

Functions of Water

- Water is an essential constituent of cell structures and provides the medium in which the chemical reactions of the body take place.
- Outside the cell, it is a vehicle for transport of substances (it carries nutritive elements to tissues and removes waste materials from tissues).
- It assists in the regulation of body temperature.
- It is a solvent for electrolytes. It helps to regulate electrolyte balance of the body.
- It acts as a lubricant in joints, pleura, conjunctiva, and peritoneum.

Distribution of Water (Fig. 22.1)

Total body water is distributed in two main compartments.
1. *Intracellular compartment*, i.e., water within the cell = 40% of body weight.
2. *Extracellular compartment*, i.e., water outside the cell = 20% of body weight. This compartment is subdivided into two:

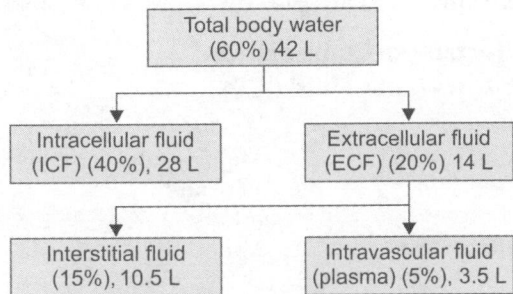

Fig. 22.1: Distribution of body water.

- Plasma = 5%, i.e., fluid part of the blood; intravascular fluid; inside the blood vessels.
- Interstitial fluid = 15%, i.e., fluid outside the blood vessel; extravascular fluid. Includes connective tissue, cartilage bone, cerebrospinal fluid (CSF), lymph, eyes, skin, salivary gland, mucous membrane.

Water Balance

In the normal adult, water content of the body is well balanced. Quantity of water taken inside is balanced by the water eliminated from the body. Both water intake and output depend on climate, physical activity, etc.

Water Intake

☐ Plain water and drinks (beverages)	= 1,500 mL
☐ Water in food	= 700 mL
☐ Oxidation of food stuff (metabolic water)	= 300 mL
Total	**= 2,500 mL**

Water Output

- Urine (kidneys) = 1,500 mL
- Perspiration (skin) = 500 mL
- Expired air (lung) = 400 mL
- Feces (intestine) = 100 mL
- Total = 2,500 mL

ELECTROLYTES

Electrolytes are inorganic substances or compounds which disassociate in solution and exist as ions—positively (cation) and negatively (anion) charged particles, e.g., Na^+, K^+, Cl^-, HCO_3^-. They can conduct electricity. They maintain equilibrium of body fluids. Their concentration is expressed as mEq/L.

Electrolyte Composition: Intracellular Fluid (ICF)

Cations:	mEq/L	Anions:	mEq/L
Major: K^+	148	Major: Proteins	54
Mg^{++}	40	PO_4^- and others	136
Minor: Na^+	10	Minor: Cl^-	2
Ca^{++}	2	HCO_3^-	8
Total	200		200

(K^+ is the major cation in intracellular fluid).

Extracellular Fluid (ECF)

Plasma (plasma electrolyte levels can be assumed to be the representation of extracelluar fluid as a whole).

Cations:	mEq/L	Anions:	mEq/L
Major: Na^+	142	Major: Cl^-	103
Minor: K^+	5	Minor: HCO_3^-	27
Ca^{++}	5	PO_4^- SO_4^-	3
Mg^{++}	3	Proteins	16
		Organic acids	6
Total	155		155

(Na^+ is the major cation in the extracellular fluid).

REGULATION OF WATER AND ELECTROLYTE BALANCE

Volume and composition of various body fluid compartments should be regulated within physiological limits in order to maintain normal health. It is done by the following mechanisms:

- *Neural mechanism (thirst mechanism):* The intake of fluid is regulated by the thirst mechanism under hypothalamic control.
- *Antidiuretic hormone:* Increased plasma osmolality stimulates hypothalamus to release ADH. ADH effectively increases water reabsorption by the kidney.
- *Aldosterone:* A fall in ECF volume is sensed by the juxtaglomerular apparatus of nephron which secretes renin. Renin acts on angiotensinogen to produce angiotensin I which is converted to angiotensin II. The latter stimulates the release of aldosterone from adrenal cortex. Aldosterone increases Na^+ reabsorption by the kidney resulting in the retention of Na^+ in the body.

ADH and aldosterone coordinate with each other to maintain the normal fluid and electrolyte balance.

Disorders

Negative Water Balance

Dehydration: When the loss of water is more than intake, body's water content is reduced and is said to be in negative water balance. This condition is called as dehydration.

Causes: Vomiting, diarrhea, excessive sweating, adrenocortical dysfunction deficiency of ADH (diabetes insipidus).

Symptoms: Thirst, sunken eyeballs, mental confusion, lethargy, low BP, shock.

Treatment: Intake of plenty of water orally (or) intravenously an isotonic solution (or) ORT.

Positive Water Balance

Water intoxication (overhydration): It is due to accumulation of interstitial fluid in the body. Body is unable to excrete sodium in sufficient quantity.

Causes: Renal failure, protein deficiency, overproduction of ADH, excessive administration of fluids.

Symptoms: Headache, nausea, convulsions, delirium, coma.

Treatment: Restriction of water intake and administration of hypertonic saline.

Laboratory Diagnosis of Water and Electrolyte Disorders

- Serum electrolytes – Na^+, K^-, Cl^- and HCO_3^-
- Serum urea and creatinine, osmolality
- Urine: Volume, osmolarity, Na^+ level

Related Terms

- **Normal saline** = 0.9 g%
- **Oral rehydration therapy (ORT):** It is a type of effective fluid replacement used to prevent and treat dehydration during cholera and diarrheal diseases. It consists of drinking water modest amounts of sugar and salts especially sodium and potassium.

> **Note**
> It is also available commercially as readymade preparation.

WHO formula of oral rehydration solution (ORS):
- NaCl = 3.5 g
- KCl = 1.5 g
- $NaHCO_3$ = 2.5 g
- Glucose = 20.05 g
- Drinking water = 1 L

- **Osmolality:** It is a measure of the solute particles present in the fluid medium.
Osmolality of plasma = 285–295 mmol/kg

It can be measured by:
- Osmometer
- Calculation: 2 × plasma Na mmol/L.

23 Acid–Base Balance

Chapter Outline

- Sources of Acids in the Blood
- Sources of Bases in the Blood
- Mechanisms for Maintaining Acid–Base Balance
- Disturbances in Acid–Base Balance (Acid–Base Imbalance)

The normal pH of blood is 7.35–7.45 (average 7.4, slightly alkaline). Any deviation in this pH range will result in acidosis or alkalosis, i.e., acid–base balance will be disturbed. Therefore, it is essential that pH of blood should be maintained within the normal range. It is an important homeostatic mechanism in the body.

■ SOURCES OF ACIDS IN THE BLOOD

During normal metabolic processes, fairly large amounts of acids are produced. The acid adds up H^+ ions to the blood. Large quantities of CO_2 are produced in the body due to cellular oxidation and it dissolves in H_2O to give carbonic acid.

$$CO_2 + H_2O \rightarrow H_2CO_3 \text{ (carbonic acid)}$$

Other acids are also produced.

Inorganic Acids

Sulfuric acid, phosphoric acid, hydrochloric acid.

Organic Acids

Lactic acid, pyruvic acid, uric acid, acetoacetic acid, β hydroxybutyric acid.

The diet also contains some acids which enter the blood (nonvegetarian diet adds more acids).

■ SOURCES OF BASES IN THE BLOOD

Food also provides a little quantity of basic compound (less than acid substances). As OH^- ions are not primary products of metabolism, bases are of little importance in the body (vegetarian food produces more alkali).

■ MECHANISMS FOR MAINTAINING ACID–BASE BALANCE

Both acidic and basic compounds reach blood which may disturb pH of blood unless removed promptly.

The body has three important mechanisms for maintenance of acid–base balance of blood.
1. Blood buffers
2. Respiratory mechanism
3. Renal mechanism

Blood Buffers

Buffer systems are most important in the control of pH of body fluids. Buffer systems present in the extracellular fluid and erythrocytes maintain normal pH during the transport of acids from the site of their formation (cells) to the site of their excretion (lungs and kidneys).

The buffer systems present in:

Plasma		Erythrocytes	
$\dfrac{NaHCO_3}{H_2CO_3}$	(Bicarbonate buffer)	$\dfrac{K Hb}{H Hb}$	(Hemoglobin buffer)
$\dfrac{Na\, Protein}{H\, Protein}$	(Protein buffer)	$\dfrac{KHbO_2}{HHbO_2}$	(Hemoglobin buffer)
$\dfrac{Na_2HPO_4}{NaH_2PO_4}$	(Phosphate buffer)	$\dfrac{K_2 HPO_4}{K H_2 PO_4}$	(Phosphate buffer)

Of all these buffer systems, only few are present in high concentration and significant in maintaining pH of body fluids.

Ratio of acid-base of any buffer system in blood must be kept constant if pH of blood is to be maintained within normal limits.

In case of $\dfrac{\text{Bicarbonate (NaHCO}_3\text{)}}{\text{Carbonic acid (H}_2\text{CO}_3\text{)}}$ system, a ratio of $\dfrac{20}{1}$ must exist between bicarbonate (alkali reserve) and carbonic acid in order to maintain pH within normal limits.

Any increase or decrease in H^+ ion concentration will be met by an adjustment in this ratio. But when this ratio is altered, acid-base balance of blood will be disturbed.

Bicarbonate Buffer System

It is the most important buffer in the blood since bicarbonate acts against:
- Volatile acids (carbonic acid)
- Nonvolatile acids (fixed acids)

It neutralizes 50% of all acids formed. It acts against acids (e.g., lactic acid) as follows:

For example, Lactic acid $\rightleftharpoons H^+$ + Lactate

$$HCO_3^- + H^+ \rightleftharpoons H_2CO_3$$

$$H_2CO_3 \rightleftharpoons H_2O + CO_2 \uparrow$$

The same buffer systems will act against alkali (NaOH) as follows:

$$NaOH \rightleftharpoons Na^+ + OH^-$$

$$H_2CO_3 + OH^- \rightleftharpoons HCO_3^- + H_2O$$

Hemoglobin Buffer System

Two hemoglobin buffers are:
1. $\dfrac{KHb}{HHb}$
2. $\dfrac{KHbO_2}{HHbO_2}$

It has been found that 85% of buffering action takes place in the red blood cells by hemoglobin buffer system (60%) and phosphate buffer system (25%).

Chloride Shift

CO_2 produced in tissues reach plasma and from plasma to erythrocytes.

Inside the red cell, CO_2 combines reversibly with water in the presence of the enzyme carbonic anhydrase to form H_2CO_3. H_2CO_3 dissociates to form H^+ and HCO_3^-. Some of these bicarbonate ions combine with K^+ to form $KHCO_3$ (potassium bicarbonate) while the other diffuse into the plasma due to concentration gradient. The electroneutrality of plasma, disturbed by the entrance of HCO_3^- ions from red cells, is balanced by the shift of equal number of chloride ions to red cells. This process is called as chloride shift.

The bicarbonate ions in plasma combine with freely available Na^+ ions to form $NaHCO_3$. The bicarbonate so formed ($KHCO_3$ in red cells and $NaHCO_3$ in plasma) is carried to lungs where they decompose to give CO_2.

Respiratory Mechanism

It provides a rapid mechanism for maintenance of pH as a short-term regulatory process. The lungs can deal with volatile acids, such as H_2CO_3. Respiratory center is highly sensitive to changes in pH and pCO_2.

When there is an increase in H^+ concentration (and also pCO_2) in blood, there will be increase in pulmonary ventilation. This increased respiration helps removal of excess CO_2 from extracellular fluids into expired air. When there is a fall in H^+ ion concentration (and also pCO_2), there will be hypoventilation and so CO_2 is retained in the blood. These two processes will continue until blood regains normal pCO_2 and restoration of pH.

Thus, ratio of $\dfrac{\text{Bicarbonate}}{\text{Carbonic acid}} = \dfrac{20}{1}$ is maintained in the extracellular fluids by the respiratory mechanism.

Renal Mechanism

Kidneys provide the most important final defense mechanism for maintenance of acid-base balance of the blood. Three renal mechanisms operate to preserve the acid-base balance.

1. *Phosphate mechanism* (**Fig. 23.1**): It takes place in the distal tubular cells of kidney. Phosphate buffer though present in small concentration is the most important buffer system in urine.

$$\frac{Na_2HPO_4}{NaH_2PO_4}$$

CO_2 is rapidly converted to H_2CO_3 by the enzyme carbonic anhydrase.

H_2CO_3 immediately undergoes ionization to H^+ and HCO_3^-.

H^+ ions formed pass into the lumen of the tubule (and at the same time equal number of Na^+ ions (liberated from Na_2HPO_4) pass into the cell. H^+ ions in the lumen combine with $NaHPO_4$ to form NaH_2PO_4.

$$NaHPO_4 + H^+ \rightarrow NaH_2PO_4$$

Na^+ ions are absorbed into blood along with HCO_3^-. NaH_2PO_4 (acid sodium phosphate) formed in the lumen is excreted in urine.

2. *Bicarbonate mechanism* (**Fig. 23.2**): It operates in proximal tubular cells.

At normal plasma bicarbonate level, all the bicarbonate filtered at the glomeruli is reabsorbed by the tubules.

In this condition, H^+ ions formed from carbonic acid, convert $NaHCO_3$ to H_2CO_3 and Na^+ ions are liberated into cell. These Na^+ ions are reabsorbed along with HCO_3^- into blood and therefore there is no excretion of bicarbonate in the urine.

3. *Ammonia mechanism* (**Fig. 23.3**): Under normal conditions, an adult excretes about 30–50 mEq of ammonia daily. Ammonia is produced by deamination of glutamine and also by oxidative deamination of some amino acids. NH_3 thus formed in the distal tubular cells diffuse into lumen. Here it combines

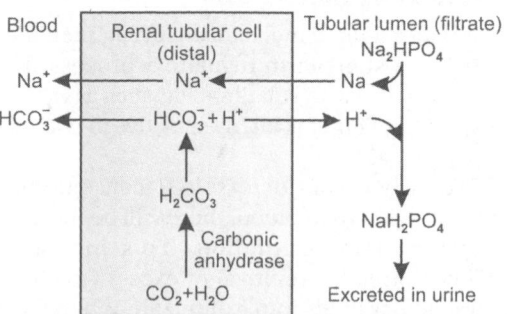

Fig. 23.1: Phosphate mechanism.

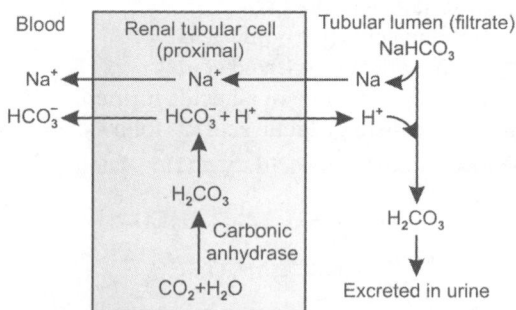

Fig. 23.2: Bicarbonate mechanism.

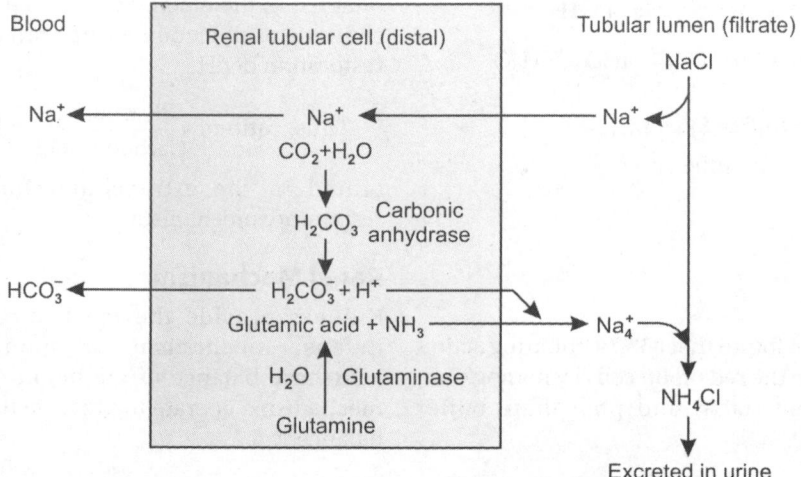

Fig. 23.3: Ammonia mechanism.

with H⁺ liberated from ionization of carbonic acid to form NH₄ (ammonium ion). NH_4^+ combines with Cl⁻ to form ammonium salt (e.g., NH₄Cl) which is excreted in urine. The conserved Na⁺ is reabsorbed along with HCO_3^- into the blood.

DISTURBANCES IN ACID–BASE BALANCE (ACID–BASE IMBALANCE)

Disturbances in acid-base balance are known as acidosis and alkalosis. These occur due to abnormalities of respiratory system or metabolism. They are classified in **Figure 23.4** and **Table 23.1**.

Compensatory Mechanism of Acid–Base Disorders

The body uses its homeostatic mechanism to counter the acid-base disorders and restore the pH to normal level (pH 7.35–7.45). This is known as compensatory mechanism. It may be complete or partial. Sometimes, compensatory mechanisms may not work.

- During acute metabolic disorders (due to changes in HCO_3^-) respiratory mechanism (compensation) sets in and regulates H_2CO_3 (i.e., CO_2) by hyperventilation or hypoventilation.
- During acute respiratory disorders (due to charges in H_2CO_3), the renal mechanism (compensation) occurs to maintain HCO_3^- level by increasing or decreasing its concentration.

Diagnosis of Acid–Base Balance and Imbalance

It can be done using blood gas analyzer by measurement of the following parameters:

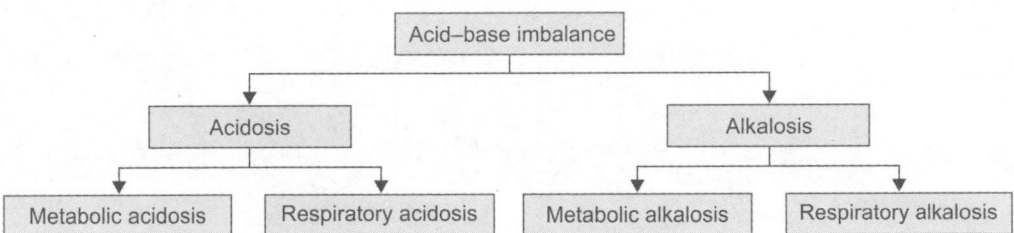

Fig. 23.4: Acid–base imbalance.

Causes	Changes	Compensation
Table 23.1: Acid-base disorders.		
	Metabolic Acidosis	
Uncontrolled diabetes mellitus (diabetic ketoacidosis), renal failure, diarrhea, lactic acidosis	Deficiency of bicarbonate in blood, low pH (H⁺ increased)	*Primary:* Respiratory
		Secondary: Renal
	Respiratory Acidosis	
Pneumonia	Elevation of H_2CO_3 in blood	*Primary:* Renal
Asthma	Low pH (H⁺ increased)	*Secondary:* Respiratory
Hypoventilation, cardiac arrest		
	Metabolic Alkalosis	
Peptic ulcer, Hypokalemia	Increased bicarbonate in blood	*Primary:* Respiratory
Intestinal obstruction, IV bicarbonate	High pH (H⁺ decreased)	*Secondary:* Renal
	Respiratory Alkalosis	
Hypoxia, hyperventilation	Decrease in H_2CO_3 in blood	*Primary:* Renal
High altitude, salicylate poisoning	High pH (H⁺ decreased)	*Secondary:* Respiratory

- Blood gas analyses (PO_2, PCO_2)
- Bicarbonate level in blood
- pH of blood
- Other laboratory investigations

Anion Gap

Definition: It is defined as the difference between the total concentrations of measured cations (Na^+ and K^+) and that of measured anions (Cl^- and HCO_3^-)

Anion gap = (Na^+ and K^+) − (Cl^- and HCO_3^-)

It actually represents unmeasured anions in the plasma (protein, phosphate, etc.).

Calculation: $[Na^+] + [K^+] - [Cl^-] + [HCO_3^-]$
$(138 + 4) − (102 + 25)$
$= 15\ mEq/L$

Normal value: 8 – 18 mEq/L (Average 15 mEq/L)

Clinical Importance

Concentration of anions and cations in plasma must be equal to maintain electrical neutrality.

Acid–base disorders are associated with alterations in the anion gap.

Increased in: Metabolic acidosis.

24. Organ Function Tests

Chapter Outline

- Liver Function Tests
- Renal Function Tests
- Pancreatic Function Tests
- Thyroid Function Tests
- Gastric Function Tests
- Cardiac Function Tests

INTRODUCTION

Organ function tests are specific tests performed to assess the functional status of organ(s).

The following are the important organ function tests:
- Liver function tests (LFTs)
- Renal function tests (RFTs)
- Pancreatic function tests
- Thyroid function tests
- Gastric function tests
- Cardiac function tests

LIVER FUNCTION TESTS

Liver is a complex organ which performs diverse functions (*refer* below). Damage to the liver or biliary tract may affect any or all of these functions. They are most often employed to determine:
- The presence of liver disease
- The type of liver disease
- The extent and progression of liver disease

Classification

They can be classified according to the functions performed by the liver.
- Tests based on heme metabolism
  - van den Bergh reaction
  - Serum bilirubin estimation
  - Bile pigments in urine
  - Bile salts in urine
  - Urobilinogen in urine and feces
- Test based on carbohydrate metabolism
  - Galactose tolerance test
- Tests based on lipid metabolism
  - Cholesterol estimation
  - Determination of stool fat
- Tests based on protein metabolism
  - Protein estimation
  - Albumin/globulin (A/G) ratio
- Test based on detoxification function
  - Hippurate test
- Test based on excretory function
  - Bromsulfthalein test
- Tests based on enzyme activity
  - Serum glutamic oxaloacetic transaminase (SGOT), aspartate aminotransferase, (AST)
  - Serum glutamic pyruvic transaminase (SGPT), alanine aminotransferase (ALT)
  - Alkaline phosphatase (ALP)
  - Lactate dehydrogenase (LDH)
- Tests based on synthetic function
  - Prothrombin time
  - Protein—albumin estimation

Tests Based on Heme Metabolism

van den Bergh's reaction: It is one of the liver function tests. It is used to differentiate three types of jaundice due to increase in serum bilirubin.

Procedure

- Serum + Diazotized sulfanilic acid (Sulfanilic acid in HCl + Sodium nitrite)

Three types of responses are observed:
1. *Direct positive reaction:* Purple color develops within 30 seconds. It indicates obstructive jaundice.

2. *Indirect positive reaction:* Purple color develops within 30 minutes after adding methyl alcohol. It is due to hemolytic jaundice.
3. *Biphasic reaction:* Purple color appears immediately and gets intensified on adding methyl alcohol. It is due to hepatic jaundice.

> **Note**
> - Normal serum gives negative reaction
>   - Test for bile pigments in urine: Fouchet's test
>   - Test for bile salts: Hay's test
>   - Test for urobilinogen in urine: Ehrlich's test
>   - Estimation of bilirubin in serum: Colorimetric method
> - Tests to differentiate three types of jaundice (*refer* Chapter 16)

Tests Based on Carbohydrate Metabolism

Galactose tolerance test: Test based on galactose tolerance is considered to be more useful than oral glucose tolerance test. Galactose is converted into glucose in the liver. Impairment of hepatic function leads to galactose intolerance. In the oral galactose tolerance test, 40 g galactose dissolved in 250 mL of water is ingested by the patient after an overnight fast. Blood galactose is determined at half an hour and an hour later. Normally, the one hour value is below 60 mg/100 mL. A value in excess of this indicates hepatocellular damage.

Tests Based on Lipid Metabolism

☐ *Estimation of free and ester cholesterol:* The esterification of cholesterol is a function of the liver. Hence, the determination of free and ester cholesterol is useful in the assessment of liver function. Proportion of esterified cholesterol decreases in parenchymatous liver disease.

☐ *Determination of stool fat*: The esterification and absorption of fat depends among other things on the availability of bile salts. But during impaired liver function, particularly in obstructive jaundice, bile salt is reduced causing more of the fat to pass out in feces. Hence, the determination of stool fat may be used as a liver function test.

Tests Based on Protein Metabolism

Albumin, fibrinogen and some α and β globulins are synthesized in liver. Serum albumin is usually decreased in parenchymatous liver disease and impaired hepatic function. This is often accompanied by a rise in serum globulins. Consequently, the ratio of serum albumin and globulin (A:G ratio) is decreased and sometimes even reversed.

Decrease in serum albumin and increase in serum globulin as seen in parenchymatous liver disease can also be detected by certain flocculation tests, e.g., cephalin-cholesterol flocculation, zinc sulfate turbidity and thymol turbidity tests. Abnormal pattern of electrophoresis of serum proteins often occurs in liver diseases. In cirrhosis, serum albumin is reduced and there is an increase in ϒ globulin.

Tests Based on Detoxification Function

The liver removes noxious materials or renders them harmless by detoxification mechanisms.

$$\text{Benzoic acid} + \text{Glycine} \rightarrow \text{Hippuric acid}$$

The liver removes benzoic acid from the system by combining with glycine to form hippuric acid which is excreted in urine. The amount excreted in urine in a fixed interval after giving benzoic acid or sodium benzoate gives the ability of the liver for detoxification.

Tests Based on Excretory Function

Bromsulfthalein (BSP) test: The ability of the liver to excrete certain dyes is used in the bromsulfthalein test. BSP is conjugated in the liver and excreted in bile. After an overnight fast, 5% solution of the dye (5 mg/kg body weight) is injected intravenously. A blood sample is collected after exactly 45 minutes and concentration of dye is estimated. In normal subjects, 5% of the dye should remain in the blood at the end of 45 minutes. More dye retention shows impaired liver function.

Tests Based on Enzyme Activity

The serum enzymes which are usually measured to help in the diagnosis of hepatic disorders are:

AST (SGOT)	Increased in hepatitis
ALT (SGPT)	Highly increased in liver disease
Alkaline phosphatase (ALP)	Markedly increased in obstructive jaundice
LDH (especially LDH5)	Increased in hepatitis
γ-glutamyl transferase (γ-GT)	Increased in alcoholic liver disease

Tests Based on Synthetic Function
- *Prothrombin time:* Prothrombin is synthesized in the liver. Prothrombin time is prolonged in hepatocellular diseases, due to decreased synthesis of prothrombin.
- *Protein:* Albumin estimation in serum. It is used to know the synthetic capacity of liver for protein and albumin.

Liver Function Tests in Clinical Practice

The following LFTs only are usually performed in blood and urine in clinical practice to assess liver functions.
- *Urine:* Detection of bile salts and bile pigments
- *Blood:* Estimation of—
  - Bilirubin: Total, direct, indirect
  - Enzymes: SGPT, SGOT, rGT, ALP, LDH
  - Prothrombin time
  - Protein (total), albumin, A/G ratio

■ RENAL FUNCTION TESTS

Kidney is a vital organ which functions to:
- Remove the waste products of metabolism
- Remove the foreign and nonendogenous substances
- Maintain water and electrolyte balance
- Maintain acid-base balance

Classification
- Tests based on glomerular filtration
  - Urea clearance test
  - Creatinine clearance test
  - Inulin clearance test
- Tests based on tubular function
  - Urine concentration test
  - Urine dilution test
  - Phenolsulfonphthalein (PSP) excretion test
- Test to measure renal plasma flow (RPF)
  - Para-aminohippurate test (PAH)

Tests for Glomerular Filtration

Under normal circumstances about 700 mL. of plasma (contained in 1,300 mL of blood) flows through the kidneys per minute and 120 mL of fluids are filtered into Bowman's capsule. The volume of the filtrate may be reduced in extra-renal conditions such as dehydration, cardiac failure, etc. If the volume of glomerular filtrate is lowered below a certain point, the kidneys are unable to eliminate waste products which accumulate in blood.

Clearance tests

The following tests are performed to assess the glomerular filtration. These tests are called as 'clearance' tests.

Clearance is defined as the volume of blood or plasma which contains the amount of the substance that is excreted in urine in one minute. To express quantitatively the rate of excretion of a given substance by the kidneys, its clearance is frequently measured.

Urea clearance test

Urea clearance is defined as the volume of blood or plasma cleared of urea per minute.

Procedure

A light breakfast with two glasses of water is given to the patient to ensure adequate urine flow. The bladder is emptied and this urine specimen is discarded. Urine is collected exactly after one our and the volume is noted. Blood is also withdrawn. A second sample of urine is collected at the end of second hour and volume is noted. Urea in blood and urine (2 samples) are estimated by a standard method (e.g., diacetyl monoxime method). Average value of two specimens of urine is used for assessing the quantity and urea content of urine.

Maximum urea clearance

If volume of urine excreted per minute is 2 mL or more, urea clearance is maximum. In this case, the following formula is used to calculate volume of blood cleared of urea per minute (maximum urea clearance cm)

$$\frac{U \times V}{B}$$

where,
- U = Concentration of urea in urine (mg/100 mL)
- V = Volume of urine in mL/min
- B = Concentration of urea in blood (mg/100 mL)
- Normal maximum urea clearance is 75 mL/per minute.

Standard urea clearance

If urine volume is less than 2 mL/min, urea clearance is reduced. In this case, the following formula is used to calculate volume of blood cleared of urea per minute (standard urea clearance C_s).

$$\frac{U \times \sqrt{V}}{B}$$

Normal standard urea clearance is 54 mL/minute.

Result of urea clearance test is expressed as percent of the normal maximum urea clearance or normal standard urea clearance.

$$\text{Percentage clearance} = \frac{\text{Test value}}{\text{Normal value}} \times 100$$

Clinical Importance

- 70% or more of urea clearance = Normal glomerular function
- 40–70% of urea clearance = Mild impairment
- 20–40% of urea clearance = Moderate impairment
- Less than 20% of urea clearance = Severe impairment

Creatinine clearance test

Definition

Creatinine clearance is defined as the number of mL of plasma which is cleared of creatinine in 1 minute.

It is the convenient test to measure glomerular filtration rate (GFR), because:
- Creatinine is a normal metabolite in the body.
- It does not require the intravenous administration of any test material.
- Creatinine is neither reabsorbed nor significantly secreted by the tubules.
- Creatinine is purely endogenous.
- It is a simple procedure.

Procedure

- 24-hour urine sample is collected accurately and its volume is measured.
- Collect a blood sample.
- Estimate the creatinine in blood and urine by a standard method (e.g., Jaff's method).

Calculation

$$\text{Creatinine clearance} = \frac{U \times V}{P}$$

where,
- U = Urine creatinine (mg/100 mL)
- P = Plasma/serum creatinine (mg/100 mL)
- V = Volume of urine (mL/minute)

Clinical Importance

- Normal creatinine clearance = 90–125 mL/minute.
- It gives accurate GFR. It is decreased in renal diseases.

Inulin clearance test

Inulin clearance is defined as the number of ml of plasma which is cleared of inulin in one minute. It is equivalent to GFR.

Normal inulin clearance is 100–150 mL/min. It is decreased in renal diseases.

Tests of Tubular Function

Kidneys play an important role in maintaining the fluid balance of the body. Healthy kidneys can get rid of excess water, and can conserve water when the water content of the body diminishes. Concentration or dilution of the urine in accordance with the requirements of the body is a function of the renal tubules.

- *Urine concentration test:* The patient is given a meal with high protein content and 200 mL of water to drink in the evening. No more meal or drink is allowed until next morning. Discard the urine passed during night. On the following morning, collect three samples of urine as follows:
  - 8.00 AM: Urine sample I
  - 9.00 AM: Urine sample II
  - 10.00 AM: Urine sample III
    - Measure the specific gravity of each specimen with urinometer. Take specific gravity of at least one specimen. It should be 1.022 to 1.030. Impairment of tubular function leads to a fall in specific gravity.
- *Urine dilution test:* The patient is not allowed to take water after midnight. The bladder is emptied at 7.00 AM and 1,200 mL of water is given within ½ hour. The bladder is emptied at an interval of 1 hour at 8.00 AM, 9.00 AM, 10.00 AM, 11.00 AM, and thus four samples are collected. The volume and specific gravity is measured in each specimen. The specific gravity of one of the samples should fall to 1.003 or less. Almost all the water drunk (1,200 mL) should be excreted within these 4 hours. Failure to do so is a sign of impaired tubular function.

- *Phenolsulfthalein (PSP) excretion test:* Kidneys are able to remove PSP from blood when introduced parenterally. After intravenous injection of the dye, its concentration in urine sample is measured. Excretion of <15% of the injected dose in 15 minutes and <50% in 70 minutes indicate impairment of tubular function.

Renal Function Tests in Clinical Practice

The following examination and estimations are done in blood and urine to assess kidney functions in clinical practice.
- Routine examination of urine
- Estimation of urea and creatinine in blood
- Creatinine clearance test

■ PANCREATIC FUNCTION TESTS

The functions of pancreas may be divided into:
- *Exocrine function tests:* The exocrine secretions of the pancreas into the intestine are water, bicarbonate, and enzymes namely amylase, lipase and trypsin (a) They can be studied by directly determining them in the content obtained by duodenal intubation before and after stimulation of the pancreas by injection of secretin. (b) They can also be studied indirectly by determining the enzymes in serum and urine, the fat and nitrogen in feces and the sodium chloride in sweat. Serum amylase and lipase are increased in acute pancreatitis.
- *Endocrine function tests:* The tests are performed to assess the status of the beta cells of islets of Langerhans, which secrete the hormone insulin. The endocrine secretions control blood glucose concentration. It is discussed in detail under the title 'Blood Sugar Regulation' (*refer* Chapter 11).

■ THYROID FUNCTION TESTS

Thyroid is an endocrine gland which secretes the hormones.
- Thyroxine [Tetraiodothyronine (T_4)]
- Triiodothyronine (T_3)

They are necessary for normal growth and maturation. Abnormal levels of T_3 or T_4 in plasma occur in numerous diseases (hyperthyroidism/hypothyroidism).

Thyroid function is assessed by the following tests:
- *Basal metabolic rate (BMR):* It can be measured by spirometer. It is a tedious procedure and now replaced by other tests. It is low in hypothyroidism and high in hyperthyroidism.
- *Serum cholesterol:* It is high in hypothyroidism and low in hyperthyroidism.
- *Serum protein bound iodine (PBI):* Its normal value is 4–8 µg/100 mL serum. It can be estimated by a chemical method. It is low in hypothyroidism and high in hyperthyroidism.
- *^{131}I uptake by thyroid gland:* The patient is given orally a known quantity of ^{131}I. The radioactivity in 24 hours urine of patient is determined using γ counter. Normally 30% of the given radioactivity is the uptake by the thyroid gland and 60% is excreted in urine. In hypothyroidism, uptake is low and in hyperthyroidism it is high.
- *Assay of T_3–T_4 and TSH in serum:* They can be determined by:
  - Radioimmunoassays
  - Nonisotopic assays

■ GASTRIC FUNCTION TESTS

Composition of Gastric Juice

The gastric juice is a clear pale yellow, odorless fluid having a pH around 1. It contains 98–99% water and 1–2% solids. The solids include mucin, digestive enzymes—pepsin, renin and lipase, and inorganic salts. Hydrochloric acid is an important constituent of gastric juice.

Gastric juice is the combined secretion of three different types of cells in the gastric mucosa. The chief cells secrete pepsin, the parietal cells secrete hydrochloric acid and mucous cells secrete mucus.

The chemical examination of gastric contents yields valuable information regarding the secretory and motor functions of stomach and also may reveal the presence of abnormal substances indicating pathological conditions.
1. Fractional test meal analysis
2. Augmented histamine test
3. Pentagastrin test

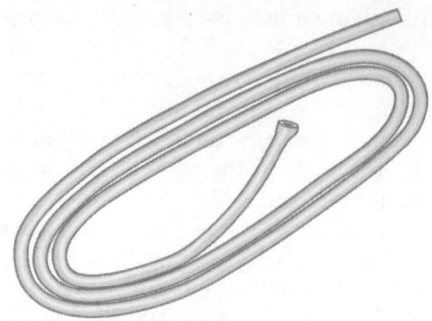

Fig. 24.1: Ryle's tube.

Fractional Test Meal Analysis (FTM)

Procedure
After an overnight fast, the stomach contents are completely removed by aspiration using *Ryle's tube* (**Fig. 24.1**). This is known as the resting juice. About 450 mL of oat meal is then given. The gastric juice is aspirated as before for every ¼ hour up to 2 hours. Thus a total of 9 samples are collected including the resting juice.
- Physical examination of each sample is done with regard to color, reaction, smell, etc.
- Qualitative tests: These are performed with each sample to find out the presence of starch, bile, blood, mucus, lactic acid.

Volume
In most cases, after a night fast, only a small quantity (20–50 mL) of resting juice is obtained. Volume above 100 mL may indicate abnormality. An increased volume may be due to hypersecretion of gastric juice as in duodenal ulcer or delayed emptying of the stomach as in pyloric obstruction or malignant diseases of stomach.

Blood
It should not be present normally. Continued presence of blood in many specimens may be due to gastric carcinoma or active gastric ulcer.

Starch
It is not present in the resting juice normally. It is present in duodenal ulcer with delayed emptying of stomach and pyloric obstruction.

Bile
It may be found occasionally, but is not usually of particular significance. A small quantity of bile may be regurgitated from the duodenum into the stomach as a result of nausea which some people experience during swallowing the tube.

Quantitative analysis
Amount of total acidity, free acidity and combined acidity in each sample of gastric juice is quantitatively estimated by titration. The total acidity and free acidity are plotted against time intervals in a graph.

Comments
Normal value
- Total acidity = 20–55 clinical units
- Free acidity = 10–40 clinical units
- Combined acidity = 10–15 clinical units

Abnormalities
Hyperchlorhydria
When the free acidity is above 50 clinical units, the condition is hyperchlorhydria. Hyperacidity is seen in duodenal ulcer. Zollinger-Ellison syndrome.

Hypochlorhydria
This condition occurs due to hypoacidity, e.g., carcinoma of stomach, chronic gastritis.

Achlorhydria
It occurs due to absence of hydrochloric acid in the stomach, e.g., cancer of stomach.

Achylia gastrica
It indicates absence of HCl and pepsin as in pernicious anemia.

Augmented Histamine Test
Histamine is a powerful stimulant for HCl in stomach. After an overnight fast, gastric contents are aspirated at resting condition (7.00 AM). Gastric contents are collected at ¼ hour interval for 1 hour by a Ryle's tube. All these samples are of basal secretion (prehistamine secretion). Histamine is then administered at 08.00 AM subcutaneously (0.04 mg histamine/kg body weight). Gastric contents are aspirated for one hour at ¼ hour intervals (posthistamine secretion). Free acidity is measured by titration in all samples. Rate of acid secretion can increase about 5–10 times over basal level on histamine administration. This test is useful in assessing active parietal cell mass. In pernicious anemia, there is lack of response to histamine. This test is a guideline for the surgeon to limit acid secretion by vagotomy. It can also differentiate true achlorhydria from pseudoachlorhydria.

Pentagastrin Stimulation Test

It is also used to assess gastric function. It is performed after giving pentagastrin (synthetic peptide) and basal acid output and maximum acid output are measured. It is indicated in patients with persistent duodenal ulcer.

■ CARDIAC FUNCTION TESTS

Various biochemical tests are performed to diagnose cardiac diseases especially myocardial infarction (MI).

Group-I
- Lipid profile
- SGOT (AST)
- CPK (Total)
- LDH

Group-II
- Troponins
- Myoglobin
- CPK-MB
- Homocysteine

25 Hormones

Chapter Outline
- Definition
- Biomedical Importance/Functions
- Classification
- Individual Hormones

DEFINITION

Hormones are secretions produced by endocrine glands (ductless glands). They are liberated into blood from where they are carried to target organs on which they exert their specific effects.

The term hormone is derived from the word '*hormacin*' (Greek) meaning 'to excite'. This term was first applied by Bayliss and Starling in 1902 for secretion produced by intestinal mucosa. Study of endocrine glands is known as endocrinology **(Fig. 25.1)**. Endocrine glands and their hormones are discussed in **Table 25.1**.

BIOMEDICAL IMPORTANCE/ FUNCTIONS

- They act as chemical messengers for communication between cells.

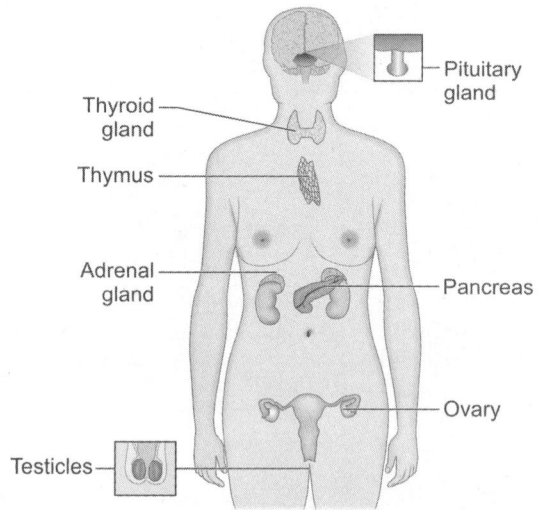

Fig. 25.1: Endocrine system.

Table 25.1: Endocrine glands and their hormones.	
Gland	*Hormones*
• Pituitary gland	
▪ Anterior pituitary	• Growth hormone (GH) • Adrenocorticotropic hormone (ACTH) • Thyroid-stimulating hormone (TSH) • Follicle-stimulating hormone (FSH) • Luteinizing hormone (LH), prolactin (PRL)
▪ Posterior pituitary	Antidiuretic hormone (ADH) (vasopressin), oxytocin
▪ Middle lobe	Melanocyte stimulating hormone (MSH)
• Hypothalamus	Hypothalamic releasing hormones
• Thyroid	Thyroxine (T_4), Triiodothyronine (T_3), Calcitonin
• Parathyroid	Parathyroid hormone (PTH), calcitonin
• Pancreas	Glucagon, insulin, somatostatin, pancreatic peptide

Contd...

Contd...

Gland	Hormones
• Adrenals	
▪ Adrenal cortex	Glucocorticoids, mineralocorticoids, sex hormones
▪ Adrenal medulla	Epinephrine, norepinephrine
• Gonads	
▪ Testes	Androgens
▪ Ovaries	Estrogens, progestins
• Placenta	Human chorionic gonadotropin (hCG)
	Placental lactogen, estrogens, progestins
• Gastrointestinal (GI) tract hormones	Gastrin, secretin, etc.
• Other glands	
▪ Thymus	Thymosin
▪ Pineal gland	Melatonin
▪ Kidney	Erythropoietin

- Hormones exert many biochemical (metabolic) effects in the body, e.g., regulation of blood glucose, calcium, phosphorous, water, and electrolyte levels.
- They are involved in several physiological functions, e.g., development and maintenance of secondary sexual characteristics, menstruation and pregnancy.
- They are used clinically as contraceptive agents and anticancer agents.
- They may lead to pathological conditions due to overproduction or diminished synthesis.

CLASSIFICATION

Hormones can be classified in different ways:

Based on the Chemical Nature

Hormones are divided into three groups according to their chemical nature.

Type	Examples
Protein/peptide hormones	Insulin, glucagon, ADH, oxytocin, growth hormone, tropins, prolactin
Steroid hormones	Sex hormones, glucocorticoids, mineralocorticoids
Amino acid derivatives	Epinephrine, norepinephrine, triiodothyronine (T_3), thyroxine

Based on the Mechanism of Action

Hormones are classified into two major groups.

Type	Examples
• Group I	
▪ Hormones that bind to intracellular receptors	Androgens, estrogens, progestins, calcitriol, glucocorticoids, mineralocorticoids, thyroid hormones (T_3, T_4)
• Group II	
Hormones that bind to cell surface receptors (hormones that act through second messengers)	
▪ cAMP as second messenger	ACTH, ADH, FSH, LH, hCG MSH, TSH, PTH, glucagon, somatostatin, calcitonin
▪ cGMP as second messenger	Atrial natriuretic factor
▪ Calcium or phosphatidylinositol as second messenger	Gastrin, oxytocin, thyrotropin-releasing hormone (TRH)
▪ Kinase or phosphatase cascade as second messenger	Insulin, growth hormone, prolactin, erythropoietin

Mechanism of Action of Steroid Hormones and Thyroid Hormones (Group I Hormones) (Fig. 25.2)

Steroid hormones and thyroid hormones diffuse through the cell membrane to reach cytosol.

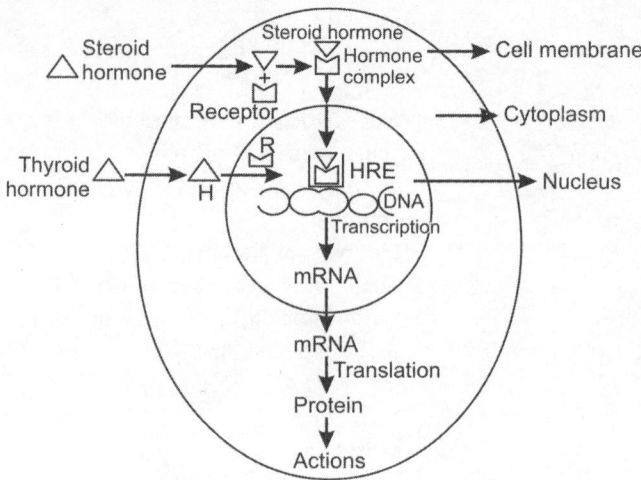

Fig. 25.2: Mechanism of action of steroid and thyroid hormones.

They may then enter the nucleus in different ways:
- From cytosol, thyroid hormones directly enter the nucleus. Inside the nucleus, it combines with the receptor, forming hormone-receptor complex.
- In the cytosol itself steroid hormone combines with the receptor forming hormone-receptor complex, which then enters nucleus.
- Hormone-receptor complex then binds to a specific region [Hormone response element (HRE)] of a DNA strand and activates a gene.

Thus mRNA is formed by transcription and it reaches cytosol. mRNA is translated into a specific protein which brings about metabolic and physiologic effects.

Mechanism of Action of Protein/Peptide Hormones (Group II Hormones) (Fig. 25.3)

cAMP (Cyclic AMP)

The hormone (first messenger) binds to specific receptor site on the cell membrane. This hormone receptor combination stimulates G-protein which activates the inner membrane

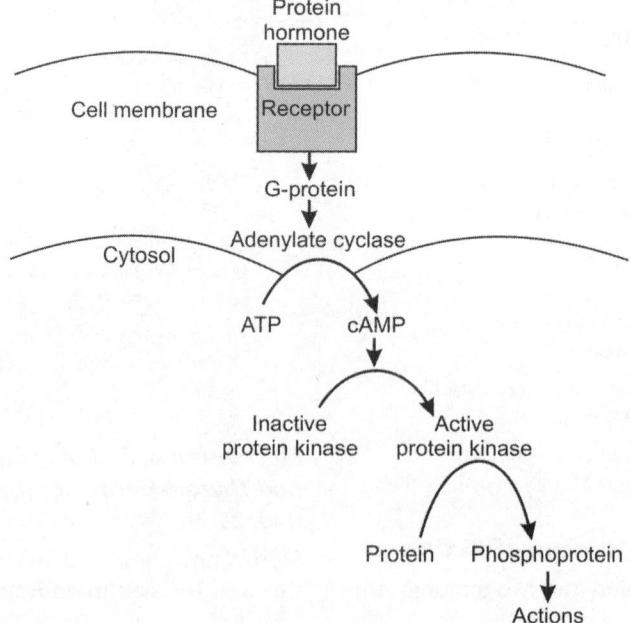

Fig. 25.3: Mechanism of action of protein/peptide hormones through cAMP.

bound enzyme namely adenylate cyclase (adenyl cyclase). Adenylate cyclase catalyzes the conversion of ATP to cAMP (cyclic AMP). cAMP (second messenger), thus formed, has several important actions, out of which the main one is to stimulate the phosphorylation of proteins. Phosphoprotein causes biochemical actions.

Note
Other second messengers are given under classification.

Regulation of hormone secretion
Secretion of hormones may be controlled by several mechanisms:
- Neuroendocrine control mechanism
- Feedback control mechanism
- Endocrine rhythms

■ INDIVIDUAL HORMONES

Hormones of Pituitary Gland
Pituitary gland (hypophysis) lies in the sella turcica at the base of the brain and is connected with the hypothalamus by pituitary (hypophyseal) stalk.

It consists of three lobes:
1. Anterior pituitary (adenohypophysis)
2. Posterior pituitary (neurohypophysis)
3. Middle lobe (pars intermedia)

Hormones of Anterior Pituitary Gland
Anterior pituitary gland is the master endocrine gland. It secretes two types of hormones:
1. Growth hormone
2. Tropic hormones

Growth hormone
Chemistry: It is a single polypeptide containing 191 amino acids. Its molecular weight is 21,500.

Control of secretion is regulated by:
- Hypothalamic releasing factors, such as growth hormone-releasing hormone (GHRH) and somatostatin
- Status of nutrition or stress

Mechanism of action
It acts by binding to specific membrane receptors on its target cells.

Functions
- *Biochemical*
  - Carbohydrate metabolism: It produces hyperglycemia.
  - *Lipid metabolism:* It increases ketogenesis.
  - *Protein metabolism:* It promotes protein synthesis.
  - *Mineral metabolism:* It increases absorption of calcium and helps to retain calcium, phosphate, sodium, and potassium.
- *Physiological:* It stimulates growth of skeletal frame and all tissues of the body.

Abnormalities
- *Hypersecretion:* Excess growth (gigantism in children and acromegaly in adults).
- *Hyposecretion:* Retardation of growth (dwarfism).

Tropic hormones (tropins)
Tropic hormone is the one which influences the activities of other endocrine glands.

Pituitary tropic hormones control the functional activities and the structural integrity of other important endocrine glands namely thyroid, adrenals, and gonads or influence the metabolic reactions in other target tissues. Pituitary tropic hormones are:
- *Thyroid-stimulating hormone (TSH):* It is a glycoprotein, it has two polypeptide chains with high cysteine content. It stimulates biosynthesis of T_3 and T_4. Its release is governed by a negative feedback mechanism by T_3, T_4 and TRH (thyrotropin-releasing hormone).
- *Adrenocorticotropic hormone (ACTH):* It is a straight chain polypeptide with 39 amino acids. It stimulates the synthesis and release of adrenal cortical hormones. It increases the secretion of mineralocorticoids and glucocorticoids. It stimulates protein synthesis. It is controlled by corticotropin releasing-hormone (CRH). Its excess production leads to Cushing's syndrome.
- *Gonadotropins:* These influence maturation and function of the testis and ovary. There are two types of gonadotropins.
  1. *Follicle-stimulating hormone (FSH):* It is a glycoprotein. Its functions are:
     - *In females:* It promotes follicular growth. It enhances the production of estrogens.
     - *In males:* It stimulates testosterone production required for spermatogenesis. It also promotes growth of seminiferous tubules and testes.

2. *Luteinizing hormone (LH):* It is also a glycoprotein. Its functions are:
   - *In female:* It stimulates production of progesterone from corpus luteum.
   - *In males:* It stimulates production of testosterone from Leydig cells. (FSH and LH are responsible for the development and maintenance of secondary sexual characters in male).
- *Prolactin (PRL): Alternative names—*lactogenic hormone, luteotropic hormone, mammotropin.

Chemistry

It is a protein containing 199 amino acids. Its molecular weight is 23,000.

Regulation

Its secretion is mainly regulated by prolactin release inhibiting hormone (PRIH).

Effects
- It stimulates mammary growth and the secretion of milk.
- It is involved in carbohydrate and lipid metabolism.
- It promotes growth of corpus luteum and stimulates production of progesterone.

Abnormalities (Hypersecretion)

- *Women:* Amenorrhea (cessation of menses) galactorrhea (discharge of milk)
- *Men:* Gynecomastia (breast development)

Hormones of Posterior Pituitary Gland

The posterior lobe of pituitary secretes two hormones.

Antidiuretic hormone (ADH)

- *Alternative name:* Vasopressin
- *Chemistry:* It is a cyclic polypeptide containing 9 amino acids.
- *Mechanism of action:* Its action is mostly mediated through cAMP.

Effects
- Its main function is regulation of water balance in the body. It promotes reabsorption of water from the kidneys by distal tubules and reduces urine volume.
- It causes rise in systemic blood pressure.
- It increases intracellular calcium concentration.

Abnormalities

Hyposecretion of ADH leads to diabetes insipidus. It is characterized by excretion of large volumes of dilute urine (polyuria).

Oxytocin

Chemistry

It is also a cyclic polypeptide containing 9 amino acids with disulfide linkages. But oxytocin and ADH differ at 3rd and 8th amino acids.

Mechanism of action: Its action is mediated through membrane receptors present in the uterus and mammary gland.

Actions
- It promotes milk ejection from the mammary gland.
- It causes contraction of uterine smooth muscle for childbirth.

Hormones of Middle Lobe of Pituitary

Melanocyte stimulating hormone (MSH)

It exists in three forms:
1. α-MSH
2. β-MSH–secreted in nonhuman species
3. γ-MSH–secreted in humans. All are polypeptides.

Functions

It stimulates skin pigmentation by deposition of melanin, which darkens the skin.

Abnormalities

Patients suffering from Addison's disease have hyperpigmentation associated with increased plasma MSH activity.

Hormones of Hypothalamus

Secretion of hormones from the pituitary is, in part, regulated by hypothalamic releasing factors (hypothalamic releasing hormones).

Hormones of Thyroid Gland

Thyroid gland is closely attached to the anterior and posterior aspects of the upper part of the trachea. Its weight is about 20 g in adults. It has two lobes connected by isthmus (bridge tissue). It has numerous follicles containing colloid with iodinated thyroglobulin.

Hormones Produced

Major hormones
1. *Thyroxine (T_4)*
2. *Triiodothyronine (T_3):* Produced by follicular cells.

Hypothalamic releasing factors	Pituitary hormone affected
Corticotropin-releasing hormone (CRH)	ACTH
Gonadotropin-releasing hormone (GnRH)	LH, FSH
Growth hormone-releasing hormone (GHRH)	GH
Growth hormone-releasing inhibiting hormone (GHRIH)	GH
Thyrotropin-releasing hormone (TRH)	TSH
Prolactin-release-inhibiting hormone (PPIH)	PRL

Others
Calcitonin: Produced by C-cells (parafollicular cells) found between follicular cells.

Thyroxine (T_4) and triiodothyronine (T_3)
Chemistry
Thyroxine (T_4) and Triiodothyronine (T_3) are iodinated amino acid tyrosine derivatives.

Structure (Figs. 25.4A and B)

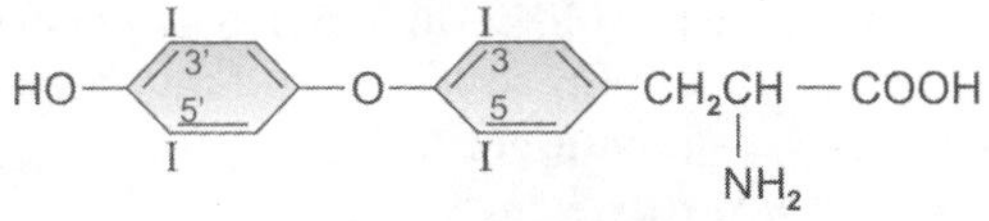

A Thyroxine (T_4)
(3, 5, 3', 5' - Tetraiodothyronine)

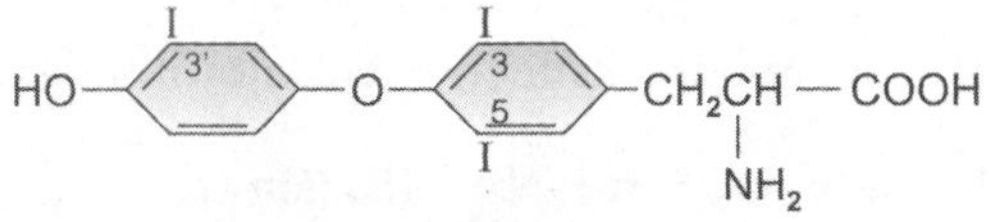

B 3, 5, 3', Triiodothyronine (T_3)

Figs. 25.4A and B: Structure of (A) thyroxine and (B) triiodothyronine.

Biosynthesis
Two components are required by the thyroid gland to synthesize thyroid hormones.
1. *Thyroglobulin:* It is a glycoprotein present in the colloid of follicles of thyroid gland.
2. *Iodine:* It is an inorganic element supplied through diet.

Pathway
Thyroid hormones are synthesized by the iodination of tyrosine residues of thyroglobulin.
- *Trapping of iodide:* The thyroid concentrates (inorganic) iodide by transporting it from the circulation to the colloid present in its follicles.
- *Oxidation of iodide to iodine:* (Inorganic) iodide is oxidized to organic or active iodine inside the follicular cells by the enzyme peroxidase.
- *Iodination of tyrosine:*
  - Active iodine combines with tyrosine residues of thyroglobulin. It occurs first in 3rd position of tyrosine to form monoiodotyrosine (MIT).
    Iodine + Tyrosine → Monoiodotyrosine.
  - Monoiodotyrosine is next iodinated in the 5th position to form diiodotyrosine (DIT).
    Monoiodotyrosine + Iodine → Diiodotyrosine.
- *Coupling of iodotyrosine:*
  - Two molecules of diiodotyrosine undergo oxidative condensation to form thyroxine (T_4) catalyzed by thyroperoxidase.
    Diiodotyrosine + Diiodotyrosine → Thyroxine (T_4) + Alanine
  - One molecule of monoiodotyrosine undergoes oxidative condensation with diiodotyrosine to form triiodothyronine (T_3).
    Monoiodotyrosine + Diiodotyrosine → Triiodothyronine (T_3).

Regulation of secretion
Secretion of thyroid hormones is controlled by the following factors:
- Thyroid-stimulating hormone (TSH)
- Negative feedback mechanism
- Supply of iodine in the diet
- Hypothalamus

Transport in blood
Within plasma, T_3 and T_4 are mostly transported in association with two proteins namely thyroxine binding proteins.
1. Thyroxine binding globulin (TBG)
2. Thyroxine binding prealbumin (TBPA)

Storage
Thyroid hormones are stored along with thyroglobulin in the colloids.

Mechanism of action

Thyroid hormones are transported into their target cells by a "carrier mediated" active transport system of the cell membrane. Their target organs include liver, kidneys, adipose tissue, cardiac tissue, neurons, lymphocytes, etc.

Actions

- *Biochemical*
  - *Carbohydrate metabolism:* They induce hyperglycemia and glycosuria by:
    - Increasing intestinal glucose absorption and decreasing its utilization
    - Inducing glycogenolysis and gluconeogenesis
  - *Lipid metabolism:* They increase lipid turnover and utilization. Plasma cholesterol level is increased in hypothyroidism and decreased in hyperthyroidism.
  - *Protein metabolism:* They increase amino acid transport, RNA and protein synthesis.
  - *Basal metabolism:* They affect basal metabolic rate (BMR). BMR is higher in hyperthyroidism and lower in hyperthyroidism.
- *Physiologic:* Regulates general growth and development

Agents Inhibiting Thyroid Function

Antithyroid drugs: Drugs inhibiting thyroid function are known as antithyroid drugs, e.g.,
- Thiourea
- Thiouracil
  - Aminobenzenes
  - Propranolol

Thyroid function tests (*refer* Chapter 24)

The tests used to assess the function of the thyroid gland are:
- Determination of BMR
- Estimation of PBI, cholesterol in blood
- Determination of uptake of ^{131}I by thyroid gland
- Estimation of T_3, T_4 and TSH

Goitrogens (Fig. 25.5)

Naturally occurring substances which produce goiter are known as goitrogens, e.g., cabbage, mustard seeds, etc.

Abnormalities

- *Hyperthyroidism (thyrotoxicosis):* It occurs due to oversecretion of thyroid hormones or Grave's disease (exophthalmic goiter).

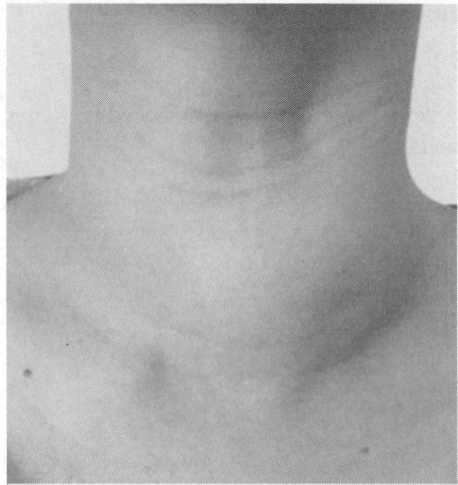

Fig. 25.5: Goiter.
(For color version, see Plate 4)

- *Biochemical changes:*
  - Low cholesterol level
  - High BMR
  - Hyperglycemia
  - Glycosuria
  - Reduced glucose tolerance
  - Increased T_3, T_4 in blood
- *Clinical symptoms:* Rapid heart rate, nervousness, irritability, anxiety, loss of weight despite increased appetite, weakness, excess sweating, sensitivity to heat, inability to sleep, and protrusion of eyeballs.
- *Hypothyroidism:* It occurs due to less secretion of thyroid hormones. It is associated with cretinism (in children) and myxedema in adults; endemic goiter.
  - *Biochemical changes*
    - High cholesterol level
    - Reduced BMR, decreased T_3, T_4 in blood
  - *Clinical symptoms:* Slow heart rate, weight gain, sluggish behavior, sleepiness, constipation, sensitivity to cold and dry skin.

Hormones of Parathyroid Gland

Parathyroid gland contains four lobes; two embedded in superior poles and two in inferior poles of thyroid gland. It secretes two hormones.
1. Parathyroid hormone (PTH)
2. Calcitonin

Parathyroid Hormone

- *Chemistry:* PTH is a linear polypeptide consisting of 84 amino acids.

- *Biosynthesis:* PTH is initially synthesized in the chief cells of parathyroid gland as a prohormone (Pro PTH). It is then converted to mature PTH by trypsin like enzyme.

    PrePro PTH → ProPTH → PTH

Regulation of secretion
PTH secretion is regulated by circulating ionic calcium. Low ionic calcium levels stimulate whereas high ionic calcium levels inhibit PTH secretion. Phosphates have no effect on PTH secretion.

Mechanism of action
PTH acts through a membrane receptor on the target cell.

Storage
It is not stored in the gland. Thus it is synthesized and secreted continuously.

Actions
- *Biochemical*
    - Intestinal mucosa: It increases the absorption of calcium and phosphorus from the intestine.
    - Bones: It mobilizes calcium and phosphorus from bones.
        - It stimulates demineralization by osteoclasts which affect resorption of bones.
    - Kidneys:
        - It decreases urinary excretion of calcium and increases excretion of phosphorus.
        - It activates vitamin D to form calcitriol in renal tissue.
- *Others:* It elevates serum alkaline phosphatase. It increases serum calcium and serum phosphorus.

Abnormalities
Hyperparathyroidism
It occurs due to oversecretion of PTH.

Types and causes
- *Primary hyperparathyroidism:* May be due to hyperplasia or a tumor
- *Secondary hyperparathyroidism:* Due to chronic renal disease.

Clinical symptoms
- Extensive resorption of bone
- Kidney stone formation, urinary tract infection, decreased renal function.

Biochemical changes
Calcium↑ Phosphate↓ Magnesium↓ Alkaline phosphatase↑

Hypoparathyroidism
This condition is due to diminished secretion of PTH.

Types and causes
- *Primary hypoparathyroidism:* It occurs due to autoimmune destruction of the gland.
- *Secondary hypoparathyroidism:* It occurs due to thyroidectomy or accidental damage.
- *Idiopathic hypoparathyroidism:* It occurs due to unknown cause (pseudohypoparathyroidism inherited disorder).

Clinical symptoms
- Tetany
- Denser bones
- Mental retardation

Biochemical changes
Calcium↓, Phosphate↑

Calcitonin
It is synthesized by parafollicular cells found in thyroid gland and also by parathyroid gland and thymus gland. It is a single chain polypeptide containing 32 amino acids.

Regulation
It is regulated by the level of blood calcium.

Action
It is a calcium regulating hormone. Its action on calcium level is antagonistic to that of PTH.
- *On bones:* It inhibits bone resorption and mobilization of calcium and phosphorus from bone.
- *On kidneys:* It decreases tubular reabsorption of calcium and phosphorus.
- *On intestinal mucosa:* It decreases calcium absorption from intestine.

Hormones of Adrenal Glands
Adrenal glands are two pyramidal structures each one lying on upper pole of both the kidneys. They are also known as suprarenal glands.

Each gland consists of two separate parts, namely:
1. Adrenal cortex
2. Adrenal medulla

Section 4: Miscellaneous Topics of Biochemical Importance

Hormones of Adrenal Cortex

Adrenal cortex occupies outer peripheral portion of adrenal gland. Histologically, it consists of three layers or zones of cells:
1. Zona glomerulosa (outer layer)
2. Zona fasiculata (middle layer)
3. Zona reticularis (innermost layer)

The hormones secreted by these cells are steroid hormones.

Classification

Adrenal cortical hormones (adrenocorticosteroids) can be divided into three groups, according to their function.
1. Glucocorticoids
2. Mineralocorticoids
3. Sexcorticoids

Structural Features of Steroid Hormones

All the steroid hormones have the cyclopentanoperhydrophenanthrene ring. They differ in number and type of substituted groups, number and location of double bonds, and stereochemical configuration. They are derived from cholesterol (**Fig. 25.6**).

They are divided into three groups based on structural feature:
1. *C-21 steroids:*
   - Contain total 21 carbon atoms
   - Contain two carbon side chain and an -OH group at position 17 of D ring
   - Possess glucocorticoid and mineralocorticoid effects.
   - Also known as 17-OH corticoids or 17-OH corticosteroids
2. *C-19 steroids:*
   - Contain 19 carbon atoms
   - No side chain but only O group at position 17
   - Possess androgenic activity
   - Also called as 17-oxosteroids or 17-ketosteroids
3. *C-18 steroids:*
   - Contain 18 carbon atoms
   - Possess estrogenic activity

Glucocorticoids

Glucocorticoids are C-21 group steroids. They are so-called because they exhibit an important effect in increasing the blood glucose concentration.

Biosynthesis (Fig. 25.6)

Glucocorticoids are synthesized from cholesterol in the zona fasiculata cells as follows:
Cholesterol → Glucocorticoids

Important members
- Cortisol
- Corticosterone
- Cortisone

Cortisol: It is the most important glucocorticoid.

Regulation of secretion: Regulation of cortisol secretion is mediated by—
- Neurohormonal mechanism
- Feedback mechanism

Mechanism of action: It acts through nuclear receptors such as other steroid hormones.

Transport: It is transported in plasma in combination with proteins.

Metabolism: It is metabolized mainly in the liver and conjugated with glucuronic acid and is excreted in urine.

Actions

- *Biochemical*
  - *Carbohydrate metabolism:* Overall effect is in increasing blood glucose level (hyperglycemic). In liver, it increases gluconeogenesis. In peripheral tissues, it decreases glucose uptake and utilization.
  - *Lipid metabolism:* Its net effect is to increase free fatty acids in plasma and also glycerol.
  - *Protein metabolism:* In liver, it increases protein synthesis. In peripheral tissues, it

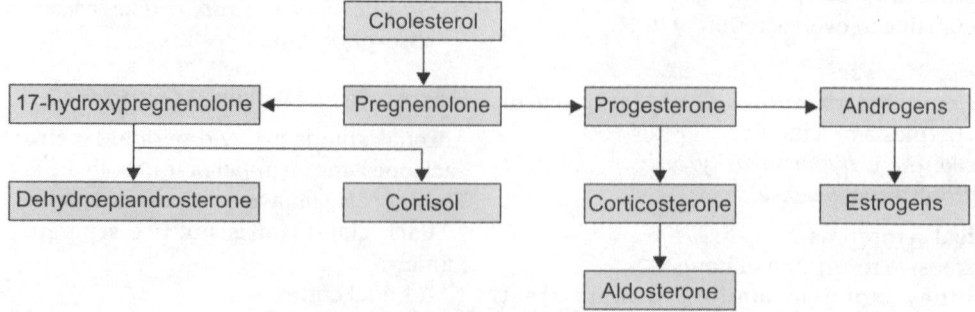

Fig. 25.6: Synthesis of steroid hormones.

increases protein degradation leading to increased amino acids in plasma.
- *Water and electrolyte balance:* It is mediated through ADH.
❑ Others
  - It has anti-inflammatory effect
  - It has also immunosuppressive effect.

Abnormalities
❑ *Hyperadrenocorticism:* Cushing's syndrome
❑ *Hypoadrenocorticism:* Addison's disease

Mineralocorticoids
Mineralocorticoids are synthesized from cholesterol in zona glomerulosa cells only. They are C-21 steroids. They mainly influence metabolism of sodium and potassium.

Important members
❑ Aldosterone
❑ Corticosterone

Aldosterone: It is the most potent mineralocorticoid.

Biosynthesis (Fig. 25.6): It is synthesized from cholesterol
$$\text{Cholesterol} \rightarrow \text{Aldosterone}$$

Regulation of secretion: Production of aldosterone is primarily regulated by renin-angiotensin system. Sodium, ADH and neural mechanism are also involved.

Transport in blood: Aldosterone is carried weakly bound to serum albumin.

Mechanism of action: They act through nuclear receptor like other steroid hormones.

Actions:
❑ *Metabolic effect*
  - *Effect on fluid volume:* They increase extracellular fluid volume by increasing circulating blood volume and urinary output.
  - *Effect on kidneys:* They increase the absorption of sodium and chloride by the renal tubules.
  - *Effect on glands and organs:* They decrease the absorption of sodium and chloride by the sweat glands, salivary glands, and gastrointestinal tract.

Abnormalities
❑ *Hypersecretion:* Hyperaldosteronism
  - Primary aldosteronism (Conn's syndrome)
  - Secondary aldosteronism
❑ *Hyposecretion:* Hypoaldosteronism

Sexcorticoids (Cortical Sex Hormones)
(For more details, *refer* page 263)
These are secreted in small amounts by zona fasciculata and zona reticularis. They are C-19 and C-18 steroids.

Biosynthesis (Fig. 25.6)
They are synthesized from cholesterol in small amounts.
$$\text{Cholesterol} \rightarrow \text{Sexcorticoids}$$

Important members
❑ Male sex hormones (androgens) (C-19 steroids):
  - Androsterone
  - Dehydroepiandrosterone
❑ Female sex hormones (C-18 steroids)
  - Estrogens
  - Progesterone

Adrenocortical function tests
The adrenocortical functions can be assessed by estimating the following:
❑ Plasma cortisol
❑ Plasma ACTH
❑ Urinary 17 ketosteroids

Hormones of adrenal medulla
Adrenal medulla occupies inner portion of the adrenal gland. It secretes two hormones:
1. Epinephrine (adrenaline) **(Fig. 25.7A)**
2. Norepinephrine (noradrenaline) **(Fig. 25.7B)**

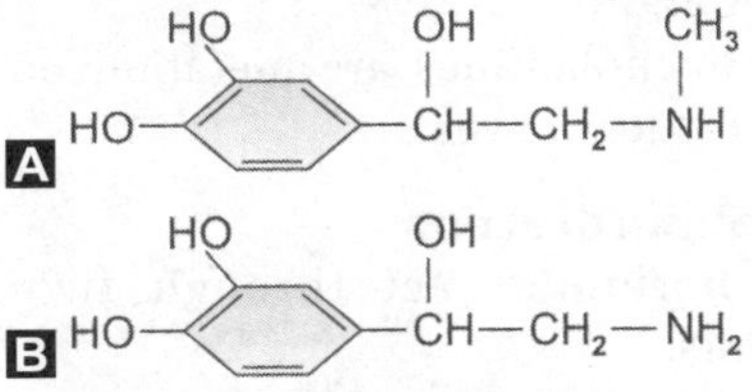

Figs. 25.7A and B: Structure: (A) Epinephrine (adrenaline); (B) Norepinephrine (noradrenaline).

Chemistry
Both epinephrine and norepinephrine are the derivatives of amino acid tyrosine. They are

catecholamines. They are produced in response to fight, fright and flight.

Both have same structures, but epinephrine has one methyl group that is absent in norepinephrine.

Biosynthesis

Both epinephrine and norepinephrine are formed from the amino acid tyrosine. Norepinephrine is synthesized from tyrosine in the chromaffin cells of the adrenal medulla (and also in sympathetic nervous system). Epinephrine is then formed by methylation of norepinephrine (*refer* Chapter 13).

Tyrosine → DOPA → Dopamine → Norepinephrine → Epinephrine

Regulation

Their secretion is controlled at the levels of synthesis, uptake, storage, and catabolism.

Storage

They are stored in the form of granules in adrenal medulla and in adrenergic neurons.

Release

Neural stimulation of adrenal medulla results in release of epinephrine and norepinephrine from storage granules. This process is calcium dependent. It is stimulated by cholinergic and β-adrenergic agents and inhibited by α-adrenergic agents.

Transport

It is transported in blood bound to plasma proteins mainly albumin. Catecholamines do not cross the blood-brain barrier.

Degradation

The catecholamines are metabolized in the target tissues or liver.

Mechanism of action

Both hormones act through two major receptors:
1. α-adrenergic receptors
2. β-adrenergic receptors

Actions

❒ *Biochemical*
- *Glycogenolysis:* Epinephrine stimulates glycogenolysis in liver and muscle producing hyperglycemia.
- *Lipolysis:* Both epinephrine and norepinephrine increase breakdown of triglycerides in adipose tissue.
- *Gluconeogenic action:* Epinephrine increases hepatic gluconeogenesis
- *Action on insulin release:* Epinephrine has a direct inhibitory action on insulin release from cells of pancreas.

❒ *Physiological:* They increase cardiac output, blood pressure and oxygen consumption.

Adrenergic Blocking Agents

These compounds antagonize epinephrine and norepinephrine. They do not interfere with the formation and release of catecholamines but prevent their action, e.g., ergotamine, phentolamine.

Abnormalities

❒ *Hypersecretion:* It results in pheochromocytoma (tumor of chromaffin cells of adrenal medulla). Estimation of VMA in urine is helpful in diagnosis.
❒ *Hyposecretion:* Not established well.

Hormones of the Pancreas

Pancreas performs two types of functions:
1. *Exocrine function:* The acinar portion of pancreas secretes into the duodenum, the enzymes and ions used for the digestive process.
2. *Endocrine function:* The endocrine function of pancreas is localized in the 'Islets of Langerhans' which consist of different types of cells. Each type of cells produces a different hormone. Totally four types of hormones are produced which have different actions.

Types of cells	Hormones produced
α cells	Glucagon
β cells	Insulin
δ cells	Somatostatin
F cells	Pancreatic polypeptide

Glucagon

Chemistry

It is a single chain polypeptide containing 29 amino acids. Histidine is the N-terminal amino acid and threonine is at the C-terminal. Its molecular weight is 3485.

Biosynthesis

It is synthesized in the α-cells of islets of Langerhans of pancreas. It is produced from a prohormone.

Proglucagon $\xrightarrow{\text{Peptidase}}$ Glucagon
(prohormone)   (hormone)

Mechanism of action

It acts through specific receptors in the cell membrane.

Effects

Generally actions of glucagon are opposite to those of insulin.

- **Biochemical**
  - *Carbohydrate metabolism:* Net effect of glucagon is to increase blood sugar level (hyperglycemic)

    This occurs by:
    - Increasing glycogenolysis in the liver
    - Increasing gluconeogenesis in the liver
  - *Lipid metabolism:*
    - It increases breakdown of triglycerides to produce free fatty acids and glycerol
    - It reduces fatty acid synthesis
  - *Protein metabolism:*
    - It reduces protein synthesis
    - It stimulates protein catabolism
  - *Mineral metabolism:* It increases K^+ release from the liver
- **Others**
  - It increases heat production and rise in BMR.
  - It has a positive inotropic effect on heart.

Uses: It is used in the treatment of hypoglycemia, heart failure, etc.

Abnormalities

Disorders due to high or low secretion of glucagon are very rare. Excessive secretion may lead to cancer of the α cells.

Insulin

It is the only hypoglycemic hormone produced in the body. It is secreted by β cells of islets of Langerhans of pancreas.

Discovery: The link between it and diabetes mellitus was proved in 1921 by Best and Banting.

Chemistry

Insulin is a polypeptide with 51 amino acids. It consists of two polypeptide chains (A and B) connected by two sulfide linkages, A7 to B7 and A20 to B19 amino acids. A third intrachain disulfide bridge connects, 6th and 11th amino acids of the A chain **(Fig. 25.8)**.

Chain	Total amino acids	N-terminal	C-terminal
A Chain	21	Glycine	Asparagine
B Chain	30	Phenylalanine	Threonine

Molecular weight of insulin is 5734.

> **Note**
> Human insulin differs from insulin of other species.

Biosynthesis

Insulin is synthesized from its precursor as given below:

Preproinsulin → Proinsulin → Insulin
(Preprohormone) → (Prohormone) → (Hormone)

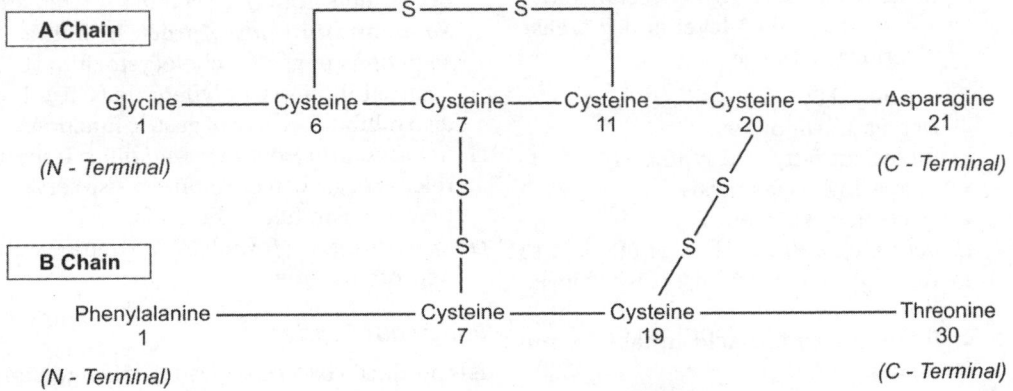

Fig. 25.8: Structure of human insulin.

Regulation
Various factors affect secretion of insulin:
- Glucose
- Hormonal factors
- Pharmacological agents, etc.

Transport
Insulin has no plasma carrier protein.

Mechanism of action
Insulin binds to its membrane receptor and produces one or more transmembrane signals. These signals modulate a wide variety of intracellular events.

Metabolism (degradation)
Insulin is mainly catabolized in the liver, kidneys and placenta. It may be degraded by an insulin specific protease or hepatic glutathione insulin transhydrogenase and is finally hydrolyzed by proteolysis.

Actions
- *Biochemical*
  - *Carbohydrate metabolism:* The net effect of insulin action on carbohydrate metabolism is to lower blood glucose and increase glycogen stores. This is achieved as follows:
    - Increases glucose uptake from extracellular fluid by various tissues.
    - Increases glycolysis.
    - Increases conversion of pyruvate to acetyl-CoA
    - Stimulates glycogenesis
    - Decreases gluconeogenesis
    - Decreases glycogenolysis
    - Increases HMP shunt
  - *Lipid metabolism:* The net effect is to lower free fatty acid (FFA) level and increase triglyceride (TG) store.

  It is achieved by:
    - Decreasing lipolysis
    - Increasing fatty acid synthesis
    - Increasing TG synthesis
    - Decreasing ketogenesis
  - *Protein metabolism:* The net effect is to increase protein synthesis. It is achieved as given below.
    - Increases amino acid uptake by the tissues.
    - Retards protein degradation.
  - Influences the synthesis of many specific proteins in inducing corresponding change in mRNA.
  - *Mineral metabolism:* Decreases concentration of potassium and inorganic phosphorus.
- *Others:*
  - *Growth:* Insulin stimulates growth and also cell proliferation.

Commercial forms of insulin
Various insulin preparations are available for therapeutic purpose:
- Soluble insulin
- Lente insulin
- Protamine insulin

Abnormalities (*refer* Chapter 11)
- *Hyposecretion:* Hyperglycemia (DM)
- *Hypersecretion:* Hypoglycemia

Somatostatin

Chemistry
It is a cyclic peptide containing 14 amino acids.

Biosynthesis
It is formed from various sources:
- S cells of islets of Langerhans of pancreas
- Gastrointestinal (GI) tract
- Hypothalamus
- Central nervous system (CNS)

Functions
- *Somatostatin from pancreas:* It inhibits both insulin and glucagon secretion. It also inhibits secretion of both HCO_3 and enzymes in pancreatic juice. It decreases the delivery of nutrients from GI tract into the circulation.
- *Somatostatin from GI tract:* It inhibits the secretions of gastric cholecystokinin (CCK), gastric inhibitory polypeptide (GIP). It can also inhibit a variety of gastric functions.
- *Somatostatin from hypothalamus:* It inhibits release of growth hormone. It also serves as a neurotransmitter in the brain.
- *Somatostatin from CNS:* It may act as neurotransmitter.

Pancreatic Peptide
It is produced by F cells of islets of Langerhans of pancreas. It is a polypeptide containing 36 amino

acids. It is supposed to have effects on hepatic glycogen level and gastrointestinal secretion.

Hormones of the Gonads

The gonads are bifunctional organs. They produce germ cells and the sex hormones. Germs cells are necessary for reproduction. Sex hormones control secondary sexual characteristics, the reproduction cycle and the growth and development of accessory reproductive organs.

Understanding of endocrine physiology and biochemistry of the reproductive process is the basis of contraception. Sex hormones are also required for maintenance of metabolism in skin, bone and muscle. They are of two types: (1) Male sex hormones; (2) Female sex hormone.

Male Sex Hormones

The testes are bifunctional organs that produce:
- Spermatozoa (male germ cells)
- Androgens (male sex hormones)

The functions of testes are carried out by three types of specialized cells:
1. *Spermatogonia:* Produce germ cells (spermatogenesis).
2. *Leydig cells:* Produce testosterone in response to LH.
3. *Sertoli cells:* Provide the environment necessary for germ cell differentiation and maturation.

Chemistry

They are steroids containing 19 carbon atoms with other structural features.

Important members of androgens are:
- Testosterone
- Dihydrotestosterone
- Androsterone
- Dehydroepiandrosterone

Biosynthesis (Fig. 25.6)

Synthesis of androgens occurs mainly in testes and is accelerated by gonadotropic hormones (LH and FSH) (They are also produced by adrenal cortex). Androgens are synthesized from cholesterol.

Testosterone

It is the major male sex hormone.

$$Cholesterol \rightarrow Testosterone$$

Regulation of secretion
Testicular function is regulated by several hormones. LH stimulates steroidogenesis and testosterone production. Spermatogenesis is regulated by FSH and testosterone.

Transport
It is transported in blood by binding with a plasma protein namely sex hormone binding globulin (SHBG).

Metabolism
- It is catabolized in the liver and other tissues to 17-ketosteroids (e.g., androsterone, etiocholanolone) sulfate or glucuronate and excreted in urine.
- It is also degraded to form dihydrotestosterone (DHT) in many tissues including prostate, seminal vesicles, external genitalia and some areas of skin.
- A small amount of it is converted to estradiol especially in the brain.

Mechanism of action
It acts through nuclear receptor.

Actions
Androgens mainly testosterone and dihydrotestosterone are involved in the following functions:
- *Biochemical*
  - *Carbohydrate metabolism:* They increase the fructose production by the seminal vesicles.
  - *Protein metabolism:* They stimulate protein synthesis in male accessory organs.
  - *Mineral metabolism*: They promote mineral deposition and bone growth.
- *Others*
  - Sexual differentiation
  - Spermatogenesis
  - Male pattern behavior
  - Development of secondary sexual organs

Abnormalities
- *Hyposecretion:* Hypogonadism
- *Hypersecretion:* Benign prostatic hypertrophy.

Female Sex Hormones

Ovaries are also bifunctional organs. They produce ova and female sex hormones which are of two types:
1. Estrogenic hormones
2. Progestational hormones

Estrogenic hormones (estrogens)
Chemistry
The naturally occurring estrogens are:
- Estradiol (E2)
- Estrone (E1)
- Estriol (E3)

All are steroids. They have 18 carbon atoms with other structural features of steroids.

Biosynthesis (Fig. 25.6)
They are mainly synthesized by the maturing Graafian follicles of the ovary and also in corpus luteum. They are also produced in testes, placenta and adrenal cortex in small amounts.

They are formed from cholesterol via androgens.

Cholesterol → Androgens → Estrogens

Regulation
Pituitary gonadotropins FSH, LH are involved in the regulation of estrogen secretion.

Transport
Estrogens are transported in blood by binding with SHBG.

Mechanism of action
They act through nuclear receptors.

Metabolism
They are metabolized by the liver, conjugated and excreted in the urine, feces, and bile.

Actions
- Biochemical
  - *Carbohydrate metabolism:* Increases rate of glycolysis.
  - *Lipid metabolism:* Reduces plasma cholesterol level and LDL. Thus women are protected against myocardial infarction.
  - *Protein metabolism:* Increases protein synthesis.
  - *Mineral metabolism:* Favors retention and elevation of calcium, and phosphorus.
- Physiological
  - Maturation and maintenance of female reproductive organs.
  - Development of female sexual characteristics.
  - Maintenance of menstrual cycle.
  - Provides the environment required for pregnancy, parturition, and lactation.

Synthetic estrogens
They are used in contraceptives. For example:
- Ethinyl estradiol
- Diethylstilbestrol

Abnormalities
- *Hypersecretion:* Polycystic syndrome
- *Hyposecretion:* Hypogonadism

Progestational hormones (progestins)
These are also known as gestagens or luteal hormones.

Progesterone is one of the important progestational hormones.

Progesterone
Chemistry
It is a C-21 steroid.

Biosynthesis (Fig. 25.6)
It is mainly synthesized in the corpus luteum. It is also formed by the placenta, adrenal cortex, and testes. It is produced from cholesterol.

Cholesterol → Progesterone

Transport
Most of it is transported in blood in binding with corticosteroid binding globulin (CBG).

Mechanism of action
It acts through nuclear receptor.

Metabolism
It is mainly degraded in the liver. Its main metabolite is pregnanediol which is excreted in urine as its glucuronide.

Actions
It produces characteristic changes in the estrogen primed endometrium.
- Biochemical
  - Causes an increase in glycogen, fat and mucin in the lining epithelial cells.
  - It increases BMR
  - It is an intermediate compound for the synthesis of androgens, estrogens, and adrenocortical hormones.
- Physiological
  - Causes extensive development of endometrium and prepares uterus for embedding of embryo. Stimulates growth of mammary glands.
  - Suppresses estrus ovulation and production of LH.

Synthetic analogues
1. Norethindrone
2. Norethynodrel

Hormones of Placenta
- *Relaxin:* It is mainly produced by corpus luteum and also by placenta. It is a peptide. It is involved in relaxation of pelvic tissues and cavity operating in conjunction with other factors.
- *Human chorionic gonadotropin (hCG):* It is a glycoprotein. It increases in blood and urine shortly after implantation. This is detected as a diagnostic test for pregnancy.
- *Placental lactogen:* It is a peptide hormone.
- *Progestin and estrogen:* These steroid hormones are also produced by placenta.

Gastrointestinal Hormones (Table 25.2)
Gastrointestinal tract secretes several peptide hormones. They assist in the gastric functions *and also exert different effects.*

Hormones of Other Endocrine Glands
- *Thymus:* Thymosin
- *Kidney:* Erythropoietin
- *Pineal gland:* Melatonin

Additional Information
Differences between enzymes, vitamins, and hormones are discussed in **Table 25.3**.

Modern Concept (POMC)
The hormones of anterior pituitary gland are classified into three groups.

Table 25.2: Gastrointestinal hormones.

Hormone	Location	Actions

• Gastrin family
  ▪ Gastrin
  ▪ Cholecystokinin (CCK)
	• Stomach, duodenum
	• Duodenum, jejunum
		• Gastric acid and pepsin secretion
		• Pancreatic amylase secretion

• Secretin family
  ▪ Secretin
  ▪ Gastric inhibitory polypeptide (GIP)
  ▪ Vasoactive intestinal polypeptide (VIP)
	Duodenum, jejunum
	Duodenal mucosa
	
	Pancreas
		Pancreatic bicarbonate secretion
		Inhibits gastric acid secretion
		Enhances insulin release. Stimulates pancreatic bicarbonate secretion.
		Smooth muscle relaxation

• Neurocrine peptides
  ▪ Neurotensin
  ▪ Substance P
  ▪ Somatostatin
	Ileum
	Gastrointestinal tract
	Stomach, duodenum, pancreas
		Not known
		Not known
		Inhibitory effects

Table 25.3: Differences between enzymes, vitamins, and hormones.

Sl. No.	Features	Enzymes	Vitamins	Hormones
1.	Origin	Body	Diet	Body
2.	Chemical nature	Organic	Organic	Organic
3.	Mechanism of action	Act as catalysts in reaction	Some vitamin act as coenzymes in reactions	Act as chemical messengers
4	Energy production	Nil	Nil	Nil

1. Growth hormone—prolactin group
   a. Growth hormone
   b. Prolactin
2. Glycoprotein hormones
   a. TSH
   b. FSH
   c. LH
3. Proopiomelanocortin (POMC) peptide family
   a. Adrenocorticotropic hormone (ACTH)
   b. Lipotropin
   c. Melanocyte-stimulating hormone (MSH)
   d. Neuromodulators (endorphins and encephalins)

Oral Contraceptives (Birth Control Pills)

These are a class of synthetic steroid hormones–ethinyl estradiol (estrogen) and norethindrone (progestin) that suppresses release of FSH and LH from the anterior lobe of pituitary gland in female.

Section 5: Applied Biochemistry

26 Molecular Biology

Chapter Outline

- Definition
- Historical Background
- Nucleus
- Gene
- Cell Cycle
- Central Dogma of Molecular Biology
- Replication (DNA Synthesis)
- DNA Replication in Prokaryotes
- DNA Replication in Eukaryotes
- DNA Damage
- DNA Repair
- Mutations
- Transcription (RNA Synthesis)
- Transcription in Prokaryotes
- Post-transcriptional Modifications (mRNA in Eukaryotes)
- Transcription in Eukaryotes
- Genetic Code
- **Translation (Protein Biosynthesis)**
- Translation in Prokaryotes
- Translation in Eukaryotes
- Regulation of Gene Expression
- Molecular Biological Techniques
- Human Genome Project

■ DEFINITION

Molecular biology is the field of life science that deals with the structure, properties and functions of macromolecules (nucleic acids and proteins) essential to life **(Fig. 26.1)**.

■ HISTORICAL BACKGROUND

The history of molecular biology started in the 1930s with the combination of various previously distinct biological and physical disciplines—biochemistry, genetics, microbiology, virology and physics. The term molecular biology was coined by Warren Weaver of the Rockefeller Foundation in 1938 based on the physical and chemical explanations of life. Molecular biology's classical period began in 1953 with James Watson and Francis Crick's discovery of the double helical structure of deoxyribonucleic acid (DNA). It focusses on the interactions between the various systems of the cell including the interrelationship of DNA, RNA, and protein synthesis and their regulations. It deals with the molecular basis of diseases in medical sciences. It has also wide applications in other fields.

■ NUCLEUS

It is the center of heredity as, DNA the primary genetic material, is located in it. It is a spherical structure bound by nuclear membrane and contains nuclear sap with nucleolus. In undivided cells, thread-like structures, are seen in the nucleus. These are known as chromatin. During cell division, chromatin becomes condensed to form chromosomes. A chromosome is a long stretch of DNA in association with special proteins called histones. This collective structure is known as nucleosomes and they look like beads surrounded by a string. This arrangement stabilizes DNA.

■ GENE

It is a segment of DNA. It has a particular sequence of nucleotides which codes for a specific amino acid. A chromosome contains several thousands of genes. Genes are the units of heredity (Genes were earlier called by the term 'factors' coined

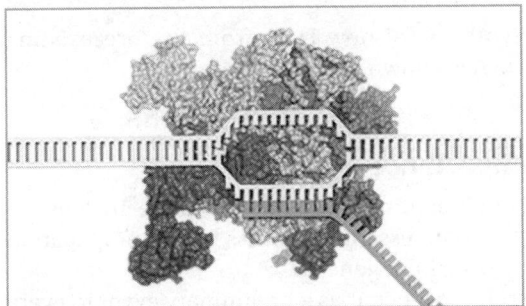

Fig. 26.1: Molecular biology.
(For color version, see Plate 4)

by the Geneticist Mendel) A cistron will code for a specific polypeptide chain.

CELL CYCLE

It refers to the sequence of events occurring during the period between two mitotic divisions in the lifecycle of an individual cell. The total cell cycle is about 20–22 hours in mammalian cells (Fig. 26.2).

It is divided into two phases:
1. *Mitotic (M) phase:* Cell division occurs in this phase. It is the shortest phase which lasts for about 1 hour. The daughter cells then enter into G_0 phase (dormant/undividing) or re-enter the cell cycle for growth.
2. *Interphase:* It consists of three subphases:
   - G_1 *phase:* The period starting from end of mitosis and the beginning of S phase is G_1 phase. It lasts for about 12 hours. Active protein synthesis occurs in this phase.
   - *S phase:* It occurs after G_1 phase. In this phase, DNA synthesis (DNA replication) occurs which lasts for 6–8 hours.
   - G_2 *phase:* The duration following S-phase till the beginning of mitosis is G_2 phase. It lasts for about 4–5 hours. In this phase, there is cytoplasmic enlargement and DNA repair.

Importance

- DNA synthesis (replication) occurs during S phase of cell cycle.
- Cell cycle is controlled by cyclins.
- Excessive division of cells occurs in cancer

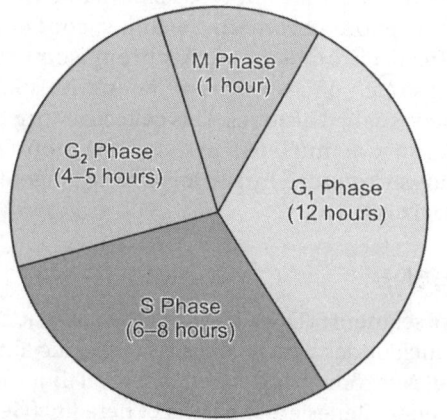

Fig. 26.2: Cell cycle.

CENTRAL DOGMA OF MOLECULAR BIOLOGY (FIGS. 26.3 AND 26.4)

It refers to the flow of genetic information from DNA to RNA and then from RNA to protein. This concept was first proposed by Francis Crick in 1958. Later on synthesis of DNA from existing DNA (replication) was included under this concept. It can be represented as follows:

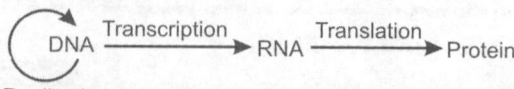

Fig. 26.3: Central dogma of molecular biology.

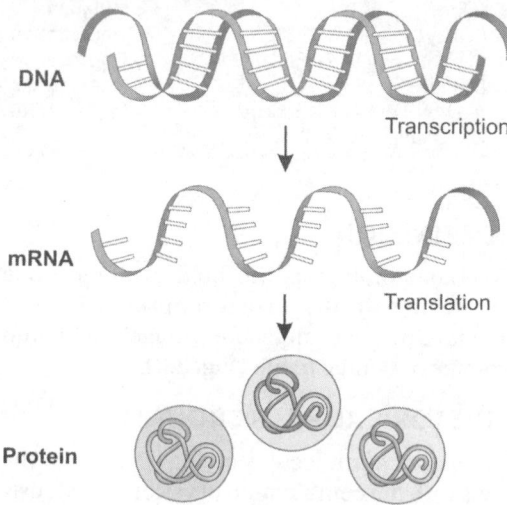

Fig. 26.4: Transfer of genetic information.

Note
Replication, transcription, and translation differ between prokaryotes and eukaryotes.

REPLICATION (DNA SYNTHESIS)

Definition

Synthesis of new DNA from the pre-existing DNA is known as replication.

$$DNA \xrightarrow{Replication} DNA$$

Importance

- It is an important function of the nucleus.
- It is an essential process for the propagation of cellular genes.
- It must occur as a preliminary event to every cell division.
- It is carried out with high fidelity.

Type

Semiconservative mechanism **(Fig. 26.5)**.

One DNA molecule gives two daughter identical DNA molecules. One strand (template strand) of each parent DNA molecule is conserved and other strand (complementary strand) is the newly formed strand.
❏ *Proposed by:* Arthur Kornberg
❏ *Proved by:* Meselson and Stahl

DNA REPLICATION IN PROKARYOTES

❏ *Site:* Nucleus
❏ *Process:* It is divided into three stages
❏ Requirements of replication:
- DNA
- Deoxyribonucleotides
- DNA helicase
- SSB and DNA A (proteins)
- DNA gyrase
- RNA primer
- DNA polymerase I, II, III
- DNA ligase
- DNA topoisomerase

Steps

Initiation

❏ *Recognition of origin of replication:* Replication begins at a specific site in DNA known as replication origin.
❏ *Strand separation:* Some specific proteins (DNAA, SSB proteins) and enzymes such as DNA helicases separate the parent strands and unwind the double helix. This forms a replication fork. At this region, both strands of parent DNA serve as templates for the DNA synthesis.
❏ *RNA priming:* RNA primer (a small fragment of RNA with a free hydroxyl group) is needed for DNA synthesis. It is synthesized by RNA primase (a specific RNA polymerase) on DNA template.
❏ *Synthesis of new DNA strands:* Synthesis of two new DNA strands occurs simultaneously in the opposite directions catalyzed by DNA polymerase III (i) one strand (leading strand) is continuous in 5'-3' direction towards the replication fork. (ii) another strand (lagging strand) in 5'-3' direction away from the replication fork discontinuously as small fragments (okazaki fragments) **(Fig. 26.6)**.

Elongation

DNA strand is elongated by DNA polymerase III by adding all the four types of deoxyribonucleotides to RNA primer one by one complementary to the one in the template (parent strand). RNA is removed by DNA polymerase I using its exonuclease activity. Okazaki fragments are linked by DNA ligase.

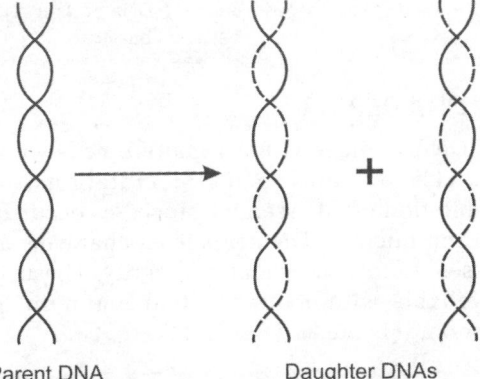

Fig. 26.5: Semiconservative replication.

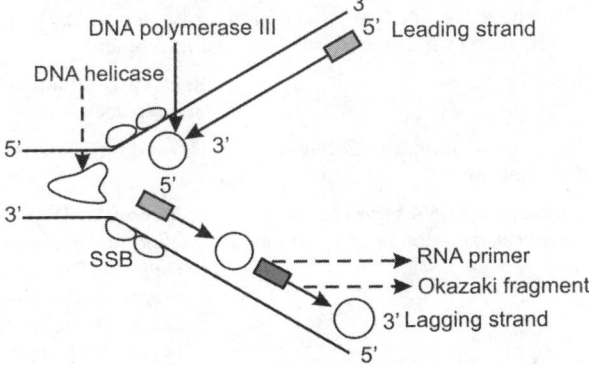

Fig. 26.6: Replication (DNA synthesis).

Termination

A specific protein (ter binding proteins) binds to ter binding sequence and prevents further unwinding of DNA. This facilitates the termination of replication.

Telomeres and Telomerase

Telomeres are repetitive DNA sequences (TTAGGGG) present at the ends of all chromosomes. At the end of each round of replication, the cell loses more telomeres resulting in shortened DNA molecules. This is prevented by the enzyme telomerase.

Note: DNA polymerase-II involved in DNA repair.

Inhibitors

- Novobiocin
- Ciprofloxacin
- Nalidixic acid

DNA REPLICATION IN EUKARYOTES

- Replication begins at several sites simultaneously.
- Replication protein A keeps the two strands apart.
- Five types of DNA polymerase are found (α, β, γ, δ, ε).
  - Primase activity with DNA polymerase α.
  - DNA polymerase β is involved in DNA repair.
  - DNA polymerase γ is responsible for mitochondrial DNA replication.
- Lagging strand is synthesized by DNA polymerase δ and proof reading.
- Polymerase ε is involved in proof reading and leading strand synthesis.

Inhibitors:
- Adriamycin
- Doxorubicin
- Nucleotide analogues

DNA DAMAGE

DNA is exposed to several physical, chemical, and environmental agents which cause damage. DNA damage is of different types (**Table 26.1**).

Table 26.1: DNA damage.

Sl. No.	Types	Causes
1.	Single-base alteration	a. Insertion or deletion of nucleotides b. Depurination c. Deamination d. Base alkylation e. Analogue incorporation
2.	Two-base alteration	UA light induced pyrimidine dimer alteration
3.	Chain-breaks	Ionizing radiation
4.	Cross-linkages	Between DNA and protein, between bases

DNA REPAIR

If DNA damage is not repaired, cells would quickly die due to lethal mutations and inhibition of all essential processes occurring in the nucleus. DNA repair mechanisms are essential for survival and integrity. These are available within the cell that maintain the genome (**Table 26.2**).

Table 26.2: DNA repair.

Sl. No.	Mechanism	Problem	Repair
1.	Base excision repair	Damage to a single base by chemical or radiation or spontaneously	Base removal by N-glycosylase, and replacement
2.	Mismatch repair	Copying errors	Removal of strand by exonuclease, digestion and replacement
3.	Double strand break repair	Ionizing radiation, chemotherapy, free radicals	Unwinding, alignment ligation
4.	Nucleotide excision repair	Damage to a DNA segment by chemical, radiation or spontaneously	• Removal of DNA segment (30 nucleotide oligomer) and replacement • Defective DNA removal, nucleotide resynthesis and ligation • Defect in nucleotide excision repair leads to xeroderma pigmentosum (*see* below **Fig. 26.7**).

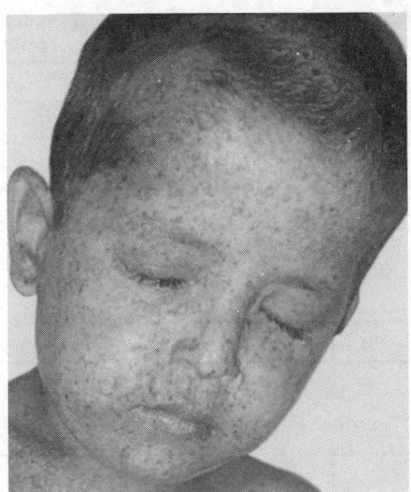

Fig. 26.7: Xeroderma pigmentosum.
(For color version, see Plate 4)

Clinical Importance
Several diseases may occur due to deficiency or loss of DNA repair mechanism, e.g., *Xeroderma pigmentosum*. It occurs due to defective nucleotide excision repair process. It is an autosomal recessive genetic disease. Patients suffering from this disorder show marked sensitivity to sunlight which leads to multiple skin cancers and premature death **(Fig. 26.7)**.

■ MUTATIONS

Definition: It refers to a change in base sequence of a triplet in the gene. It results in alteration of the genetic material.

Causes: It occurs due to faulty replication or repair of DNA in somatic cells or germ cells.

Recognized by: Morgan

Classification: It is mainly of two types **(Fig. 26.8)**.
1. Point mutations
2. Frame-shift mutation

Point mutation may cause:
- Silent mutation: Changed base codes for same amino acid (degeneracy of genetic code)
- Missense mutation: Changed base codes for different amino acid (e.g., sickle cell anemia)
- Nonsense mutation: Codon with changed base may become a termination (stop) codon.

Frame-shift nutation may cause: Several altered amino acids and/or premature proteins.

Effects

Harmful
- Level of particular enzyme may be reduced
- Increased enzyme activity (G-6PD variant) occurs
- Protein formed may be inactive
- Can lead to cancer
- Sickle cell anemia (HbS) occurs due to point mutation (missense mutation)

Beneficial
- Better evolution process
- Study of cell metabolism

Causative Agents (Mutagens)
- *Natural:* Spontaneous
- *Artificial* (induced)
  - Physical: X-rays, radiation
  - Chemical: Mustard gas, formaldehyde, benzene
  - Biological: Viruses

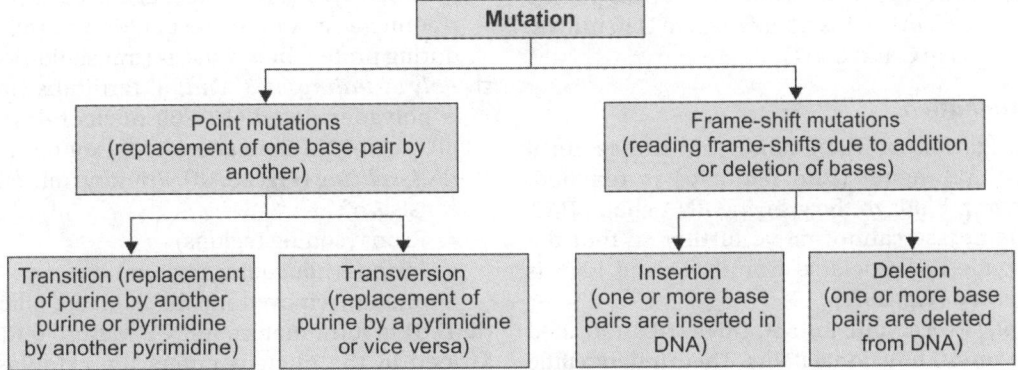

Fig. 26.8: Mutation.

■ TRANSCRIPTION (RNA SYNTHESIS)

Definition
The process by which RNA is synthesized from DNA is known as transcription.

$$DNA \xrightarrow{Transcription} RNA$$

Importance
❏ Genetic message from DNA is copied to the messenger RNA
❏ All the three types of RNA are formed from DNA in the nucleus.

■ TRANSCRIPTION IN PROKARYOTES
❏ *Site:* Nucleus
❏ *Proposed by:* Roger Kornberg, et al.
❏ *Process:* It consists of three steps.
❏ *Requirements:*
  • Template DNA strand
  • Nucleotides
  • RNA polymerases
  • Transcription factors
  • Termination factors

Steps

Initiation

The enzyme RNA polymerase and sigma(σ) factor bind at a specific region called promoter region (Pribnow box/Tata box) on the template strand of DNA (noncoding strand).

Elongation

RNA polymerase moves along the DNA template strand. RNA is synthesized as 5' - 3' strand (antiparallel to DNA template strand). Ribonucleotides are added in the nascent mRNA one by one according to the base pairing rule, i.e., A in DNA is transcribed to U in mRNA; T to A; G to C and C to G.

Termination

Elongation of RNA chain continues until terminal signal (Rho factor-ρ) is reached. When it binds to the growing RNA chain, RNA polymerase cannot move further so that the enzyme is dissociated from DNA and RNA is released **(Fig. 26.9)**.
(*Note:* Procaryotic mRNA, tRNA, rRNA formed are almost functional RNAs. They undergo little post-transcriptional modifications).

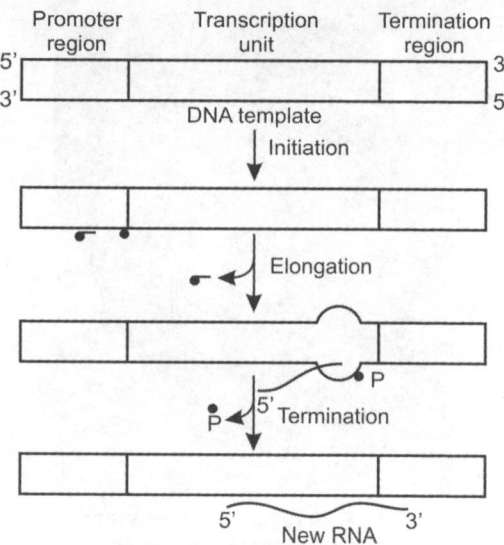

Fig. 26.9: Transcription (RNA synthesis).

But RNAs synthesized in eukaryotes undergo post-transcriptional modifications.
❏ mRNA: *See* below
❏ tRNA: tRNA folds into a clover leaf structure
❏ rRNA: rRNA undergoes modification to form 80s unit which splits into 40s and 60s subunits.

■ POST-TRANSCRIPTIONAL MODIFICATIONS (mRNA IN EUKARYOTES)

The mRNA synthesized and released from the DNA template is known as primary transcript (hnRNA). It undergoes modification (RNA editing and processing) and becomes mature mRNA.
❏ *Capping at 5' end:* mRNA is capped at the 5' terminus by the addition of methylated guanine. This is to protect against attack by ribonuclease and for recognition of mRNA during protein biosynthesis (translation).
❏ *Poly A tailing at 3' end:* 3' terminus (tail) is polyadenylated (10–200 nucleotides) to protect mRNA from attack of 3' exonuclease.
❏ *RNA-splicing* **(Fig. 26.10)**: Primary transcript consists of:
  • Exons (coding regions)
  • Introns (noncoding regions)
Introns are removed and the exons are spliced (linked) to form mature mRNA. Mature mRNA formed in the nucleus enters the cytoplasm through the nuclear membrane.

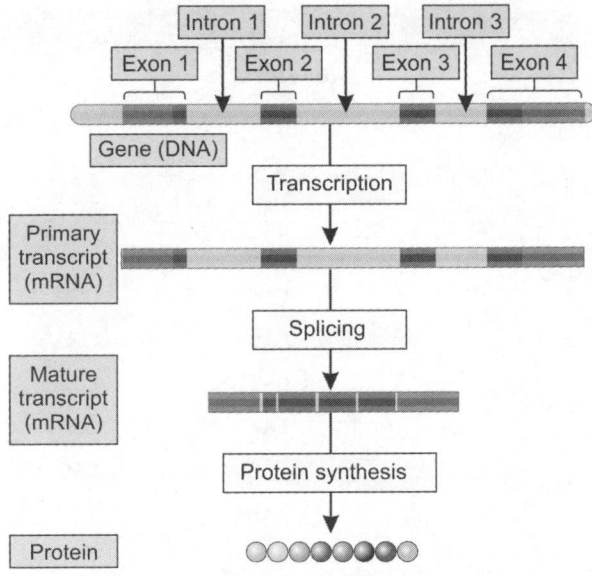

Fig. 26.10: RNA splicing.

RNA Inhibitors

- Actinomycin D (anticancer drug)
- Rifampicin (antituberculosis drug)
- Anthracyclin

TRANSCRIPTION IN EUKARYOTES

- Promoter region is complex which binds RNA polymerase with other transcription factors.
- Three distinct RNA polymerases (rRNA I, mRNA II, tRNA III) are found, one for each type of RNA.
- Introns are normally present in the primary transcript.
- Post-transcriptional modifications occur in all three types of RNA.
- Inhibitors: Actinomycin D, α amanitin, anthracycline

Reverse Transcription

The formation of DNA from RNA is known as reverse transcription. This process is catalyzed by reverse transcriptase (Discovered by Temin and Baltimore in 1970, N.P 1975).

$$RNA \xrightarrow{\text{Reverse transcription}} DNA$$

Retroviruses possess RNA as the genetic material. They cause cancer and are known as oncogenic viruses. HIV causing AIDS is a retrovirus.

GENETIC CODE

Definition

The sequences of three nucleotide bases (codons) in mRNA which contain the information for synthesis of protein molecule is known as genetic code (**Table 26.3**).

Codon

The sequence of three nucleotide (triplet) bases in mRNA which codes for a single amino acid.

Scientists who deciphered genetic code: Marshall Nirenberg, HG Khorana, et al.

Characteristics of Genetic Code

- *Count:*
  - Total codons = 64
  - Codons specifying amino acids = 61
  - Initiating codon = 1 (1 in 61), i.e., AUG (Sometimes GUG)
  - Termination codons/nonsense codons/stop codons = 3 (64–61): UAA, UAG, UGA.
- *Triplet:* Each codon in the genetic code is a sequence of three nucleotide bases specifying a single specific amino acid, e.g., UUU codes for phenylalanine.
- *Universality:* The same codons code for the same amino acids in all organisms.

Table 26.3: Genetic code-table.

1st base	Second base								3rd base
	U		C		A		G		
U	UUU	Phe	UCU	Ser	UAU	Tyr	UGU	Cys	U
	UUC		UCC		UAC		UGC		C
	UUA	Leu	UCA		UAA	Stop	UGA	Stop	A
	UUG		UCG		UAG	Stop	UGG	Trp	G
C	CUU	Leu	CCU	Pro	CAU	His	CGU	Arg	U
	CUC		CCC		CAC		CGC		C
	CUA		CCA		CAA	GLn	CGA		A
	CUG		CCG		CAG		CGG		G
A	AUU	Ile	ACU	Thr	AAU	Asn	AGU	Ser	U
	AUC		ACC		AAC		AGC		C
	AUA		ACA		AAA	Lys	AGA	Arg	A
	AUG	Met	ACG		AAG		AGG		G
G	GUU	Val	GCU	Ala	GAU	Asp	GGU	Gly	U
	GUC		GCC		GAC		GGC		C
	GUA		GCA		GAA	Glu	GGA		A
	GUG		GCG		GAG		GGG		G

- *Ambiguity (specificity):* A particular codon always codes for the same amino acid, e.g., UGG is the codon for tryptophan.
- *Degenerate:* A single amino acid may be specified by many codons, e.g., glycine has 4 codons. Codon degeneracy can be explained by Wobble hypothesis as proposed by Crick.
- *Nonoverlapping:* Each codon is an independent set of three bases. No base functions as a common member of two consecutive codons.
- *Commaless:* Each codon is immediately followed by the next codon.

Importance

- Knowledge of genetic code made us to understand biosynthesis of proteins, mutations and inherited diseases.
- It can be regarded as dictionary of nucleotide bases.

TRANSLATION (PROTEIN BIOSYNTHESIS)

■ TRANSLATION IN PROKARYOTES

Definition

The process by which RNA is converted to protein is known as translation.

$$RNA \xrightarrow{Translation} Protein$$

Importance

- Process of translation is based on genetic code
- Alteration in nucleotide sequence may produce defective proteins
  - *Site:* Ribosomes (cytoplasm)
  - *Proposed by:* Paul Zamecnik et al.
  - *Requirements of translation:*
    - 20 standard amino acids
    - Ribosomes (rRNA - protein)

- mRNA
- tRNA
- Energy (ATP + GTP)
- Factors—initiation, elongation, and releasing
- Enzymes—aminoacyl tRNA synthetase, peptidyl transferase (ribozyme)
- *Process:* It can be divided as follows:
  - Activation of amino acids
  - Initiation
  - Elongation
  - Termination
  - Post-translational modifications

Steps

Activation of Amino Acids

- Amino acid is first converted to enzyme-AMP-amino acid complex in presence of ATP. This reaction is catalyzed by aminoacyl tRNA synthetase specific for each of 20 amino acids.
- Then each enzyme–AMP-amino acid complex is attached to 3' end of tRNA to form aminoacyl tRNA.

```
                    Aminoacyl
                  tRNA synthetase
Amino acid ─────────────────────► Enzyme – AMP – Amino acid
                    ATP
                                            │
                                           tRNA
                                            │
                                            ▼
                          Aminoacyl tRNA + Enzyme + AMP
```

Initiation

70S ribosomes of prokaryotes contain two subunits, 30S subunits and 50S subunits.

- Initiation factors IF-1, IF-2, IF-3 bind to 30S subunit to form 30S initiation complex. It contains the bound mRNA and formyl methionine-tRNA (fmet–tRNA) bound to the initiation codon AUG (in mRNA) recognized through Shine Dalgarno sequence. This reaction occurs in presence of GTP.
- 50S ribosome subunit [which contain P site (peptidyl site) and A site (aminoacyl site)] associates with 30S subunit to form 70S initiation complex. During this process initiation factors are released and GTP is hydrolyzed to GDP and Pi.

Elongation

- *Binding of new aminoacyl tRNA:* The initiator tRNA with anticodon UAC recognizes the initiation codon AUG in mRNA and starts protein synthesis. The initiator tRNA first occupies 'P' site of ribosome. The next amino acid (as aminoacyl tRNA) corresponding to the codon in mRNA binds to A site. The process requires elongation factors (EF) and energy released from hydrolysis of GTP.
- *Formation of peptide bond (Transpeptidation):* Amino group of amino acid at 'A' site forms a peptide bond with carboxyl group of the aminoacyl tRNA at 'P' site. This reaction is catalyzed by the enzyme peptidyl transferase (ribozyme).
- *Translocation:* The free tRNA at the P site is released from the ribosome. Ribosome moves from 5-end to the next codon (three bases) in mRNA towards 3' end. The peptidyl tRNA is translocated to P site. Now A site is ready to receive another aminoacyl tRNA possessing the appropriate anticodon. This process requires EF-G and GTP. The elongation process is repeated till a polypeptide chain is synthesized **(Fig. 26.11)**.

Termination

Ribosome reaches the termination codon sequence (UAA, UAG or UCA) on the mRNA.

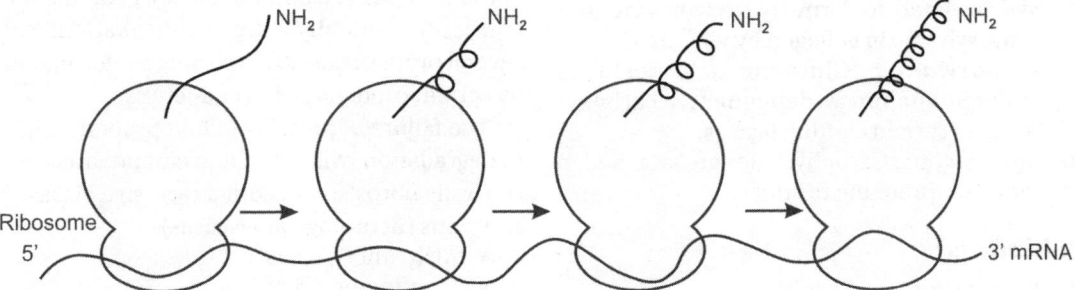

Fig. 26.11: Growing polypeptide chain.

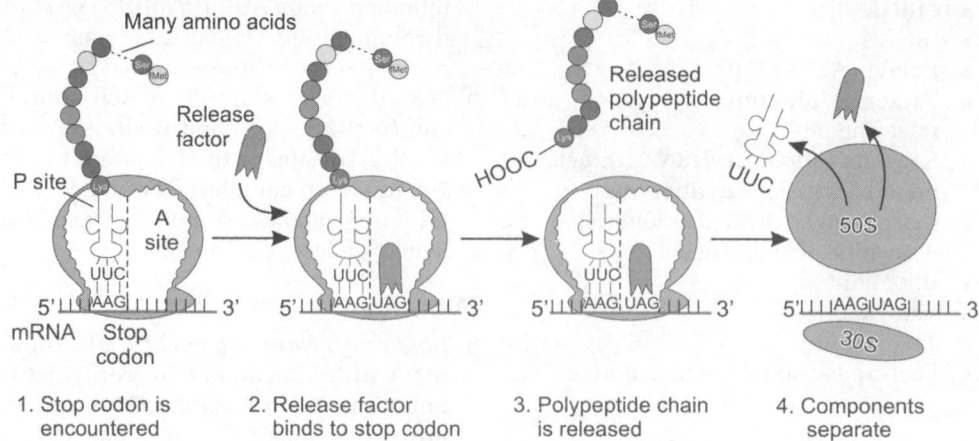

Fig. 26.12: Protein biosynthesis (translation)–termination.

These codons do not have specific tRNAs to bind with them. Thus A site is free. The releasing factors (RF) bind with A site, and hydrolyze the peptide chain from tRNA at P site. The completed polypeptide chain is released. Ribosome dissociates into 30S and 50S subunits to start translation fresh **(Fig. 26.12)**.

Post-translational Modifications

The proteins formed in translation are not functional. Several modifications occur after translation to make them functional. These are known as post-translational modifications.

Proteolytic Degradation

- Proinsulin is converted to insulin
- Trypsinogen is converted to trypsin

Covalent Modifications

- *Phosphorylation:* Hydroxy amino acids, such as tyrosine and serine undergo phosphorylation.
- *Hydroxylation:* Proline and lysine are hydroxylated to form hydroxyproline and hydroxylysine in collagen by vitamin C.
- *Carboxylation:* Glutamic acid residues undergo vitamin K dependent γ carboxylation in certain clotting factors.
- *Glycosylation:* Carbohydrates are attached to serine or threonine residues.

Inhibitors

- Tetracycline
- Chloramphenicol
- Erythromycin
- Streptomycin

TRANSLATION IN EUKARYOTES

- Ribosomes are 80S in size which consist of 40S and 60S subunits.
- mRNA is monocistronic and contains poly A tail.
- met-tRNA is not formylated.
- At least ten initiation factors (IFs) are known to participate.
- Two elongation factors are required (EF1 and EF2).
- Only one releasing factor is required (eRF).

Inhibitors of Translation in Eukaryotes

a. Tetracycline
b. Chloramphenicol
c. Cycloheximide
d. Diphtheria toxin

Protein Folding

Some proteins can spontaneously generate the correct functionally active conformation. But several proteins can attain correct conformation by certain proteins called chaperons.

The failure of proteins to fold properly leads to degradation which result in certain diseases:
- Cystic fibrosis: Autosomal recessive disease
- Prions (neurological diseases)
  - Alzheimer's disease
  - Huntington's disease
  - Mad cow disease

Protein Targeting

Proteins synthesized by translation have to reach their destination to exert their biological function. It is carried out by a process called protein targeting (protein sorting) through different mechanisms, e.g., Golgi bodies.

> **Note**
> - Ribosome assembly is the protein synthesis machinery in the cell
> - Liver is the major organ for protein synthesis
> - RBCs cannot synthesize proteins
> - Mitochondria also possess DNA (mt DNA). It is double stranded circular in nature and resembles prokaryotic DNA. It synthesizes very few proteins only. It is inherited from mother. Mutation in mtDNA may cause.
>   - Mitochondrial myopathies
>   - Leber's hereditary optic neuropathy

■ REGULATION OF GENE EXPRESSION

Gene expression refers to the synthesis of a gene product namely RNA or protein under the influence of the gene. Gene regulation refers to several mechanisms used by the cells to control the amount of each gene product they produce.

Purpose

Regulation of gene expression is required for development, differentiation, and adaptation. The action of genes is regulated. Regulation is necessary because not all the genes are required to function all of the time.

Mode of Gene Regulation

Activities of genes are controlled in various ways so that only those genes which are required at specific time are actually produced.

Types

There are two types of gene regulation:
1. *Positive regulation (induction):* Gene expression is increased by a regulatory element (positive regulator).
2. *Negative regulation (repression):* Gene expression is decreased through a regulatory element (negative regulator).

Gene Regulation in Prokaryotes

In bacteria, the major mechanism depends on whether the enzymes act in catabolic (degradative) or anabolic (synthetic) pathways. Jacob and Monod in 1961 proposed a theory (Lac operon) to explain the regulation of lactose metabolism in *E.coli* by induction or repression. Operon is a unit of genetic expression consisting of:
- Structural genes
- Regulator/inhibitor gene
- Promoter and operator areas
- Control elements

Gene Regulation in Eukaryotes

The eukaryotes utilize diverse mechanisms to achieve the regulation of gene expression.
- Regulation at the level of genome (DNA/gene), e.g., gene amplification, gene rearrangement
- Regulation at transcriptional level, e.g., synthesis of primary RNA transcript and processing
- Regulation at translational level, e.g., degradation of mRNA
- Post-translational control

Importance

Regulation of gene expression studies is important for understanding diseases, such as cancer in which abnormal expression of genes leads to uncontrolled growth.

■ MOLECULAR BIOLOGICAL TECHNIQUES

Recombinant DNA Technology

It is a molecular biological technique. It plays a major role in medicine, biology and other fields **(Fig. 26.8)**.

Definition

The technique by which altered DNA is inserted into an existing DNA by enzymatic or chemical method is called recombinant DNA technology.
- *Developed by:* Paul Berg, Daniel Nathan
- *Alternative names:* Genetic engineering, rDNA technology, gene cloning.

Steps (Figs. 26.13 and 26.14)

1. Generation of DNA fragments and selection of the desired piece of DNA of a human gene by restriction enzymes.

Section 5: Applied Biochemistry

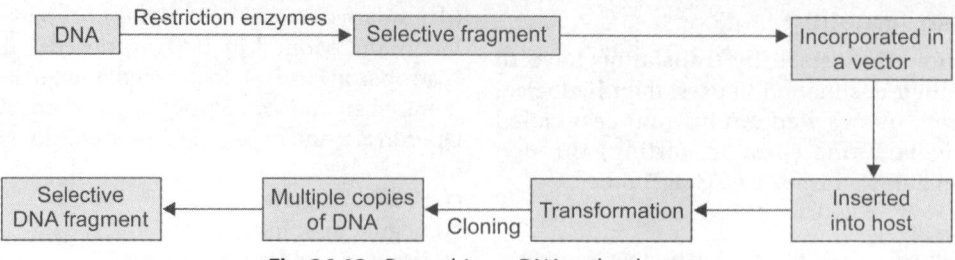

Fig. 26.13: Recombinant DNA technology.

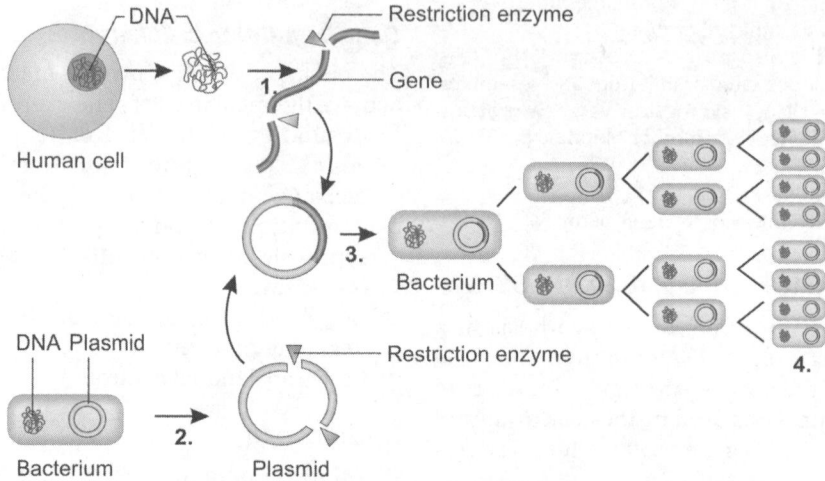

Fig. 26.14: rDNA technology process.

2. Insertion of the selected DNA into a cloning vector (plasmid) by lipofection electroporation, etc.
3. Introduction of the recombinant vector into host cells (bacteria)
4. Multiplication and selection of clones containing the recombinant molecules.
5. Expression of the gene to produce the desired product.

Applications

It has wide applications in various fields.

Medicine

Diagnosis
- To understand the molecular basis of a number of diseases, e.g., familial hypercholesterolemia.
- To apply in forensic medicine (finger printing technique).

Therapy
- To produce proteins, e.g., insulin.
- To produce vaccines, e.g., hepatitis B
- To apply gene therapy for sickle cell disease, thalassemias
- To produce new antibiotics

Industrial applications

Gene manipulations of microorganisms have been exploited in industrial biotechnology.
- It is used to improve conventional fermentation methods.
- Engineered waste is converted into highly proteineous for animal feed and also for human consumption.

Agriculture

To transfer gene to improve the yield, give resistance to pests, herbicide, and pathogens.

Veterinary

To transfer important gene traits to improve milk yield.

Hazards

- Highly toxic chemicals may be produced
- There is possibility of production of oncogenic virus, monster or dangerous animal, etc.

- New pathogenic forms produced may create new disease for the mankind.
- Unnatural microorganisms may lead to biological warfare.
- Genetic manipulation of plants might bring ecological catastrophe.

Thus, genetic engineering should be governed by social and ethical regulations in the interest of human health and society.

Polymerase Chain Reaction

Definition
Polymerase chain reaction (PCR) is an in vitro method of amplifying a target (desired) sequence of DNA. It is the basic tool for the molecular biologist (**Fig. 26.15**).

Invented by
Kary Mullis in 1984 (Nobel Prize 1993).

Steps (Fig. 26.16)
- Target DNA is heated to separate into single strands.
- Single DNA strands are cooled and allowed to anneal with primers complementary to the flanking sequences.
- New DNA strand occurs on the addition of deoxyribonucleotide triphosphates and enzyme Taq DNA polymerase.
- Cycle is repeated again and again.

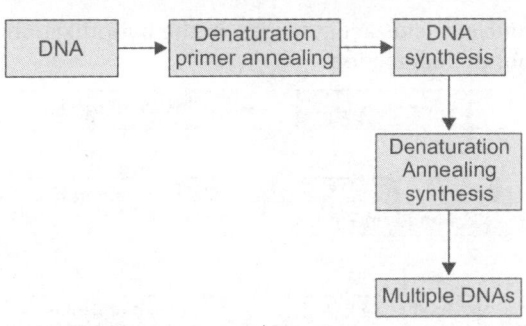

Fig. 26.15: Polymerase chain reaction.

Applications
- To generate large quantities of a specific DNA
- To detect infectious agents
- To detect polymorphism
- To apply in forensic medicine
- To make prenatal genetic diagnosis
- To apply in tissue typing for transplants
- To study evolution from DNA of archeologic samples
- To detect virally induced cancers
- Used for DNA sequencing

Blotting Techniques (Fig. 26.17)
Blotting techniques are the important analytical methods used for the identification of desired DNA, RNA fragments or proteins. It involves immobilization of nucleic acid on solid support (nylon membrane or nitrocellulose). The blotted

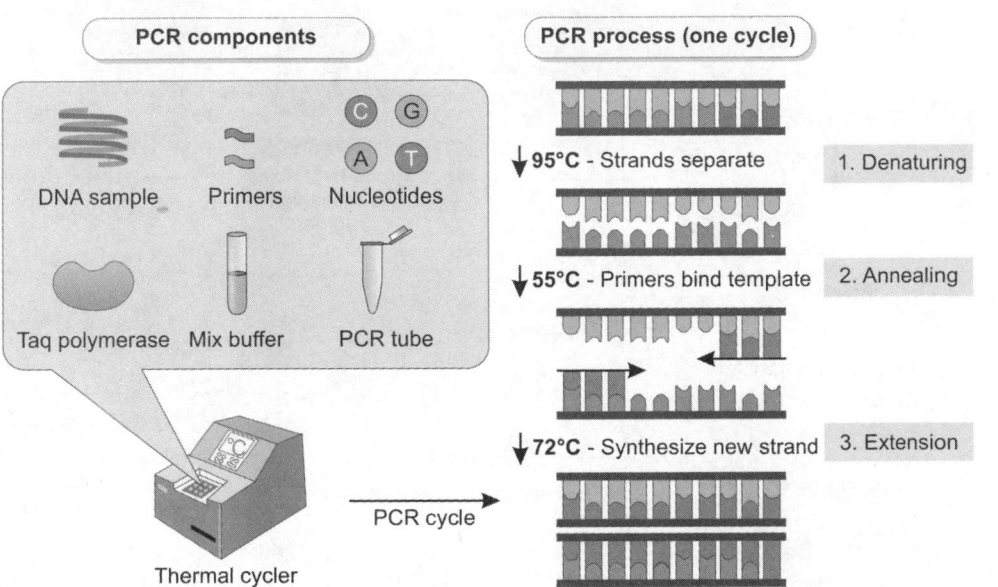

Fig. 26.16: PCR technique.

nucleic acids act as targets in the hybridization for their detection.

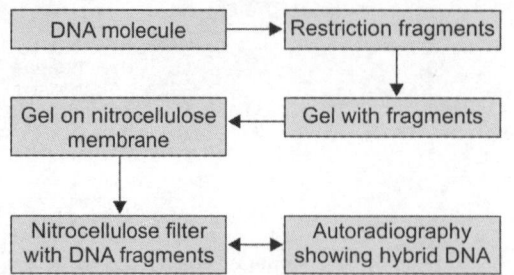

Fig. 26.17: Blotting techniques.

Types

☐ *Southern blotting (Fig. 26.18):* It was developed by Southern in 1975. It is used to detect specific DNA sequences. It is used in gene analysis, DNA cloning, identification of parenthood, thieves, etc., in forensic science, and restriction fragment length polymorphism (RFLP).

Steps:
a. Genomic DNA (isolated from cells) is digested with restriction enzyme(s).
b. This mixture is loaded into a well in a agarose gel and subjected to electrophoresis.
c. DNA (negatively charged) moves towards positively charged (anode) electrode.
d. Separated DNA molecules are denatured by mild alkali and transferred to nitrocellulose or nylon paper. This produces exact replica of the pattern of DNA fragments on the gel.
e. DNA can be annealed to the paper on exposure to heat at 80°C.
f. Nitrocellulose or nylon paper is exposed to labelled cDNA probe.
g. These probes hybridize with compliments of DNA molecules on paper.
h. Paper is washed and exposed to X-ray film to develop autoradiograph.
i. This reveals specific bands corresponding to the DNA fragments recognized by CDNA probe.

☐ *Northern blotting:* It is used to identify specific RNA molecules. It is applied to determine the number of genes present in DNA.

☐ *Western blotting:* It is used to identify the specific proteins in a tissue thereby indicating the expression of a particular gene.

DNA Sequencing

Determination of nucleotide sequence in a DNA molecule is called DNA sequencing. It is done by several methods, e.g., Maxam and Gilbert technique, dideoxynucleotide method,

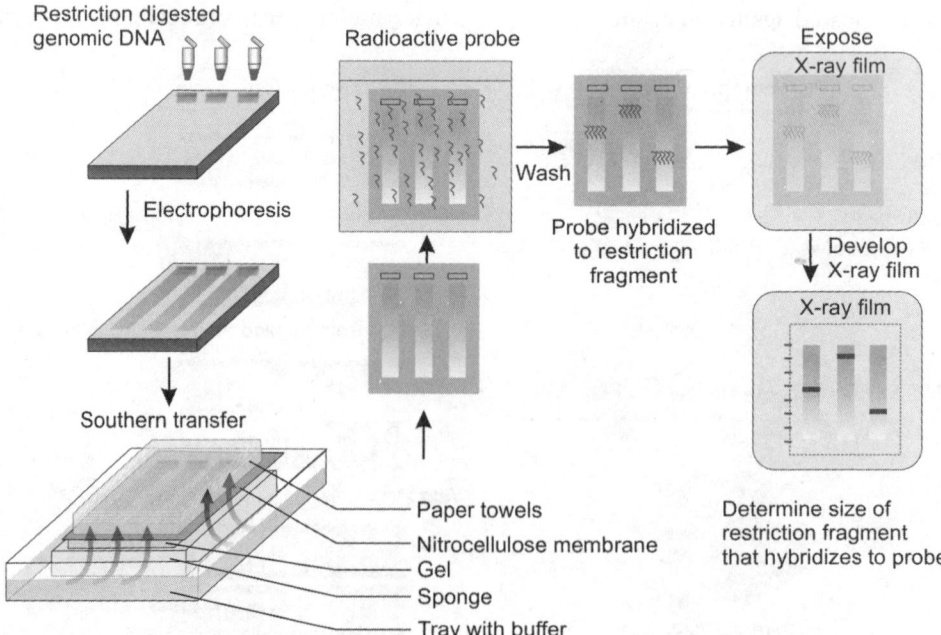

Fig. 26.18: Southern blotting.

automated sequencing, etc. This technique is important to understand gene functions and manipulation, DNA cloning and genetic disorders.

DNA Finger Printing

It is the genetic detective in medical forensics. This technique is the analysis of the nitrogenous base sequence in the DNA of an individual. It uses minute quantities of DNA from blood strains, body fluid, skin fragments, or hair fiber.

Applications
- Settlement of paternity disputes
- Identification of thieves, criminals and rapists, etc.
- Immigration cases and disputes

Gene Therapy

Artificial repair of the defective gene or introduction of a functional gene that can replace the defective gene is called gene therapy.

Types
- Somatic cell gene therapy
- Germline gene therapy

Methods
- Physical methods
- Viral vectors

Steps
- Isolate the healthy gene with the sequence controlling its expression.
- Incorporate this gene into a vector (carrier) as an expression gene.
- Finally deliver the vector into the target cells.

Defective cell
↓ Defective gene removed
Vector with new gene
↓ Introduced into cell
Patient with normal cell

Gene therapy has been accomplished in the following disorders.
- Severe combined immunodeficiency (SCID)
- Cystic fibrosis
- Hemophilia
- Sickle cell anemia

Uses/Applications/Targets
- Single gene disorders
- Cancer
- Cardiovascular diseases
- AIDS

■ HUMAN GENOME PROJECT

This project was undertaken in 1990 by the US Department of Energy and US National Institutes of Health and 16 centers all over the world collaborated with it. Its purpose was to decode the whole human genome and to sequence the whole human DNA. James Watson was the first Director of the project. The final version was announced in November 2002 by Francis Collins and Craig Venter.

Steps for Genome Sequencing
- DNA sequencing
- Use of DNA probes
- Hybridization
- PCR
- Cloning vectors
- Data analysis

Benefits
- Identification of human genes and their functions
- Improved diagnosis of genetic disorders
- Improvement in gene therapy
- Improved knowledge on mutations
- Understanding complex social trait

> **Note**
> Human genome contains about 30,000 genes.

Risks
- May discriminate individuals with substandard genome sequences
- May promote racial discrimination

27 Immunology

Chapter Outline
- Definitions
- Organization of the Immune System
- Monoclonal Antibodies

DEFINITIONS

- *Immunology:* It is the study of process by which the body defends itself from the invasion and attack of foreign organisms (Fig. 27.1).
- *Immunity:* It is the sum of all naturally occurring defense mechanisms that protect humans from infectious diseases.
- *Types of immunity:* It is of two types:
    1. *Innate immunity (nonspecific):* It refer to the immediate defense against the pathogenic organisms (not specific to any particular microbe), e.g., skin, secretions of mucus, phagocytic white blood cells (WBCs) (macrophages and neutrophils).
    2. *Acquired immunity (specific/adaptive):* It specifically recognizes and eliminates the invading microorganisms and foreign molecules (antigens). It is of two subtypes:
        a. *Cell-mediated immunity:* It is mediated by T-lymphocytes (T cells). They develop in thymus. They defend the body from the invasion of fungi, parasite, foreign substances, etc.
        b. *Humoral immunity:* It is mediated by a specific group of proteins called immunoglobulins (antibodies). These are produced by B-lymphocytes (B cells).

Antigen

An antigen can be defined as a substance capable of generating antibody on introduction into a suitable host. They may be proteins, carbohydrates, lipids, and nucleic acids.

Antibodies

These are immunoglobulins. They are immunologically active proteins and are glycoproteins. They are present in the γ-globulin fraction of serum. They are formed in response to an antigen and react specifically with that antigen. They are formed by B-lymphocytes which are found in serum, body fluids, and tissues. Their general function is to give immunity to the body.

Types of Immunoglobulins

There are five types of immunoglobulins (*refer* Chapter 4).

ORGANIZATION OF THE IMMUNE SYSTEM (FIG. 27.2)

It consists of several organs of the body (lymphoid organs).

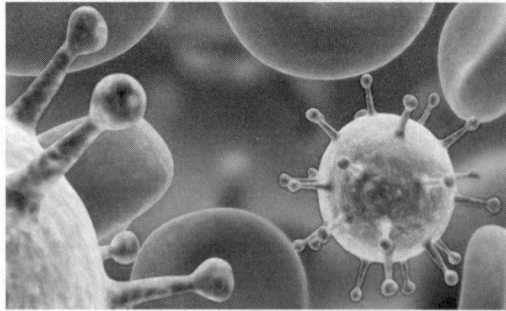

Fig. 27.1: Immunology.
(*For color version, see Plate 5*)

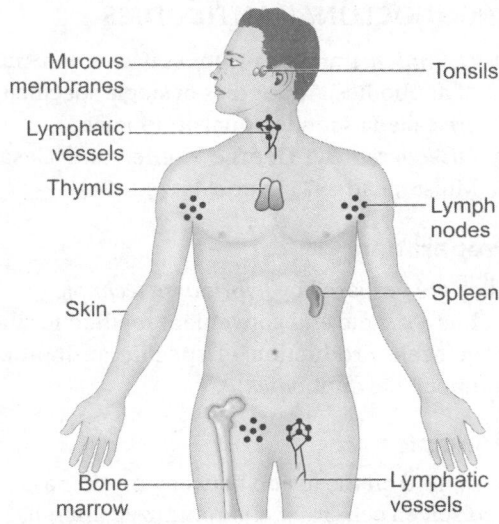

Fig. 27.2: Immune system.

1. Primary lymphoid organs:
   - Thymus—involved in cell-mediated immunity
   - Bone marrow—involved in humoral immunity.
2. Secondary lymphoid organs: For example spleen, tonsil, lymph nodes, appendix, intestine. They serve as sites for the initiation of an immune response.

Cells involved in the immune systems: Various types of white blood cells (leukocytes) carryout the immune response. Among them, the following two types of cells only act as major cells. All blood cells of the immune system originate in bone marrow stem cells.
- *T-lymphocytes:* T-lymphocytes also originate in the bone marrow, but their maturation occurs in the thymus. T-cells are involved in cell-mediated immunity.
  Types of T-cells:
  - Inducer T-cells
  - Cytotoxic T-cells
  - Helper T-cells
  - Suppressor T-cells
- *B-lymphocytes:* B-lymphocytes undergo development and maturation in the bone marrow. They recognize specifically each antigen and produce antibodies (immunoglobulins). They are involved in humoral immunity.

The Complement System

It refers to a group of immunologically distinct proteins present in the plasma and body fluids. It is the humoral mediator of antigen-antibody reactions. They are formed in liver. There are at least 20 complement proteins (c_1 to c_{20}). Their general functions are:
- Lysis of the cell membrane of foreign invading cells
- Phagocytosis of foreign cells
- Stimulation of local inflammatory reaction
- Clearance of antigen-antibody complexes from the body

Major Histocompatibility Complex

Major histocompatibility complex (MHC) refers to a cluster of proteins which occur on the cell surface of T-lymphocytes responsible for immune response transplantation antigens and proteins of the complement system. Their general functions are:
- Production of human leukocyte antigen (HLA) and immune associated antigens.
- Control of the levels of complement components
- T-cell recognition
- Graft rejection
- Genetic markers

Cytokines

The cells of the immune system and nonimmune cells release a group of proteins which bring about communication between different types of cells involved in immunity, e.g., interleukins, interferons. They are used in the treatment of cancer and immunodeficiency diseases.

Clinical Aspects of Immunology

Clinical aspects of immunology deal with man and his diseases. The immune system is primarily concerned with protection, but it can occasionally go wrong and be the cause of:
- *Hypersensitivity:* It refers to increased reactivity to an antigen. It is known as allergy.

- *Immunodeficiency:* It indicates susceptibility to an infection. It is due to the defect in the immunosystem resulting in the depression or hypofunction of the immune system.
- *Autoimmune diseases:* Autoimmune disorders occur when the immune system mistakenly targets the body's own cells or tissues. For example:
  - Rheumatoid arthritis
  - Celiac disease
  - Myasthenia gravis
  - Multiple sclerosis

Applications of Immunology

In Medicine
- Transplantation immunology
- Diagnosis (cancer, AIDS)
- Immunization (vaccination)
- Immunotherapy

Others
- Genetics
- Evolution

Immunological Techniques

These are based on in vitro antigen-antibody reactions.
- *Conventional techniques:* Widal test, Venereal disease research laboratory (VDRL) test, etc.
- *Isotopic and nonisotopic techniques:* Radioimmunoassay (RIA) and enzyme linked immunosorbent assay (ELISA) respectively (*refer* Chapter 28).
- *Molecular techniques*, e.g., hybridoma technology (*refer* below).
- *Others:* Immunoelectrophoresis.

MONOCLONAL ANTIBODIES

- *Definition:* Immune response is a random mix of antibodies. Antibodies of single specificity are called as monoclonal antibodies.
- *Discovered by:* George Kohler and Cesar Millstone in 1975 (Nobel Prize 1984).

Preparation

They are prepared by *hybridoma technology*.

It is a simple and convenient method for the large scale production of specific antibodies (monoclonal antibodies).

Principle

It is based on the fusion between myeloma cells and spleen cells from an immunized animal.

Method

- The appropriate animal is immunized with antigen under study.
- Suitable drug resistant myeloma cells are fused with plasma cells obtained from the spleen of the immunized animal.
- From the growing hybrid cells, individual clone can be selected, which produces specific antibodies and cloned.

Applications

Monoclonal antibodies produced by hybridoma technology are used for:
- Early detection of pregnancy
- Treatment of autoimmune diseases
- Detection and treatment of cancer
- Diagnosis of leprosy

28 Clinical Biochemistry

> **Chapter Outline**
> - Definition
> - Historical Background
> - Instrumentation and Techniques in Clinical Biochemistry
> - Types of Biochemical Tests
> - Refer: Other Topics Related to Clinical Biochemistry
> - Normal Values (Reference range)

■ DEFINITION

Clinical biochemistry **(Fig. 28.1)** is the study of biochemical processes associated with health and disease. It includes the measurement of substances in the body fluids [blood, urine, cerebrospinal fluid (CSF), etc.] or tissues to facilitate diagnosis of disease and monitoring of treatment.

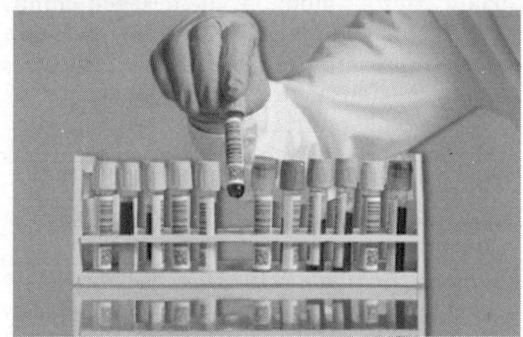

Fig. 28.1: Clinical biochemistry.
(For color version, see Plate 5)

Alternative Names

- Clinical chemistry
- Chemical pathology

■ HISTORICAL BACKGROUND

The field of clinical biochemistry had its real inception in the 20th century with the development of organic chemistry and biochemistry. Significant progress was made in measurement of biochemical constituents but was hindered by the lack of precise and reliable techniques. The development of instrumentation (colorimeter, pH meter, etc.) led to accurate quantitative techniques within reasonable time for analysis. With automation devised by Dr Leonard Skeggs in 1957, clinical biochemistry laboratory (CBL) was able to provide timely information on the ever-growing number of samples. Various automated instruments aided by computer driven systems to be used in clinical biochemistry were invented in the later part of the 20th century and the progress still continues in the 21st century. Thus, clinical biochemistry laboratory is an indispensable partner in medicine, contributing to the diagnosis and treatment of patients.

Branches

Clinical biochemistry is a branch of biochemistry. It has wider applications in several areas of medicine. It is the major division of the clinical laboratory services in the hospital **(Fig. 28.2)**.

Scope

- To study the levels of the constituents of the blood, urine, and CSF, etc., in normal state and their changes in diseases.

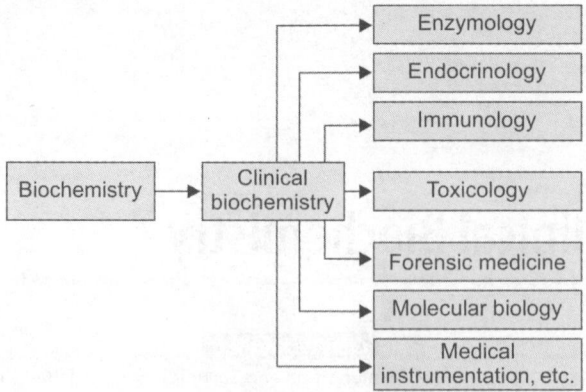

Fig. 28.2: Clinical biochemistry branches.

- To apply the suitable treatment and monitor it by estimating the relevant parameters at required intervals.

INSTRUMENTATION AND TECHNIQUES IN CLINICAL BIOCHEMISTRY

The following instruments and techniques are used in clinical biochemistry laboratory according to their needs (*refer* Chapter 29):
- Colorimeter
- Spectrophotometer
- pH meter
- Electrolyte analyzers (flame photometer/ISE)
- Blood gas analyzer
- Hormone analyzer
- Autoanalyzers
- Centrifuge
- Electrophoresis
- Chromatography
- Enzyme-linked immunosorbent assay (ELISA)
- Glucometer

Management

The clinical biochemistry laboratory is managed by clinical biochemists maintaining strict quality control and technicians work under their supervision.

Quality Control in Clinical Biochemistry Laboratory

Quality control in the clinical biochemistry laboratory (CBL) refers to the reliability of investigations. It can be defined as the sources of variation and procedures used to identify and rectify them.

Sources of Variation

- Preanalysical errors
- Analytical errors
- Post-analytical errors

Results from a laboratory that do not maintain quality control cannot be relied. Hence various steps/factors in the laboratory to maintain quality control are given importance. It involves four interrelated factors as given below.

1. *Precision:* Reproducibility of the result when the sample is analyzed on different occasions by same person.
2. *Accuracy:* Closeness of the estimated result to the true value.
3. *Specificity:* Ability of the analytical method to specifically determine a particular parameter.
4. *Sensitivity:* Ability of a particular method to detect small quantities of the measured constituent.

Methods of Quality Control

There are two methods usually employed to maintain quality control in the clinical biochemistry laboratory.
1. *Internal quality control:* It means the analysis of the same pooled sample on different days in a laboratory and the results may vary within a narrow range.
2. *External quality control:* It refers to the analysis of a sample received from external sources (quality control centers) and comparing the results.

External quality control centers:
- Christian Medical College, Vellore, Tamil Nadu
- Biorad company

Anticoagulants

Chemical agents that prevent coagulation of blood are known as anticoagulants. They are used for performing biochemical tests or hematological examination.

1. *Heparin:* It converts prothrombin to thrombin. It is an ideal anticoagulant because it does not cause any change in composition of blood. It is used for estimating Na^+, K^+, Cl^- in plasma. But it is costlier to use.
2. *Potassium oxalate-sodium oxalate:* These substances precipitate calcium and inhibit blood coagulation.
3. *Potassium oxalate sodium fluoride:* This mixture of two anticoagulants are used for collecting blood to estimate glucose. Sodium fluoride inhibits glycolysis and preserves blood glucose level.
4. *Ethylenediaminetetraacetate (EDTA):* It chelates with calcium and prevents coagulation. It is mostly used for hematological examinations.

Analysis of Body Fluids

Healthy individuals have normal range of constituents in body fluids. But once affected by a disease or abnormality, chemical composition of body fluids may change (mostly increased and rarely decreased). It can be considered as an indication of abnormal or pathological defect which can be diagnosed by analysis of body fluids.

Collection of Blood (Fig. 28.3)

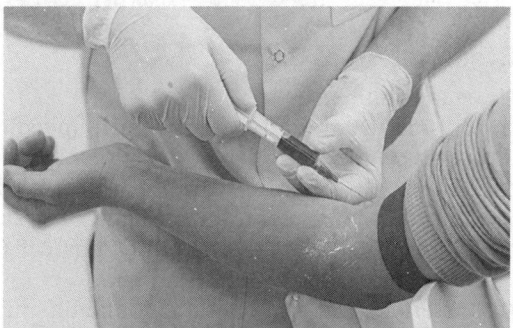

Fig. 28.3: Blood collection.
(For color version, see Plate 5)

Venous Blood

Using a sterile needle and syringe, blood is drawn from antecubital vein or some other prominent veins of the forearm under aseptic conditions. Venous blood is mostly used for biochemical investigations.

Arterial Blood

Arterial blood is collected from radial artery or femoral artery. It is mostly required for analysis of blood gases.

Capillary Blood

It is collected from tip of the thumb or finger after pricking with a lancet. It is used for instant estimation of blood sugar by glucometer in biochemistry and hematological examination.

Separation of Plasma or Serum from Blood

Blood drawn by venipuncture is collected into a sterile test tube.

Whole Blood

Collect the blood into a test tube with a proper anticoagulant. It is used for estimating hemoglobin, sugar, urea, lactate, NH_3.

Plasma

Collect the blood into a test tube with a proper anticoagulant. It is centrifuged at 3,000 rpm for 5 minutes. Plasma is collected carefully into another test tube with a dropper. It is mostly used for the estimation of glucose, fibrinogen, electrolytes.

Serum

Collect the blood into a plain sterile test tube. Keep it in a slanting position for 30–45 minutes and centrifuge at 3,000 rpm for 5 minutes. Collect the serum (supernatant) into another test tube with a dropper. Most of the parameters are estimated in serum, e.g., proteins, cholesterol, creatinine, bilirubin, uric acid, electrolytes, enzymes, etc.

> **Note**
> ☞ Nowadays color coded vacutainer tubes are used according to the specimen type required (serum/plasma/blood) **(Fig. 28.4)**.
> ☞ Utmost care should be taken to avoid hemolysis if serum or plasma is used for biochemical analysis.

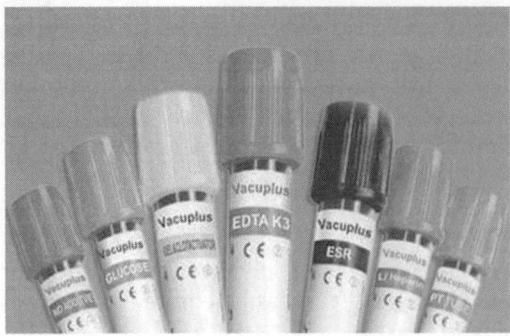

Fig. 28.4: Vacutainer tubes.
(For color version, see Plate 5)

Collection of Cerebrospinal Fluid

CSF is a colorless clear fluid of the nervous system. It is formed by selective dialysis of the plasma by choroid plexuses of the ventricles of the brain. Total volume of CSF is about 130 mL. For analysis it is collected from spinal canal by lumbar puncture by well trained physician. It is examined for sugar, protein, and chloride in biochemical laboratory (*refer* Appendix G: Normal value chart).

Collection of Urine

Urine is an excretory waste product of the body formed in the kidneys. The physical and chemical analysis of urine is an important part of the routine urine analysis. Properties and composition of urine gives an insight to various diseases. Detection of abnormal constituents is done for suspected renal pathology and systemic diseases.
- Urine samples should be voided directly into clean and dry containers **(Fig. 28.5)**.

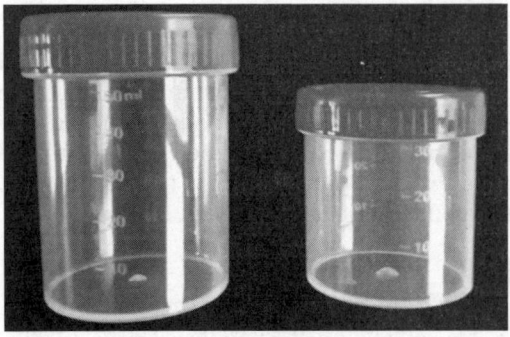

Fig. 28.5: Urine containers.
(For color version, see Plate 5)

- Initial stream of voided urine is discarded to avoid contamination with organisms in the distal urethra. Then midstream urine is collected.
- A random urine sample is satisfactory for routine investigation. First morning sample is desirable for normal analysis.
- 24 hours urine is preferable for determination of protein, creatinine, calcium, uric acid. For this, the patient is instructed to collect the urine sample from 8 AM to next day 8 AM in a clean and dry container with a proper preservative.

Preservation of Urine

- Urine analysis must be done within 1–2 hour of collection of urine
- Urine standing for long time may undergo several changes.

For example, lysis of blood cells, changes in pH, urinary decomposition, turbidity due to bacterial growth, precipitation of phosphates, etc.

Preservatives

Various preservatives are used for collection of 24 hours urine sample, for example:
- Hydrochloric acid (10 mL): For estimation of creatinine, calcium, ammonia and 17-keto steroids.
- Thymol (few crystals): For determination of sodium, potassium chloride, bicarbonate, protein, etc.
- Toluene
- Formalin

Note
Collected urine must be preserved in the refrigerator at 4°C with chemical preservative, if analysis is delayed.

Examination of Urine

Urine is examined as:
- Physical examination (color, pH, specific gravity, etc.)
- Chemical examination [normal and abnormal constituents (*refer* Chapter 19)]
- Microscopic examination (RBC, pus cells, etc.)
- Bacteriological examination (contaminants, etc.)

Table 28.1: Types of biochemical tests.

Type of tests	Purpose
Routine tests	Common clinical biochemistry tests: To assess general health, e.g., estimation of glucose (sugar), urea, cholesterol, etc.
Specific tests	Hormone analysis, T_3, T_4, TSH, stone analysis, etc.
Biochemical profile	A group of tests rather than a single test to get information about a particular disease status. For example, renal profile—urea, creatinine, etc., lipid profile, protein A/G ratio SGPT, γGT, bilirubin etc., for LFT
Function tests	To assess the functions of specific organ. For example, liver function tests, renal function tests
Screening tests	To identify the inborn errors of metabolism. For example, phenylketonuria, galactosemia, etc.
Emergency tests	To perform on urgent basis to help the clinician to decide the course of the treatment. For example, estimation of glucose, urea creatinine and electrolytes in the blood

Note: Clinical biochemistry tests are performed in the laboratory of diagnostic. Division of the hospital attached to medical colleges.
Names of the tests: Refer Appendix G: Normal value chart.

TYPES OF BIOCHEMICAL TESTS

The tests performed in the clinical biochemistry laboratory is shown in **Table 28.1**.

REFER: OTHER TOPICS RELATED TO CLINICAL BIOCHEMISTRY

1. Water (fluid) and electrolyte balance (Chapter 22)
2. Acid base balance (Chapter 23)
3. Organ function tests (Chapter 24)
4. Inborn errors of metabolism (respective Chapter/Appendix C)
5. Diagnostic enzymes (Chapter 7)
6. Tumor markers (Chapter 34)
7. Blood sugar regulation (Chapter 11)
8. Blood calcium regulation (Chapter 17)
9. Abnormal urine (Chapter 19)
10. Plasma proteins (Chapter 4)

Diseases

Various diseases occur due to biochemical abnormalities (selective list only is given below).
1. Diabetes mellitus (Chapter 11)
2. Atherosclerosis (Chapter 12)
3. Gout (Chapter 15)
4. Jaundice (Chapter 16)
5. Vitamin deficiency diseases (Chapter 8)
6. Mineral deficiency diseases (Chapter 17)
7. Hormone (endocrine) disorders (Chapter 25)
8. Nutritional disorders (Chapter 21)
9. Immunological disorders (Chapters 3 and 27)
10. Molecular diseases (Chapter 26)

Biochemical changes and abnormalities are summarized in **Table 28.2**.

Table 28.2: Abnormalities and biochemical changes.

Sl. No.	Diseases/ abnormalities	Biochemical changes
1.	Diabetes mellitus	Blood glucose and HbA_1C increased
2.	Nutritional disorders	Serum albumin is low in kwashiorkor (protein malnutrition)
3.	Endocrine function	TSH is low in hyperthyroidism and high in hypothyroidism
4.	Organ function tests	Liver failure—serum bilirubin and SGPT (ALT) increased
5.	Genetic diseases	Ammonia (NH_3) increased in urea cycle disorders phenylalanine increased in phenylketonuria (IEM)
6.	Myocardial infarction (MI)	CPK, SGOT (AST), and cardiotroponin I in serum elevated

Contd...

Contd...

Sl. No.	Diseases/ abnormalities	Biochemical changes
7.	Cancer	Tumor markers increased in serum, PSA in prostate cancer
8.	Acidosis and alkalosis	Changes in blood pH
9.	Inflammation/ infection	C-reactive protein increased
10.	Poisons	Serum butyl cholinesterase decreased in organophosphorus poisoning

NORMAL VALUES (REFERENCE RANGE)

Laboratory tests are procedures wherein a sample of blood, urine or other body fluid are checked to assess a person's health. The results of the test will show if a person is within the normal laboratory values. Normal values are based on several factors:

- Method employed
- Time of collection of blood
- Age, sex
- Ethnic group
- Laboratory conditions

In a healthy population, the range that includes 95% of target population is considered to be the reference range. Statistically, a mean of ± 2 S D is considered to be normal range. The values of the analyte outside the reference range are considered to be abnormal values.

(*Refer* Appendix G: Normal value chart)

29. Instrumentation and Techniques in Biochemistry

Chapter Outline

- Colorimetry
- Spectrophotometer
- Electrolyte Analyzer
- Autoanalyzers
- Glucometer
- Blood Gas Analyzers
- Hormone Analyzers
- pH meter
- Clinical Centrifuge
- Chromatography
- Electrophoresis
- Radioimmunoassay
- Enzyme-linked Immunosorbent Assay
- **Biochemical Laboratory Instruments**

INTRODUCTION

Various instruments and techniques are being used/applied in the diverse areas of biochemistry and clinical biochemistry. Some of these instruments are manually operated and others are electrically operated with/without computer control.
- *Analytical biochemistry:* To analyze cell constituents, e.g., ultracentrifugation, homogenizer, etc.
- *Clinical service:* To analyze the constituents of body fluids [blood, urine, cerebrospinal fluid (CSF), etc.] in the diagnosis and prognosis of disease, e.g., colorimeter, autoanalyzer, etc.
- *Research:* To analyze the molecular basis of disease, e.g., chromatography electrophoresis, blotting techniques, etc.

COLORIMETRY

Colorimetry (photometry) is the technique used to find out the concentration of the substances accurately based on the principle of absorption of light by the molecules in solution. The following are the instruments based on this principle/technique.

Colorimeter (Fig. 29.1)

Colorimeter works on the principle of Beer-Lambert law.
- *Beer's law:* The intensity of the color is directly proportional to the concentration of the absorbing molecules in solution.
- *Lambert's law:* The amount of light absorbed by a colored solution depends on the length of the column or the depth of the liquid through which the light passes.
- *Beer-Lambert's law:* It combines these two laws and is expressed as follows:

The amount of light absorbed by a colored solution is directly proportional to its concentration and the depth of the liquid through which light passes. It is operative in the visible range (400–700 nm).

Parts of a Colorimeter (Figs. 29.1A to F)

- Tungsten lamp (light source) **(Fig. 29.1A)**
- Condenser lens (to provide parallel beam) **(Fig. 29.1B)**
- Cuvettes (made up of special glass tube to hold solution) **(Fig. 29.1C)**
- Filter (to select monochromatic light) **(Fig. 29.1D)**

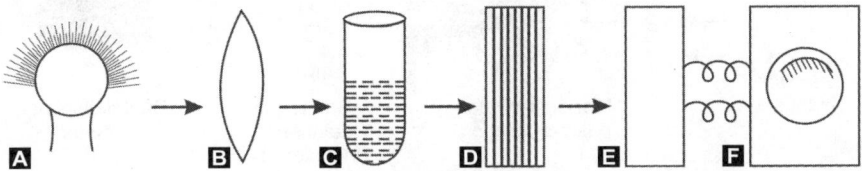

Figs. 29.1A to F: Parts of a colorimeter.

- Photocell (detector) **(Fig. 29.1E)**
- Galvanometer (digital or analogue meter) **(Fig. 29.1F)**

Operation of a Colorimeter

- The instrument is connected to the main.
- Instrument is first adjusted to zero optical density (OD) or 100% transmission (T) after keeping the proper filter and the cuvette with water (blank).
- The substance to be measured is prepared as a colored derivative, taken in the cuvette and placed in the colorimeter and measured (test OD).
- Similarly, a standard solution containing the known concentration of the same substance is treated and measured (standard OD).
- The concentration of the substance can be calculated as follows:

$$\frac{\text{Test OD}}{\text{Standard OD}} \times \text{Concentration of Standard}$$

Applications

- Most of the clinical biochemistry estimations (blood sugar, urea, cholesterol, etc.) are performed using colorimeters.
- They give more accurate results compared to other quantitative estimations.

■ SPECTROPHOTOMETER

Parts (Fig. 29.2)

- Source of light
  - Tungsten lamp—emits visible light (400–700 nm)
  - Deuterium lamp—emits UV radiation (200–400 mm)
- Monochrometer by diffraction grating
- Cuvettes—quartz cuvettes
- Photocell
- Galvanometer

Working

It mostly resembles operation of a colorimeter, but uses various ranges of wavelength through diffraction gradings.

Advantages

- Used to estimate the concentration of substance in both colored and colorless solution.
- Quick and accurate results than colorimeter
- Measurement at both visible and UV region
- More sophisticated than colorimeter
- Minute quantities of substances can be estimated

■ ELECTROLYTE ANALYZER

Flame Photometer

It is used for quantitative analysis of electrolytes (sodium, potassium, chloride, etc.) in the blood and urine. It operates on the principle of measurement of emitted light. The fluid or solution after proper dilution is sprayed on the flame of a burner. It evaporates in the flame and light of characteristic wavelength is emitted by the atoms. The intensity of the emitted light is measured by a galvanometer and it is proportional to the concentration of the electrolyte being estimated.

Parts (Fig. 29.3)

- *Flame (burner):* It is present within the instrument needed for temperature control and the heatup the solution.
- *Nebulizer:* It breaks up the sample into atoms.
- *Mixing chamber:* It mixes the relevant solution with the sample.
- *Color filters:* Specific filter for analytes.
- *Photodetector:* It shows which metal the sample contains and to what concentration level.

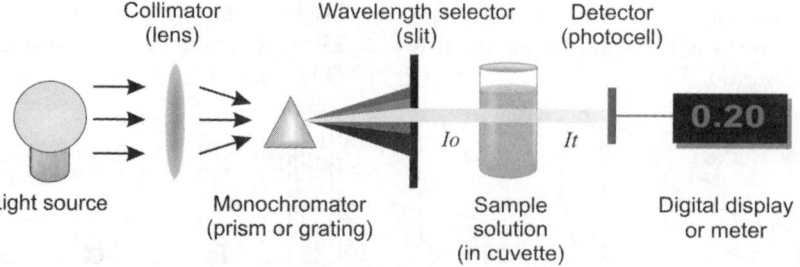

Fig. 29.2: Parts of spectrophotometer.

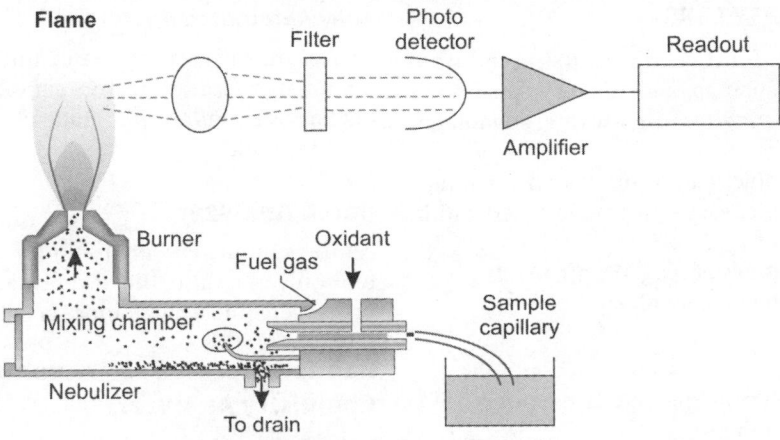

Fig. 29.3: Parts of flame photometer.

Ion Selective Electrode/Electrolyte Analyzer

Ion selective electrode (ISE) is a transducer (sensor) which converts the activity of a specific ion dissolved in solution into an electrical potential which is measured by a voltmeter. ISE is the modern analytical tool for the fast and direct ion activity determination of sample solution/body fluids **(Fig. 29.4)**.

Parts

- Reference electrode probe
- Specific ion probe
- Voltmeter, display, cable wires
- Case housing both electrodes
- Internal buffer
- Ion selective membrane

Advantages

- Easy to operate
- Wide concentration measurement
- Unaffected by sample color or turbidity
- Fast results than flame photometer
- Used for the diagnosis of fluid and electrolyte disorders by measurement of Na^+, K^+, Cl^- in plasma/urine.

Model

Figure 29.4 shows ion selective electrode (ISE).

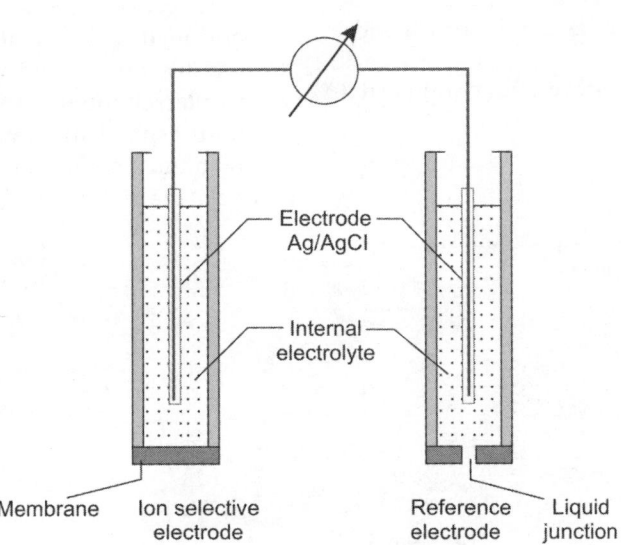

Fig. 29.4: Ion selective electrode (ISE).

AUTOANALYZERS

Analysis of blood samples using manual instruments, such as colorimeter takes longer time. But autoanalyzers offer several advantages as follows:
- Several samples can be processed at a time
- Very accurate results can be obtained within a short time
- Microquantities of reagents are used
- Minimum labor is involved

Types

They are broadly divided into two types:
1. Semiautoanalyzers
2. Fully automated analyzers

Semiautoanalyzers

The initial part of the procedure, (i.e., pipetting of reagents and specimen mixing and incubation) is carried out manually. Rest of the procedure, i.e., setting of the incubation temperature (kinetic determination), zero setting, photometric readings, results display, automatic printing and data management and processing is carried out by the analyzers.

Advantages

- Semiautoanalyzers are cheap and compact compared to fully automated analyzers
- Reagents are not corrosive and less quantity of reagents and samples are used
- Minimum labor is required
- Though it can process one parameter at a time, several samples can be processed at faster rate.
- Accurate results obtained compared to colorimeter results.

Model

See **Figure 29.5**.

Fully Automated Analyzers

There are different types of fully automated autoanalyzers. Starting from sample pipetting to display of results are automatically done without manual work.

Batch Analyzer

All the samples are analyzed for one constitutent only at a time. But several samples can be processed quickly with more accuracy.

Random Access Fully Automated Chemistry Analyzers

Fully Automated Analyzers

A fully automated analyzer is a medical laboratory instrument designed to measure different substances in a number of biological samples quickly with minimum human assistance when compared to semiautoanalyzers **(Fig. 29.6)**.

Discovered by: Leonard Skeggs in 1957, (Technicon Corporation USA)

Parts

- Sampler
- Proportionating pump
- Dialyzer
- Constant temperature
- Flow through colorimeter
- Recorder

Working

- All reagents necessary for the tests to be performed are kept in the proper cups.
- Samples are loaded into the cap of the sampler channels of the proportionating pump, aspirate them and dilute them
- The diluted serum samples are led through one of the dialyzer unit.

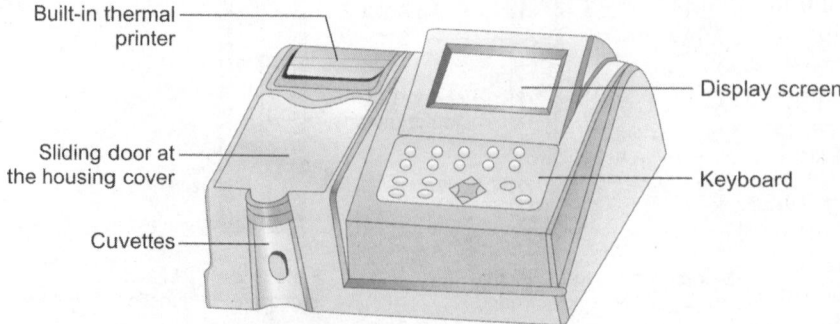

Fig. 29.5: Semiautoanalyzer parts.

Chapter 29: Instrumentation and Techniques in Biochemistry

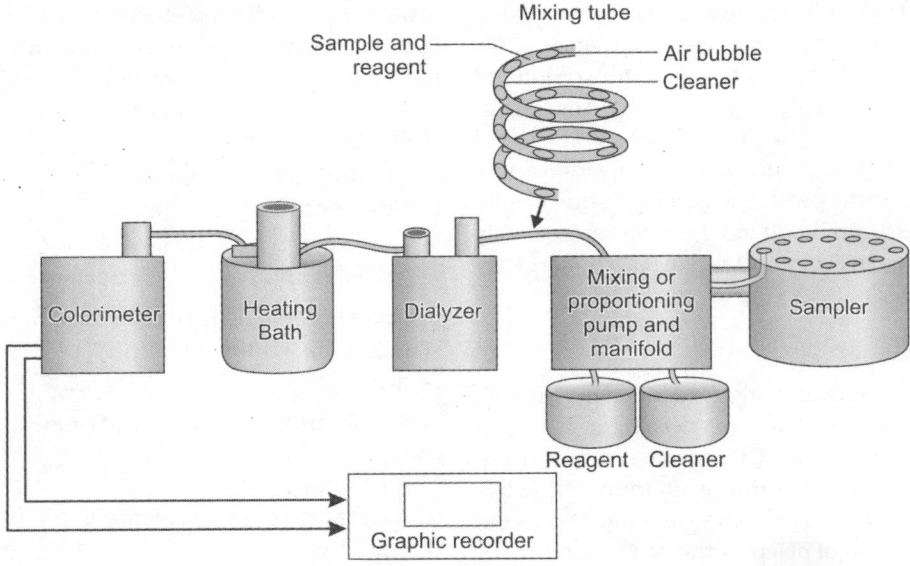

Fig. 29.6: Autoanalyzer parts.

- The pump introduces suitable reagents through other side of the dialyzer.
- A portion of dialyzable constituents of serum passes across the membrane to the reagent stream.
- Further treatment, such as incubation at suitable temperature is given in the constant temperature bath.
- The intensity of the color developed is measured in a colorimeter and recorded in the recorder.

Types
- Continuous flow autoanalyzers
- Centrifuge autoanalyzers
- Discrete autoanalyzers
- Dry chemistry autoanalyzers

Application/uses
- Speed and accuracy of results
- Very minimum labor involved
- Processing several parameters in a single sample at a time
- Increased quantum of clinical biochemical analysis
- Easy operation—automatic

Models (Fig. 29.6)
- Cobas fully automated biochemistry analyzers.
- Mindray fully automated biochemistry analyzers

Dry Chemistry Analyzer
The reagents used for the reaction are embedded on a plastic matrix. The color developed by addition of the sample to the matrix is measured by reflectance spectrophotometer. Glucometer used to measure blood sugar at home is also dry chemistry analyzer.

GLUCOMETER
Glucometer is a medical device for determining the concentration of glucose in the blood. It is mostly used for home monitoring of blood glucose level and for on the spot checking for hyperglycemia (diabetes mellitus) or hypoglycemia (coma). It was developed by Leland Clark and Ann Lyons in USA. At present several models of glucometers are available. A small drop of blood obtained by pricking the skin with a lancet is placed on a disposable test strip containing glucose reagents. The meter reads and calculates. The blood glucose level is displayed in units as mg/dL mmol/within few seconds.

BLOOD GAS ANALYZERS
Blood gas analyzers (ABG) are used to measure combinations of pH, blood gases (i.e., pO_2 and pCO_2) and related parameters from whole blood (mostly arterial blood). It gives indications about

the status of the lungs, heart, and kidneys during critical conditions (acid–base disorders).

ABG should be readily available and blood should be immediately accessible for urgent transfusion. An ABG test requires that a small volume of blood be drawn from the radial artery or femoral artery with a syringe and a thin needle and inject into blood gas analyzer immediately without delay. They are used in ICUs, emergency departments, operating theaters.

Principle

Electrodes are constructed of a permeable membrane and are bathed in a solution that allows H^+, O_2, CO_2 to pass through the membrane, react with the solution and cause a current or voltage change that equates to the measurement of pH, pO_2 and pCO_2.

Model

Radiometer blood gas analyzer.

■ HORMONE ANALYZERS

Nowadays hormone assays are performed by chemiluminescence immunoassay hormone analyzers than RIA. They are useful to assess the hormone status of the human body—infertility, diagnosis, metabolic studies, e.g., LH, FSH, GH, insulin, T_3, T_4, TSH, etc. Random sampling and continuous access sampling are two ways a hormone analyzer can process a sample.

Models

☐ Mindray hormone analyzer
☐ Vidas hormone analyzer

■ pH METER

pH meter is an electric device used to measure strength of acidity/alkalinity of a solution (Fig. 29.7).

The complete system of pH measurement consists of:
☐ A potentiometer
☐ A reference calomel electrode
☐ A glass electrode
☐ A solution of known pH

Modern pH meters are digital meters for accurate measurements.

pH of a solution can be determined more accurately by potential measurement of certain electrodes electrically. The common electrical method for determination of pH depends upon the use of glass electrode. It is based on the principle that when a glass membrane separates two different solutions differing in pH, a potential difference is found to exist between two surfaces

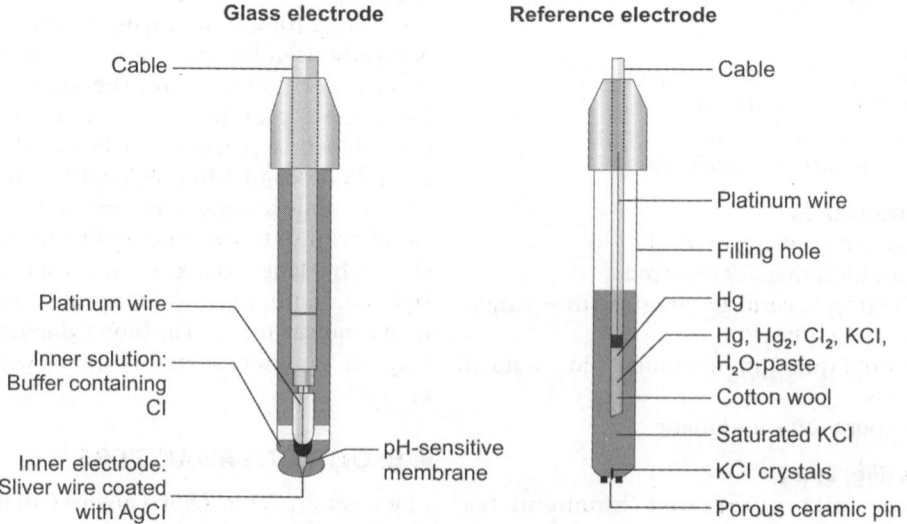

Fig. 29.7: Parts of pH meter.

of the glass. The potential is measured against a standard calomel electrode.

Uses/Applications: To Measure

- pH of fluids
- pH of soil in agriculture
- pH of water in water supplies
- pH of alcoholic drinks in brewing industry
- pH of different solutions in pharmaceuticals

■ CLINICAL CENTRIFUGE

Centrifuge is a laboratory equipment driven by a motor which spins liquid samples at high speed (rpm). Clinical centrifuge is used to separate serum/plasma from blood and to precipitate protein from a liquid mixture.

Ultracentrifuge

It is an important instrument for the isolation of high molecular weight compounds and subcellular organelles.

Principle: It is based on the sedimentation of particles or macromolecules at high centrifugal force (Svedberg units).

Developed by: Swedish scientist Svedberg (1923).

Process

- The biological sample containing the material to be isolated is subjected to required centrifugal force.
- At specific time, subcellular organelles are sedimented.
- They are separated by differential centrifugation.
  - 700 g × 10 min: Nuclear fraction sedimented
  - 15,000 g × 15 min: Mitochondrial fraction sedimented
  - 1,00,000 g × 60 min: Microsomal fraction sedimented.

Applications

- For isolation of subcellular organelles, e.g., ribosomes, mitochondria, etc.
- For isolation of proteins, lipoproteins and nucleic acids.
- For determination of molecular weights of macromolecules.

■ CHROMATOGRAPHY

Definition

Chromatography is an analytical technique by which members of a group of similar substances are separated by a continuous distribution between two phases namely stationary phase and mobile phase.

Uses

- To separate different amino acids/sugars from a mixture
- To purify enzymes, drugs, etc.
- To identify and separate the preservatives and additives added in the food items.

Introduced by: Tswett in 1906.

Types: It is divided into different types depending on the mode of separation and principles involved **(Fig. 29.8)**.

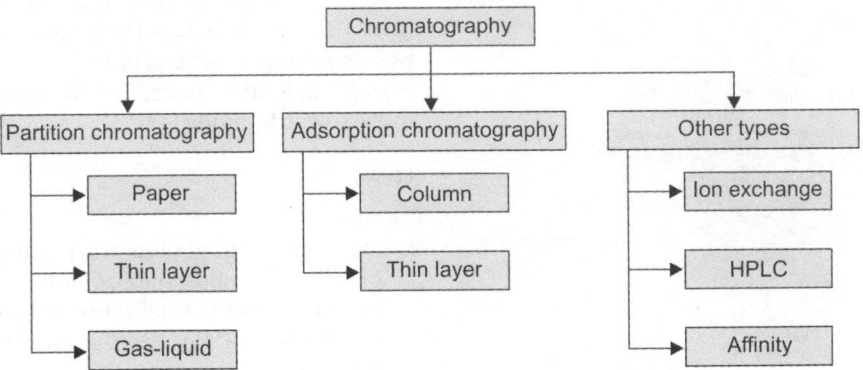

Fig. 29.8: Types of chromatography.
(HPLC: high performance liquid chromatography)

- Paper chromatography: It is of two types:
  1. *Ascending chromatography:* The mixture to be separated is applied as a small spot at one corner of the Whatman filter paper (2 cm from the edge) **(Fig. 29.9)**. It is dipped in the solvent system which usually consists of butanol-acetic acid and water (4:1:5 ratio) kept in a glass trough. Water is held back in the paper and is called as stationary phase. The organic solvent moving across is known as mobile phase. Run time is about 16 hours. Paper is removed, dried and developed as colored spots using spraying reagent (ninhydrin reagent for amino acids).

     The ratio of the distance travelled by the solute front divided by the distance travelled by the solvent front is known as Rf value (Ratio of fronts).

     $$Rf = \frac{\text{Distance travelled by the solute}}{\text{Distance travelled by the solvent front}}$$

     Each compound has a definite Rf value which helps in the identification of various amino acids, sugars, etc.
  2. *Descending chromatography:* In this type of paper chromatography, the solvent moves downwards. The details are almost similar to that of ascending paper chromatography.
- *Thin layer chromatography (TLC):* An inert substance (cellulose) is used instead of paper. It is spread as thin layer on glass or plastic plate. Separation is very rapid.
- *Gas liquid chromatography (GLC):* It is applied mainly for the separation of volatile substances and biological substances, such as lipids, drugs, etc.

Adsorption Chromatography

An absorbent (silica gel/alumina) is packed as a column into a glass tube (stationary phase). The sample mixture is loaded on this column. The components present in the mixture get differentially absorbed on the adsorbent and removed by a buffer (mobile phase) and identified.

Other Types

- *Ion exchange chromatography:* It involves the separation of molecules based on their electrical charges using ion exchange resins.
- *High pressure liquid chromatography (HPLC):* In this technique, high pressure in the range of 5,000–10,000 psi is applied to provide fine separation at a faster rate.
- *Affinity chromatography:* It is based on the property of specific and noncovalent binding of enzymes to other molecules (ligands) such as substrates or cofactors.

■ ELECTROPHORESIS

It is a widely used analytical (separation) technique in clinical diagnosis and research **(Fig. 29.10)**.

Definition

It refers to the migration of charged particles (ions) in an electrical field. Molecules with positive charge (cations) move towards cathode (–) and negative charged molecules (anions) move towards anode (+).

Uses

To separate:
- Different fractions of serum/plasma proteins, immunoglobulins, lipoproteins.
- Different types of isoenzymes of lactate dehydrogenase (LDH), creatine phosphokinase (CPK), etc.
- Different classes of hemoglobins
- Used for diagnosis of certain diseases, e.g., nephritic syndrome, multiple myeloma, etc.

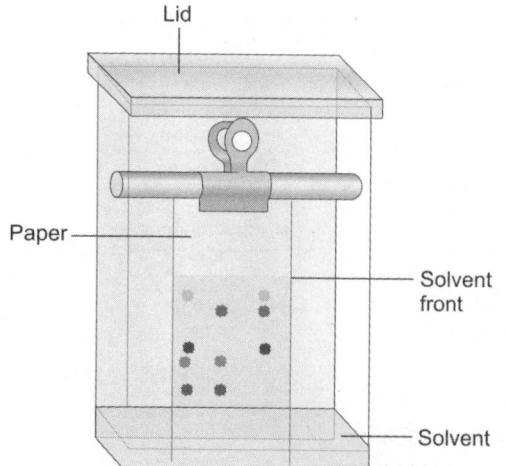

Fig. 29.9: Ascending chromatography.

Chapter 29: Instrumentation and Techniques in Biochemistry

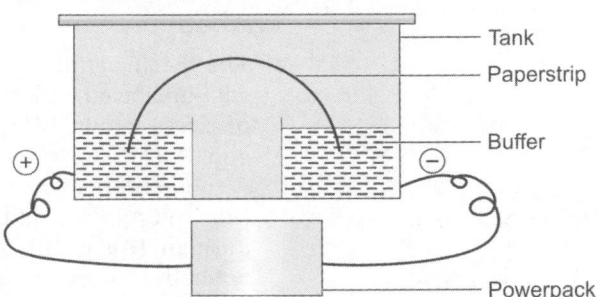

Fig. 29.10: Electrophoretic apparatus.

Types

- Moving boundary electrophoresis (discovered in 1937 by Tiselius).

  In this type, no support medium is used and separation occurs at boundary.

- Zonal electrophoresis (discovered in 1946 by Consoley).

  In this type, different types of support medium can be used on which sample is applied and gets separated, e.g:
  - Paper electrophoresis
  - Agar (agarose) electrophoresis
  - Disc electrophoresis
  - Immunoelectrophoresis

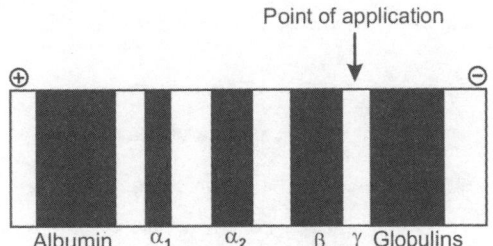

Fig. 29.11: Electrophoretic pattern.

Paper Electrophoresis

Serum proteins can be separated into albumin and different fractions of globulins by electrophoresis on paper as support medium. This process depends on the size of their molecular weight and charge **(Fig. 29.11)**.

It consists of two parts:
1. Electrophoresis powerpack
2. Electrophoresis tank

The filter paper strip is placed in an inverted V position hanging from a glass rod. The two ends of filter paper strip are made to dip in the barbitone buffer (pH 8.6) kept at two compartments. Apply 10 µL of serum on the paper strip. Buffer tank is closed with the lid. Switch on the current and allow to run for 3–4 hours. The paper is removed from the tank, dried at 80°C, stained with bromophenol blue and then destained with 5% acetic acid. It is again dried at room temperature for 1 hour. The separated protein fractions appear as blue colored bands and visualized as albumin and α_1, α_2, β and γ globulins. These bands which represent different fractions of protein can be quantitatively evaluated by elution with 40% NaOH or through scanning densitometer **(Figs. 29.12A and B)**. Normal pattern and abnormal pattern is shown in **Figure 29.13** and **Table 29.1**.

Agar (Agarose) Electrophoresis

The gel prepared in a buffer is spread on microscopic slide and cooled. A small quantity of sample is applied by cutting into the gel with a sharp edge. Serum proteins are separated within 1½ hour.

Table 29.1: Abnormal pattern—serum proteins.		
Protein fractions	**Normal %**	**Changes in disease**
Albumin globulins	55–65	Nephrotic syndrome–albumin decreased, α_2-globulin elevated
α_1	2–4	Multiple myeloma-M band appears in γ-globulin fraction
α_2	6–12	Chronic infection-γ-globulin is increased
β	8–14	Liver cirrhosis–albumin is decreased
γ	12–22	β-globulin is wide or fused with γ-globulins

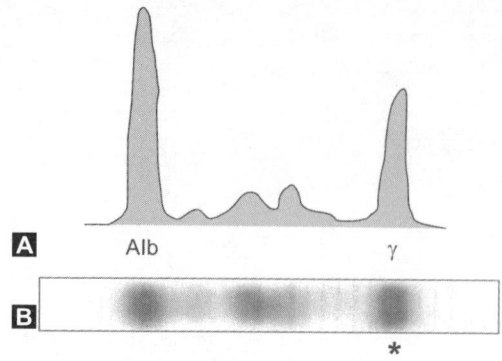

Figs. 29.12A and B: Electro pattern—normal.

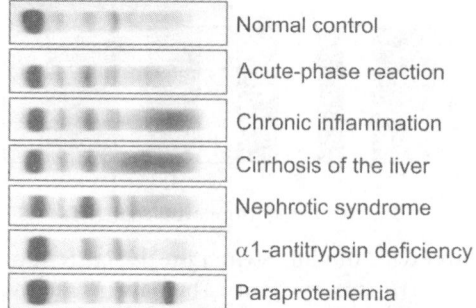

Fig. 29.13: Abnormal electrophoretic pattern.

Disc Electrophoresis (PAGE)

It depends on the separation of molecules based on their size as well as electrical charge. Isoenzymes of LDH and CPK are separated by this technique.

Immunoelectrophoresis

In this specific technique, electrophoretic separation is followed by an antigen-antibody reaction. It separates serum proteins into more than 40 bands.

■ RADIOIMMUNOASSAY

Radioimmunoassay (RIA) is a highly sensitive analytical technique. It is used for the estimation of several substances in biological fluids which are present in micro quantities, e.g., hormones.

Developed by: Solomon, Benson and Rosalyn Yalow in 1959.

Principle

It is based on the competition between the labeled and unlabeled antigen (substance to be estimated) to bind with antibody to form antigen antibody complex.

Method

- The specific antibody (Ab) is made to react with unlabeled antigen (Ag) in the presence of excess amount of isotopically labeled (^{131}I) antigen (Ag$^+$) with known radioactivity.
- A competition occurs between the antigens (Ag$^+$ and Ag) to bind the antibody. Labeled antigen (Ag$^+$) will bind more with the antibody.
- The labeled antigen-antibody (Ag$^+$-Ab) complex is precipitated and the radioactivity of ^{131}I present in Ag$^+$ Ab is determined.

Applications

- Estimation of hormones, drugs, proteins, nucleic acids
- Used in diagnosis of hormonal disorders, cancer, etc.
- Widely used in biomedical research.

■ ENZYME-LINKED IMMUNOSORBENT ASSAY

Enzyme-linked immunosorbent assay (ELISA) is a nonisotopic immunoassay. It is equally sensitive to RIA. Also there is no risk of radiation hazard **(Fig. 29.14)**. It was first described by Engvall and Perlmann in 1971.

Principle

It is based on the immunochemical principle of antigen-antibody reaction.

Method

- The biological specimen containing the protein to be estimated is applied on the antibody coated surface.
- The protein–antibody complex is then made to react with a second protein specific antibody to which an enzyme (e.g., peroxidase) is covalently linked.
- The unbound antibody linked enzyme is washed. The activity of the enzyme bound to the second antibody complex is assayed which is related to the concentration of protein to be estimated.

> **Note**
> Several types of ELISA are available **(Fig. 29.14)**:
> ☞ Direct
> ☞ Indirect
> ☞ Sandwich
> ☞ Competitive

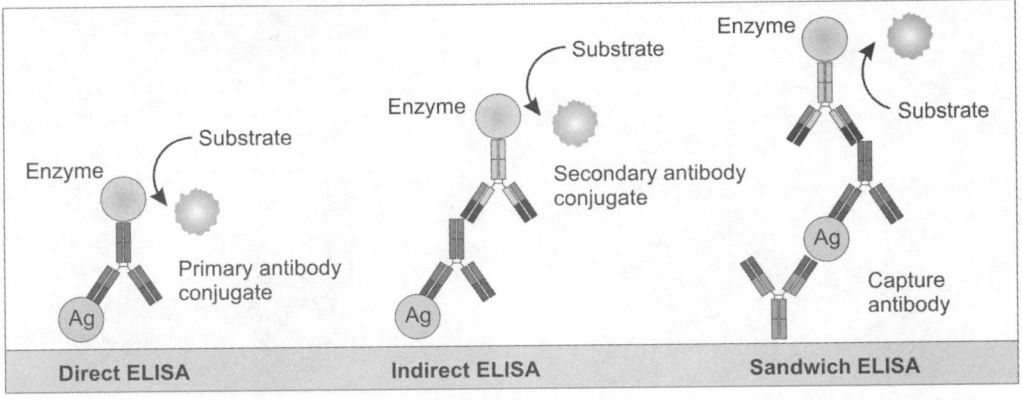

Fig. 29.14: ELISA steps.

Applications

- To determine small quantities of biological substances, e.g., hormones, antigen, antibodies, proteins, etc.
- To detect pregnancy within few days after conception. It is by detecting human chorionic gonadotropin (hCG) in urine
- To diagnose AIDS

Note
- Hybridoma technology: *Refer* Chapter 27.
- Blotting techniques: *Refer* Chapter 26.

BIOCHEMICAL LABORATORY INSTRUMENTS (FIGS. 29.15 TO 29.23)

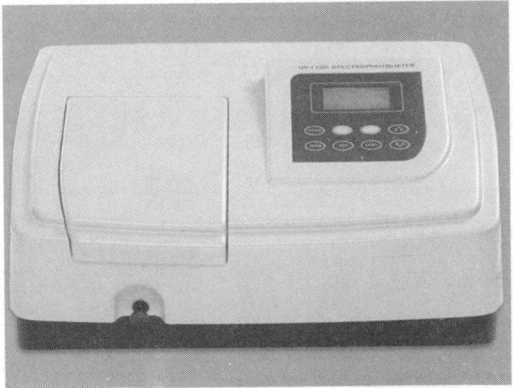

Fig. 29.16: Spectrophotometer.
(For color version, see Plate 6)

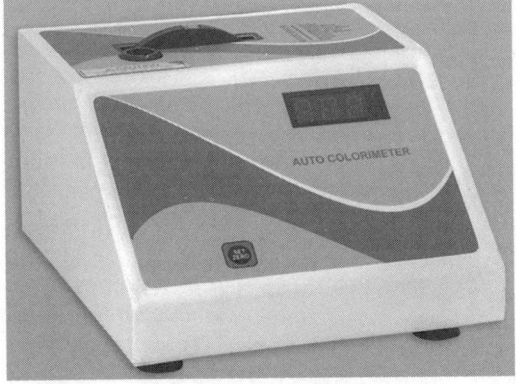

Fig. 29.15: Colorimeter.
(For color version, see Plate 5)

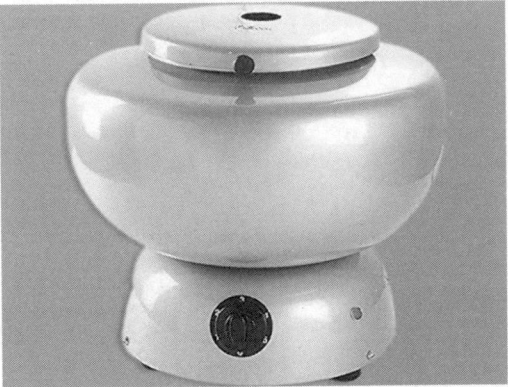

Fig. 29.17: Clinical centrifuge.
(For color version, see Plate 6)

Section 5: Applied Biochemistry

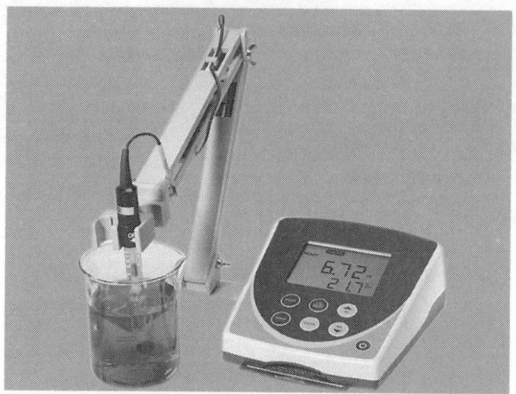

Fig. 29.18: pH meter.
(For color version, see Plate 6)

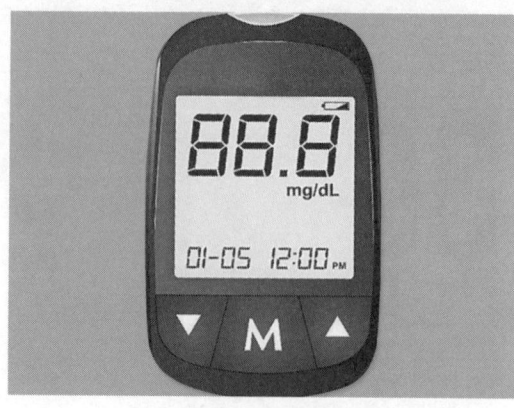

Fig. 29.21: Glucometer.
(For color version, see Plate 6)

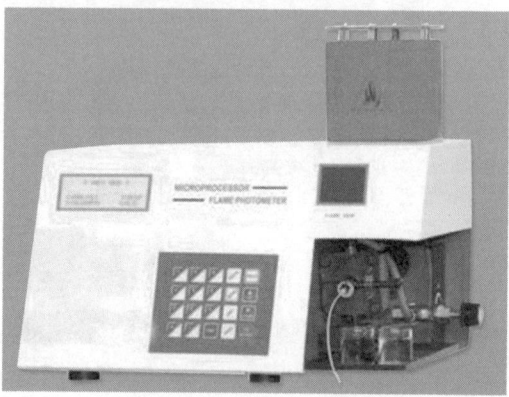

Fig. 29.19: Flame photometer.
(For color version, see Plate 6)

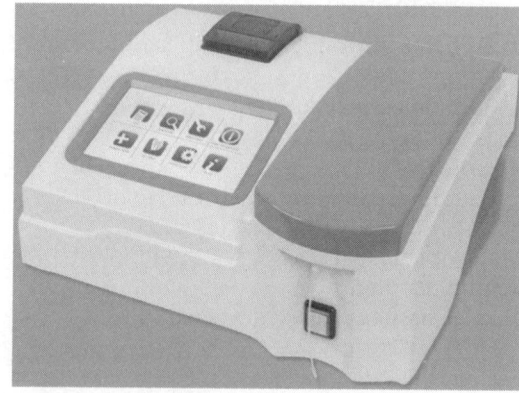

Fig. 29.22: Semiautoanalyzer.
(For color version, see Plate 7)

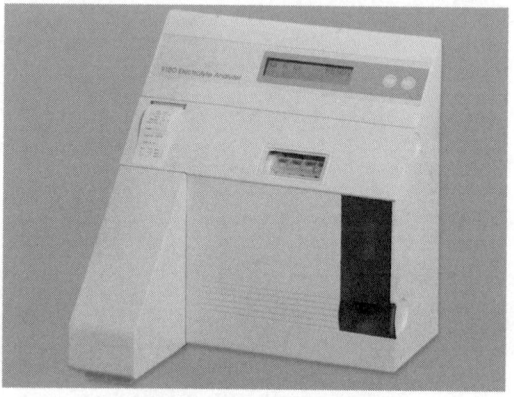

Fig. 29.20: Electrolyte analyzer.
(For color version, see Plate 6)

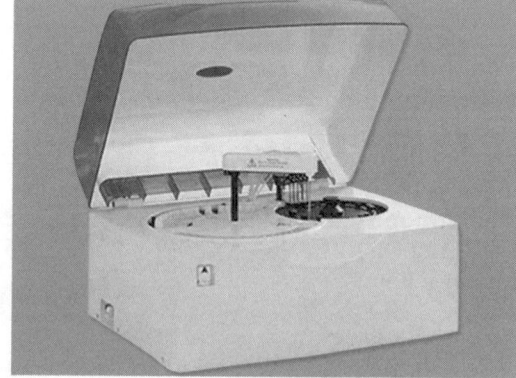

Fig. 29.23: Fully automatic analyzer.
(For color version, see Plate 7)

30 Biochemistry in Medical and Paramedical Specialties

Chapter Outline
- Definition
- Historical Background
- Objectives
- Branches
- Biochemistry in Medicine
- Biochemistry in Paramedical Specialties (Allied Health Sciences Courses)

DEFINITION

Biochemistry is the science which describes the chemical basis of life. It is one of the branches of chemistry applied to living systems.

HISTORICAL BACKGROUND

Biochemistry started as a young science in 19th century through the investigation of plant and animal tissues, fermentation, respiration and analysis of naturally occurring substances. It was earlier called as physiological chemistry. The term 'Biochemistry' was introduced in 1903 by a renowned German chemist Carl Neuberg. Biochemistry matured into a distinct science in the 20th century with the discovery of metabolic pathways, vitamins, hormones, etc. Twentieth century was the remarkable period of progress in biochemistry through discovery of nucleic acids, research techniques, and instrumentation. Many of the Nobel Prize winners in medicine and physiology are biochemists. Progress of biochemistry and the list of achievements continue in the 21st century as evident from mapping of human genome.

OBJECTIVES

The objectives of biochemistry are to study:
- The structures, properties, and functions of compounds constituting the cells and tissues (biomolecules).
- The metabolism of compounds utilized for energy or other functions of the body (metabolism).
- The nutrition which deals with diet and its relation to health (clinical nutrition).
- The chemistry of genetics (molecular biology)
- The role of biochemistry in medicine in health and disease (clinical biochemistry).

BRANCHES

Biochemistry can be broadly divided into the following branches (**Fig. 30.1**).

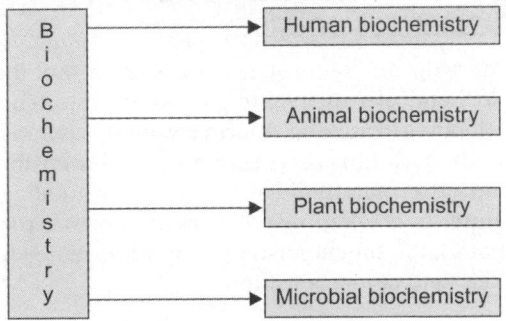

Fig. 30.1: Biochemistry branches.

BIOCHEMISTRY IN MEDICINE

Biochemistry is perhaps the most rapidly developing subject in medicine. Biochemistry influences:
- Medicine in presenting normal chemical composition and metabolic processes of the human beings.
- Explaining the causation, diagnosis, and treatment of diseases.

Many disciplines of medical sciences, dentistry and paramedical sciences have

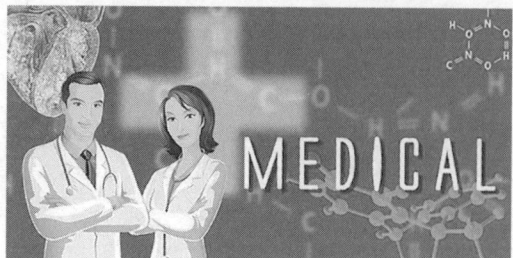

Fig. 30.2: Medical.
(For color version, see Plate 7)

also been widely influenced by biochemistry. Biochemistry is the major tool in medical research **(Fig. 30.2)**.

Human biochemistry deals with the following aspects of the human body **(Fig. 30.3)**.

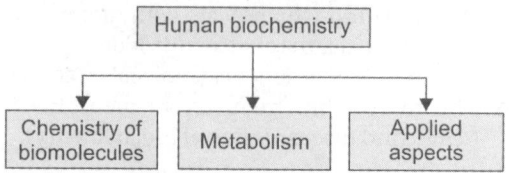

Fig. 30.3: Human biochemistry parts.

BIOCHEMISTRY IN PARAMEDICAL SPECIALTIES (ALLIED HEALTH SCIENCES COURSES)

The scope of the present book is to present the biochemical principles to paramedical students belonging to nursing, pharmacy, physiotherapy, medical laboratory technology, nutrition and other paramedical courses. Paramedical students are supposed to read their course material in biochemistry giving importance to their field of specialization.

Biochemistry in Nursing (Fig. 30.4)

Nursing profession is the important paramedical profession as the nursing care is needed for the alleviation of the suffering and rehabilitation to normal life. Nurses must have a good understanding of biochemistry in general and clinical biochemistry in particular. They should possess a sound knowledge of the various biochemical reactions normally taking place in the body and their alteration in diseases to facilitate effective patient care. Practically they must know the significance of the various biochemistry tests as part of diagnosis. Based

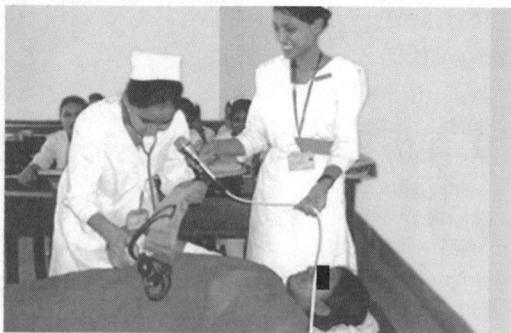

Fig. 30.4: Nursing.
(For color version, see Plate 7)

on the test results, they will be able to assess the patients' needs and plan for patient care.

Biochemistry in Pharmacy (Fig. 30.5)

Students of pharmacy are supposed to know basic biochemistry and metabolism of biochemical compounds, such as carbohydrates, lipids, proteins, etc., which are influenced by drugs. A better knowledge of biochemistry in normal and abnormal state of health is necessary for proper understanding of living organisms. Correlation between biochemistry and pharmacy has been mentioned in some selective topics. In the chapter on detoxification, excretion of toxic drugs has been explained taking few examples, such as aspirin, and pharmaceutical compounds such as phenol, benzoic acid, etc. A brief role of application of enzymes in pharmaceutical chemistry has also been given. The role of some drugs which are used in cancer, and other diseases are also referred, e.g., methotrexate, monoamine oxidase (MAO) inhibitors, etc.

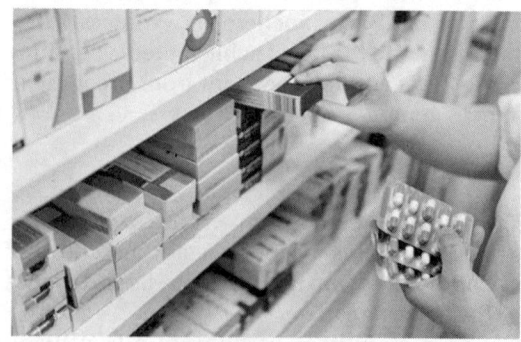

Fig. 30.5: Pharmacy.
(For color version, see Plate 7)

Biochemistry in Physiotherapy (Fig. 30.6)

Physiotherapists have to be well-versed with biophysical principles, basic biochemistry and the metabolic pathways and apply to the study of muscle biochemistry and physiology. They must also be able to correlate various biochemical parameters and their changes in muscle disorders and apply suitable methods to control them. They must also understand biochemical events in muscle contraction in normal state and during exercise.

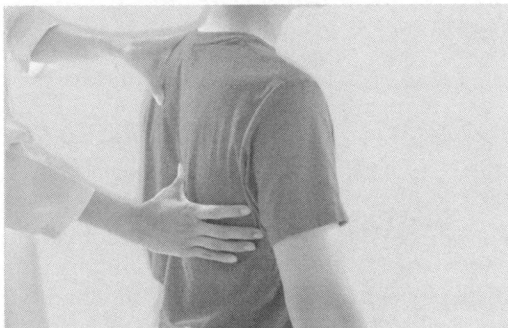

Fig. 30.6: Physiotherapy.
(For color version, see Plate 7)

Biochemistry in Medical Laboratory Technology (Fig. 30.7)

Students studying medical laboratory technology should be trained at handling various instruments which are used for processing of blood, urine, Cerebrospinal fluid (CSF), etc. for diagnosis of disease. For this, they must learn theoretical principles in basic biochemistry in addition to getting practical training in clinical biochemistry. They must know the normal values (reference values) of biochemical parameters in body fluids. They provide the results for the specimens of patients sent to the laboratory by the clinicians.

Biochemistry in Nutrition and Dietetics (Fig. 30.8)

Normal health gives happiness and self-satisfaction in life and is the way for long lifespan of an individual. To achieve and maintain normal health, proper nutrition must be given. Dieticians provide the solution for this purpose. There is a close relationship between biochemistry and nutrition. Dieticians must undergo a basic course in biochemistry and learn the principles of nutrition related to the well-being of an individual. They are taught to devise the balanced diet in normal state and in various disease states in consultation with the clinician.

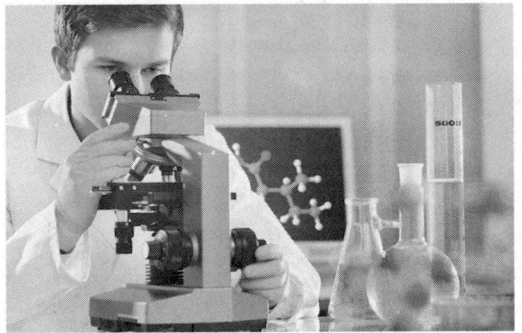

Fig. 30.7: Medical laboratory technology.
(For color version, see Plate 8)

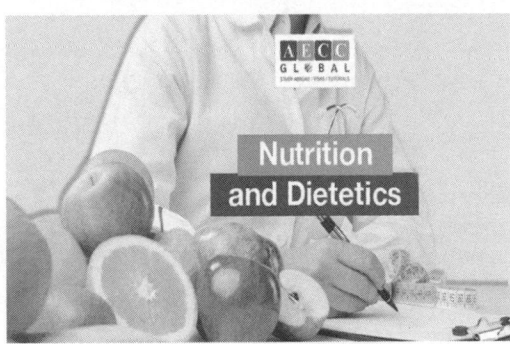

Fig. 30.8: Nutrition and dietetics.
(For color version, see Plate 8)

> **Note**
>
> Students of several other paramedical courses and dental students also study biochemistry with special emphasis in their field of specialization.

Section 6: Special Topics

31. Eicosanoids (Prostaglandins)

Chapter Outline
- Definition
- Classification
- Examples
- Functions

■ DEFINITION

Eicosanoids are the derivatives of C_{20} fatty acids. They are formed from arachidonic acid and other C_2O polyunsaturated fatty acids. They act as local hormones which perform several physiologically and pharmacologically important functions.

■ CLASSIFICATION

Eicosanoids are divided into two major classes which are further subclassified **(Fig. 31.1)**.

Prostanoids

Prostaglandins

Prostaglandins (PG) are a group of eicosanoids which are naturally occurring substances.

Discovery

They were first discovered in human semen in 1970 by ulf von Euler who thought that they were synthesized by prostate and hence the name prostaglandins. They are present in several tissues of the body.

Structure

They are derived from a C_{20} fatty acid namely prostanoic acid which has a cyclopentane ring and two side chains with carboxyl group on one side. They differ in their structure due to presence of substitute group and double bond on cyclopentane ring.

Examples

They are divided into four main groups. The number in subscript indicates the number of double bond and the Greek letter, the isomeric form:

1. PG-E-Group: PGE_1, PGE_2
2. PG-F-Group: PGF_α, $PGE_{2\alpha}$
3. PG-A-Group
4. PG-B-Group

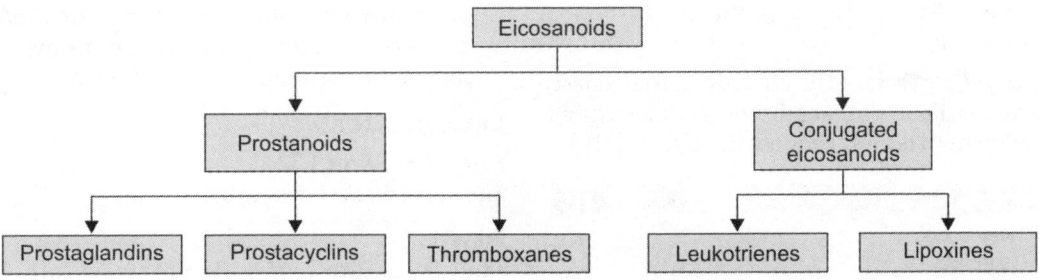

Fig. 31.1: Classification of eicosanoids.

Mechanism of action
They act through second messenger (cAMP) to exert their biochemical effects.

Synthesis
Refer Chapter 13.

Functions
Prostaglandins act as local hormones. They are the most potent biologically active compounds. The actions of PGs differ in different tissues.

Reproduction:
- PG_s (PGE_2, PGF_2) have stimulating effect on contraction of uterus and hence used to induce labor.
- They are used as contraceptives to prevent conception.
- They are involved in spermatogenesis, sperm maturation, and transport.

Regulation of BP: PGs (PGA, PGE) cause vasodilatation and increased blood flow thus lowering blood pressure. Hence they are used in the treatment of hypertension.

Gastric function: They (PGE_1, PGE_2) inhibit gastric secretion and hence used to treat gastric ulcers. They also increase intestinal motility and cause loose motion.

Respiratory function: PGE is a bronchodilator. PGF is a constrictor of bronchial smooth muscle. PGE_1 and PGE_2 are used for the treatment of asthma patients.

Renal function: PGA and PGE increase GFR and promote urine output.

Inflammation: They (PGE_1, PGE_2) are natural mediators of inflammatory reaction, i.e., induce symptoms of inflammation. Corticosteroids are used to treat them.

Platelet aggregation and thrombosis: PGE_2 promotes platelet aggregation and blood clotting which may lead to thrombosis.

Pain and fever: Pyrogens promote biosynthesis of PGs.

Metabolic effects: PGE increases glycogenesis, decreases lipolysis and promotes calcium mobilization from bones. They act through cAMP.

> **Clinical Importance**
> PGs are used:
> - To induce labor
> - In medical termination of pregnancy
> - As contraceptive to prevent conception
> - In the treatment of hypertension, gastric ulcer, thrombosis
> - As effective nasal decongestant (inhibitors of PG synthesis are used to control pain, fever, e.g., aspirin).

Side effects
- Gastrointestinal disturbances leads to cramping and diarrhea.
- PGE_2 cause pain and coughing due to vibration of mucosal lining of the throat.

Prostacyclins (PGI)
Examples: PGI_2, PGI_3
Site of synthesis: Blood vessel walls

Functions
They inhibit platelet aggregation and produce vasodilatation to prevent thrombosis.

Thromboxanes (TX)
Examples: TXA_2, TXA_3
Site of synthesis: Platelets

Functions
Promotes platelet aggregation and thrombosis.

> **Note**
> Prostacyclins and thromboxanes are antagonists in their action. PGI_2 is a vasodilator whereas TXA is a vasoconstrictor.

Conjugated Eicosanoids
Leukotrienes (LT)
Example: LTC_4, LTD_4, LTE_4
Site of synthesis: Leukocytes, mast cells, platelets, and macrophages.

Funtions
- A mixture of leukotrienes is a potent constrictor of the bronchial airway musculature.
- They are important regulators in many diseases involving inflammatory or hypersensitivity reactions such as asthma.

Lipoxines (LX)
Examples: LXA4, LX4
Site of synthesis: Leukocytes

Function
They play an anti-inflammatory role in vasoactive and immunoregulatory function.

32. Lipid Peroxidation—Free Radicals and Antioxidants

Chapter Outline
- Definition
- Formation
- Mechanism of Lipid Peroxidation
- Assessment
- Harmful Effects
- Antioxidants
- Types

■ DEFINITION

Free radical is an atom or a molecule which contains one or more unpaired electrons.

Alternative name: Reactive oxygen species (ROS).

■ FORMATION

Free radicals may be generated mainly from two sources.

Cellular Metabolism

Cellular metabolism is due to:
- Lipid peroxidation in membranes
- Phagocytosis
- Electron transport chain
- Oxidation of heme to bile pigments
- Oxidative enzymes

Environmental Effects

Environmental effect is due to:
- Ionizing radiation on tissues (e.g., X-rays)
- Drug metabolism
- Cigarettes, alcohol, and trace metals

Example: O_2, H_2O_2, OH—singlet oxygen (O_2), hydrogen peroxide radical, (HCOO–, NO⁻, lipid peroxide radial (ROO–) etc.

■ MECHANISM OF LIPID PEROXIDATION

Free radicals are formed during peroxide formation from naturally occurring polyunsaturated fatty acids. It occurs in three stages.

1. Initiation
2. Propagation
3. Termination

■ ASSESSMENT

Estimation of malondialdehyde (MDA) is the marker to assess oxidative stress and free radical damage to the body.

■ HARMFUL EFFECTS

- Free radicals can damage almost all types of biomolecules and destroy cells leading to several diseases, cancer, diabetes mellitus, etc.
- They are also responsible for deterioration of foods (rancidity).
- They are also involved in biochemical and morphological changes during ageing.
- They also play a key role in muscle dystrophy, Parkinson's disease, Alzheimer's disease.

■ ANTIOXIDANTS

They are used to control and reduce lipid peroxidation. They are considered as scavengers of free radicals.

■ TYPES

They can be classified in different ways.

According to Mode of Action

- *Preventive antioxidants:* They reduce the rate of chain reaction, e.g., catalases, peroxidases, ceruloplasmin, ethylenediaminetetraacetic acid (EDTA).

- *Chain breaking antioxidants:* They interfere with chain propagation, e.g., phenols, aromatic amines, vitamin E and selenium, superoxide dismutase.

According to In vitro/In vivo Use

- *In vitro antioxidants:* Used to prevent lipid peroxidation in food (rancidity), e.g., prophylgallol, butylated hydroxyl toluene.
- *Natural (in vivo) antioxidants:* Occur in the body, e.g., beta carotene, vitamin A, vitamin E, and vitamin C, selenium (nutritional antioxidants).

Metabolic Antioxidants

- Glutathione
- Ceruloplasmin
- Transferrin

33 Environmental Biochemistry

Chapter Outline
- Definition
- Classification
- General Effects
- Types

Environment is the collective term for the conditions in which organism lives. It includes all social, biological, physical, and chemical factors.

DEFINITION

Study of substances present in the environment which may produce abnormality in the metabolism or alter the health of the organism is known as environmental biochemistry. They may enter through respiratory or dermal route.

CLASSIFICATION

Environmental pollutants are of various types:
- Corrosives, irritants, and heavy metal poisons
- a. Air pollutants
  b. Noise pollutants
- Occupational/industrial hazardous agents
- Radiations
- Biological agents
- Drugs
- Dietary factors
- Water
- Chemical carcinogens
- Climate

GENERAL EFFECTS

- Toxic
- Deposited in adipose tissue
- Inhibit enzymes in metabolism
- Produce neurological, respiratory, gastrointestinal, renal problems, etc.

TYPES

1. a. *Corrosives*
   - Strong acids : H_2SO_4, HCl, HNO_3
   - Strong alkalies : NaOH, NH_4OH
   - Salts : Potassium cyanide

   b. *Irritants*
   - Metallic : Arsenic, mercury, lead etc.
   - Nonmetallic : Halides, phosphorus
   - Organic : Castor oil, croton oil
   - Mechanical : Powdered glass, diamond dust

   c. *Heavy metal poisons*
   - Lead : From exhaust of vehicles
   - Mercury : From dental amalgam, paints
   - Tin : From tin coated vessels
   - Aluminum : From packing materials
   - Arsenic : From rat poisons, fruit sprays

2. a. *Air pollutants (atmospheric pollutants):* A contaminant that occurs in the atmosphere in sufficiently high concentration to cause an adverse effect is called air pollutant.

   Types

   Natural sources of air pollution:
   - Forest fires, volcanic eruption, dust storms, air born particles
   - Biological contaminants: Fungi, bacteria, viruses, pollen grains

   Artificial sources of air pollution:
   - Emissions from automobiles, industries, etc.
     - CO_2, CO

- Hydrocarbons, lead
- Nitrogen dioxide (NO_2)—reduces O_2 supply to tissues
- Sulfur dioxide (SO_2)—affects respiratory system
  (*Note*: $NO_2 + SO_2$ = Acid rain)

- Smog: Mixture of smoke, fog, air, and other chemicals.
- Ozone layer: It is formed from atmospheric oxygen and absorbs harmful ultraviolet radiations of sun. But it is prevented by release of gases from refrigerators and aeroplanes.

Effects
- Respiratory disorders
- Cardiovascular disorders

b. *Noise pollution:* Noise is the major urban environment pollutant. A noise above 150 decibels may affect hearing and produce neuromuscular tension, irritability, etc.

3. *Industrial (or) occupational pollutants*

Sl. No.	Causative industry	Agent	Symptom/disorder
1.	Rubber, explosives, plastics	Acid fumes	Mucous membrane irritant
2.	Refrigeration, fertilizers	Ammonia	Chronic bronchitis
3.	Electroplating	Cyanide	Respiratory arrest
4.	Paper, textile, disinfectant	Halides	Mucous membrane irritant
5.	Resin, leather	Formaldehyde	Carcinoma
6.	Oil, petroleum	Hydrogen sulfide	Chronic bronchitis
7.	Arc welding, photochemical	Ozone	Eye irritant
8.	Explosives, rocket fuel	Nitrogen dioxide	Chronic bronchitis, emphysema, reduces supply of O_2 to tissues

4. *Radiations*
   - Ultraviolet radiations—solar
   - Ionizing radiation—α, β, γ rays
   - Electromagnetic radiations—power lines, cell phones

5. *Biological agents*
   - Viruses
   - Bacteria

6. *Drugs:* Drugs which have carcinogenic potential or component, e.g., *diethylstilbestrol*.

7. a. *Toxic substances in food stuffs*
   - Toxins normally present in plants, e.g., goitrogens, neurotoxins
   - Contamination occurring during cultivation. e.g., pesticides, insecticides
   - Products of post harvest period (storage), e.g., aflatoxins (hepatic carcinogen)
   - Chemical contaminants during food processing, e.g., mineral oils
   - Food adulterants, e.g., mustard oil, monosodium glutamate (aginomoto)
   - Toxins entering after cooking.

b. *Pesticides and insecticides:* Widely used in agricultural practice:
   - DDT (Dichloro-diphenyl-trichlorethane)
   - Cyclic halogenated hydrocarbons, e.g., aldrin
   - Organophosphorus compounds, e.g., parathion, malathion
   - Carbamates, e.g., baygon.

8. *Water pollution:* Generally water contains many impurities such as inorganic and organic compounds.
   - Inorganic:
     - Carbonates, bicarbonates, sulfates and chlorides of calcium and magnesium add to hardness and/or alkalinity.
     - Iron oxide adds red coloration to water
     - Excess sodium fluoride may cause dental fluorosis
     - Lead present in water, air, foods, soils, affect central nervous system.
   - Organic:
     - Decayed leaves and animals
     - Organic waste liberate methane, H_2S and ammonia into the environment
     - Pesticides (DDT) may cause nervous irritability, convulsions.

9. *Carcinogens:* Carcinogen is a chemical or agent which produces cancer. Carcinogen may be considered as part of environmental biochemistry.

Environmental carcinogens (chemicals)	Occupation	Cancer
Aniline	Dye industry	Urinary bladder
Arsenic	Insecticide, manufacturers and users, miners	Skin, lung, liver
Benzene	Rubber and cement workers, dye users	Acute myloid leukemia
Beryllium	Miners	Lung
Cadmium	Miners, processors	Lung, prostate, kidney
Nickel	Miners and processors	Lung, nasal sinus

Contd...

Environmental carcinogens (chemicals)	Occupation	Cancer
Pesticides	Farmers or other users	Non-Hodgkin's lymphoma, lung
Uranium	Miners and processors	Lung
Vinyl chloride	Plastic industry	Lung

10. *Climate:*
- Exposure to cold may cause shivering to produce extra heat generated by hydrolysis of ATP.
- Exposure to heat may produce heat stroke due to failure of heat regulatory system.

34 Cancer

Chapter Outline
- Definition
- Types
- Causative Factor of Cancer
- Chemical Carcinogens
- Oncogenes
- Tumor Markers

DEFINITION

Cancer is a group of diseases involving abnormal cell growth which may invade local tissues or spread to other parts of the body. It is the second most common cause of death in the developing countries.

Alternative names: Tumor, neoplasm

TYPES

Depending on its origin of tissue/organ, cancer is of different types.
- Skin cancer
- Breast cancer
- Prostate cancer
- Brain cancer
- Lung cancer
- Oral cancer, etc.

Note

Histologically, it is divided into:

☞ Carcinoma	☞ Melanoma
☞ Lymphoma	☞ Leukemia
☞ Sarcoma	☞ Hepatoma

CAUSATIVE FACTORS OF CANCER

Various factors contribute to the incidence of cancer.
- Predisposable factors:
  - Age
  - Heredity
  - Environmental factors
- Agents causing cancer:
  - Physical:
    - Ionizing radiations (α, β, γ, rays)
    - Ultraviolet radiations (solar)
  - Chemical:
    - Industrial agents
    - Diet related chemicals
  - Biological:
    - Viruses
    - Parasitic infections
    - Chronic infections

CHEMICAL CARCINOGENS

Chemicals which cause cancer are known as chemical carcinogens. Process by which cancer is produced by chemicals is known as carcinogenesis. It is a multistep process.

$$\text{Normal cell} \xrightarrow{\text{Initiation}} \text{Altered cell} \xrightarrow{\text{Promotion}} \text{Cancer cell}$$

For example:
- Aromatic amines
- Nitrosamines
- Aromatic hydrocarbons
- Diethylstilbestrol (drug)
- Naturally occurring compounds, e.g., aflatoxin
- Inorganic compounds (*refer* below Table)

Occupational Carcinogens

Sl. No.	Carcinogen	Occupation	Cancer
1.	Aniline	Dye industry	Urinary bladder
2.	Asbestos	Fabrication	Lung
3.	Arsenic	Mining	Skin, lung, liver
4.	Benzene	Rubber worker, dye users	Leukemia
5.	Vinyl chloride	Plastic industry	Liver
6.	Nickel	Miners	Lung, nasal sinus
7.	Uranium	Miners, processors	Lung
8.	Pesticides	Farmers	Lung

Test for Carcinogenicity of Chemicals: Ames Test

Clinical Manifestations (Symptoms) of Cancer

- Indigestion or difficulty in swallowing
- A sore that does not heal
- Persistent cough or cough with blood
- Change in a wart or mole
- Unusual bleeding or discharge
- Lump or thickening in breast/testis

Biochemical Changes of Cancer Cells

- Increased glycolysis
- Increased protein biosynthesis
- Synthesis of fetal antigens
- Reduced levels of some minerals (selenium, zinc, etc.) and vitamins (A, C, E)

General Changes

- Unrestrained growth
- Round shape
- Form multilayer
- Metastasis (move to other cells/organs)

Factors which Favor Production of Cancer

- Saturated fats
- Refined carbohydrates
- Salt
- Pickled vegetables
- Alcohol
- Fried foods
- Oncogenes

Factors which Inhibit Production of Cancer

- Fruits
- Vegetables
- Vitamin A, C, E (antioxidants)
- Minerals (selenium, zinc, etc.)
- Immune stimulants
- Tumor suppressor genes (antioncogenes)

Oncogenes

Oncogenes cause cancer by multiplication of cells. They are of two types.
1. *Viral oncogenes:* Present in viruses, e.g., RNA viruses, DNA viruses.
2. *Cellular oncogenes:* Present in normal cells. They are known as protooncogenes and are activated to oncogenes by various mechanisms to induce cancer, e.g., Tyrosin protein kinase.

Normal genes → proto-oncogenes → Oncogenes (by Mutation, gene amplification / Chromosome abnormalities) → Cancer

Antioncogenes (Tumor Suppressor Genes)

There are some genes in the normal cells which can prevent cancer.
a. RB
b. P^{53}

Diagnosis

Cancer can be detected by tumor markers.

Tumor Markers

Definition

Tumor markers are substances present in the blood, urine or tissues which are synthesized by cancer cells. They are used as biomarkers to detect one or more types of cancer.

Type

They are of different types depending on their chemical nature or function.

Examples

Sl. No.	Chemical nature	Example	Cancer
1.	Enzymes	Prostatic acid phosphatase	Prostate
2.	Hormone	Human chorionic gonadotropin (hCG)	Chorionic carcinoma
3.	Proteins	Immunoglobulins, prostate specific antigen (PSA)	• Multiple myeloma • Prostate
4.	Oncofetal antigens	α fetoprotein (AFP), CA – 125	• Liver • Germ cells
5.	Oncogenes	Ras	Colon, rectum, lung, kidney, pancreas

Drugs for Treatment of Cancer

- Methotrexate
- 6-mercaptopurine
- Mitomycin C
- Cyclophosphamide
- Monoclonal antibodies
- Other: Vaccines, gene therapy

35 Acquired Immune Deficiency Syndrome

Chapter Outline
- Causes
- Epidemiology
- Structure of HIV
- Abnormal Activities
- Clinical Symptoms
- Diagnosis
- Treatment
- Corona Viruses

Acquired immune deficiency syndrome (AIDS) is the fastest leading cause of death in USA. It was first reported in 1981.

CAUSES

It is caused by human immunodeficiency virus (HIV). It is a retroviral disease. Isolation of this virus was done independently by Robert Gall (USA). Mantaigneir (France).

EPIDEMIOLOGY

It has been reported in 2016 that about 40 million people worldwide (5 million in India) are infected with HIV. Its transmission is mainly through three routes: (1) sexual contact (2) parental inoculation (3) infected mothers to infants.

STRUCTURE OF HIV

HIV is a spherical virus. It contains a core surrounded by a lipid layer derived from the plasma membrane. The core contains two strand of RNA and four core proteins.

ABNORMAL ACTIVITIES

AIDS primarily produces immunological abnormalities by affecting cell-mediated immune system due to reduction in CD4 cells of the lymphocytes and impairment in the function of surviving CD4 cells. It also exhibits abnormalities in antibody production by B-lymphocytes (abnormal immunity). It also infects the cells of the central nervous system.

CLINICAL SYMPTOMS

Due to repression by HIV, various clinical symptoms are observed in the AIDs patients: Fever, diarrhea, weight loss, multiple opportunistic infections, lymphadenopathy, neurological complications, secondary neoplasm, etc.

DIAGNOSIS

HIV infection can be detected by the following laboratory tests.
- *Enzyme-linked immunosorbent assay (ELISA):* It detects antibodies in the circulation.
- *Western blot:* It is used to confirm ELISA positive cases.
- *Polymerase chain reaction (PCR):* It is used to detect the presence of HIV genome in the peripheral blood lymphocytes.

TREATMENT

There is no cure for AIDS. But certain drugs are used to prolong the life of AIDS patients. (a) zidovudine (b) didanosine (c) vaccine: till date it has not been possible to develop a vaccine against AIDS because HIV exhibits genetic heterogenetics.

Note
Corona viruses (COVID-19) which caused infections in millions of people throughout the world during 2019-2021 are also RNA viruses (Retro virus).

36 Biotechnology

Chapter Outline
- Definition
- Historical Development
- Branches (Divisions)
- Scope/Importance
- Process
- Applications
- Risks, Hazards, and Ethics
- Related Terms in Molecular Biology

It is a multidisciplinary applied science. It is high technology of the 21st century.

■ DEFINITION

Various definitions have been put forward. It can be defined as "the application of scientific and engineering principles to the processing of materials by biological agents to produce goods and services".

■ HISTORICAL DEVELOPMENT

- I Phase: Pre-Pasteur era
- II Phase: Pasteur era
- III Phase: Fleming era
- IV Phase: Watson–Crick era

■ BRANCHES (DIVISIONS)

- Medical biotechnology
- Veterinary biotechnology
- Agricultural biotechnology
- Pharmaceutical biotechnology

■ SCOPE/IMPORTANCE

Biotechnology can produce greater impact on several aspects of our life. There are rapidly increasing opportunities for the application of biotechnology to the manufacture of medical, veterinary and agricultural products, etc.

■ PROCESS

Biotechnology involves the conversion of relatively cheap raw material into highly valuable products or services. Thus, it involves microbial, animal or plant cells and enzymes to synthesize, degrade or transform materials. The most commonly used technique in biotechnology is genetic engineering which is otherwise known as recombinant DNA technology.

■ APPLICATIONS

Biotechnology has wide application in different fields.

Medical Field

The impact of pharmaceuticals on human health care is an area where biochemical innovations lead to commercial realization.
- Therapeutic products (antibiotics, hormones, etc.)
- Vaccines
- Immunodiagnostics and DNA probes for identification of disease
- Gene therapy, etc.

Veterinary Field

Biotechnology could greatly increase the speed and range of selective breeding of animals which represents a major source of food production worldwide. Transgenic animals are produced for this purpose.

Agriculture

Agricultural biotechnology will lead to high quality plants with lower cost of production. The main improvements include improved strain to insects, pests and microbial diseases.

Foods

Food biotechnology encompasses a wide range of options for improved quality, nutrition and safety of food, e.g., fermented foods and beverages.

Environment and Energy

Due to urbanization and industrialization, much attention is paid to improving the environment through:
- Waste water and sewage treatment
- Composting
- Bio-remediation

■ RISKS, HAZARDS, AND ETHICS

Biotechnology is a globally important complex issue. Many risks and hazards including serious health safety, environmental and socioeconomic changes are associated with it. Notwithstanding the above difficulty biotechnology will have an increasingly important role to play in our society. It has greater scope for the future.

■ RELATED TERMS IN MOLECULAR BIOLOGY

- *Genome:* Total DNA present in an organism or a cell.
- *Genomics:* Study of the genome and its actions.
- *Proteome:* Sum of all proteins expressed by the genome of an organism.
- *Proteomics:* Study of all proteins expressed by genes of a cell or an organism.
- *Bioinformatics:* Combined science of biology and information technology.
- *Transgenic animal:* Transgenic animals are genetically modified organisms.
- *Cloning:* It is the process of producing genetically identical individuals of an organism either naturally or artificially, e.g., Little Nicks.
  Meaning: Cloning make identical copy/replicate.
- *Apoptosis*: Programmed cell death.

■ STEM CELLS

Stem cells are special human cells that have the ability to develop into many different cell types.

Sources
- Embryonic stem cells
- Tissue specific stem cells, etc.

Uses
- Used to replace lost or damaged cells that our body cannot replace naturally.
- Used to treat diseases, e.g., macular degeneration diseases.

■ MITOCHONDRIAL DNA (mtDNA/mDNA)

Refer page 277.

Appendices

APPENDIX A: QUESTIONS (CHAPTER-WISE)

SECTION 1: INTRODUCTION TO BIOCHEMISTRY

Chapter 1

Essay Questions   *10–15 marks each**

1. Name the subcellular organelles. Give a brief description of any three of them and their biochemical functions.
2. Mention the different biophysical phenomena occurring in the body. Write briefly on any three.
3. Describe the various transport mechanisms in the body.

Short Notes   *3–5 marks each**

1. Structure and biochemical functions of each of the following subcellular organelles:
   a. Mitochondria
   b. Nucleus
   c. Ribosomes
2. Structure of cell membrane (or) Fluid mosaic model of cell membrane.
3. Membrane transport/active transport
4. Radioactive isotopes
5. Colloids

Minor Questions   *1–2 marks each**

1. What is the marker enzyme of:
   a. Mitochondria   b. Lysosomes
2. Define:
   a. Acid   b. Base
   c. Buffer   d. pH
3. Define:
   a. Osmosis
   b. Surface tension
   c. Sodium pump
4. Name two pathways by which macromolecules are transported through cell membrane.
5. Mention two differences between prokaryotic and eukaryotes.

---
* Applicable to all chapters

Multiple Choice Questions (MCQs)
                                                1 mark each*

1. The powerhouse of the cell is:
   a. Nucleus
   b. Ribosomes
   c. Mitochondria
   d. Endoplasmic reticulum
2. The technique to isolate the cell organelles is:
   a. Dialysis
   b. Ultracentrifugation
   c. Electrophoresis
   d. Chromatography
3. Lysosomes mostly contain:
   a. Synthesis   b. Isomerases
   c. Hydrolases   d. Catalase
4. Which of the following is a radioactive isotope?
   a. 141_I b. 20_p
   c. 131_I d. 10_N
5. The major complex organic biomolecules are:
   a. Protein   b. DNA and RNA
   c. Polysaccharides   d. All of the above

SECTION 2: CHEMISTRY OF BIOMOLECULES

Chapter 2

Essay Questions

1. What are carbohydrates? Classify them giving important examples. Write their biomedical importance/functions.
2. Write the important physical and chemical properties of monosaccharides.
3. Describe the mucopolysaccharides (Glycosaminoglycans) with examples.

Short Notes

1. Mutarotation
2. Glycosides
3. Physiologically important disaccharides

4. Homopolysaccharides
5. Heteropolysaccharides
6. Glycosaminoglycans/mucopolysaccharides
7. Osazones
8. Isomerism

Minor Questions
1. What is the use of dextrose in medicine?
2. Name two ring structures of glucose.
3. What are the hydrolytic products of starch?
4. What is meant by inversion of sugar?
5. Write the principle and application of Benedict's test.
6. Define:
   a. Epimer   b. Anomer
   c. Optical isomer d. Osazone
   e. Stereoisomers   f. Aldose/ketose
   g. Glycosidic bond
7. Write two differences between
   a. Amylose and amylopectin
   b. Starch and glycogen

Multiple Choice Questions
1. All the following are reducing sugars, *except*:
   a. Galactose   b. Lactose
   c. Sucrose   d. Fructose
2. Amino sugar containing drug is:
   a. Erythromycin   b. Streptomycin
   c. Ouabain   d. None of the above
3. Blood sugar refers to:
   a. Fructose   b. Glucose
   c. Glycogen   d. Lactose
4. The polysaccharide used to determine glomerular filtration rate (GFR) is:
   a. Starch   b. Insulin
   c. Heparin   d. Inulin
5. Invert sugar is:
   a. Glucose
   b. Fructose
   c. Sucrose
   d. A mixture of glucose and fructose

Chapter 3

Essay Questions
1. Define lipid. How are they classified? Give suitable examples. Write their biomedical importance/functions.
2. Write the physical and chemical properties of fats (or) fatty acids.
3. What are phospholipids? Mention their different classes. Write the structural components, sources and important functions of any three phospholipids.
4. Give an account or eicosanoids/prostaglandins.

Short Notes
1. Lipid peroxidation/free radicals/antioxidants
2. Rancidity
3. Phospholipids
4. Glycolipids
5. Lipoproteins
6. Cholesterol
7. Essential fatty acids/ω-fatty acids
8. Prostaglandins/eicosanoids
9. Amphipathic lipids

Minor Questions
1. Name two polyunsaturated fatty acids (PUFA).
2. Define:
   a. Saponification number
   b. Iodine number
   c. Emulsification
3. What is the cause of respiratory distress syndrome?
4. Name the compounds formed from cholesterol.
5. Define:
   a. Eicosanoids   b. Micelles
   c. Liposomes   d. Neutral lipids
6. Name two methods to assess the purity of oils.
7. Name two tests to detect cholesterol.

Multiple Choice Questions
1. An example for simple lipid:
   a. Fatty acid
   b. Lecithin
   c. Glycerol
   d. Triglyceride (triacyl glycerol)
2. Cholesterol contains:
   a. Corrin ring
   b. Purine ring
   c. Cyclopentanoperhydrophenanthrene ring
   d. Ionone ring
3. Lipoproteins can be separated into different fractions by:
   a. Electrophoresis
   b. Ultracentrifugation
   c. Both of the above
   d. Dialysis
4. Hydrolysis of fat by alkali is known as:
   a. Emulsification b. Esterification
   c. Peroxidation   d. Saponification

5. Prostaglandins are synthesized from:
   a. Arachidonic acid   b. Palmitic acid
   c. Stearic acid   d. Glycine

Chapter 4
Essay Questions
1. What are proteins? Classify them based on their composition and solubility giving suitable examples. Write their biomedical importance/functions.
2. Write the important physical and chemical properties of proteins.
3. Give the classification of amino acids providing examples. Write their biomedical importance/functions.
4. Write the important physical and chemical properties of amino acids.
5. Describe the different levels of structures of proteins.

Short Notes
1. Structural organization of proteins
2. Denaturation of proteins
3. Chromatography
4. Electrophoresis
5. Essential amino acids
6. Biologically important peptides
7. Plasma proteins
8. Immunoglobulins
9. Lipoproteins
10. Glycoproteins
11. Apoproteins/Apolipoproteins
12. Glutathione
13. Collagen

Minor Questions
1. How many types of amino acids are present in proteins?
2. Mention two:
   a. Globular proteins
   b. Fibrous proteins
   c. Structural proteins
   d. Functional proteins
   e. Semiessential amino acids
3. What is meant by coagulation? Name two coagulable proteins.
4. Define:
   a. Zwitter ion
   b. Peptide bond
   c. Isoelectric point
   d. Ampholytes
   e. Proteoglycans
5. Name a method to separate:
   a. Amino acids   b. Plasma proteins
6. Name two color reactions of proteins.

Multiple Choice Questions
1. Glutathione is a:
   a. Dipeptide
   b. Tripeptide
   c. Protein
   d. Glycoside
2. An example for derived protein is:
   a. Albumin   b. Gelatin
   c. Casein   d. Protamine
3. Number of different amino acids present in proteins are:
   a. 10   b. 20
   c. 150   d. 250
4. Two semiessential amino acids are:
   a. Arginine and glycine
   b. Histidine and alanine
   c. Arginine and histidine
   d. Proline and methionine
5. A method to separate amino acids is:
   a. Dialysis   b. Chromatography
   c. Filtration   d. Electrophoresis

Chapter 5
Essay Questions
1. Give an account of the structure, properties, and functions/biomedical importance of DNA.
2. Write the types, structure, properties, and functions/biomedical importance of RNA.

Short Notes
1. DNA double helix
2. Transfer RNA (tRNA)/Messenger RNA (mRNA)
3. Differences between DNA and RNA
4. Biologically important nucleotides
5. Nucleoproteins
6. Cyclic AMP/ATP

Minor Questions
1. What is the difference between nucleoside and nucleotide?
2. Name the four types of:
   a. Ribonucleotides
   b. Deoxyribonucleotides
3. What is cyclic AMP? What is its importance?
4. What is Chargaff rule?
5. Name two synthetic nucleotides/nucleosides/nucleobases used in medicine.

Multiple Choice Questions

1. The base present in DNA but absent in RNA is:
   a. Guanine b. Thymine
   c. Uracil d. Cytosine
2. Which compound has double helical structure?
   a. Ribonucleic acid
   b. Collagen
   c. Deoxyribonucleic acid
   d. Hemoglobin
3. Which RNA has clover leaf structure?
   a. tRNA b. rRNA
   c. mRNA d. hnRNA
4. Nucleotide is:
   a. Base-sugar
   b. Base-amino acid
   c. Base-sugar-phosphate
   d. Base-sugar-alcohol

Chapter 6

Essay Question

Describe the structure, properties, and functions of normal hemoglobins.

Short Notes

1. Porphyrins
2. Normal hemoglobins
3. Abnormal hemoglobins/hemoglobinopathy
4. Hemoglobin derivatives
5. Sickle cell anemia/sickle cell disease
6. Thalassemia
7. Oxygen dissociation curves of hemoglobin
8. Myoglobin
9. Hemoproteins/hemoenzymes
10. Transport of O_2/CO_2

Minor Questions

1. What is Bohr effect?
2. What is the defect in methemoglobinemia?
3. What is glycosylated hemoglobin?
4. Which abnormal hemoglobin causes sickle cell anemia?
5. What is the use of spectroscope?

Multiple Choice Questions

1. Hemoglobin is a:
   a. Derived protein
   b. Simple protein
   c. Conjugated protein
   d. Mucoprotein
2. The instrument used to detect hemoglobin derivatives in blood is:
   a. Spectroscope b. Colorimeter
   c. Calorimeter d. Spectrophotometer
3. Normal range of hemoglobin in adult male is:
   a. 1–2 g% b. 6–8 g%
   c. 13–17 g% d. 9–11 mg%
4. An example for abnormal hemoglobin is:
   a. HbO b. HbS
   c. HbT d. HbX

Chapter 7

Essay Questions

1. What are enzymes? Classify them according to IUB system. Give two examples for each class and one reaction catalyzed by each.
2. Discuss the various factors affecting enzyme activity (velocity of reaction/rate of reaction). Add a note on k_m.
3. Describe the various types of enzyme inhibition.

Short Notes

1. Mechanism of enzyme action/theories
2. Enzyme specificity
3. Coenzymes
4. Enzyme inhibition/competitive enzyme inhibition
5. Enzymes of clinical importance (diagnostic enzymes)
6. Isoenzymes
7. Regulation of enzymes

Minor Questions

1. What is the difference between zymogen and zymase?
2. Define:
   a. Apoenzyme
   b. Holoenzyme
   c. Ribozyme
   d. Lysozyme
3. Mention two enzymes which are increased in acute pancreatitis/liver diseases/MI.
4. What are allosteric enzymes?
5. Give two therapeutic applications of enzymes.
6. What are
   a. Plasma specific enzymes
   b. Plasma nonspecific enzymes
7. What is multienzyme complex? Give two examples.

Multiple Choice Questions

1. Normal level of SGOT (AST) at 37°C is:
   a. 5–45 IU/L
   b. 0–80 IU/L
   c. 60–80 IU/L
   d. 100–250 IU/L
2. Number of isoenzymes of LDH in serum is:
   a. 2
   b. 3
   c. 5
   d. 6
3. All the enzymes are increased in myocardial infarction, *except:*
   a. CPK
   b. SGOT
   c. LDH
   d. Alkaline phosphatase
4. Enzymes are classified into how many major classes?
   a. 2
   b. 4
   c. 6
   d. 10
5. All these following are coenzymes, *except:*
   a. TPP
   b. NAD⁺
   c. SGPT (ALT)
   d. Pyridoxal phosphate

Chapter 8

Essay Questions

1. Write the sources, chemistry, biochemical functions, daily requirement (RDA) and deficiency symptoms (manifestations) of each of the following vitamins:
   a. Vitamin A
   b. Vitamin D
   c. Vitamin C
   d. Thiamine (B_1)
   e. Riboflavin (B_2)
   f. Niacin (B_3)
   g. Pyridoxine (B_6)
   h. Folic acid (B_9)
   i. Vitamin B_{12}
   j. Pantothenic acid (B_5)

Short Notes

1. Wald's visual cycle (rhodopsin cycle)
2. Vitamin E
3. Vitamin K
4. Biotin
5. Calcitriol
6. Hypervitaminosis A and D
7. Antivitamins
8. Scurvy
9. Beriberi
10. Pellagra
11. Vitamin K cycle
12. Rickets
13. Absorption, transport, and storage of vitamin A/vitamin B_{12}
14. Write the sources and functions of vitamin A/C.
15. Write the sources and coenzyme functions of vitamin niacin/pyridoxine.
16. Write the sources and deficiency symptoms/manifestations of vitamin A/D.

Minor Questions

1. Name three vitamins which function as antioxidants.
2. Write two differences between fat-soluble vitamins and water-soluble vitamins.
3. Name two coenzyme forms of:
   a. Riboflavin
   b. Niacin
   c. Vitamin B_{12}
4. Name two sulfur containing vitamins.
5. What is methyl trap (folate trap)?
6. What is:
   a. FIGLU
   b. Osteomalacia
   c. Avidin
   d. Lipoic acid

Multiple Choice Questions

1. Which one is a water-soluble vitamin?
   a. Vitamin A
   b. Vitamin E
   c. Biotin
   d. Vitamin K
2. RDA (daily requirement) of vitamin A for an adult is:
   a. 100 IU/day
   b. 1000 IU/day
   c. 5,000 IU/day
   d. 15–20 mg/day
3. Deficiency of niacin causes:
   a. Pellagra
   b. Osteomalacia
   c. Beriberi
   d. Scurvy
4. A rich source of vitamin C is:
   a. Egg
   b. Lemon
   c. Rice
   d. Milk
5. Antivitamin is:
   a. Tocopherol
   b. Digoxin
   c. Aminopterin
   d. Calcitriol

■ SECTION 3: METABOLISM

Chapters 9 and 10

Essay Question

1. Define 'Electron transport chain' (ETC). Give its diagrammatic representation. Mark its parts and mention the sites of ATP production. Describe briefly how electrons from reducing equivalents are transported through it.

Short Notes
1. Enzymes of biological oxidation
2. Electron transport chain
3. Oxidative phosphorylation
4. Chemiosmotic theory
5. Two methods to investigate metabolism

Minor Questions
1. Name two:
   a. Inhibitors of electron transport chain
   b. Uncouplers oxidative phosphorylation
2. Name two:
   a. High-energy compounds
   b. Low-energy compounds
3. Mention four groups of enzymes involved in biological oxidation.
4. Explain oxidation reduction with one example.
5. Define:
   a. Anabolism   b. Catabolism
   c. Amphibolism   d. Bioenergetics
6. Write two differences between substrate level phosphorylation and oxidative phosphorylation.

Multiple Choice Questions
1. Electron transport chain (respiratory chain) is located in:
   a. Nucleus   b. Mitochondria
   c. Lysosomes   d. Ribosomes
2. Oxidative phosphorylation is the process for:
   a. Phosphorylation of glucose
   b. Generating creatine phosphate
   c. Generating ATP
   d. Utilizing ATP
3. An example for high-energy compound:
   a. GMP
   b. Glucose-6-phosphate
   c. ATP
   d. AMP
4. Energy is liberated during:
   a. Anabolism   b. Conjugation
   c. Catabolism   d. Transamination

Chapter 11

Essay Questions
1. Give a detailed account of digestion and absorption of carbohydrates.
2. Describe glycolysis (Embden–Meyerhof pathway). Add a note on its energetics and importance.
3. Write the reactions of citric acid cycle/TCA cycle/Krebs cycle. Add a note on its energetics and importance.
4. Give a brief account of glycogen metabolism (or) gluconeogenesis.
5. Describe the hexose monophosphate (HMP) shunt. What is its importance?
6. Discuss the regulation of blood sugar (or) glucose homeostasis (or) maintenance of blood sugar.

Short Notes
1. Glycogen storage diseases
2. Glycogenesis
3. Glycogenolysis
4. Uronic acid pathway
5. Lactose intolerance
6. Fructose metabolism
7. Galactose metabolism
8. Galactosemia
9. Diabetes mellitus
10. Glucose tolerance test (GTT)
11. Glycosuria

Minor Questions
1. Name the two glucose transporters.
2. What is Rapoport Luebering cycle?
3. What is Cori cycle?
4. What is lactic acidosis?
5. Which enzyme is deficient in:
   a. von Gierke's disease
   b. Essential pentosuria
6. What is renal glycosuria?
7. What is hypoglycemia?

Multiple Choice Questions
1. All the following enzymes are involved in the digestion of carbohydrates, *except:*
   a. Pancreatic amylase
   b. Isomaltase
   c. Pepsin
   d. Salivary amylase
2. ATP yield (current concept) in citric acid cycle per turn is:
   a. 2   b. 8
   c. 10   d. 20
3. Normal fasting level of glucose in plasma is:
   a. 15–45 mg%
   b. 70–110 mg%
   c. 150–220 mg%
   d. 60–160 mg%

4. Pyruvate is converted to acetyl-CoA by:
   a. Oxidation
   b. Oxidative decarboxylation
   c. Reduction
   d. CO_2 fixation
5. Enzyme deficient in von Gierke's disease:
   a. Glycogen synthase
   b. Glucose 6-phosphatase
   c. Glucokinase
   d. Phosphorylase

Chapter 12
Essay Questions
1. Describe the digestion and absorption of lipids (Fats).
2. Discuss β-oxidation of fatty acids. Add a note on its energetics and regulation.
3. Describe the de novo biosynthesis (extramitochondrial pathway) of fatty acids.
4. Name the ketone bodies. How are they formed and utilized in the body?
5. Write the steps in the biosynthesis of cholesterol. Mention the factors which affect cholesterol level in blood.
6. Discuss lipoprotein metabolism.

Short Notes
1. Lipid storage diseases
2. Fatty liver and lipotropic factors
3. Bile acids
4. Reverse cholesterol transport (HDL metabolism)
5. Enterohepatic circulation of bile salts
6. Atherosclerosis
7. Diabetic ketoacidosis

Minor Questions
1. What is fatty acid synthase complex?
2. What is meant by:
   a. α-oxidation of fatty acids
   b. ω-oxidation of fatty acids
3. Name the compound accumulating in:
   a. Gaucher's disease
   b. Nieman–Pick disease
   c. Tay–Sach's disease
4. What is the normal level of cholesterol in serum? Name two conditions in which it is elevated.
5. What is the defect in familial hypercholesterolemia?
6. What is brown adipose tissue?
7. Name the types of hyperlipoproteinemia.
8. BMI
9. What is lipid profile?

Multiple Choice Questions
1. Malabsorption of fat results in:
   a. Lactose intolerance
   b. Gaucher's disease
   c. Steatorrhea
   d. Lactic acidosis
2. Good cholesterol is:
   a. VLDL cholesterol
   b. HDL cholesterol
   c. Chylomicrons
   d. LDL cholesterol
3. Prostaglandins are formed from:
   a. Palmitic acid   b. Linoleic acid
   c. Stearic acid   d. Arachidonic acid
4. β-oxidation of fatty acids takes place in:
   a. Mitochondria
   b. Cytosol
   c. Endoplasmic reticulum
   d. Lysosomes
5. All the following are ketone bodies, *except*:
   a. Acetone   b. Acetic acid
   c. Acetoacetate   d. β-hydroxybutyrate

Chapter 13
Essay Questions
1. Describe the digestion and absorption of proteins.
2. Describe the reactions involved in urea cycle/Krebs–Henseleit cycle. Add a note on its metabolic disorders.
3. Describe the metabolism of each of the following amino acids.
   a. Glycine
   b. Sulfur-containing amino acids
   c. Aromatic amino acids
   d. Branched-chain amino acids

Short Notes
1. Transamination
2. Urea cycle
3. Phenylketonuria
4. Alkaptonuria
5. Albinism
6. Hartnup disease
7. Maple syrup urine disease
8. Transmethylation
9. One carbon metabolism
10. Ammonia intoxication/Toxicity

11. Nitric oxide (NO)
12. GABA
13. Serotonin

Minor Questions

1. Name one:
   a. Endopeptidase
   b. Exopeptidase
2. What are the symptoms of ammonia intoxication?
3. What is the normal level of urea in the blood?
4. Name three amino acids which form creatinine. What is its importance?
5. Mention two:
   a. Catecholamines
   b. Indoleamines
   c. Polyamines
6. Name
   a. Glucogenic amino acids
   b. Ketogenic amino acids
   c. Both
7. What is Meister cycle (γ-glutamyl cycle)?

Multiple Choice Questions

1. Milk protein is digested in the stomach by:
   a. Trypsin   b. Renin
   c. Rennin   d. Lactase
2. Urea cycle occurs mainly in:
   a. Muscle   b. Liver
   c. Kidneys   d. RBCs
3. Histidine can be converted to histamine by:
   a. Oxidation   b. Reduction
   c. Decarboxylation d. Transamination
4. All the following are formed from glycine, *except:*
   a. Heme   b. Serotonin
   c. Purine   d. Creatinine
5. Alkaptonuria occurs due to deficiency of:
   a. Tyrosinase
   b. Phenylalanine hydroxylase
   c. Arginase
   d. Homogentisate oxidase

Chapter 14

Essay Question

1. What is meant by integration of metabolism? Discuss the metabolic changes occurring in the body during starvation or fed state.

Short Notes

1. Metabolic changes in starvation
2. Metabolic changes in fed state
3. Role of liver in metabolic integration

Minor Questions

1. Name the catabolic pathways/anabolic pathways of metabolism.
2. Name the compounds formed from acetyl-CoA.
3. What is the main storage organ for energy?
4. What is the importance of integration of metabolism?

Multiple Choice Questions

1. The metabolic pathway of integration:
   a. Electron transport chain
   b. Glycolysis
   c. β-oxidation
   d. Krebs cycle
2. Main energy source of brain during prolonged starvation:
   a. Fatty acids   b. Glucose
   c. Ketone bodies   d. Fructose

Chapter 15

Essay Questions

1. Describe the synthesis and catabolism of purine nucleotides.
2. Describe the synthesis and catabolism of pyrimidine nucleotides.

Short Notes

1. Digestion and absorption of nucleoproteins
2. Uric acid metabolism/uric acid formation
3. Hyperuricemia
4. Gout

Minor Questions

1. Name the sources of nitrogen and carbon atoms in:
   a. Purine ring   b. Pyrimidine ring
2. Write the salvage pathway for synthesis of:
   a. Purine nucleotide
   b. Pyrimidine nucleotide
3. Write enzyme deficiency and symptoms of Lesch–Nyhan syndrome.
4. What is xanthinuria?
5. What is uricotelic organism?

Multiple Choice Questions

1. The major end product of purine catabolism in humans is:
   a. Xanthine   b. Uric acid
   c. Allantoin   d. Urea
2. A drug which is used to treat gout is:
   a. Rifampicin   b. Aspirin
   c. Allopurinol   d. Digoxin
3. Uric acid is formed from xanthine by the action of:
   a. Xanthine oxidase   b. Tyrosinase
   c. Arginase   d. LDH
4. Which one of the following is an inborn error of pyrimidine metabolism?
   a. Orotic aciduria
   b. Gout
   c. Lesch–Nyhan syndrome
   d. Methylmalonic aciduria

Chapter 16

Essay Questions

1. Describe the synthesis of hemoglobin. Add a note on its regulation and inhibition.
2. Describe the catabolism of hemoglobin (or) Discuss the formation of bilirubin and its excretion.

Short Notes

1. Porphyria
2. Jaundice
3. Van den Bergh reaction
4. Neonatal jaundice (physiologic jaundice)

Minor Questions

1. Name two bile pigments.
2. Write the normal level of:
   a. Total bilirubin
   b. Direct bilirubin
   c. Indirect bilirubin
3. What is icteric index?
4. Mention two conditions for hyperbilirubinemia
5. What is Gilbert syndrome?
6. What are urobilinogen and stercobilinogen?

Multiple Choice Questions

1. Synthesis of hemoglobin mainly occurs in:
   a. Mature erythrocytes
   b. Kidney
   c. Spleen
   d. Liver and immature erythrocytes
2. Which enzyme in heme synthesis is inhibited by lead poisoning?
   a. Ferro chelatase
   b. Uroporphyrinogen decarboxylase
   c. ALA dehydratase
   d. ALA synthase
3. Catabolism of hemoglobin produces:
   a. Acetyl-CoA   b. Bile acids
   c. Bile pigments   d. Pyruvic acid
4. Normal level of bilirubin (total) in serum is:
   a. 0.2–1 mg%   b. 0.5–1.5 mg%
   c. 0.2–0.4 mg%   d. 1–2 mg%
5. Jaundice occurs due to increased concentration of:
   a. Bile acids   b. Ketone bodies
   c. Bile pigments   d. None of the above

Chapter 17

Essay Questions

1. Name the two major groups of minerals. Give examples. Write the sources, functions and abnormalities of any one mineral in each group.
2. Write the sources, absorption, and functions of calcium in the body. Add a note on the regulation of calcium.
3. Write the sources, distribution, absorption, transport, and functions of iron in the body.

Short Notes

1. Electrolytes
2. Iodine metabolism
3. Goiter
4. Anemia
5. Wilson's disease
6. Fluorosis
7. Deficiency and toxicity symptoms of:
   a. Iron   b. Calcium
   c. Iodine   d. Sodium
8. Calcium homeostasis
9. Iron absorption and transport

Minor Questions

1. Name two:
   a. Macrominerals
   b. Microminerals (trace elements)
2. Mention one condition for:
   a. Hyponatremia   b. Hyperkalemia
   c. Hypocalcemia   d. Hemochromatosis
3. Name two copper-containing proteins.

4. What is the cause of:
   a. Menke's disease   b. Bronze diabetes
   c. Tetany   d. Osteoporosis
5. Name the element present in:
   a. Carbonic anhydrase
   b. Cytochrome oxidase
6. What is glucose tolerance factor?
7. What are the function of:
   a. Zinc   b. Magnesium

Multiple Choice Questions

1. Normal level of sodium in serum/plasma is:
   a. 95–105 mEq/L   b. 135–145 mEq/L
   c. 3.5–5 mEq/L   d. 22–28 mEq/L
2. All the following are trace elements, *except*:
   a. Selenium   b. Potassium
   c. Zinc   d. Copper
3. The element present in most abundance in human body is:
   a. Iron   b. Phosphorus
   c. Calcium   d. Sodium
4. Manganese is a constituent of the enzyme:
   a. Arginase
   b. Lactate dehydrogenase
   c. Xanthine oxidase
   d. Enolase
5. All the following are goitrogenic substances, *except*:
   a. Cabbage   b. Sea foods
   c. Radish   d. Cauliflower

Chapter 18

Essay Question

1. What is meant by detoxication? Mention its different mechanisms. Give two examples of each (or) Discuss the various mechanisms of metabolism of xenobiotics with examples.

Short Notes

1. Detoxication
2. Detoxication by conjugation

Minor Questions

1. Explain how the following are detoxified?
   a. Aspirin   b. Phenol
   c. Bilirubin   d. Picric acid
2. What is cytochrome P 450?
3. Name the conjugating agents used in detoxication.

Multiple Choice Questions

1. The principal organ where detoxication takes place is:
   a. Kidney   b. Liver
   c. Intestine   d. Spleen
2. Which of the following compounds is detoxified by oxidation?
   a. Methyl alcohol   b. Picric acid
   c. Bilirubin   d. Benzoic acid
3. Aspirin is detoxified by:
   a. Oxidation   b. Conjugation
   c. Reduction   d. Hydrolysis
4. Phase I detoxication includes:
   a. Hydrolysis   b. Reduction
   c. Oxidation   d. All of the above

Chapter 19

Essay Question

1. Describe the various routes of excretion. Write examples of excretion products of human body.

Short Notes

1. Normal constituents of urine
2. Abnormal constituents of urine

Minor Questions

1. Name:
   a. Four inorganic constituents
   b. Four organic constituents of normal urine.
2. Name the abnormal constituents of urine. Name one condition when each one appears in the urine.
3. Name the test to detect:
   a. Glucose
   b. Albumin
   c. Bile pigments in the abnormal urine.
4. Write the biochemical composition of:
   a. Feces   b. Sweat
5. What is steatorrhea?

Multiple Choice Questions

1. Total volume of urine excreted daily by a normal adult is:
   a. 500–1000 mL   b. 700–1200 mL
   c. 800–1500 mL   d. 2–3 L
2. All the following are abnormal constituents of urine, *except*:
   a. Creatinine   b. Ketone bodies
   c. Bile pigments   d. Glucose

3. Most abundant constituent of sweat is:
   a. KCl   b. CaCl$_2$
   c. NaCl   d. MgCl$_2$

SECTION 4: MISCELLANEOUS TOPICS OF BIOCHEMICAL IMPORTANCE

Chapter 20

Essay Question

1. What is meant by basal metabolic rate (BMR)? How will you measure it? Name three conditions in which BMR is (a) Increased, (b) Decreased

Short Notes

1. Respiratory quotient (RQ)
2. Specific dynamic action (SDA) of foods
3. Basic metabolic rate (BMR)
4. How will you calculate daily calorie requirement of a student?

Minor Questions

1. Name the instrument to measure the calorific value of foods.
2. Define:
   a. Respiratory quotient
   b. Specific dynamic action of foods
   c. BMR
   d. Calorie
3. Name three factors to take into account when calculating daily energy requirement of an individual.
4. Which type of physical activity requires maximum energy?
5. Name the instrument to measure BMR.

Multiple Choice Questions

1. The unit of energy is:
   a. Calorie (C)
   b. Joule (J)
   c. Both of the above
   d. Entropy (s)
2. Oxidation of which substance in the body yields more calories per gram?
   a. Carbohydrate   b. Fats
   c. Plant proteins d. Animal proteins
3. Normal BMR of an adult is:
   a. 10 C/sq m/hr   b. 20 C/sq m/hr
   c. 40 C/sq m/hr   d. 60 C/sq m/hr
4. Daily caloric requirements of an adult is:
   a. 1,000 C   b. 2,500 C
   c. 3,000 C   d. 3,500 C

Chapter 21

Essay Question

1. What are primary foods? Write their sources and nutritional significance/functions.

Short Notes

1. Biological value of proteins
2. Nitrogen balance
3. Protein-caloric malnutrition
4. Dietary fiber
5. Balanced diet
6. Kwashiorkor

Minor Questions

1. Name the energy giving dietary nutrients.
2. What is:
   a. Glycemic index   b. BMI
   c. Food pyramid   d. RDA
3. Name the body building compounds.
4. What is meant by supplementation of amino acids?
5. Mention one:
   a. Complete protein
   b. Incomplete protein
6. Define:
   a. Kwashiorkor   b. Marasmus
7. Name two:
   a. Under-nutritional disorders
   b. Overnutritional disorders

Multiple Choice Questions

1. Proportion of carbohydrates, fat, and protein in the balanced diet is:
   a. 1:1:4   b. 1:4:1
   c. 4:1:1   d. 1:2:4
2. Disease due to overnutrition is:
   a. Marasmus   b. Hartnup disease
   c. Atherosclerosis d. Wilson's disease
3. Milk is rich in all the following, *except*:
   a. Iron   b. Phosphorus
   c. Calcium   d. Sodium
4. Kwashiorkor occurs due to dietary deficiency of:
   a. Minerals
   b. Carbohydrates
   c. Proteins
   d. Vitamins

Chapter 22

Essay Question

1. Write the composition of fluid compartments of the body. How is fluid and electrolyte balance maintained?

Short Notes

1. Electrolytes
2. Regulation of fluid and electrolyte balance

Minor Questions

1. Name the major electrolytes in plasma. What are their normal levels in plasma?
2. Mention one condition for:
   a. Dehydration
   b. Overhydration

Multiple Choice Questions

1. The major cation present in the intracellular fluid is:
   a. Potassium   b. Sodium
   c. Magnesium   d. Calcium
2. Which hormone regulates electrolyte balance?
   a. Cortisol   b. Insulin
   c. Oxytocin   d. ADH

Chapter 23

Essay Questions

1. What is the normal pH of blood? How is it maintained? Discuss the various mechanisms by which acid–base balance is regulated.
2. Name the various acid–base disorders. Mention their causes, changes, and compensatory mechanisms.

Short Notes

1. Blood buffers and their role in acid–base balance.
2. Respiratory mechanism of acid–base balance.
3. Renal mechanism of acid–base balance.
4. Acidosis/metabolic acidosis.
5. Alkalosis/respiratory alkalosis.
6. Anion gap.

Minor Questions

1. What is the normal pH of blood? Name two conditions when it is altered.
2. Name three mechanisms which regulate (maintain) pH of blood.
3. Write the Henderson–Hasselbalch equation. What is its importance?
4. Give two causes for:
   a. Metabolic acidosis
   b. Respiratory acidosis
   c. Metabolic alkalosis
   d. Respiratory alkalosis
5. What is chloride shift? Write its importance.
6. What is alkali reserve?
7. Mention the normal levels of acid–base parameters in blood.

Multiple Choice Questions

1. Normal pH of arterial blood is:
   a. 6.35–6.45
   b. 7.35–7.45
   c. 4.35–4.45
   d. 6.95–7.25
2. The ratio between bicarbonate and carbonic acid in the blood is:
   a. 10:1   b. 20:1
   c. 1:1   d. 2:1
3. Mechanism for regulation of acid–base balance includes:
   a. Renal mechanism
   b. Respiratory mechanism
   c. Blood buffers
   d. All of the above
4. Metabolic acidosis occurs due to:
   a. Renal failure   b. Diarrhea
   c. Diabetes mellitus   d. All of the above

Chapter 24

Essay Questions

1. Name the liver function tests. Describe any three of them.
2. Mention the renal function tests. Describe the clearance tests based on measurement of glomerular filtration rate (GFR).

Short Notes

1. Van den Bergh test
2. Creatinine clearance test
3. Urea clearance test
4. Gastric function tests
5. Thyroid function tests

Minor Questions

1. Name three types of jaundice.
2. Name the enzymes used to assess the function of the liver.

3. Name two tests to measure glomerular filtration rate (GFR).
4. Name two gastric function tests. Which device is used to aspirate gastric juice?
5. Name two enzymes which are increased in acute pancreatitis/which are used to assess pancreatic function.
6. Name the cardiac biochemical markers.

Multiple Choice Questions

1. Which one is not liver function test?
   a. Galactose tolerance test
   b. Prothrombin time
   c. Urea clearance test
   d. Bromsulfthalein test
2. Normal creatinine clearance is:
   a. 1–2 mL/min   b. 50–60 mL/min
   c. 90–120 mL/min   d. 150–200 mL/min
3. Gastric function can be assessed by:
   a. BSP excretion test
   b. Xylose excretion test
   c. Hippuric acid synthesis test
   d. Fractional test meal analysis
4. Test to detect jaundice in urine:
   a. Benzidine test   b. Fouchet test
   c. Rothera's test   d. Molisch test

Chapter 25

Essay Questions

1. What are hormones? Classify them according to their mechanism of action. Give their important functions.
2. Name the hormones secreted by adrenal medulla. Write their metabolic actions.
3. Write the structure, functions, regulation, and abnormalities of insulin.
4. Describe the synthesis, functions, and abnormalities of thyroid hormones.
5. Mention the pituitary hormones. Write their functions.

Short Notes

1. Glucagon
2. Prolactin
3. Thyroxine/cortisol
4. Insulin
5. Gastrointestinal hormones
6. Gonadal hormones
7. Mechanism of action of peptide (protein) or steroid hormone
8. Second messengers

Minor Questions

1. Name two:
   a. Protein hormones
   b. Steroid hormones
2. What are second messengers? Name the second messenger of:
   a. Glucagon   b. Insulin
3. Name the hormones secreted by:
   a. Posterior pituitary gland
   b. Pancreas
4. Write the causes and symptoms of:
   a. Cushing's syndrome
   b. Addison's disease
   c. Pheochromocytomas
   d. Cretinism
5. Write the importance of 17-ketosteroids

Multiple Choice Questions

1. The hormones produced by α cells of islets of Langerhans of pancreas is:
   a. Insulin   b. Glucagon
   c. Aldosterone   d. ADH
2. All steroid hormones are formed from:
   a. Acetyl-CoA   b. Glycerol
   c. Arachidonic acid   d. Cholesterol
3. Hyperthyroidism results in:
   a. Grave's disease
   b. Cushing's syndrome
   c. Addison's disease
   d. Pheochromocytoma
4. All the following are peptide/protein hormones, *except*:
   a. GH   b. Insulin
   c. Cortisol   d. Prolactin
5. Diabetes insipidus occurs due to deficient secretion of:
   a. Oxytocin   b. ADH
   c. Glucagon   d. Gastrin

■ SECTION 5: APPLIED BIOCHEMISTRY

Chapter 26

Essay Questions

1. Define 'replication'. Describe its mechanism in 'prokaryotes'. How does it differ from that of eukaryotes?
2. Define 'transcription'. Describe how does it occur?
3. Define 'translation'. Describe it in detail (or) Describe the process of protein biosynthesis.
4. Discuss recombinant DNA technology.

5. Name the molecular biological techniques. Describe any two in detail.

Short Notes

1. Cell cycle
2. Post-translational modifications
3. Genetic code
4. Blotting techniques/southern blot
5. Polymerase chain reaction (PCR)
6. Recombinant DNA technology
7. Biotechnology
8. Human genome project
9. Gene therapy
10. Mutation

Minor Questions

1. Define:
   a. Gene
   b. Cistron
   c. Genome
   d. Nucleosome
2. What is central dogma of molecular biology?
3. What do you mean by reverse transcription?
4. Mention four mechanisms of DNA repair. What is xeroderma pigmentosum?
5. What are restriction endonucleolases? Give one example.
6. What is:
   a. Finger-printing technique
   b. RFLP
   c. Northern blot
   d. Western blot
   e. Cloning

Multiple Choice Questions

1. Replication is the synthesis of:
   a. DNA from RNA
   b. DNA from DNA
   c. RNA from DNA
   d. Protein from RNA
2. Method to detect DNA is:
   a. Western blot
   b. Southern blot
   c. Northern blot
   d. Hybridoma technology
3. Total number of codons in the genetic code is:
   a. 3   b. 61
   c. 64   d. 74
4. Cell cycle occurs in:
   a. Cytosol   b. Nucleus
   c. Lysosomes   d. Ribosomes
5. Protein biosynthesis (translation) mainly occurs in:
   a. Nucleus   b. Mitochondria
   c. Ribosomes   d. Cell membrane

Chapter 27

Essay Questions

1. Give an account of various plasma proteins and their functions.
2. What are immunoglobulins? Give their origin, structure, and functions.

Short Notes

1. Structure and functions of immunoglobulin G.
2. Monoclonal antibodies
3. Hybridoma technology

Minor Questions

1. Name the five types of immunoglobulins.
2. Name the technique to separate immunoglobulins.
3. Name two autoimmune diseases
4. Define:
   a. Antigen   b. Antibody

Multiple Choice Questions

1. Immunoglobulins belong to which fraction of plasma protein?
   a. Albumin   b. α-globulins
   c. β-globulins   c. γ-globulins
2. Immunoglobulin which can cross-placental barrier to fetus is:
   a. Immunoglobulin E
   b. Immunoglobulin G
   c. Immunoglobulin D
   d. Immunoglobulin A
3. All the following are immunoglobulins, *except:*
   a. IgD   b. IgE
   c. IgS   d. IgG

Chapter 28

Essay Questions

1. Mention ten important substances of biochemical importance present in the blood. Give their normal range. Name two conditions in which each one is increased.
2. Mention ten important substances present in the urine. Write their normal range. Name two conditions in which each one is increased.

Short Notes

1. Diagnostic enzymes/plasma proteins
2. Diabetes mellitus
3. Electrolytes
4. Types of tests in clinical biochemistry
5. Electrophoresis of serum proteins
6. Abnormal urine

Minor Questions

1. Define: Normal range (normal value/reference value)
2. Write the normal values of
    a. Fasting sugar
    b. Postprandial sugar
    c. Random sugar in plasma
3. Name any four important instruments used in clinical biochemistry laboratory.
4. Name any two important techniques used in clinical biochemistry laboratory.
5. What is renal glycosuria?

Multiple Choice Questions

1. Normal level of total protein in serum is:
    a. 3.2–5.8 g% b. 5–7.5 g%
    c. 6–8 g%   d. 7.5–8.5 g%
2. Urinary excretion of creatinine per day is:
    a. 300–700 mg b. 1–2 g
    c. 10–15 g   d. 15–30 g
3. Diabetes mellitus can be detected by which test using urine specimen?
    a. Hay's test   b. Benedict's test
    c. Rothera's test d. Benzidine test
4. Which fraction of plasma proteins is increased in nephrotic syndrome?
    a. Albumin   b. α_2-globulins
    c. β-globulin d. γ-globulin

Chapter 29

Essay Question

1. Name the different techniques instruments used in biochemistry laboratory. Describe any two of them.

Short Notes

1. Chromatography
2. Electrophoresis
3. Enzyme-linked immunosorbent assay (ELISA)/RIA
4. Hybridoma technology
5. Centrifuge/glucometer
6. Colorimeter
7. Spectrophotometer
8. Flame photometer/electrolyte analyzer
9. pH meter
10. Autoanalyzers

Minor Questions

1. Name the technique to separate:
    a. Amino acids
    b. Plasma proteins
2. What is Beer–Lambert's Law?
3. Name the instrument to measure:
    a. Blood gases
    b. Hormones
    c. Electrolytes
4. Name the instrument to measure:
    a. Specific gravity of urine
    b. Specific gravity of milk

Multiple Choice Questions

1. Which instrument is used for quantitative estimation of constituents of blood in the clinical biochemistry laboratory?
    a. Calorimeter   b. Colorimeter
    c. pH meter   d. Centrifuge
2. Device used to collect gastric juice:
    a. Spectroscope b. Folin Wu tube
    c. Ryle's tube   d. None of the above
3. Paper chromatography is used to separate:
    a. Proteins   b. Nucleic acids
    c. Amino acids   d. Enzymes

Chapter 30

Essay Question

1. Describe the role of biochemistry in medical and paramedical specialties.

Short Notes

1. Role of biochemistry in medicine
2. Role of biochemistry in paramedical specialties.

Minor Questions

1. How is biochemistry important for nursing speciality?
2. Why pharmacy students are advised to learn biochemistry?
3. Why biochemistry is important for physiotherapist?
4. Biochemistry is the backbone of medical laboratory technology. Explain.

Appendices

SECTION 6: SPECIAL TOPICS

Chapters 31 to 36

Essay Questions

1. What are eicosanoids. Describe the sources, types and functions of prostaglandins.
2. Discuss lipid peroxidation. Add a note on antioxidants.
3. Narrate the different types of environmental pollutants. Add a note on chemical carcinogens.
4. What is meant by biotechnology? Name its branches. List its applications in various fields.

Short Notes

1. Eicosanoids
2. Prostaglandins
3. Synthesis of prostaglandins
4. Lipid peroxidation
5. Antioxidants
6. Environmental pollutants
7. Cancer
8. Tumor markers
9. Viruses
10. Biotechnology

Minor Questions

1. What are eicosanoids? Give four examples.
2. Mention the types of prostaglandins.
3. Write any two functions of prostaglandins.
4. What is meant by: (a) Lipid peroxidation; (b) Free radicals; (c) Rancidity; (d) Antioxidant.
5. Name four environmental pollutants/chemical carcinogens.
6. What is cancer? Give its alternative names.
7. Mention the causative agents of cancer.
8. Name four tumor markers.
9. What are the biochemical effects of cancer?
10. Mention two viruses.
11. What are (a) Oncogens (b) Antioncogens?
12. Mention two application of Biotechnology.

ANSWERS FOR MCQs

Ch. 1	1. c	2. b	3. c	4. c	5. d
Ch. 2	1. c	2. a	3. b	4. d	5. d
Ch. 3	1. d	2. c	3. c	4. d	5. a
Ch. 4	1. b	2. b	3. b	4. c	5. b
Ch. 5	1. b	2. c	3. a	4. c	--
Ch. 6	1. c	2. a	3. c	4. b	--
Ch. 7	1. a	2. c	3. d	4. c	5. c
Ch. 8	1. c	2. c	3. a	4. b	5. c
Ch. 9	1. b	2. c	3. c	4. c	--
Ch. 10	1. b	2. c	3. c	4. c	--
Ch. 11	1. c	2. c	3. b	4. b	5. b
Ch. 12	1. c	2. b	3. d	4. a	5. b
Ch. 13	1. c	2. b	3. c	4. b	5. d
Ch. 14	1. d	2. c	--	--	--
Ch. 15	1. b	2. c	3. a	4. a	--
Ch. 16	1. d	2. c	3. c	4. a	5. c
Ch. 17	1. b	2. b	3. c	4. c	5. b
Ch. 18	1. b	2. a	3. d	4. d	--
Ch. 19	1. c	2. a	3. c	--	--
Ch. 20	1. c	2. b	3. c	4. b	--
Ch. 21	1. c	2. c	3. a	4. c	--
Ch. 22	1. a	2. d	--	--	--
Ch. 23	1. b	2. b	3. d	4. d	--
Ch. 24	1. c	2. c	3. d	4. b	--
Ch. 25	1. b	2. d	3. a	4. c	5. b
Ch. 26	1. b	2. b	3. c	4. b	5. c
Ch. 27	1. d	2. b	3. c	--	--
Ch. 28	1. c	2. b	3. b	4. b	--
Ch. 29	1. b	2. c	3. c	--	--

APPENDIX B: CLINICAL CASES

1. A 10-year-old boy was suffering from abdominal discomfort, bloating, increased urination, and diarrhea after taking milk.
   a. What is the probable diagnosis?
   b. What is it due to?
   c. Suggest to relieve the symptoms.
2. A patient's blood on investigation showed an abnormal hemoglobin (Hbs).
   a. What is your diagnosis?
   b. What is its cause?
3. A 45-year-old male with history of alcoholism had fatty liver on examination and investigation.
   a. What is fatty liver?
   b. What are two types of fatty liver?
   c. Name two lipotropic factors.
4. Blood glucose level of a person in postprandial state was 145 mg/100 mL. Benedict test with urine was positive.
   a. Mention the clinical condition.
   b. What is it due to?
5. A newborn baby developed yellowish discoloration of the skin and conjunctiva three days after birth. He was given phototherapy.
   a. What is the type of clinical condition?
   b. Why phototherapy is given?
   c. Name the investigations to diagnose the condition.
6. A 3-year-old boy with retarded growth was brought to the hospital with complaint of diarrhea. On examination, he was found to have cataract in both eyes.
   a. What is the probable diagnosis?
   b. What is the biochemical basis of this disorder?
7. Comment on the acid–base status of the patient on the following data.
   pH: 7.15
   pCO_2: 39 mm Hg
   Plasma bicarbonate: 16 mEq/L
   a. What is your diagnosis?
   b. Write the normal levels of the above parameters in blood.
   c. What is the instrument to measure them?
8. A sample of urine for routine analysis from a child turned dark. Urine reduced Benedict's reagent and test for homogentisic acid was positive.
   a. What is this disorder?
   b. Why does it happen?
9. A patient aged 55 years was admitted with the complaint of acute pain in the abdomen on laboratory investigation, serum amylase and lipase were highly elevated.
   a. What is your diagnosis?
   b. What are their normal levels in serum?
10. A patient came to O.P of the hospital with chest pain.
    a. What are the biochemical investigations you will suggest?
    b. Which one is the most preferable?
11. Calculate the creatinine clearance from the values given below.
    Plasma creatinine: 0.8 mg/100 mL
    Volume of 24 hours urine: 1,500 mL/day
    Urine creatinine: 90 mg/100 mL
    a. What is your interpretation?
    b. Mention the normal levels of the above.
12. A 30-year-old man presented with spongy bleeding gums and loose teeth.
    a. What is the disease the patient is suffering from?
    b. What is the biochemical basis of this disease?
13. A 20-year-old boy had generalized edema of the body with puffiness of the face in the morning.
    a. What is your diagnosis?
    b. What are the changes in the serum electrophoretic pattern of this patient?
14. A lean 10-year-old boy was brought to the OP with the complaint of passing urine frequently. His laboratory report is:
    Urine sugar: +++
    Blood glucose (F): 190 mg
    Blood glucose (PP): 420 mg
    a. What is the probable diagnosis?
    b. What is it due to?
15. A 20-year-old female patient came for ophthalmic examination. She was found to have Kayser-Fleischer rings around the cornea in both eyes.
    a. What is the disease the patient is suffering from?
    b. What are the biochemical abnormalities of this disease?

16. A 5-year-old boy had bone deformities such as bow legs, pigeon chest. He had delayed eruption of teeth. He was a pure vegetarian and used to take less amount of milk.
    a. What is the diagnosis?
    b. What are the biochemical investigations to confirm it?
17. A man aged 55 years came to the hospital with history of recurrent attacks of joint pain especially at big toe. His joints were swollen and tender.
    a. What is your diagnosis?
    b. What is the biochemical cause?
18. A child aged 4 years presented with generalized edema, moon face and muscle wasting.
    a. What is your probable diagnosis?
    b. What is the cause and treatment?
19. A 12-year-old boy was brought to the hospital with the history of mental retardation, stunted growth and swelling in the neck. He was diagnosed to have hypothyroidism.
    a. Which mineral is deficient in the patient?
    b. Mention the clinical symptoms of this disease.
20. Following are the results of oral GTT performed on a 60- year-old man.
    a. Interpret the results.
    b. Mention the normal levels of FBS and PPBS.

Time (hour)	Blood glucose (mg %)	Urine sugar
0 (F)	195	Green
1/2	270	Orange
1	350	Brick red
1 1/2	325	Brick red
2	290	Orange

ANSWERS

1. Lactose intolerance
2. Sickle cell anemia
3. Fatty liver
4. Renal glycosuria
5. Neonatal jaundice
6. Galactosemia
7. Metabolic acidosis
8. Alkaptonuria
9. Acute pancreatitis
10. Myocardial infarction (MI)
11. Use the formula $\dfrac{U \times V}{P}$
12. Scurvy
13. Nephrotic syndrome
14. Diabetes mellitus type-I (IDDM)
15. Wilson's Disease
16. Rickets
17. Gout
18. Kwashiorkor
19. Hypothyroidism
20. Diabetes mellitus type-II (NIDDM)

APPENDIX C: INBORN ERRORS OF METABOLISM

DEFINITION

Inborn errors of metabolism (IEM) are genetic (inherited) disorders which are caused by deficiency of enzymes/proteins involved in metabolic pathways. They produce a wide variety of symptoms. They can be diagnosed by screening tests.

$$\text{Substrate} \xrightarrow{\text{Enzyme}} \text{Product}$$

Details: *Refer* respective pages

Sl. No.	IEM	Enzyme deficiency/metabolic defect
I.	*Carbohydrate metabolism*	
1.	Glycogen storage diseases	*Refer* p. 142
2.	Essential fructosuria	Fructokinase
3.	Fructose intolerance	Aldolase B
4.	Galactosemia	Galactose 1-phosphate uridyl transferase
5.	Pentosuria	Xylitol dehydrogenase
6.	G6PD deficiency	Glucose-6 phosphate Dehydrogenase (G6PD)
II.	*Lipid metabolism*	
1.	Gaucher's disease	β-glucosidase
2.	Niemann-Pick disease	Sphingomyelinase
3.	Tay-Sachs disease	Hexosaminidase A
4.	Familial hypercholesterolemia	Defective LDL receptors
5.	Hyperlipoproteinemia Hypolipoproteinemia	*Refer* p. 162
III.	*Protein metabolism*	
1.	Glycinuria	Defective renal reabsorption
2.	Primary hyperoxaluria	Glycine transaminase
3.	Cystinuria	Defective renal reabsorption
4.	Cystinosis	Defective lysosomal function
5.	Homocystinuria type I (classic)	Cystathionine synthase
6.	Maple syrup urine disease	Branched chain α-ketoacid dehydrogenase
7.	Histidinemia	Histidase
8.	Hyperprolinemia type I	Proline oxidase
9.	Phenylketonuria (classic)	Phenylalanine hydroxylase
10.	Alkaptonuria	Homogentisate oxidase
11.	Albinism	Tyrosinase
12.	Hartnup disease	Defective intestinal absorption of tryptophan
13.	Urea cycle disorders	*Refer* p. 169

Contd...

Contd...

Sl. No.	IEM	Enzyme deficiency/metabolic defect
IV.	***Nucleotide metabolism***	
1.	Gout	Deficiency of HGPRT and superactive PRPP synthetase
2.	Lesch–Nyhan syndrome	Deficiency of HGPRT
3.	Orotic aciduria	Deficiency of orotate phosphorisbosyl transferase and orotate decarboxylase
4.	Xanthinuria	Deficiency of xanthine oxidase
V.	***Hemoglobin metabolism***	
1.	Porphyria	*Refer* page 197
2.	Crigler–Najjar syndrome type-I	UDP–glucuronyl transferase
3.	Crigler–Najjar syndrorme type-II	UDP–glucuronyl transferase
VI.	***Mineral metabolism***	
1.	Wilson's disease	Mutation in ATP7B gene Accumulation of copper in liver, brain, etc.
2.	Menke's disease	Defective absorption of copper
VII.	***Molecular biology***	
1.	Xeroderma pigmentosum	Defect in DNA repair mechanism (nucleotide excision repair)

APPENDIX D: ISOMERISM

ISOMERISM (REFER CHAPTER 2)

Compounds having same molecular formula but different structures are called as isomers. The phenomenon of existence of isomers is known as isomerism. They differ in physical and chemical properties.

Basically, isomerism is divided into two types and subtypes **(Fig. A1)**:

Structural Isomerism

Due to difference in the arrangement of atoms in the molecule.
- *Chain isomerism:* Due to variation in carbon chains.
- *Position isomerism:* Due to difference in the position of functional groups.
- *Functional isomerism:* Due to difference in both molecular chains and functional groups.

Note

Tautomerism is a type of structural isomerism which occurs due to migration of atom or group from one position to other.

Stereoisomerism

Same structural formula but differ in a spacial arrangement of atoms or groups in the molecule.

Geometrical Isomerism (Cis-trans isomerism)

It occurs in molecules having double bonds.
- *Cis isomerism:* Similar groups occur on the same side.
- *Trans isomerism:* Similar groups occur on opposite side.

For example:

$$H-C-COOH \qquad H-C-COOH$$
$$H-C-COOH \qquad HOOC-C-H$$

Malic acid (Cis)   Fumaric acid (Trans)

Optical Isomerism

It occurs due to the presence of an asymmetric carbon atom (chiral carbon). A carbon is chiral (asymmetric) that is attached to four different groups. Their mirror images cannot be superimposed e.g., right hand is the mirror image of left hand. Compounds having optical isomerism are called as optical isomers. They differ in their optical activity to rotate the plane polarized light.

- Dexorotatory (d or +)
  Optical isomer rotates the plane polarized light to right.
- Levorotatory (1 or –)
  Optical isomer rotates the plane polarized light to left.
- Racemic mixture
  It contains equal concentration of d and l forms and cannot rotate the plane polarized light.

Measurement: Optical rotation can be measured by polarimeter.

Formula to calculate the number of optical isomers: 2^n

Where n refers to number of chiral carbons (For more details, *refer* Chapter 2)

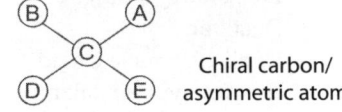

Chiral carbon/asymmetric atom

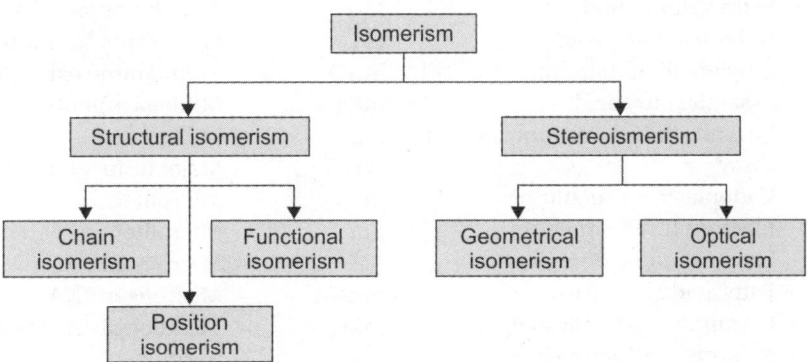

Fig. A1: Isomerism.

APPENDIX E: ABBREVIATIONS USED IN THIS BOOK

A/G	– Albumin/globulin (ratio)	FMN	– Flavin mononucleotide
ACTH	– Adrenocorticotropic hormone	FSH	– Follicle-stimulating hormone
ADH	– Antidiuretic hormone	FTM	– Fractional test meal
ADP	– Adenosine diphosphate	GABA	– γ-aminobutyric acid
AFP	– α-fetoprotein	GAG	– Glycosaminoglycans
AIDS	– Acquired immunodeficiency syndrome	GGT (rGT)	– γ-glutamyl transferase
		GLUT	– Glucose transporters
ALP	– Alkaline phosphate	GMP	– Guanosine monophosphate
ALT	– Alanine transaminase	g	– Gram
AMP	– Adenosine monophosphate	HBA_1C	– Glycosylated hemoglobin
AST	– Aspartate transaminase	HbA1	– Adult hemoglobin
ATP	– Adenosine triphosphate	HbF	– Fetal hemoglobin
BMR	– Basal metabolic rate	HbO_2	– Oxyhemoglobin
BPG	– Bisphosphoglycerate (2, 3-BPG)	HbS	– Sickle-cell hemoglobin
		Hb	– Hemoglobin
BUN	– Blood urea nitrogen	hCG	– Human chorionic gonadotropin
Cal	– Calorie	HDL	– High density lipoproteins
cAMP	– 3', 5'-cyclic adenosine monophosphate (cyclic AMP)	HGPRT	– Hypoxanthine guanine phosphoribosyltransferase
CEA	– Carcinoembryonic antigen	HIAA	– Hydroxyl indole acetic acid
CMP	– Cytidine monophosphate	HIV	– Human immunodeficiency virus
CNS	– Central nervous system	HLA	– Human leukocyte antigen
CoA	– Coenzyme A	HMP	– Hexose monophosphate
COHb	– Carboxyhemoglobin	HPLC	– High performance liquid chromatography
CoQ	– Coenzyme Q (ubiquinone)		
CPK (CK)	– Creatine phosphokinase (creatine kinase)	HRE	– Hormone responsive element
		IDDM	– Insulin-dependent diabetes mellitus
CPS	– Carbamoyl phosphate synthase		
CSF	– Cerebrospinal fluid	Ig	– Immunoglobulin
DAM	– Diacetyl monoxime	IMP	– Inosine monophosphate
ΔG	– Free energy change	IU	– International unit
dl	– Deciliter	IV	– Intravenous
DNA	– Deoxyribonucleic acid	LDH	– Lactate dehydrogenase
DOPA	– Dihydroxyphenylalanine	LDL	– Low density lipoproteins
ECF	– Extracellular fluid	LFT	– Liver function tests
EC	– Enzyme commission	LH	– Luteinizing hormone
EDTA	– Ethylenediaminetetraacetic acid	MAO	– Monoamine oxidase
EFA	– Essential fatty acids	mEq	– Milliequivalents
ELISA	– Enzyme-linked immunosorbent assay	mg	– Milligram
		MHC	– Major histocompatibility complex
ER	– Endoplasmic reticulum	μL	– Microliter
ETC	– Electron transport chain	μm	– Microliter
FAD	– Flavin adenine dinucleotide	μM	– Micromoles
FAS	– Fatty acid synthase	mRNA	– Messenger RNA
FIGLU	– Formiminoglutamic acid	MSH	– Melanocyte-stimulating hormone
fMet	– N-formylmethionine		

mtDNA	– Mitochondrial DNA	rDNA	– Recombinant DNA
NAD$^+$	– Nicotinamide adenine dinucleotide	RER	– Rough endoplasmic reticulum
		Rf	– Ratio of fronts
NADH	– Reduced NAD$^+$	RIA	– Radioimmunoassay
NADP$^+$	– Nicotinamide adenine dinucleotide phosphate	RNA	– Ribonucleic acid
		RQ	– Respiratory quotient
NADPH	– Reduced NADP$^+$	rRNA	– Ribosomal RNA
NMR	– Nuclear magnetic resonance	SAM	– S-adenosylmethionine
NPN	– Non-protein nitrogen	SCID	– Severe combined immunodeficiency
OD	– Optical density		
PABA	– Para aminobenzoic acid	SDA	– Specific dynamic action
PAGE	– Polyacrylamide gel electrophoresis	SGOT	– Serum glutamate oxaloacetate transaminase
PBI	– Protein bound iodine	T$_3$	– 3, 5, 3'-triiodothyronine
pCO$_2$	– Partial pressure of CO$_2$	T$_4$	– 3, 5, 3', 5-tetraiodothyronine (thyroxine)
PDH	– Pyruvate dehydrogenase		
PEM	– Protein-energy malnutrition	TCA	– Tricarboxylic acid
PER	– Protein efficiency ratio	TIBC	– Total iron binding capacity
PGA	– Pteroylglutamic acid	TLC	– Thin layer chromatography
PG	– Prostaglandins	TMP	– Thymidine monophosphate
pH	– Negative log of (H$^+$)	TPP	– Thiamine pyrophosphate
Pi	– Inorganic phosphate	tRNA	– Transfer RNA
pO$_2$	– Partial pressure of O$_2$	UDPG	– Uridine disphosphate
POMC	– Proopiomelanocortin	UMP	– Uridine monophosphate
PRPP	– Phosphoribosyl pyrophosphate	UTP	– Uridine triphosphate
		UV	– Ultraviolet
PTH	– Parathyroid hormone	VLDL	– Very low density lipoproteins
PT	– Prothrombin time	VMA	– Vanillyl mandelic acid
PUFA	– Polyunsaturated fatty acids		

APPENDIX F: LIST OF PARAMEDICAL COURSES (ALLIED HEALTH SCIENCE COURSES) [BSc (UG) LEVEL]

1. BSc Nursing
2. B. Pharm
3. BSc Medical Laboratory Technology
4. BSc Nutrition and Dietetics
5. BPT
6. BOT
7. BSc Optometry/B.Sc Ophthalmic Technology.
8. BSc Perfusion Technology
9. BSc Dialysis Technology
10. BSc Renal Science
11. BSc Neuro Science
12. BSc Biomedical Sciences
13. BSc Anaesthesia Technology
14. BSc Dialysis Technology
15. BSc Radiology and Imaging
16. BSc Radiotherapy Technology
17. BSc X-ray Technology
18. BSc Operation Theater Technology (OTT)
19. BSc Emergency and Trauma Care Technology
20. BSc Respiratory Care Technology
21. BSc Biochemistry
22. BSc Molecular Biology
23. BSc Biotechnology
24. BSc Medical Genetics
25. BSc Medical Record Technology
26. BSc Audiology and Speech Technology
27. BSc Cardiac Technology
28. BSc Cathlab Technology
29. BSc Blood Bank Technology
30. BSc Public Health
31. BSc Physician Assistant
32. BSc Medical Bionano Technology
33. B Tech Biomedical Engineering
34. BSc Clinical Research
35. BSc Medical Technology
36. AUSH
37. BSc Forensic Science
38. BSc Radiology
39. BSc Paramedical Science Course
40. BSc Allied Health Science Course

APPENDIX G: NORMAL VALUE CHART

NORMAL VALUES/REFERENCE RANGE

Parameter	Normal values
Blood (Serum/plasma)	
Bilirubin	
Total	0.2–1 mg/dL
Direct	0–0.2 mg/dL
Indirect	0.2–0.8 mg/dL
Cholesterol	
Total	150–200 mg/dL
HDL	30–60 mg/dL
LDL	80–150 mg/dL
VLDL	20–40 mg/dL
Calcium	9–11 mg/dL
Creatinine	0.6–1.2 mg/dL
Glucose	
Fasting (F)	70–110 mg/dL
Postprandial (PP)	<140 mg/dL
Random (R)	70–170 mg/dL
Phosphorus	3–4.5 mg/dL
Protein	
Total	6–8 g/dL
Albumin	3.5–5 g/dL
Globulins	2.5–3.5 g/dL
A/G ratio	1.2–1.5 : 1
Triglycerides	50–175 mg/dL
Urea	15–40 mg/dL
Urea nitrogen (BUN)	8–20 mg/dL
Uric acid	
Male	4–7 mg/dL
Female	3.5–6 mg/dL
Enzymes	
Amylase	50–125 IU/L
Acid phosphatase	0–12 IU/L
Alkaline phosphatase	40–150 IU/L
Creatine kinase (CK)	10–50 IU/L
γ-Glutamyl transferase (γGT)	5–40 IU/L
Lactate hydrogenase (LDH)	50–200 IU/L

Contd...

Contd...

Parameter	Normal values
Lipase	30–150 IU/L
SGOT (AST)	5–45 IU/L
SGPT (ALT)	5–40 IU/L
Electrolytes	
Sodium	135–145 mEq/L
Potassium	3.5–5 mEq/L
Chloride	95–105 mEq/L
Bicarbonate	22–28 mEq/L
Hormones	
Cortisol	5–20 µg/dL
Estradiol (Female)	10–45 ng/dL
Insulin	6–25 µu/mL
Prolactin	1–25 ng/dL
Testosterone (Male)	300–800 ng/dL
Thyroid-stimulating hormone (TSH)	5–10 µu/mL
Triiodothyronine (T_3)	110–180 ng/dL
Thyroxine (T_4)	5–12 µg/dL
Blood Gases	
pO_2	85–100 mm Hg
pCO_2	35–45 mm Hg
Blood pH	7.35–7.45
Urine	
Sodium	130–200 mEq/L
Potassium	40–65 mEq/L
Chloride	170–250 mEq/L
Calcium	100–300 mg/day
Phosphorus	0.5–1.5 g/day
Urea	15–30 g/day
Creatinine	1–2 g/day
Uric acid	200–500 mg/day
Albumin	<30 mg/day
Specific gravity	1.010–1.025
Cerebrospinal fluid (CSF)	
Sugar	50–75 mg/dL
Protein	15–45 mg/dL
Chloride	120–130 mEq/L

APPENDIX H: BIOCHEMISTRY PRACTICAL GUIDE

PMS/AHS students undergo a practical course in Biochemistry (personal performance or observation) based on their syllabi in Biochemistry. Hence, a practical outline guide is given below for reference.

■ QUALITATIVE ANALYSIS

Carbohydrate Practicals

Sl. No.	Name of the test	To detect
1.	Molisch test	General test for all carbohydrates
2.	Iodine test	Polysaccharides
3.	Benedict's test	All reducing sugars (glucose, fructose, maltose, lactose)
4.	Barfoed's test	Monosaccharides
5.	Seliwanoff's test or Foulger's test	Ketosugars (fructose)
6.	Hydrolysis test	Nonreducing sugar (sucrose)
7.	Osazone test	Glucose/fructose/maltose/lactose

Protein Practicals

A. Precipitation reactions/tests

Sl. No.	Name of the test	To detect
1.	Lead acetate test	All proteins
2.	Sulfosalicylic acid test	All proteins
3.	Heat coagulation test	Heat coagulable proteins (albumin)
4.	a. Saturation test (Half) b. Saturation test (Full)	Casein, gelatin Albumin
5.	Organic solvent test	All proteins
6.	Isoelectric precipitation test	Casein

B. Color reactions/tests

Sl. No.	Name of the test	To detect
1.	Biuret test	General test for proteins
2.	Ninhydrin test	α-amino acids
3.	Xanthoproteic test	Aromatic amino acids
4.	Millon's test	Tyrosine

Contd...

Contd...

Sl. No.	Name of the test	To detect
5.	Hopkins–Cole test (aldehyde test)	Tryptophan
6.	Sakaguchi test	Arginine
7.	Sulfur test	Sulfur containing amino acides cystine and cysteine only (not methionine)
8.	Pauly's test	Histidine
9.	Neumann's test	Casein
10.	Molisch test	Glycoprotein (egg albumin)

Non-protein Nitrogenous Substances (NPN) Practicals

Sl. No.	Name of the test	To detect
1.	a. Alkaline hypobromite test	Urea
	b. Specific urease test	Urea
2.	a. Schiff's test	Uric acid
	b. Benedict's uric acid test (or) Phosphotungstic acid test	Uric acid
	c. Murexide test	Uric acid
3.	Jaffe's reaction/test	Creatinine

Analysis of Normal Urine

A. Physical examination
1. Appearance
2. Odor
3. Color
4. pH
5. Specific gravity by urinometer

B. Chemical examination/tests

Sl. No.	Name of the test	To detect
A.	**Inorganic constituents**	
1.	Silver nitrate test	Chloride
2.	Sulkowitch test	Calcium
3.	Neumann's test	Phosphorus
4.	Litmus test	Ammonia
5.	Precipitation test	Sulfates (inorganic)

Contd...

Appendix H: Biochemistry Practical Guide

Contd...

Sl. No.	Name of the test	To detect
B.	**Organic constituents**	
1.	Precipitation test	Sulfates (organic)
2.	a. Alkaline hypobromite test	Urea
	b. Specific urease test	Urea
3.	a. Schiff test	Uric acid
	b. Benedict's uric acid test (phosphotungastic acid test)	Uric acid
	c. Murexide test	Uric acid
4.	Jaffe's test/reaction	Creatinine

Analysis of Abnormal Urine

A. Physical examination
1. Appearance
2. Color
3. Odor
4. pH
5. Specific gravity by urinometer

B. Chemical examination/tests

Sl. No.	Name of the test	To detect
1.	Benedict's test	Reducing sugars (glucose)
2.	Sulfosalicylic acid test, Heller's test	Proteins
3.	Heat coagulation test	Albumin
4.	Benzidine test/ Tolidine test	Hemoglobin/blood
5.	Rothera's test	Ketone bodies (acetone, aceto acetic acid, β-hydroxybutyric acid)
6.	Hay's test	Bill salts (sodium/ potassium salts of taurocholic acid/ glycocholic acids)
7.	Fouchet's test/ Gmelin test	Bile pigments (bilirubin/biliverdin)
8.	Ehrlich's test	Urobilinogen

■ QUANTITATIVE ANALYSIS

Instrument used: Colorimeter/Autoanalyzers

Sl. No.	Estimations	Specimen	Method
1.	Glucose (blood sugar)	Blood/ plasma/ serum	1. Glucose oxidase-Peroxidase (GOD-POD) method 2. O-Toluidine method 3. Folin–Wu method
2.	Urea	Blood/ plasma/ serum	1. Diacetyl-monoxime (DAM) method 2. Enzymatic method
3.	Cholesterol	Plasma/ serum	1. Zak method 2. Enzymatic method
4.	Total protein	Plasma/ serum	Biuret method
5.	Creatinine	a. Plasma/ serum	Jaffe's method
		b. Urine	Jaffe's method

■ MISCELLANEOUS EXPERIMENTS

A. Tests for lipids
1. To detect saturation
2. To detect oily nature (grease test)
3. To detect cholesterol: (a) Salkowski test, (b) Lieberman–Burchard test

B. Analysis of gastric juice
Device to take out gastric juice: Ryle's tube
Normal constituents
1. Topfer's test ⎱ To detect HCl
2. Gunzberg test ⎰
Abnormal constituents
1. Iodine test: To detect starch
2. Benzidine test: To detect blood
3. Hay's test: To detect bile salts
4. Fouchet's test: To detect bile pigments
5. Uffelmann test: To detect lactic acid

C. Analysis of milk
1. Lactometer: To find out specific gravity
2. Indicator paper: To find out pH
3. Precipitation test: To detect calcium
4. Neumann's test: To detect phosphorus
5. Heat coagulation test: To detect albumin
6. Benedict's test: To detect lactose (milk sugar)

D. Analysis of cerebrospinal fluid (CSF)
1. Sugar: As for blood
2. Protein: Sulfosalicylic acid method/ Pondy's test
3. Chloride: Titration/electrolyte analyzer

Index

Page numbers followed by 'f' refer to figure, and 't' refer to table

A

Abetalipoproteinemia 162
Absorption 9, 98, 100, 101, 103, 104, 106, 108–111, 127, 148, 156, 158, 159, 165, 189
   band 76
Acetoacetate-fumarate pathway 174
Acetoacetyl-CoA 131, 153, 155
Acetyl pyridine 116
Acetylation 85
Acetyl-CoA
   action of 109
   two molecules of 153
Achlorhydria 248
Achylia gastrica 248
Acid 6, 57
   action of 77
   base balance 205, 238, 241
      diagnosis of 241
      disturbances in 241
   base disorders 241t
      compensatory mechanism of 241
   base imbalance 241, 241f
   inorganic 238
   number 35
   organic 238
Acidic amide 172
Acidosis
   metabolic 241
   respiratory 241
Acquired immune deficiency syndrome 316
Active folate, formation of 114
Acyl carrier protein 155
Acyl derivatives, formation of 51
Acyl phosphates 125
Acyl-CoA 150, 151
   synthetase thiokinase 150
Addison's disease 203, 226, 259
Adenine nucleotides 70
Adenosine
   diphosphate 70, 125
   monophosphate 65, 70, 125, 190
   triphosphate 3, 70
Adenyl cyclase 253
Adenylate 65
Adenylic acid 65
Adipose tissue 134, 187
Adrenal cortex 134
   hormones of 258
Adrenal glands, hormones of 257
Adrenal medulla 260
   hormones of 259
   neural stimulation of 260
Adrenaline 175, 259f

Adrenergic blocking agents 260
Adrenocortical function tests 259
Adrenocorticotropic hormone 253
Adriamycin 270
Adsorption chromatography 298
Aerobic glycolysis 129, 130t
Aflatoxins 312
Agar electrophoresis 299
Air pollution
   artificial sources of 311
   natural sources of 311
Alanine 49, 170
   aminotransferase 166
   transferase 90
Albinism 58, 81, 176
Alcohol 42, 44, 56, 94, 157, 219
Aldehydes 219
   formation 42
Aldosterone 236, 259
Aldotriose 14
Aldrin 312
Alkaline phosphatase 199, 214
Alkalis 57
   action of 19, 77
   hydrolysis 33
Alkalosis
   metabolic 241
   respiratory 241
Alkaptonuria 175
Allopurinol 71, 191
Allosteric enzymes 90
Alpha-alanine 170
Alpha-amino levulinic acid 109
Alpha-ketoglutarate dehydrogenase complex 120
Alzheimer's disease 217, 276
Ambiguity 274
Ames test 315
Amethopterin 112, 116
Amides, formation of 51
Amino acid 47, 48, 166, 169, 221
   acidic 48
   activation of 275
   basic 49
   biosynthesis of 186
   branched chain 179
   catabolism of 47
   classification of 48, 48f
   C-terminal 51
   degradation of 186
   derivatives 251
   essential 43, 49, 176
   formation of 167
   glucogenic 139, 171, 172, 174
   ketogenic 49, 174
   metabolism 108, 109, 114, 165
   mutual supplementation of 233

   neutral 48
   nonessential 50, 169
   N-terminal 51
   pool 165, 166f
   semi-essential 49
   separation of 51
   standard 47
Amino group
   disposal of 167
   removal of 166
Aminolevulinic acid 108
Aminopeptidase 164
Aminopterin 112, 116
Aminosugars 22
Ammonia
   direct excretion of 167
   intoxication 168
   mechanism 240, 240f
   metabolism 167
   toxicity 168
Ampholytes 50, 56
Amylase 91
Amyloidosis 56
Amylopectin 26, 26t
Amylose 26, 26t
Anabolism 119, 128, 138, 165
Anaerobic glycolysis 129, 130
Andersen's disease 142
Androsterone 263
Anemia 115, 217
   hemolytic 79
   pernicious 113
Anion gap 242
Anomers 18
Anorexia 107
Antagonists 102, 104, 105, 107–110, 112
Anterior pituitary gland, hormones of 253
Antibiotics 13
Antibody 282
   monoclonal 284
   specific 300
Anticoagulant 13, 25, 28, 287
Anticodon arm 69
Antifolate drugs 190
Antigen 282
   antibody complex 300
Antimycin A 124
Antioncogenes 315
Antioxidants 34, 96, 100, 115, 309, 315
   chain breaking 310
   metabolic 310
   natural 310
   nutritional 310
   preventive 309
   types 309

Antiport system 11
Antithyroid drugs 256
Antivitamins 102, 104, 105, 107–110,
    112, 116, 116t
Apolipoprotein 62, 162
Apoprotein 62, 162
Arachidonic acid 156
Arginase 169
Arginine 49, 176
    cleavage of 168
Argininosuccinate
    cleavage of 168
    synthesis of 168
Argininosuccinic aciduria 169
Artificial sweetener 30
Ascorbic acid 23, 102
Asparaginase 91
Asparagine 49, 50, 172
Aspartame 30
Aspartate
    aminotransferase 166
    transaminase 90
Aspartic acid 49, 50, 171
Atherosclerosis 31, 40, 160, 162, 162f
Atmospheric oxygen 42
Atmospheric pollutants 311
Augmented histamine test 247, 248
Autoanalyzers 294
    advantages 294
    parts 295f
    types 294
Autoimmune diseases 284
Auto-oxidation 34
Azathioprine 71

B

Bacteria 68
Balanced diet 230
    composition of nutrients of 231
    construction of 230
Barbiturates 124
Barfoed's test 20
Basal metabolic rate 224, 247
Batch analyzer 294
Beer-Lambert's law 291
Bees wax 35
Benedict's test 20, 222
Benzidine 226
    test 222
Benzoic acid 244
Berczeller theory 218
Beriberi 103, 104
Beta-carotene 310
Betaine 158
Beta-oxidation 150f, 152f
Beta-thalassemias 79
Bial's test 136
Bicarbonate
    buffer 6
    system 239
    mechanism 240, 240f
Bile 248
    acids 47, 160
        biosynthesis of 161f

precursors of 45
synthesis of 114
pigments 197
    excretion of 196, 197
    formation of 196
    salts 8, 46
Bilirubin 343
Biochemical 1, 10, 100
    compounds 13, 31
    tests, types of 289, 289t
Biochemistry 1
    branches 303f
    instrumentation in 291
    international union of 83
    objectives of 303
    techniques in 291
Bioenergetics 121, 124
Bioflavonoids 115
Biogenic amines 184, 185t
Biological fluids 9
Biological oxidation 42, 121
    enzyme involved in 121
Biomedical functions 200, 210
Biomolecules 303
    chemistry of 13
Biophysical aspects 5
Biosynthesis 95, 98, 100, 101, 103, 104,
    106, 108–112, 114, 159, 255,
    257, 260, 261, 263
Biotechnology 81, 317
    agriculture 317
    applications 317
    branches 317
    environment and energy 318
    ethics 318
    foods 318
    hazards 318
    historical development 317
    medical field 317
    risks 318
    scope 317
    veterinary field 317
Biotin 85, 102, 110
    structure of 110f
    sulfonic acid 110
Birth control pills 266
Bisphosphoglycerate 76, 130
Bitot's spots 96
Blood 248, 285
    acids in 238
    arterial 287
    buffer 73, 238
    calcium, regulation of 204, 205f
    capillary 287
    coagulation 36, 58 102, 203
    collection of 287, 287f
    disorder, hereditary 78
    gas 343
        analyzers 295
    glucose, regulation of 251
    group substances 30
    iodine level in 212
    level, normal 206
    normal level of hemoglobin in 80
    pressure, regulation of 308

sugar regulation 144
    disorders of 146
    transport in 255, 259
    viscosity of 8, 58
Blotting techniques 279, 280f
B-lymphocytes 283
Body
    building foods 228
    fluids 285
        analysis of 287
    mass index 163, 233
    water, distribution of 235f
Bone 257
    formation 96
    mineralization of 99, 203, 205
Brain 187, 188
Branched chain amino acids 179
    catabolism of 180f
Bridge tissue 254
Bromsulfthalein test 244
Brownian movement 9
Brush border enzymes 127
Buffer 6

C

Caffeine 226
Calcitonin 257
Calcitriol 98
    biosynthesis of 98, 98f
Calcium 12, 99, 203
    binding proteins 102
    homeostasis 204
Calorie, small 223
Calorigenic action 225
Camp, structure of 70f
Cancer 314
    brain 314
    breast 314
    causative factors of 314
    cells 315
        biochemical changes of 315
    drugs for treatment of 315
    favor production of 315
    inhibit production of 315
    lung 314
    oral 314
    prostate 314
    skin 314
    stomach 248
    symptoms of 315
    types 314
Carbaminohemoglobin, formation
    of 76
Carbamoyl phosphate synthase 168,
    169
Carbohydrates 13, 27, 30, 186, 227, 228
    absorption of 126
    biosynthesis of 47
    chemistry of 13
    classification of 14f
    dietary 126
    digestion of 126
    effect of 228

Index

metabolism 103, 106, 108, 109, 119, 126, 186-188, 256, 258, 261–264, 337
    tests based on 244
    protein sparing action of 233
    respiratory quotient of 224
Carbon 12
    atoms 25
        asymmetric 17
        numbering of 40, 40t
    chain isomerism 85
    dioxide, transport of 76
    metabolism 111
    monoxide 124
    skeleton, disposal of 168
Carbonic acid 240
Carbonic anhydrase 214
Carbonyl carbon atoms 18
Carboxyhemoglobin 78
    formation of 76
Carboxyl group 42
Carboxylases 84
Carboxypeptidase 164, 214
Carcinogens
    environmental 313
    hepatic 312
    occupational 314
Cardiac function tests 249
Cardiolipin 38
Cardiovascular disease 162
Carnauba wax 35
Carnitine deficiency 151
Catabolic pathway 167
Catabolism 47, 119, 128, 149, 156, 158, 160, 166, 169-174, 175f, 176–179, 180f, 181f, 182, 183, 184f, 191, 192f, 96, 194, 194f, 198f
Catalases 9, 80, 83, 122, 309
Catalyze
    hydrolysis 83
    isomerization 83
Catecholamines 184
Celiac disease 284
Cell 1, 83t, 134, 156
    cycle 268, 268f
    membrane 1, 5, 30
        structure of 5f
    organelle 12
    permeability 204
    types of 260
Cellular metabolism 217, 309
Cellular oncogenes 315
Cellulose 28
Central nervous system 152
Cephalin 37
Cerebral symptoms 107
Cerebrocuprein 212
Cerebronic acid 42
Cerebrosides 38, 158
Cerebrospinal fluid 235, 285, 305, 343
    analysis of 345
    collection of 288
Ceruloplasmin 212, 309
Chaulmoogric acid 42

Chemical
    carcinogens 314
    coupling hypothesis 123
    test for carcinogenicity of 315
Chemiosmotic theory 123, 124f
Chitin 30
Chloride 8, 12, 203, 221
Cholecalciferol 99
Cholecystokinin 148
Cholesterol 44, 46, 160, 162
    biosynthesis of 159f
    crystals 45f
    degradation of 160f
    metabolism of 149, 159
    oxidase 92
    structure of 45f
Choline 115, 158
Chromaffin cells 260
Chromatography 28
    affinity 298
    ascending 298, 298f
    descending 298
    gas liquid 298
    ion exchange 298
    thin layer 298
    types of 297f
Chromium 216
Chylomicrons 161, 162
Chylothorax 149
Chyluria 149
Chymotrypsin 164
Cis-trans isomerism 339
Citric acid cycle 83, 128, 131, 132, 132f, 133, 134t, 186
Citrulline, synthesis of 168
Citrullinemia 169
Clinical biochemistry 285, 285f, 289
    branches 285, 286f
    instrumentation in 286
    laboratory, quality control in 286
    management 286
    scope 285
    techniques in 286
Clinical centrifuge 297, 301f
Clofibrate 163
Clover leaf structure 69
Cobalamin 102, 112
Cobalt 215
Cobamide coenzymes 85
Codon 273
Coenzyme 84, 103, 106, 108, 110, 111, 113, 121
    A 71, 85
    component of 206
    nucleotides 71
Collagen 62
    synthesis 114
Colloids 8
    protective 9
Color tests 45
Colorimeter 291, 301f
    operation of 292
    parts of 291, 291f
Complete blood count 80
Compound lipids 35

Conjugation 219, 220
Consciousness, loss of 77
Constipation 107
Copper 12, 212
    metabolism, inborn errors of 213
Coprosterol 46
Cori's cycle 139, 139f
Cori's disease 142
Corneal transparency 25, 28
Corrin ring system 112
Cortisol 258
Cotransport system 11
COVID-19 316
Cow's milk, composition of 232t
Creatine
    kinase 91, 92
    phosphokinase 91, 92, 92f
Creatinine 47, 170, 176, 221
    clearance test 246
    formation of 177f
    synthesis of 170
Crystalline
    compounds 19
    solid 25
    substances 50
Crystalloids 8
Cushing's syndrome 203, 259
Cyanide 124
Cyanmethemoglobin, formation of 77
Cyanopsin 96
Cyanosis 77
Cyclooxygenase pathway 156, 156f
Cyclopentano-perhydrophenanthrene ring 44f
Cysteine 49, 50, 169, 173
    dioxygenase 173
    storage disease 174
Cystinosis 174
Cystinuria 11, 174
Cytarabine 71
Cytidine
    monophosphate 65
    nucleotides 71
Cytidylate 65
Cytidylic acid 65
Cytochrome 80, 121
    oxidase 83, 121
    P 450 122
Cytokines 283
Cytoplasm 1
Cytoskeleton 4, 12
Cytosol 1, 12, 134, 150, 156, 159, 168, 195

D

D arm 69
De novo synthesis 154f
Deaminase 82, 83
Decarboxylation 85, 133, 159
Dehydration 133, 155
Dehydrocholesterol 46, 97
Dehydrogenase 82, 121
    fad-linked 121
Dementia 107

Dental fluorosis 215, 215f
Deoxyadenosine monophosphate 65
Deoxyadenosylcobalamin 113
Deoxyadenylate 65
Deoxyadenylic acid 65
Deoxycytidine monophosphate 65
Deoxycytidylate 65
Deoxycytidylic acid 65
Deoxyguanosine monophosphate 65
Deoxyguanylate 65
Deoxyguanylic acid 65
Deoxypyridoxine 116
Deoxyribonucleic acid 22, 64, 66, 267
    damage 270, 270t
    double helix 67, 67f
    finger printing 281
    repair 270, 270t
    sequencing 280
    synthesis 67, 268, 269f
Deoxyribonucleotide, structure of 66t
Deoxyribose 64
Deoxysugars 22
Deoxythymidylate 65
Deoxythymidylic acid 65
Depression 107
Desthiobiotin 110
Detoxication 48, 170, 218, 218f
    mechanism, types of 218
Detoxification function, tests based on 244
Dextrans 28
Dextrins 26
Dextrose 30
Diabetes mellitus 146, 160, 162, 163, 289, 295
    insulin dependent 146
    noninsulin dependent 146
Diabetic curve 147
Dialysis 7
Diarrhea 107, 127, 217
Diastereoisomers 30
Dichlororiboflavin 105, 116
Dietary fructose, restriction of 144
Dietetics 305f
    biochemistry in 305
Diffusion 7
Digestion 126, 148 156, 158, 159, 164, 189
Digestive system 126f
Digitonin 13
Dihydrolipoyl dehydrogenase 131
Dihydrolipoyl transacetylase 131
Dihydrothymine 194
Dihydrouracil 194
Dihydroxyacetone 14, 128
Dimercaprol 124
Dioxygenases 122
Dipeptidase 82, 164
Direct oxidative pathway 173, 173f
Disaccharidases 127
Disc electrophoresis 300
Disulfide bonds 55
Donnan membrane equilibrium 9
Dopamine 175
Doxorubicin 270

Dry chemistry analyzer 295
Dyspnea 77

E

Edema 7
Edman's reagent 51
Ehlers-Danlos syndrome 62
Eicosanoids 43, 307
    classification of 307, 307f
    conjugated 308
    metabolism of 156
    types of 44f
Elastase 164
    split peptide bonds 164
Electrolyte 56, 236, 343
    analyzer 292, 293, 302f
        advantages 293
        parts 293
    composition 236
    disorders 236
        laboratory diagnosis of 236
Electron
    carrier systems 121
    transport
        chain 102, 121, 122, 122f
        system 114
Electrophoresis 79, 80, 298
Electrophoretic apparatus 299f
Electrophoretic pattern 299f
    abnormal 300f
Embden-Meyerhof-Parnas pathway 128
Emulsions 46
Endocrine
    disorders 226
    function 260, 289
        tests 247
    glands 250t
        hormones of 265
    system 250f
Endocytosis 11, 12f
Endoenzymes 82
Endopeptidases 164
    action of 164
Endoplasmic reticulum 2, 3, 156, 159
Energetics 129, 130t, 131, 133, 134t, 136, 139, 151, 151t, 190
Energy 13, 223
    compounds 125
    expenditure 224, 224t
    generation phase 128
    intake 229
    investment phase 128
    metabolism 69, 223
    requirement 226
    yielding foods 227, 227f
Enolase catalyzes elimination 128
Environmental biochemistry 311
    classification 311
    general effects 311
    types 311
Enzymatic reaction, velocity of 86
Enzyme 52, 53, 57, 81, 90t, 92, 121, 131, 150, 265t, 343

action, mechanism of 85, 86
activity 87f, 88f
    control of 69
    expression of 90
    regulation of 89
adaptive 89
application of 90
classification of 83, 83f
commission 84
composition of 82f
concentration, effect of 86, 87, 87f
constitutional 89
deficiency 181, 337
degradation 89
diagnostic significance of 90
extracellular 82
factors affecting activity of 86
inhibitors 86, 88, 88f
    importance of 89
intracellular 82
kinetics 86
lactate dehydrogenase 129
latent 89
linked immunosorbent assay 300, 301f, 316
location of 83t
mechanism 85f
metal ion 85f
pancreatic 91
plasma specific 91
specificity 84
types of 91
Epimers 18
Epinephrine 146, 175
    structure of 259f
Epithelialization 96
Ergosterol 97
Erythrocuprein 212
Erythrocytes 134
Erythromycin 13
Esterification 45
Esters, formation of 21, 50
Estrogens 264
    synthetic 264
Ethylenediaminetetraacetate 287
Ethylenediaminetetraacetic acid 309
Etiocholanolone 263
Eukaryotes 1, 4, 68
    deoxyribonucleic acid replication in 270
    gene regulation in 277
    transcription in 273
    translation in 276
Eukaryotic cell 1, 2t
    structure of 2f
Excessive sodium chloride excretion 222
Excretion 100, 101, 103, 104, 106, 108–111, 196, 197, 211, 221
Excretory function, tests based on 244
Exergonic reaction 124
Exocrine function 260
    tests 247
Exocytosis 11, 12f
Exoenzymes, extracellular 82

Index

Exopeptidases 164
   action of 164
Extracellular fluid 5, 201, 236
Extracellular matrix 62
Extrahepatic tissues 153
   role of 145
Extramitochondrial pathway 154
Extrinsic membrane proteins 5

F

Fats 227, 228
   absorption of 8
   biosynthesis of 47
   digestion of 8
   neutral 32
   respiratory quotient of 224
Fatty acid 40, 40t, 46, 70, 148
   active 150
   beta-oxidation of 150f
   biosynthesis of 149, 154, 154f, 186
   branched chain 42
   catabolism of 149
   cyclic 42
   derivatives of 43
   metabolism of 149
   oxidation 186
   polyunsaturated 41
   saturated 41, 160
   short chain saturated 154
   synthase 155
      complex 120
   synthesis 83
      enzyme of 89
   unsaturated 41
Fatty liver 157, 157f
   disease 157
      nonalcoholic 157
   formation of 31
Feces 221
Fehling's test 20
Fermentation 21
Fever 308
Fiber, dietary 13, 228
Fibrinogen 59
Fibrinolysis 58
Fibroblasts, activities of 115
Fibrosis, cystic 222
FIGLU test 112, 177
Finger printing 80
Fischer projection 16, 17
Flame photometer 292, 302f
   parts of 293f
Flavin
   adenine dinucleotide 71, 105
   mononucleotide 71, 105
Fluid
   balance 7
   mosaic model 5, 5f
   volume, effect on 259
Fluorescence 74
Fluoride 215
Fluoroacetate 215
Folate coenzymes 85
Folate trap 113f

Folic acid 102, 111, 158
   structure of 111f
Follicle-stimulating hormone 253
Food 227
   and nutrition 233
   calorific value of 223
   components of 227f
   groups 231
   items 231t
      composition of 231
   primary 227
   protective 229
   pyramid 234, 234f
   specific dynamic action of 224, 225
   stuffs, toxic substances in 312
   toxins 231
Formiminoglutamic acid test 112
Fouchet's test 222
Fractional test meal analysis 248
Fractions, subcellular 1, 4
Frederikson's classification 162
Free ribosomes 4
Fructose
   intolerance, hereditary 144
   metabolism 143, 143f
   structure of 18
Fructosuria, essential 143
Fully automated analyzers 294, 302f
Furanose ring 16, 17

G

Galactoflavin 105
Galactosamine 30
Galactose 30
   metabolism 144, 144f
   tolerance test 244
Galactosemia 144
Gamma-aminobutyric acid 171
Gamma-glutamyl cycle 165f
Gangliosides 39, 158
Gas, transport of 73
Gastric
   function 308
   tests 247
   juice 164
      analysis of 345
      composition of 247
   phase 164
Gastritis 217
Gastrointestinal disorders 112
Gastrointestinal tract 28, 262
   hormones 251
Gaucher's disease 31, 39
Geiger-Muller counter 9, 119
Gene 267
   amplification 277
   analysis 80
   expression 96
   regulation of 277
   regulation, mode of 277
   therapy 281
      steps 281
      types 281
      uses 281

Genetic 163
   carrier 67
   code 273, 274t
      characteristics of 273
   diseases 289
   disorders 78
   information, transfer of 268f
Genome sequencing, steps for 281
Gibbs-Donnan membrane
   equilibrium 8
Gingivitis 107
Glands 250
   effect on 259
Globin 74
Globular proteins 52
Globulins 58
Glomerular filtration 221
   rate 170
   tests for 245
Glossitis 112, 113
Glucagon 145, 260
Glucocorticoids 145, 258
Glucometer 295, 302f
Gluconeogenesis 138, 138f, 186
Gluconeogenic action 260
Glucosazone 20f
Glucose 139, 224, 343
   6-phosphate dehydrogenase 136, 206
   absorption 128f
   anabolism of 128, 138
   catabolism 128
      alternative pathways of 134
   infusion 146
   metabolism of 128
   oxidase 92
   peroxidase 92
   production 145
   sources of 145f
   structure of 14
   tolerance test 146, 147f
   utilization of 145, 145f
Glucosuria 146
Glucuronic acid 219
Glutamic acid 49, 50, 169, 171
Glutamine 49-51, 172, 220
   pathway 167
Glutathione 62, 220
   synthesis of 169
Glycemic index 233
Glyceraldehyde 14, 128
Glycerol 44, 139
Glycine 49, 169, 220, 244
Glycinuria 170
Glycoconjugates 30
Glycogen 27, 28t
   metabolism 140
      disorders of 142
   phosphorylase 141
   storage diseases 142, 142t
   structure of 27f
   synthesis of 69
Glycogenesis 83, 140, 140f
Glycogenolysis 71, 83, 138, 140, 141, 141f, 260

Glycolipids 35, 38
   constituents of 13
   metabolism of 149, 158
Glycolysis 83, 128, 129f, 130, 186
Glycoprotein 61
   constituents of 13
   hormones 266
   synthesis 96
Glycosaminoglycans 28, 62
Glycosidases 83
Glycosides 21
   cardiac 13
   formation of 21
   function 22t
Glycosuria 147, 222
   alimentary 147
   diabetic 147
   renal 147
Glycosylation 276
   reaction 3
Goiter 256f
   exophthalmic 256
Goitrogenic substances 212
Goitrogens 256
Golgi bodies 277
Golgi complex 2, 3
Gonadotropins 253
Gonads 251
   hormones of 263
Gout 192f
Grave's disease 256
Gravity, specific 33, 221
Group-transfer reactions 120
Growing polypeptide chain 275f
Growth
   hormone 145, 253, 266
   retardation 112
Guanine 190
   nucleotides 71
Guanosine
   diphosphate 71
   monophosphate 65, 190
   triphosphate 71
Guanylate 65
Guanylic acid 65
Gums 217

H

Halogenation 42
Hartnup disease 11, 165, 183
Haworth projection 16, 17
Hay's test 8, 222
Headache 97, 107, 217
Healthy liver 157f
Heart
   attack 217
   disease 163
      coronary 162, 163
Heat coagulation test 222
Heavy metal
   poisons 311
   salts 57
Hematoporphyrin, formation of 77

Heme 47, 73
   metabolism, tests based on 243
   structure of 75f
   synthesis 108, 109
Hemin
   crystals 77f
   formation of 77
Hemochromatosis 211
Hemoglobin 73, 197
   abnormal 78, 78t
   biosynthesis of 195, 196f
   buffer 6
      system 239
   catabolism of 196, 198f
   chemistry of 73
   estimation of 80
   identification of 80
   metabolism of 195, 338
   normal human 75, 76
   oxygen dissociation curves of 76f
   reduced 78
   spectroscopic analysis of 78
   structure 75f
   synthesis of 195
   test for 80
Hemoglobinopathy 78
Hemoproteins 80
Hemorrhage 115
Hemorrhagic disease 102
Hemosiderosis 211
Henderson-Hasselbalch equation 6
Heparan sulfate 29
Heparin 287
Hepatic failure 144
Hepatocuprein 212
Her's disease 142
Heteroglycans 28
Heteropolysaccharides 26, 28
Hexokinase 206
Hexose monophosphate 134, 135f, 186
High-energy compounds 125
Hippuric acid 244
Histidine 49, 177
   catabolism of 177f
Histidinemia 177
Histones 267
Homeostasis 52, 81
Homocysteine 113
Homocystinuria 113
Homogentisate
   dioxygenase 122
   oxidase 122
Homopolysaccharides 26
Hormonal control 155
Hormone 52, 53, 140, 207, 250, 250t,
      251-253, 265t, 300, 343
   analyzers 296
   antidiuretic 236, 254
   biomedical importance 250
   classification 251
   constituents of 170
   corticotropin releasing 253
   estrogenic 264
   functions 250
   gastrointestinal 265, 265t

   hypothalamic releasing 254
   imbalance 163
   luteinizing 254
   major 255
   mechanism of action of 251
   parathyroid 99, 256
   progestational 264
   role of 145
   secretion, regulation of 253
   tropic 253
Human chorionic gonadotropin 265
Human genome project 281
Human immunodeficiency virus,
      structure of 316
Human insulin, structure of 261f
Human milk, composition of 232t
Huntington's disease 276
Hyaluronic acid 29
Hybridoma technology 284
Hydnocarpic acid 42
Hydrocarbon
   aromatic 219
   chain 42
Hydrogen 12, 121
   bonds 55
   sulphide, presence of 222
Hydrolysis 33, 37, 56, 219
   enzymatic 34
   part of 148
Hydrolytic processes 83
Hydrolytic rancidity 34
Hydroperoxidases 121
Hydrophobic bonds 55
Hydroxy fatty acids 42
Hydroxyindoleacetic acid 183
Hydroxykynurenine 183
Hydroxylases 122
Hydroxylation 45, 218, 276
Hyperadrenalism 226
Hyperammonemia 169
Hyperargininemia 169, 177
Hyperbilirubinemia
   conjugated 198
   unconjugated 197
Hypercalcemia 100, 205
Hyperchloremia 203
Hyperchlorhydria 248
Hypercholesterolemia 160
Hyperglycemia 145, 146, 295
Hyperkalemia 203
Hyperlipidemia 143
Hyperlipoproteinemia 40, 160, 162
   types of 162t
Hypermagnesemia 206
Hypernatremia 202
Hyperornithinemia 177
Hyperparathyroidism
   primary 257
   secondary 257
Hyperphenylalaninemia 182
Hyperphosphatemia 100, 206
Hyperprolinemia 173
Hyperproteinemia 59
Hypersecretion 254
Hypertension 163
   treatment of 308

Hyperthyroidism 160, 226, 256
Hyperuricemia 143, 191
Hypervitaminosis 93, 97, 100
Hypoadrenalism 226
Hypoalbuminemia 59
Hypocalcemia 205
Hypochloremia 203
Hypochlorhydria 248
Hypocholesterolemia 160
Hypogammaglobulinemia 59
Hypoglycemia 143-146, 295
Hypokalemia 203
Hypolipoproteinemia 40, 162
Hypomagnesemia 207
Hyponatremia 202
Hypoparathyroidism 257
  idiopathic 257
  primary 257
  secondary 257
Hypophosphatemia 206
Hypoproteinemia 59
Hyposecretions 146
Hypothalamus 262
  hormones of 254
Hypothyroidism 160, 226, 256
Hypouricemia 192
Hypoxanthine 192, 192

I

I-cell disease 4
Immune system 283f
  cells involved in 283
  organization of 282
Immunity 52, 58, 115, 282
  abnormal 316
  acquired 282
  cell-mediated 282
  humoral 282
  innate 282
  types of 282
Immunodeficiency disease, severe combined 193
Immunoelectrophoresis 300
Immunoglobulins 59, 283
  structure of 60, 60f
  types of 282
Immunology 282, 282f
  application of 284
  clinical aspects of 283
In vitro antioxidants 310
Indoleamines 184
Infantile mitochondrial myopathy 123
Inosine monophosphate 190
Inositol 115, 158
Insecticides 312
Insomnia 107
Insulation 31, 36
Insulin 145, 261
  commercial forms of 262
  deficiency of 146
  release, action on 260
Insulinoma 146
Intestinal mucosa 257

Intestinal pH 204
Intestine 148
  small 127, 189
Intracellular fluid 5, 201, 236
Inulin 28
  clearance test 246
Iodide, trapping of 255
Iodine 211, 255
  number 35
Iododeoxyuridine 71
Iodopsin 96
Iodotyrosine, coupling of 255
Ion selective electrode 293, 293f
  advantages 293
  parts 293
Ionic state 50
Iron 12, 74, 208
  absorption 210f
    factors affecting 210
  binding capacity 211
  distribution of 209f
  metabolism 114
  transport of 210, 210f
Isoelectric pH 50
Isoenzymes 91
Isoleucine 49, 179
Isomaltase 30, 127
Isomerases 83
Isomerism 17, 30, 41, 50, 339, 339f
  structural 339
Isoniazid 116
Isoriboflavin 105, 116
Isotopes 9
  nonradioactive 9
Isotopic techniques 284
Isovaleric acidemia 179

J

Jamaican vomiting sickness 151
Jaundice 144, 198, 198f
  causes of 199t
  laboratory diagnosis of 199t
  types of 199t

K

Keratomalacia 96
Ketoacidosis, diabetic 153
Ketogenesis 152, 152f
Ketolysis 152, 153, 153f
Ketone bodies
  formation of 152, 152f
  metabolism of 152
  utilization of 152, 153, 153f
Ketotriose 14
Kidney 257, 265
  damage 217
  effect on 259
Koshland's induced fit model 86, 86f
Krebs-Henesleit cycle 168
Kwashiorkor 233, 233f, 233t

L

Lactate dehydrogenase 91, 92, 92f
Lactation 108
Lactic acidosis 143
Lactosazone 24f
Lactose 23
  intolerance 24, 127
  tolerance test 127
Lambert's law 291
L-amino acid oxidase 121
Lanosterol 160
  formation of 160
Learning
  disabilities 217
  disturbances 217
Lecithinases 37
Lecithins 37
Leptin resistance 163
Lesch-Nyhan syndrome 191
Leucine 49, 179
Leukocytes 156
Leukotrienes 308
  functions 308
Leydig cells 263
Ligases 84
Lineweaver-Burk plot 87, 87f
Link reaction 131, 131f
Linoleic acid 152, 156
Lipids 31, 46, 162, 186
  absorption of 148, 149f
  amphipathic 46
  biosynthesis 69
  chemistry of 31, 46
  classification of 32f
  complex 35
  derived 31, 40
  digestion of 148, 149f
  disorders 162
    diagnosis of 163
  metabolism 106, 109, 114, 119, 148, 186-188, 253, 256, 258, 261, 262, 264, 337
    tests based on 244
  neutral 46
  peroxidation 309
    assessment 309
    formation 309
    harmful effects 309
    mechanism of 309
  simple 32
  tests for 345
Lipogenesis 154
Lipoic acid 85, 115
Lipolysis 71, 260
Lipooxygenase pathway 156, 156f
Lipoprotein 35, 39, 39t, 53, 58, 161
  high-density 162
  low-density 11, 162
  metabolism of 149, 161, 162f
  molecule 46
  production of 157
  structure 46f
  very low-density 36, 161, 162

Liposomes 46
Lipotropic factor 31, 157, 158
Lipoxines 308
    function 308
Liquid chromatography
    high
        performance 297
        pressure 298
Liver 134, 187
    cirrhosis 157
    disease 160, 166
    enzymes, elevation of 157
    function tests 243, 245
        classification 243
Long chain free fatty acids 124
Lovastatin 160, 163
Lung
    function 8
    surfactant 31
L-xylulose 136
Lyases 83
Lymphoid organs 282, 283
Lyophilic colloids 8
Lyophobic colloids 9
Lysine 49, 178
    metabolism of 178f
Lysosomes 2, 3
Lysozyme 91

M

Macrominerals 200, 201t, 230
Macromolecules, transport of 11
Macrophages 156
Mad cow disease 276
Magnesium 12, 206
Major histocompatibility complex 283
Malate dehydrogenase 139
Malonyl-CoA 155
Maltosazone 24f
Maltose 23, 24
Maltotriose 30
Mammary gland, lactating 134
Manganese 214
Marasmus 233, 233t
Mass spectrometry 12
Mast cells 156
McArdle's syndrome 142
Medical and paramedical specialties,
    biochemistry in 303
Medical laboratory technology 305f
    biochemistry in 305
Medicine, biochemistry in 303
Meister cycle 165f
Melanin 175
Melanocyte stimulating hormone
    254, 266
Melting point 33
Membrane
    fluidity 45
    ribosomes 4
    transport 10
Menkes disease 213
Mental
    confusion 217

retardation 144
status changes 217
Mercaptans 222
Messenger ribonucleic acid 68
Metabolic defect 337
Metabolic disorders, acute 241
Metabolic pathways 120
    compartmentation of 89
    regulation of 186
Metabolism 95, 98, 100, 114, 119, 149,
    159, 186, 189, 202-204, 206,
    262, 303
    inborn errors of 143, 144, 175, 337
    integration of 186, 187f
    phases of 119
Metal complex, formation of 74
Metal ions 85
Metallothionein 78, 213
Methemoglobin, formation of 77
Methemoglobinemia 77
Methionine 49, 113, 158, 179
    catabolism of 181f
Methotrexate 112, 304
Methyl malonic acid 113
Methyl malonyl-CoA 113
Methyl pantothenate 109
Methyl trap 113f
Methylation 219
Methylcobalamin 113
Methylmalonic
    acidemia 179
    aciduria 113
Mevalonate, formation of 159
Microalbuminuria 222
Microfilaments 4
Microminerals 200, 207, 230
    classification of 208f
Microsomal fraction 12
Microsomal system 155
Microsomes 12, 36, 159
Microtubules 4
Milk 231
    analysis of 345
Minamato disease 217
Mineral 221, 230
    classification of 200f
    functions 230
    metabolism 119, 200, 253,
        261-264, 338
    oils 312
    toxicity of 233
Mineralocorticoids 259
Mitochondria 2, 2f, 36, 153, 156, 168,
    195
    inner membrane of 122
Mitochondrial deoxyribonucleic acid
    318
Mitochondrial system 155
Molecular biological techniques 277
Molecular biology 267, 267f, 318, 338
    central dogma of 268, 268f
Molybdenum 214
Monoacylglycerols 148
Monoamine oxidase 304
    inhibitors 304

Monosaccharides 14, 15t
Monounsaturated fatty acids 41
    biosynthesis of 155
Mucopolysaccharides 28, 29t
    synthesis 96
Multienzyme complex 120
Multiple sclerosis 284
Muscle 145
    nerve function 204
    tremors 217
Muscular paralysis 217
Mutagens 271
Mutarotation 19
Mutation 271, 271f
Myasthenia gravis 284
Myelin sheath 36
Myocardial infarction 92, 249, 289
Myoglobin 80
Myosin kinase 204

N

N-acetyl glucosamine 30
N-acetyl neuraminic acid 39
Nausea 97, 107, 217
Nephrotic syndrome 160, 162, 226
Neuraminic acid 22
Neutral amino acid 48
    absorption of 165
Niacin 102, 105
    structure of 105f
Nicotinamide adenine dinucleotide
    71, 106
    phosphate 71, 106
Nicotinic acid 105
Niemann-Pick disease 38
Nightblindness 96
Nitric oxide 176
Nitrocellulose 279
Nitrogen 12
    balance 229
        negative 229
        positive 229
Nitrogenous bases 63, 63f
Noise pollution 312
Nonisotopic techniques 284
Nonoxidative deamination 166
Nonoxidative phase 134
Noradrenaline 175, 259f
Norepinephrine 175
    structure of 259f
Normal value chart 343
Northern blotting 280
Nucleic acids 63, 66, 189
    absorption of 189
    chemistry of 63
    constituents of 13
    digestion of 189
    metabolism of 119, 189
    types of 63f
Nucleoplasm 5
Nucleoproteins 72
Nucleosides 64, 65
    structure of 65f
    synthetic 71

Nucleotide 69, 71
  analogues 270
  metabolism 338
  structure of 66f
  synthetic 69, 71
Nucleus 1, 4, 267
Nutrition 227, 232, 305f
  biochemistry in 305
  normal 232
  parenteral 234
Nutritional disorders 232, 289
  causes 232
Nyctalopia 96
Nylon membrane 279

O

Odor 221
Okazaki fragments 269
Oligosaccharides 14, 23
Omega fatty acids 43
Omega-oxidation 152
Oncogenes 315
Oncotic pressure 7
Optical isomerism 339
Optical isomers 17
Oral cavity 115
Oral contraceptives 146, 266
Oral rehydration
  solution 237
  therapy 127, 237
Organ 134, 195
  effect on 259
  function tests 243, 289
Organic compounds, heterogeneous
    group of 31
Organic solvents 57
Ornithine
  cycle 168
  transcarbamoylase 169
Orotic aciduria 193
Osazones, formation of 20
Osmosis 7
Osmotic diuresis 7
Osmotic imbalance 8
Osmotic pressure 7, 9, 223
Osteoblasts, activities of 115
Osteomalacia 99, 100
Ouabain 127
Overhydration 236
Overnutrition 226
Oxalates 221
Oxaluria, primary 170
Oxidation 42, 45, 86, 88, 120, 133, 151,
    218, 219, 255
  reduction, mechanism of 120
Oxidative deamination 166
Oxidative decarboxylation 85, 103
Oxidative phosphorylation 123, 124
  inhibitors of 124
  uncouplers of 124
Oxidative rancidity 34
Oxidoreductases 83
Oxygen 12
  transport of 76

Oxygenases 122
Oxyhemoglobin 78
  formation of 76
Oxythiamine 104, 116
Oxytocin 254
Ozone layer 312

P

Pain 308
  abdominal 107, 217
  chest 217
Pancreas 250, 262
  hormones of 260
Pancreatic amylase 82
Pancreatic function tests 247
Pancreatic peptide 262
Pancreatic phase 164
Pantothenic acid 102, 108, 116
  structure of 109f
Pantoyl taurine 109, 116
Paper
  chromatography 298
  electrophoresis 299
Para-aminobenzoic acid 111
Paralysis 217
Parathyroid gland, hormones of 256
Parenteral therapy 234
Pellagra 107f
Penicillinase 91
Pentagastrin test 247, 249
Pentasaccharides 23
Pentose sugars 64f
Pepsin 81, 91
Peptide 60-62
  bond, formation of 275
  constituents of 47
  hormones 251, 252f
    mechanism of action of 252
Peroxidases 80, 83, 121, 309
Peroxisomes 2, 4
Pesticides 312, 313
pH 6, 221
  effect of 86, 88
  meter 296, 302f
    parts of 296f
Pharmacy 304f
  biochemistry in 304
Pharyngitis 113
Phenolsulfthalein excretion test 247
Phenylalanine 49, 174f, 181
  hydroxylase 122, 174f
Phenylketonuria 81, 175, 182
  classic 182
Phlorhizin 127
Phosphagens 125
Phosphatases 83
Phosphate 64, 221, 242
  buffer 6
  mechanism 240, 240f
  metabolism 99
Phosphatidylcholine 38
Phosphatidylethanolamine 38
Phosphocreatine 70

Phosphoenolpyruvate 129, 139
  carboxykinase 139
Phosphofructokinase 206
Phosphoglucomutase 206
Phosphoglycerides 36
Phosphoglycerokinase 206
Phosphoinositides 36, 38
Phospholipases 37
Phospholipids 35, 46, 162
  metabolism of 149, 158
  synthesis of 158f
Phosphoribosyl pyrophosphate 190
Phosphoribosyl transferase 190
Phosphoribosylamine 190
Phosphoric acid 64
Phosphorus 12, 205
Phosphorylation 159, 276
  substrate-level 125
Phosphosphingosides 36, 38
Photometry 291
p-hydroxyphenyl pyruvate,
    hydroxylation of 174
Physiotherapy 305f
  biochemistry in 305
Pigments 73
Pineal gland 265
Pituitary gland 250
  hormones of 253
Pituitary hormones, anterior 145
Pituitary tropic hormones 253
Placenta 251
  hormones of 265
Placental lactogen 265
Plasma 287
  electroneutrality of 239
  functional enzymes 91
  lipoproteins, disorders of 162
  membrane 5
  nonfunctional enzymes 91
  nonspecific enzymes 91
  normal level in 58
  proteins 58
    abnormalities in 59
  separation of 287
Plasmalogens 37
Platelet 156
  aggregation 308
Poisons, hemolytic 37
Polyacrylamide gel electrophoresis 91
Polyamines 185
Polydipsia 146
Polyhydroxy alcohols 13
Polymerase chain reaction 279, 279f,
    316
  technique 279f
Polynucleotide 65, 66f
Polysaccharides 14, 25
Polyunsaturated fatty acids 41
  biosynthesis of 155
Polyuria 146
Pompe's disease 142
Porphobilinogen 195
Porphyria 196, 197t
  acquired 196
  acute intermittent 196, 197
  congenital erythropoietic 197

cutanea tarda 197
erythrohepatic 197
erythropoietic 197
hepatic 197
variegate 197
Porphyrin 73, 74
    structure of 74f
Porphyropsin 96
Posterior pituitary gland, hormones of 254
Potassium 12, 202
    bicarbonate 239
    oxalate sodium fluoride 287
Proenzyme 82
Progesterone 264
Progestins 264
Prokaryotes 1, 1f, 4, 68
    DNA replication in 269
    gene regulation in 277
    ribosomes of 275
    transcription in 272
    translation in 274
Prokaryotic cell 2t
Proline 49, 50, 172
Propionate 139
Propionyl-CoA 152
Prostacyclins 308
Prostaglandins 156, 307
Prostanoids 307
Proteins 51, 53, 61, 162, 227, 228, 230, 242, 251, 343
    absorption of 164
    biological value of 229, 229t
    biosynthesis 186, 274, 276f
    bound iodine 212
    buffer 6
    calorie malnutrition 232
    chemistry of 47
    classification of 52f
        quality of 229
    color reactions of 57, 57t
    complete 229
    conjugated 53, 54t
    constituents of 47, 170
    contractile 53
    copper-containing 212
    denaturation of 57, 57f
    derived 53, 54t
    digestion of 164
    energy malnutrition 232
    estimation of 57
    fibrous 53
    first class 229
    folding 276
    fraction of 230
    functions 228
    incomplete 229
    influence quantity of 228
    integral membrane 5
    intrinsic membrane 5
    mechanism of action of 252, 252f
    metabolism 103, 106, 119, 164, 187, 188, 253, 256, 258, 261-264, 337
        tests based on 244
    peripheral membrane 5
    plant 229
    poor 229
    practicals 344
    protective 53
    purity of 57
    quality 228
    renaturation of 57
    respiratory quotient of 224
    second class 229
    separation of 57
    simple 53, 53t
    sorting 3
    storage of 53
    structural organization of 54
    synthesis 69, 83
    targeting 277
    transport of 53
Proteinuria 222
Proteoglycans 62
    constituents of 13
Proteolytic degradation 276
Protoporphyria 197
Protoporphyrin, synthesis of 195
Provitamin
    A 94
    D 97, 98
    D2 98
    D3 46, 98
Pseudoachlorhydria 248
Purine 47, 64
    bases 64f
    deoxyribonucleotides
        catabolism of 191
        synthesis of 191
    formation of 167
    nucleotides 69, 70
        metabolism of 189
    ribonucleotides
        biosynthesis of 189, 190f
        catabolism of 191, 192f
        ring, atoms of 190, 190f
        synthesis of 169
Pyloric obstruction 248
Pyranose ring 16
Pyridine 3-sulfonic acid 107
Pyridoxal phosphate 85, 108
Pyridoxine 102, 107
    structure of 107f
Pyrimidine 64
    base 64f
    deoxyribonucleotides 194
    formation of 167
    nucleotides 69, 71
        metabolism of 193
    ribonucleotides
        biosynthesis of 193f
        catabolism of 194, 194f
        synthesis of 193
    ring, atoms of 193, 193f
Pyrithiamine 104, 116
Pyruvate 131, 139
    carboxylase 204
    degradation of 129
    dehydrogenase 131, 204, 206
        complex 120
    kinase 204

Q

Quality control, methods of 286
Quick theory 218

R

Radiation, types of 9
Radioactive isotopes 9
Radioactive isotopic techniques 119
Radioimmunoassay 300
Rancidity 34
Rapoport Luebering cycle 130, 131f
Recombinant DNA technology 277, 278f
Red blood cell 75
    fragility of 7
Rehydration 133
Relaxin 265
Renal disease 203
Renal dysfunction 123
Renal function 308
    tests 221, 245, 247
        classification 245
Renal mechanism 239
Respiratory distress syndrome 37
Respiratory function 308
Respiratory mechanism 239
Restlessness 217
Retinal 94
Retinene reductase 214
Retinoic acid 94
Retinol 94
    binding protein 95
Retro virus 316
Rheumatoid arthritis 284
Rhodopsin cycle 95
Riboflavin 102, 104
    structure of 104f
Ribonucleases 83
Ribonucleic acid 64, 66, 68
    inhibitors 273
    splicing 273f
    synthesis 272
Ribose 64
    5-phosphate 190
Ribosomal ribonucleic acid 68, 69
    packages of 4
Ribosome 4f, 12, 275
Ribozyme 85, 275
Ricinoleic acid 42
Rickets 99f
Rothera's test 222, 153
Ryle's tube 248, 248f

S

Saccharin sucralose 30
S-adenosyl homocysteine, hydrolysis of 180
S-adenosylmethionine 70, 125
    component of 71
Salicylate 57, 146
Salivary amylase 82

Index

Salmonella infections 79
Salt 6
   formation 51
Sanger's reagent 51
Scurvy 115*f*
Secretion, regulation of 255
Selenium 216, 310
Semiautoanalyzer 294, 302*f*
   parts 294*f*
Serine 49, 170
Serotonin pathway 183
Sertoli cells 263
Serum 287
   amylase 81
   calcium, regulation of 204
   cholesterol 247
   glutamate
      oxaloacetate transaminase 81, 166
      pyruvate transaminase 81
   glutamic
      oxaloacetic transaminase 92*f*, 199
      pyruvic transaminase 199
   iron binding capacity of 211
   protein 299*t*
      bound iodine 247
Sex hormones
   cortical 259
   female 259, 263
   male 259, 263
Sexcorticoids 259
Sherwin theory 218
Sialic acid 22, 30
Sickle cell
   anemia 78
   disease 78, 78*f*
   hemoglobin 78
Sickling test 79
Siderosis, nutritional 211
Skeletal
   fluorosis 215
   muscle 187
   tissue 188
Skin symptoms 107
Small molecules, transport mechanisms for 10
Smog 312
Sodium 12, 202
   fluoride 215
   pump 11*f*
Soft tissue 235
Somatostatin 262
Sorenson's formal titration 51
Southern blotting 280, 280*f*
Spectrophotometer 292, 301*f*
   advantages 292
   parts of 292, 292*f*
Speech
   disturbances 217
   slurred 168
Spermatogonia 263
Sphingolipidoses 159
Sphingolipids 46
Sphingomyelins 38

Standard urea clearance 245
Starch 28*t*, 248
   granules 27*f*
   structure of 26*f*
Steatorrhea 149
Stem cells 318
Stereoisomerism 339
Steroid
   hormones 45, 251
      mechanism of action of 251, 252*f*
      structural features of 258
      synthesis of 258*f*
   mechanism of action of 252*f*
   neutral 161
   nucleus 44*f*
   synthesis 71
Stomach 127, 148, 189
Stomatitis 107, 113
Stool fat, determination of 244
Straight chain 18
   structures 16
Streptokinase 81, 91
Streptomycin 13
Stroke 217
Subcellular organelles 1, 2
   marker enzymes of 3*t*
Substrate strain theory 86
Successive amino acids, carboxypeptidase splits of 164
Succinyl-CoA 113
   action of 109
Sucrose 23
Sugars 17, 64
Sulfates 221
Sulfhemoglobin, formation of 77
Sulfinyl pyruvate 173
Sulfolipids 35, 40
Sulfosalicyclic acid test 222
Sulfur 207, 219
   excretion of 207
Sulfuric acid 219
Sweating 222
Symport system 11
Synovial fluid, viscosity of 8
Synthesis 71, 156, 158, 169–174, 176–179, 206
Synthesize thyroid hormones 255
Synthetic function, tests based on 245

T

Tay-Sachs disease 31, 39
T-cells, types of 283
Teeth
   formation 96
   mineralization of 203, 205
Temperature, effect of 86, 88, 88*f*
Testes 134
   functions of 263
Testosterone 263
Tetrahydrofolate 111
Tetrasaccharides 23
Thalassemia 79, 79*f*
Thermogenic action 225

Thiamine 102, 103
   pyrophosphate 85, 103, 131, 133
   structure of 103*f*
Thiosulfate 220
Threonine 49, 178
   catabolism of 178*f*
Thromboxanes 308
Thymidine monophosphate 65
Thymidylate 65
Thymine nucleotide 71
Thymus 265
Thyroglobulin 255
Thyroid 134, 146, 247, 250
   function 247
      agents inhibiting 256
      tests 247, 256
   gland 247
      hormones of 254
   hormones 175, 255, 256
   stimulating hormone 253
Thyrotoxicosis 256
Thyroxine 124, 146, 255
   structure of 255*f*
Tissue
   building 58
   oxidation 210
T-lymphocytes 283
Total acidity, amount of 248
Total calorie requirement, calculation of 226
Toxicity 97, 100, 115, 211, 212, 214
Toxicology 218
Toxins, sources of 232*t*
Trace elements 207
   essential 207, 208*t*
   nonessential 217, 217*t*
Transaldolase 83
Transamination pathway 173, 174*f*
Transfatty acids 42
Transfer ribonucleic acid 68
   structure of 69*f*
Transferrin 58
Transfusion 7
Transketolase 83, 206
   reaction 103
Transmethylation 181
Transphosphorylases 83
Tremors 168
   bone diseases 217
Triacylglycerol 32, 148, 156, 163
   increased synthesis of 157
   metabolism of 149, 156
   mixed 32
   simple 32
   synthesis of 157*f*
Triglycerides 32, 162, 163, 343
Triiodothyronine 255
   structure of 255*f*
Tripeptide 61
Trisaccharides 23
Tristearin 224
Trypsin 91, 164
Tryptophan 49, 182
   catabolism of 183, 184*f*
   dioxygenase 122
   pyrrolase 122

Tubular
    function, tests of 246
    reabsorption 221
    secretion 221
Tumor
    markers 315
    suppressor genes 315
Tyndall effect 9
Typtophan oxygenase 83
Tyrosinase 121
Tyrosine 49, 50, 174, 175f
    catabolism of 175f
    iodination of 255
    metabolism of 121
    synthesis of 174f
Tyrosinemia 176

U

Uniport system 11
Unsaturated fatty acids 41
    biosynthesis of 155
    oxidation of 152
Uranium 313
Urea 57, 221
    biosynthesis 168
    clearance test 245
    cycle 167f, 168
        disorders 169t
        metabolic disorders of 168
    formation of 167
Uric acid 221, 343
    normal level of 191
Uricotelic organisms 191
Uridine
    diphosphate glucose 136, 140
    monophosphate 65, 71
    triphosphate 140
Uridylate 65
Uridylic acid 65, 193
Urine 221, 285, 343
    abnormal 345
    collection of 288
    concentration test 246
    containers 288f
    dilution test 246
    examination of 288
    normal 344
    preservation of 288
    tests in 222

Urocanate pathway 177
Urocanic aciduria 177
Urokinase 91
Uronic acid pathway 134, 136, 137f, 186
Uroporphyrinogen synthase 195

V

Vacutainer tubes 288f
Valine 49, 179
Van den Bergh's reaction 243
Van der Waals forces 55
Ventilation, pulmonary 239
Vinyl chloride 313
Viral oncogenes 315
Viscosity 8, 56, 58
Vision, blurred 168
Visual cycle 93
Visual disturbances 217
Vitamin 93, 116t, 230, 265t
    A 93, 94, 228, 310, 315
        acid 94
        aldehyde 94
        structure of 94f
    B complex 103
        coenzyme of 69
    B_1 103
    B_{12} 112, 158
        structure of 112f
    B_2 104
    B_3 105
    B_5 108
    B_6 107
    B_7 110
    C 23, 102, 113, 231, 310, 315
        structure of 114f
    classification of 94f
    D 45, 97, 98, 161, 204, 228, 231
        D_2, structure of 97f
        D_3 98, 99
            formation of 98
            structure of 97f
    E 100, 228, 310, 315
        structure of 100f
    fat-soluble 93, 116t
    functions 230
    K 101, 228
        cycle 102, 102f
        structure of 101f

    lipid soluble 93
    non B-complex 113
    P 115
    toxicity of 233
    water soluble 93, 102, 116t
Vomiting 107, 217
Von Gierke's disease 142

W

Wald's visual cycle 95, 95f
Warburg's tissue 120
Water 235
    and electrolyte balance 235, 259
        regulation of 236
    balance 235
        negative 236
        positive 236
    disorders, laboratory diagnosis of 236
    distribution of 235
    functions of 235
    intake 235
    intoxication 236
    output 236
    pollution 312
Western blotting 280
Wilson's disease 213, 213f

X

Xanthine oxidase 121
Xanthinuria 192
Xenobiotics, metabolism of 218
Xeroderma pigmentosum 271, 271f
Xerophthalmia 93, 96, 96f

Z

Zellweger's syndrome 151
Zinc 12, 213
Zona
    fasiculata 258
    glomerulosa 258
    reticularis 258
Zymase 82
Zymogen 82